AF884579

Manual for

ONCOLOGY CLINICAL RESEARCH NURSING

Edited by
RuthAnn Gordon, MSN, RN, FNP, OCN®
John Bourgeois, DNP, MMHC, RN, CCRP, OCN®, NEA-BC

Oncology Nursing Society
Pittsburgh, Pennsylvania

ONS Publications Department
Publisher and Director of Publications: Lynn Nace, BA
Acquisitions Editor: Dave Burns, BA
Staff Editor II: Andrew Petyak, BA, PMP
Design and Production Administrator: Dany Sjoen

Copyright © 2025 by Oncology Nursing Society. All rights reserved. No part of the material protected by this copyright may be reproduced or utilized in any form, electronic or mechanical, including photocopying, recording, or by an information storage and retrieval system, without written permission from the copyright owner. For information, visit www.ons.org/publications-journals/permissions-archives, or send an email to pubpermissions@ons.org.

Library of Congress Cataloging-in-Publication Data

Names: Gordon, RuthAnn editor | Bourgeois, John editor
Title: Manual for oncology clinical research nursing/ edited by RuthAnn Gordon, MSN, RN, FNP, OCN and John Bourgeois, DNP, MMHC, RN, CCRP, OCN, NEA-BC.
Description: First edition. | Pittsburgh, Pennsylvania : Oncology Nursing Society, [2025] | Includes bibliographical references and index. |
Identifiers: LCCN 2025034884 | ISBN 9781635930719 paperback | ISBN 9781635930726 ebook
Subjects: LCSH: Cancer--Nursing
Due to a government shutdown in September 2025, this information was not finalized at the time of publication.

Publisher's Note

This book is published by the Oncology Nursing Society (ONS). ONS neither represents nor guarantees that the practices described herein will, if followed, ensure safe and effective patient care. The recommendations contained in this book reflect ONS's judgment regarding the state of general knowledge and practice in the field as of the date of publication. The recommendations may not be appropriate for use in all circumstances. Those who use this book should make their own determinations regarding specific safe and appropriate patient care practices, taking into account the personnel, equipment, and practices available at the hospital or other facility at which they are located. The editors and publisher cannot be held responsible for any liability incurred as a consequence from the use or application of any of the contents of this book. Figures and tables are used as examples only. They are not meant to be all-inclusive, nor do they represent endorsement of any particular institution by ONS. Mention of specific products and opinions related to those products do not indicate or imply endorsement by ONS. Websites mentioned are provided for information only; the hosts are responsible for their own content and availability. Unless otherwise indicated, dollar amounts reflect U.S. dollars.

ONS publications are originally published in English. Publishers wishing to translate ONS publications must contact ONS about licensing arrangements. ONS publications cannot be translated without obtaining written permission from ONS. (Individual tables and figures that are reprinted or adapted require additional permission from the original source.) Because translations from English may not always be accurate or precise, ONS disclaims any responsibility for inaccuracies in words or meaning that may occur as a result of the translation. Readers relying on precise information should check the original English version.

Printed in the United States of America

ONS
Oncology Nursing Society

Innovation • Excellence • Advocacy • Inclusivity

Contributors

Editors

RuthAnn Gordon, MSN, RN, FNP, OCN®
Nursing Director, Clinical Trials
Memorial Sloan Kettering Cancer Center
New York, New York

John Bourgeois, DNP, MMHC, RN, CCRP, OCN®, NEA-BC
Assistant Director of Clinical Services and Operations
Winship Cancer Institute of Emory University
Atlanta, Georgia
Chapter 21. Procurement, Accountability, and Administration of Investigational Agents

Authors

Amanda Brink, DNP, APRN, FNP-BC, AOCNP®
Nurse Practitioner
University of Texas MD Anderson Cancer Center
Houston, Texas
Chapter 26. Cytogenetics

Crystal D. Chu, PhD, RN
Assistant Professor
University of Virginia
Charlottesville, Virginia
Chapter 7. Legal, Regulatory, and Legislative Issues; Chapter 37. Publishing Guidance for Oncology Clinical Research Nurses

Kristen Clemens, BSN, RN, OCN®
Clinical Trials Nurse
Memorial Sloan Kettering Cancer Center
New York, New York
Chapter 11. Elements of a Protocol

Tahani Dweikat, MSN, EMHCA, RN, CCRP, AG-CNS, EBP-C, OCN®
Director (Interim), Clinical Research
Clinical Research Unit and Hematology Research
System Clinical Trials
City of Hope National Medical Center
Duarte, California
Chapter 17. Adherence and Retention in Clinical Trials

Rose Ermete, BSN, RN, OCN®, CRN-BC, CCRP
Senior Quality Assurance Nurse Auditor
SWOG Cancer Research Network
San Antonio, Texas
Chapter 36. Mentorship

Elaine Esler, MSN, RN, OCN®, NE-BC
Cancer Immunotherapy Program Nurse Supervisor
University of California, San Francisco
San Francisco, California
Chapter 9. Standard Operating Procedures

Rosilyn Gborogen, PhD, MBA, MSN, RN
Breast Oncology Nurse Navigator
Michigan Medicine – University of Michigan
Rogel Cancer Center
Ann Arbor, Michigan
Chapter 1. History and Background of Oncology Clinical Trials

Christopher Graham, BSN, RN, OCN®
Clinical Research Nurse
Gastrointestinal Cancer Center
Dana-Farber Cancer Institute
Boston, Massachusetts
Chapter 4. Types of Clinical Research: Experimental

Tasha Hall, PhD, RN
Executive Medical Affairs Director
Exelixis
Alameda, California
Chapter 30. Documentation

Alison Ivey, MS, MBA, RN, OCN®, CCRP
Associate Director for Administration
University of Florida Health Cancer Center
Gainesville, Florida
Chapter 19. Accessibility and Underserved Populations

Elizabeth A. Johnson, PhD, MS-CRM, RN
Assistant Professor
Mark and Robyn Jones College of Nursing
Montana State University
Bozeman, Montana
Chapter 14. Virtual Clinical Trials

Reneé Kurz, DNP, FNP-BC, AOCNP®
Director of Clinical Research Operations
Rutgers Cancer Institute of New Jersey
New Brunswick, New Jersey
Chapter 10. Ethics of Clinical Research

Julie McCluggage, RN, CRN-BC, OCN®
Research Nurse
University of California, San Francisco
San Francisco, California
Chapter 18. Clinical Trial Registries

Asia S. McCoy, MSN-CRN, RN, OCN®
Clinical Trials Nurse
Memorial Sloan Kettering Cancer Center
New York, New York
Chapter 15. Public and Patient Education

Madeline Merrill, MSN, AGNP-BC
Clinical Trials Nurse Practitioner and APP Education Specialist
Memorial Sloan Kettering Cancer Center
New York, New York
Chapter 25. Genetic Testing

Anita Moore, MS, BSN, RN
Nurse Consultant
Centers for Medicare and Medicaid Services
Baltimore, Maryland
Chapter 8. Good Clinical Practice

Rita Musanti, PhD, APN-BC, AOCNP®
Advanced Practice Nurse
Phase 1 Research
Rutgers Cancer Institute of New Jersey
New Brunswick, New Jersey
Chapter 35. Oncology Clinical Research Nurse Education

Elizabeth Ness, MS, RN, CRN-BC
Director, Office of Education and Compliance
Center for Cancer Research, National Cancer Institute
Bethesda, Maryland
Chapter 13. Protocol Development and Response Assessment; Chapter 22. Adverse Events

Cynthia Samborski, MSN, MHA, RN, CCRC
Clinical Research Administrator
Roswell Park Comprehensive Cancer Center
Buffalo, New York
Chapter 12. Informed Consent

Jessica Schnase, MSN, RN, OCN®, CCRP
Senior Manager, Clinical Research
Endeavor Health
Naperville, Illinois
Chapter 16. Accrual Base, Recruitment, and Promotion Strategies

Yelena Shames, MSN, ACNP-BC, CNRN
Clinical Trials Nurse Leader
Memorial Sloan Kettering Cancer Center
New York, New York
Chapter 5. Types of Clinical Research: Observational; Chapter 6. Expanded Access to Investigational Drugs

Patricia Shannon, BS, RN, OCN®
Clinical Research Nurse IV
HonorHealth Research and Innovation Institute
Scottsdale, Arizona
Chapter 23. Patient and Caregiver Education

Gary Shelton, DNP, MSN, NP, ANP-BC, AOCNP®
Nurse Practitioner, Oncology-Hematology
Mount Sinai Health System
New York, New York
Chapter 20. Gender Identification; Chapter 24. Pharmacogenetics and Pharmacogenomics

Brittany Stith, BSN, RN, OCN®, CCRP
Director, Office of Research
Tallahassee Memorial HealthCare
Tallahassee, Florida
Chapter 32. Creating and Maintaining a Regulatory File

Jazel Dolores Sugay, MSN, RN, OCN®
Senior Clinical Research Nurse
Northwestern University
Chicago, Illinois
Chapter 33. Data and Safety Monitoring Plans

Victoria Szenes, DNP, RN, CPNP
Senior Director, Clinical Development
Generate Biomedicines
Boston, Massachusetts
Pediatric Nurse Practitioner
Memorial Sloan Kettering Cancer Center
New York, New York
Chapter 2. Drug Development; Chapter 10. Ethics of Clinical Research

Monique Tarrant, MSN, MPH, RN, AGCNS-BC
Nurse Leader, Outpatient Ambulatory Services
Memorial Sloan Kettering Cancer Center
New York, New York
Chapter 27. Tumor Profiling

Gabriele Urschel, DNP, FNP-C, AOCNP®
Oncology Nurse Practitioner
Rocky Mountain Cancer Center
Longmont, Colorado
Chapter 28. Storage of Genetic Material

Ginnette Watkins-Keller, DNP, RN, NEA-BC, OCN®
Associate Director of Clinical Trials Administration
Rutgers Cancer Institute of New Jersey
New Brunswick, New Jersey
Chapter 34. Preparing for Audits, Inspections, and Monitoring Visits

Ashley Webb, MS, MN, RN, CRN-BC, OCN®
Research Nurse Lead
Institute for Cell, Gene and Immunotherapy
Masonic Cancer Center
University of Minnesota
Minneapolis, Minnesota
Chapter 31. Data Management

Laura S. Wood, MSN, RN, OCN®
Oncology Nurse Specialist
Cleveland Clinic Taussig Cancer Center
Cleveland, Ohio
University of Michigan Rogel Cancer Center
Ann Arbor, Michigan
Chapter 29. Pharmacokinetic and Pharmacodynamic Testing

Donglan Xia, PhD, RN, OCN®
Clinical Research Manager
University of Texas Southwestern Medical Center
Dallas, Texas
Chapter 3. Types of Clinical Research: Background

Disclosure

Editors and authors of books and guidelines provided by the Oncology Nursing Society are expected to disclose to the readers any significant financial interest or other relationships with the manufacturer(s) of any commercial products.

A vested interest may be considered to exist if a contributor is affiliated with or has a financial interest in commercial organizations that may have a direct or indirect interest in the subject matter. A "financial interest" may include, but is not limited to, being a shareholder in the organization; being an employee of the commercial organization; serving on an organization's speakers bureau; or receiving research funding from the organization. An "affiliation" may be holding a position on an advisory board or some other role of benefit to the commercial organization. Vested interest statements appear in the front matter for each publication.

Contributors are expected to disclose any unlabeled or investigational use of products discussed in their content. This information is acknowledged solely for the information of the readers.

The contributors provided the following disclosure and vested interest information:

Christopher Graham, BSN, RN, OCN®: Revolution Medicines, consultant or advisory role
Tasha Hall, PhD, RN: Exelixis, stock ownership
Elizabeth A. Johnson, PhD, MS-CRM, RN: American Cancer Society, Pfizer, research funding
Madeline Merrill, MSN, AGNP-BC: Horizons CME, honoraria
Victoria Szenes, DNP, RN, CPNP: Allogene Biotherapeutics, Generate Biomedicines, stock ownership
Gabriele Urschel, DNP, FNP-C, AOCNP®: Advanced Practice Providers Oncology Summit, honoraria
Laura S. Wood, RN, MSN, OCN®: AVEO Oncology, honoraria

Contents

Preface

Since the publication of the first *Manual for Clinical Trials Nursing* more than 25 years ago, the role of the oncology clinical research nurse (OCRN) has undergone a profound transformation. The earliest editions of this manual were born out of a pressing need to equip bedside nurses transitioning into research roles with essential knowledge, tools, and regulatory guidance. At that time, clinical trials were expanding rapidly, and the demand for experienced OCRNs far outpaced the supply. What began as a practical introduction has grown into an enduring, discipline-defining resource.

Now, with the release of this edition, including a title change to better reflect the OCRN role, we mark another turning point—one defined by precision medicine, digital health, and growing attention to equity in research. This edition reflects a thoughtful reimagining of structure and content, guided by a new editorial team that brings fresh insights alongside our returning contributors. A guiding principle throughout the development of this edition was to thoughtfully examine the impact of technology on every aspect of clinical research nursing. As new digital tools, platforms, and data systems reshape daily practice, the authors of this edition were tasked with considering not only foundational competencies but also the evolving digital landscape that now permeates patient care, protocol management, and regulatory oversight. This will support OCRNs in navigating a field where innovation is constant and adaptability is essential.

Among the most notable updates are the addition of new chapters that reflect the evolving complexity and inclusivity of modern clinical trials. Chapter 14. Virtual Clinical Trials explores decentralized research models and digital patient engagement; Chapter 19. Accessibility and Underserved Populations highlights a more profound commitment to equity in trial design and enrollment; and Chapter 20. Gender Identification ensures appropriate recognition and care for diverse patient identities. In addition to these new topics, the chapter sequence has been streamlined to support intuitive navigation and clearer alignment with current workflows. The manual continues to evolve to ensure the readers are up to date on both regulatory and industry standards. Some chapters and sections from previous iterations have been retired, acknowledging shifts in practice and priorities within the OCRN role.

Throughout the manual are foundational content and emerging themes that speak to the future of oncology clinical research nursing. Each chapter concludes with concise key points, and web-based references are embedded throughout to provide real-time access to evolving guidance and best practices.

It is a product of deep collaboration, rigorous review, and a shared commitment to the professional development of OCRNs. We remain grateful to the Oncology Nursing Society for its continued support and to the contributing authors for lending their voices, experience, and vision to this important work. Together, we have worked to reframe the manual for today's practice while honoring its roots. Whether you are stepping into the field for the first time or refining your practice as a seasoned OCRN, we hope this edition will inform, inspire, and empower you in the vital work ahead.

RuthAnn Gordon, MSN, RN, FNP, OCN®
John Bourgeois, DNP, MMHC, RN, CCRP, OCN®, NEA-BC

Acknowledgments

We take this opportunity to recognize and celebrate the remarkable contributions of oncology clinical research nurses. They are the critical link between scientific advancement and patient care through coordinating complex protocols, safeguarding participant safety, and bringing humanity and clarity to a highly regulated environment. Their expertise ensures research integrity; their compassion sustains the patient experience. This manual is a tribute to their work and an investment in the future of their practice.

SECTION I.
History and Foundation

CHAPTER 1

History and Background of Oncology Clinical Trials

Rosilyn Gborogen, PhD, MBA, MSN, RN

Introduction

A clinical trial is a systematic process conducted in humans to evaluate the safety and efficacy of drugs and devices in the diagnosis, treatment, and prevention of diseases or medical conditions (Kandi et al., 2021; Purna Singh et al., 2022). Clinical trials in oncology play a crucial role in enhancing the understanding of cancer and its treatment. These trials are designed to assess new therapies, diagnostic tools, treatment strategies, and supportive care interventions for various types and stages of cancer (Farah et al., 2023). Oncology clinical trials offer valuable insights into the evolution of cancer research and its impact on patient care (Unger et al., 2019). They stand as pillars in the ongoing battle against cancer, representing the culmination of scientific progress, medical expertise, and patient advocacy (American Association for Cancer Research, 2023). These trials are not just studies; they are the cornerstone of modern oncology, shaping the landscape of cancer treatment through rigorous experimentation and innovation.

It is essential to explore their history and background to comprehend the impact and significance of oncology clinical trials (National Cancer Institute [NCI], n.d.-a). From beginnings marked by limited understanding and primitive methodologies to the contemporary era of precision medicine and targeted therapies, the evolution of oncology trials mirrors the relentless pursuit of effective cancer treatments (Del Paggio et al., 2021).

The journey began centuries ago, when misconceptions and futile interventions marred early attempts to comprehend and combat cancer. Throughout history, cancer has often been viewed as an enigmatic affliction, eluding comprehension and defying conventional medical wisdom (Pohl et al., 2024). The early 20th century witnessed significant advancements in oncology trials, fueled by groundbreaking discoveries in cellular biology, genetics, and pharmacology (Falzone et al., 2018). As scientific understanding deepened, so did the realization that cancer is not a singular entity but a complex array of diseases, each with distinct characteristics and treatment requirements (Mishra, 2019). This led to the initiation of oncology clinical trials in the mid-20th century (American Cancer Society, 2014). Initially crude in design and scope, these trials were the testing grounds for emerging therapies and treatment modalities. From the first attempts at chemotherapy to the advent of targeted therapies and immunotherapy, each milestone in oncology was preceded by rigorous clinical investigation (Sharma et al., 2023).

Randomized controlled trials are universally recognized as the gold standard in clinical research, particularly in oncology, where they serve as the definitive method for assessing the efficacy and safety of new treatments (Shiely et al., 2024). This methodological innovation elevated the scientific rigor of oncology research and paved the way for evidence-based medicine. The era of precision medicine has revolutionized oncology clinical trials, ushering in personalized therapy tailored to individual patients' genetic profiles and tumor characteristics (Doroshow, 2023). This shift has led to a transition from a one-size-fits-all approach to a patient-centric model, which holds promise for improving treatment outcomes and minimizing adverse effects (Valdes, 2019). The field of oncology has experienced the advancement of treatment from preliminary cancer surgeries offering limited results to in-depth, targeted therapies increasing the overall survival and quality of life for many patients with cancer. Data show that 7.1% of patients with cancer are now enrolled in treatment trials, a significant increase from the historical rate of less than 5% (Cooner et al., 2023; Unger et al., 2024). However, efforts are ongoing to improve trial access and ensure high patient safety and trial quality (Thota et al., 2024).

Oncology clinical trials encompass a broad range of interventions, from conventional treatments such as chemotherapy and radiation to innovative therapies like targeted treatments and immunotherapies that continue to drive advancements in cancer care (Lipsick, 2023). These trials are supported by a well-established infrastructure of policies and procedures at both national and international levels (see Figure 1-1), ensuring patient safety, ethical conduct, and high standards of research (World Health Organization, 2024). The transition from the Cooperative Groups to the National Clinical Trials Network in 2014 significantly improved the infrastructure for oncology clinical trials (NCI, 2024). This change focused on enhancing collaboration between institutions, increasing trial efficiency, and broadening patient access to clinical trials (Good et al., 2020). This regulatory framework not only safeguards participants but also promotes innovation and encourages broader participation in trials, which is essential for improving outcomes in oncology. With these systems in place, understanding the historical evolution of oncology clinical trials and the key milestones that have shaped their development is crucial for appreciating the ongoing progress and challenges in the field.

This chapter will explore the historical evolution of oncology clinical trials, highlighting the key milestones that have shaped their development and their profound influence on cancer research and treatment. It will examine the journey from early attempts to modern-day precision medicine and describe the pivotal role of these trials in advancing scientific understanding, improving patient outcomes, and addressing the multifaceted challenges of cancer care.

The Historical Context of Clinical Trials

The history of clinical trials reflects humanity's enduring quest for effective treatments across various diseases, marking significant milestones in medical innovation and scientific inquiry (Karrasch, 2025; Piantadosi, 2024). Clinical trials can be traced back to ancient civilizations, where rudimentary forms of experimentation aimed to determine the efficacy of treatments (Jenkins & Hubbard, 1991). Early clinical trials often were comparative studies (see Chapter 3). In modern medicine, the evolution of clinical trials gained momentum in the 20th century, particularly after the establishment of ethical guidelines and regulatory frameworks designed to protect human participants and ensure the integrity of research. The first documented clinical trial using a matched control group, random assignment, and single blinding (see Chapter 4) occurred in 1931 when American physician James Burns Amberson and colleagues evaluated sanocrysin (sodium aurothiosulfate), a gold compound, for treating pulmonary tuberculosis at the W.H. Maybury Sanatorium in Michigan (Lilienfeld, 1982). This trial exemplified a pivotal shift toward systematic evaluation of treatments, which would become standard practice in clinical research. The 1938 Federal Food, Drug, and Cosmetic Act further solidified the need for safety in drug testing before marketing to the public (Swann, 1998).

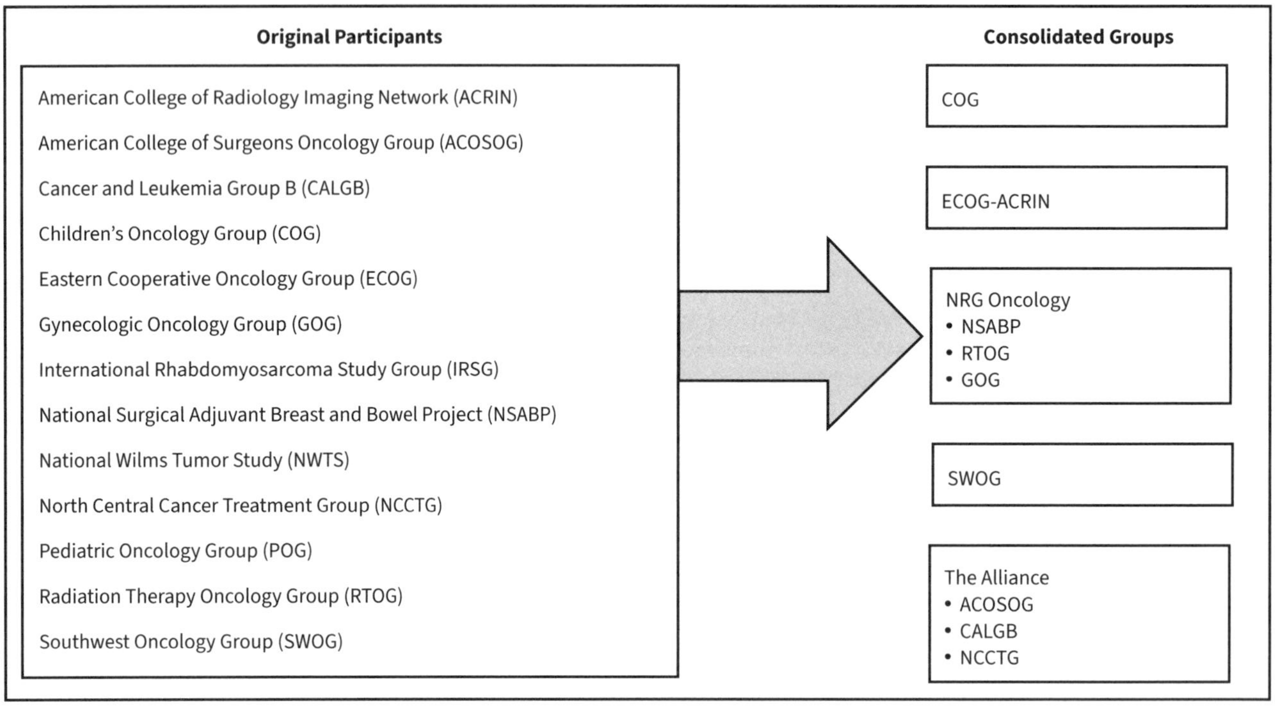

FIGURE 1-1 | U.S.-Based Clinical Trials Cooperative Group Program Members

Note. Based on information from Children's Oncology Group, n.d.; Harden, 1987; National Cancer Institute, n.d.-a.

Significant advancements continued through the decades, leading to the establishment of NCI, as part of the National Institutes of Health (NIH), in the 1930s (see Table 1-1), which provided federal support for medical research (Harden, 1987). This support fostered collaboration among researchers and institutions, paving the way for more robust and expansive clinical trial designs. As a result, the latter half of the 20th century witnessed the introduction of numerous innovations in trial methodology, including cooperative group trials that enabled broader patient participation and data collection (Cheson, 1991).

Oncologic Research

With the historical foundation of clinical trials established, oncology research emerged as a critical area of focus, particularly as cancer became a leading cause of morbid-

TABLE 1-1 | Key Milestones in the Development of U.S. Oncology Clinical Trials and Related Research

Year	Event
1747	Scottish physician James Lind conducts the first documented comparative study on patients with scurvy.
1800s	Drugs and vaccines to treat smallpox, diphtheria, and cholera are developed and tested.
1887	The National Institutes of Health (NIH) is founded.
1900s	Research on the prevention and treatment of infectious diseases begins.
1906	The Pure Food and Drug Act, regulating drug purity, safety, and labeling, is signed into law.
1937	The National Cancer Institute Act establishes the National Cancer Institute (NCI).
1938	The Federal Food, Drug, and Cosmetic Act replaces the 1906 Pure Food and Drug Act and requires that drugs be tested for safety before marketing.
1947	The Nuremberg Code establishes a basic code of ethics for experimentation on human participants.
1955	The first randomized controlled trial (RCT) in oncology is conducted, marking a significant step toward systematic and scientifically rigorous cancer research.
1962	The Kefauver-Harris Amendments to the Federal Food, Drug, and Cosmetic Act mandate preclinical testing and the provision of informed consent.
1964	The Declaration of Helsinki establishes specific guidelines for physicians conducting research involving humans.
1966	U.S. Surgeon General policy mandates an independent review of all research on human participants, proposing the establishment of institutional review boards.
1971	The National Cancer Act mandates NCI to conduct and apply basic cancer research.
1974	The National Research Act establishes the National Commission for the Protection of Human Subjects of Biomedical and Behavioral Research.
1976	NCI initiates the Cooperative Group Outreach Program.
1979	*The Belmont Report* outlines ethical principles and guidelines for the protection of human participants.
1981	Laws governing the protection of human participants in research funded by the U.S. Department of Health and Human Services are added to the Code of Federal Regulations.
1983	NCI funds Community Cancer Outreach Programs.
1986	NIH establishes policies for the inclusion of women in clinical trials.
1988	NCI establishes the High-Priority Clinical Trials Program.
1989	The U.S. Food and Drug Administration publishes guidelines for the inclusion of older adult patients in clinical trials.
1990	The Office of Research on Women's Health is created.

(Continued on next page)

TABLE 1-1 | Key Milestones in the Development of U.S. Oncology Clinical Trials and Related Research *(Continued)*

Year	Event
1991	Sixteen federal agencies adopt the federal policy for the protection of human participants, known as the Common Rule.
1993	The NIH Revitalization Act mandates the inclusion of women and minorities in NIH-sponsored clinical trials.
1996	The International Conference on Harmonization establishes guidelines for Good Clinical Practice in human participant research. U.S. Congress passes the Health Insurance Portability and Accountability Act (HIPAA).
1997	The Food and Drug Modernization Act mandates the establishment of a public resource for information on clinical trials.
1998	The NIH Policy and Guidelines on the Inclusion of Children as Participants in Research Involving Human Subjects mandate that children must be included in all NIH-sponsored research, except under certain circumstances.
2000	The World Health Organization establishes international guidelines for ethics committees involved in the review of biomedical research.
2002	The Best Pharmaceuticals for Children Act amends the Federal Food, Drug, and Cosmetic Act to improve drug safety and efficacy testing for children.
2003	The U.S. Department of Health and Human Services implements HIPAA.
2003	The Pediatric Research Equity Act requires that New Drug Applications include pediatric study plans, ensuring that children are adequately represented in clinical trials.
2004	The International Committee of Medical Journal Editors issues a statement mandating public registration of clinical trials, including a description of informed consent and ethics committee approval as prerequisites for manuscript publication.
2005	Federalwide Assurance for the Protection of Human Subjects is required for all studies funded or conducted by the Department of Health and Human Services that involve human participants.
2006	NCI initiates phase 0 clinical trials to study the pharmacokinetics and pharmacodynamics of molecular-targeted drugs.
2007	Medicare's Clinical Trials Policy is revised with updated coverage rules for Medicare.
2007	Pilot program of NCI Community Cancer Centers Program is launched and focuses efforts on cancer research, improving quality cancer care, and survivorship for patients who are treated at community hospitals.
2010	Enactment of the Patient Protection and Affordable Care Act requires insurers to cover routine costs of participation in clinical trials.
2012	Clinical Trials Cooperative Groups are consolidated from 13 groups to 5 (4 adult and 1 pediatric).
2013	The NCI Community Oncology Research Program is created to bring state-of-the-art cancer prevention, control, treatment, and imaging clinical trials, cancer care delivery research, and disparities studies to individuals in their own communities. It replaces the Community Clinical Oncology Program and the NCI Community Cancer Centers Program.
2014	Insurance coverage requirements for clinical trial participation go into effect as mandated by the Patient Protection and Affordable Care Act.
2016	The 21st Century Cures Act aims to accelerate medical product development and bring innovations to patients more quickly, emphasizing the need for modernizing clinical trial designs and regulations.
2020	The COVID-19 pandemic accelerates the adoption of decentralized and virtual clinical trial methodologies, including in oncology, to maintain research continuity and patient safety.
2021	FDA modernizes clinical trial regulations to incorporate real-world data and analytics.
2022	Oncology clinical trials begin integrating artificial intelligence and machine learning for more personalized medicine.
2023	Precision oncology trials see a rise, focusing on individualized treatment based on genetic profiles.
2024	Advancements in immunotherapy continue to redefine treatment protocols in oncology trials.

Note. Based on information from Alliance for Clinical Trials in Oncology, n.d.; National Cancer Institute, n.d.-c; Nuremberg Code, 1949; Şimşek, 2024; Singh, 2015; World Medical Association, 2013.

ity and mortality worldwide. NCI played a pivotal role in advancing oncology clinical trials and promoting cancer research funding (NCI, 2022; Pohl et al., 2024). Its formation marked the beginning of structured efforts to systematically investigate cancer treatments, leading to the development of cooperative oncology groups for clinical trials, all occurring in the context of the ethical standards established by the Nuremberg Code of 1947 (Maurya, 2024; Nuremberg Code, 1949). The 1950s saw groundbreaking advancements in cancer treatment, including the introduction of cobalt teletherapy and improvements in chemotherapy. These innovations enhanced treatment efficacy and underscored the importance of clinical trials in validating new therapies (DeVita & Rosenberg, 2012). For instance, in the mid-1970s, significant studies evaluating single-agent and combination therapies for breast cancer contributed to a decline in cancer mortality rates by the early 1990s (NCI, 2015).

The National Cancer Act of 1971 significantly increased funding for cancer research and established NCI's role in conducting basic scientific research while applying findings to clinical practice (Jenkins & Hubbard, 1991). By the 1970s, most oncology trials were conducted at NCI-designated comprehensive cancer centers. However, recognizing the need to extend trial access beyond these centers, NCI initiated outreach programs to enhance patient accrual in trials, ensuring that community oncologists could also participate in NCI-sponsored research (Cheson, 1991; Tucker et al., 2021). These programs provided funding for community physicians to participate in NCI-sponsored clinical trials (Cheson, 1991; Jenkins & Hubbard, 1991). Approximately 80%–85% of patients with cancer are now seen and treated at community cancer centers or hospitals near their home communities with access to a wide array of clinical trial opportunities (NCI, 2014; Tucker et al., 2021).

The consolidation of cooperative oncology groups in the 2000s aimed to streamline research efforts and improve operational efficiencies within clinical trials (NCI, 2005). Notably, the NCI Community Oncology Research Program, launched in 2013, sought to bring state-of-the-art cancer prevention, control, treatment, and imaging clinical trials directly to patients in their communities, thus increasing accessibility and representation in oncology research (NCI, 2019).

The introduction of initiatives such as the NIH Roadmap and the U.S. Food and Drug Administration (FDA) Critical Path Initiative in the early 2000s further advanced the field by promoting bioinnovation and translating basic research into clinical practice. These initiatives facilitated the identification of biomarkers and novel therapeutic targets, resulting in significant improvements in patient outcomes and survival rates (Kaitlin & DiMasi, 2011).

History of Drug and Trial Safety

In the late 1800s, fraudulent claims about drug safety and efficacy, as well as abuses in drug and device manufacturing, were widespread in the United States, resulting in many serious injuries and deaths (Swann, 1998) (see Chapter 10). This led to the passage of the 1906 Pure Food and Drug Act, which established the first federal standards to regulate the purity and labeling of food and drugs. FDA, originally the Bureau of Chemistry, was tasked with enforcing these regulations. By 1938, more stringent laws required drug safety testing and FDA approval before marketing, and the FDA's authority was extended to medical devices. The Kefauver-Harris Amendments of 1962, enacted in response to the thalidomide tragedy, further mandated preclinical testing, required proof of both drug efficacy and safety, and informed consent for clinical research participants (Swann, 1998).

From the mid-1800s to the mid-1900s, research on vulnerable populations, such as prisoners, minorities, and individuals with mental illness, was conducted without participant informed consent (Allen, 1994; Merkatz & Junod, 1994). After the medical atrocities revealed during World War II, the Nuremberg Code of 1947 introduced a set of ethical guidelines that emphasized voluntary consent and have since influenced modern research ethics (Merkatz & Junod, 1994; Nuremberg Code, 1949; Orphanopoulos, 2025). The Declaration of Helsinki, adopted in 1964, recognized an international ethical framework for biomedical research that included guidelines for informed consent, scientific justification, and review by an independent committee (World Medical Association, 1996).

The National Research Act of 1974 established the National Commission for the Protection of Human Subjects of Biomedical and Behavioral Research, leading to the publication of *The Belmont Report* in 1979. It outlined three core principles: respect for persons through informed consent, beneficence by minimizing harm and maximizing benefits, and justice through the fair distribution of research risks and benefits (Kimmelman, 2020). These principles shaped the development of institutional review boards and were codified into the Code of Federal Regulations in 1981 (National Commission for the Protection of Human Subjects of Biomedical and Behavioral Research, 1979; Sparks, 2002). One key regulation, the Common Rule, established measures to protect research participants, including criteria for informed consent, institutional review board guidelines, and specific protections for vulnerable populations (Protection of Human Subjects, 2017).

The International Council for Harmonisation of Technical Requirements for Pharmaceuticals for Human Use (ICH) was established initially in 1990 as the International Conference on Harmonization. In 1996, it released *ICH Harmonised Tripartite Guideline: Good Clinical Practice E6(R1)* guidelines, which streamlined regulatory standards for clinical trials worldwide (Grimes et al., 2005; ICH, 1996b). These guidelines established consistent principles for participant protection and trial conduct across multiple countries, including the United States, the European Union, and Japan (Dixon, 1998; ICH, 1996a). Moreover, the Health Insurance Portability and Accountability Act, implemented in 2003, introduced specific privacy protections for clinical research participants (NIH, 2004; Office for Human Research Protections, 2016, 2024).

Transition to Oncology-Specific Treatment and Infrastructure

In oncology, increasingly targeted therapies have driven advancements in clinical trials. A significant milestone occurred in 2014 with the transition from NCI's Cooperative Groups to its National Clinical Trials Network. This shift was designed to foster collaboration among institutions, improve trial efficiency, and expand patient access to clinical trials (Alliance for Clinical Trials in Oncology, n.d.; NCI, n.d.-c). The National Clinical Trials Network also implemented electronic data reporting systems, which have improved patient enrollment and streamlined data collection and trial protocols, enhancing the overall infrastructure of oncology research (NCI, n.d.-c). However, ethical challenges persist, especially regarding equitable representation. Historically, minority groups and women have been underrepresented in clinical trials, raising concerns about the fairness of research findings and their applicability across diverse populations.

Exclusion of Minorities and Women in Clinical Trials: Barriers to Representation

The treatment of minorities and women in oncology clinical trials has been influenced by various social, cultural, ethical, and scientific factors (Mitchell et al., 2022). Historically, these groups have been significantly underrepresented in clinical research, including cancer trials, resulting in disparities in access to innovative therapies and limiting the applicability of research outcomes across diverse populations (Lee, 2009).

Despite the increasing incidence and mortality rates of cancer in the Black community, this group has been underrepresented in clinical trials (George et al., 2014). Lack of participation by minorities in general and specifically the Black population has primarily been attributed to fears of exploitation generated by the Tuskegee syphilis experiment conducted by the U.S. Public Health Service from the 1930s to the 1970s. This study allowed Black men with syphilis to go untreated, even after curative treatment was available, to study the natural progression of the disease. Therefore, there is mistrust, fear, and a lack of confidence regarding medical establishments and research among minorities, which continues to be a barrier for many researchers (Allen, 1994; George et al., 2014).

Lack of access to state-of-the-art health care, cultural or ethnic factors, economic status, language or literacy barriers, and long-standing fear, apprehension, and skepticism have been identified as obstacles to minority participation in clinical trials (George et al., 2014). However, because 40% of the Community Clinical Oncology Program's annual referrals come from minority populations, NCI provides funding to institutions that serve a high percentage of minority groups through its Minority-Based Community Clinical Oncology Program, established in 1990 (McCaskill-Stevens et al., 2005; NCI, 2003). According to George et al. (2014), more than 30% of the U.S. population is of a racial or ethnic minority; however, racial and ethnic minorities represent less than 18% of the participants in clinical trials. Between 2000 and 2020, only 43% of trials reported race and ethnicity data, highlighting persistent underrepresentation. Still, minority enrollment has improved, rising annually by 1.7% (Turner et al., 2022).

The causes of the low participation of minority groups from the study perspective in clinical trials are complex. Reasons may be partly because of study designs or a lack of available trials in communities with highly disparate populations. Often, disparate populations lack sufficient health care, which can exacerbate disease processes. Clinical trial eligibility is frequently rigid and exclusionary of many of these comorbidities. The proportion of racial and ethnic minorities in NCI-funded clinical trials increased from 14% in 1999 to 25% in 2019, with the Minority-Based Community Clinical Oncology Program enrolling 10% of these participants (Haynes & Smedley, 1999; Ong, 2020).

In 1977, women were excluded from participation in clinical trials because of concerns about the potential teratogenic effects of untested drugs on a developing fetus, partially because of severe birth defects caused by the drug thalidomide (effective in preventing nausea in pregnant women). This FDA-mandated exclusion applied to phase 1 clinical trials involving the use of untested drugs in pregnant women or women of childbearing potential (Merkatz & Junod, 1994). However, in practice, it was extended to all women in all phases of clinical trials (Bush, 1994).

These policies severely limited knowledge about gender- and race-related differences in drug safety and efficacy (Allen, 1994; Merkatz & Junod, 1994; Millon-Underwood et al., 1993). The AIDS epidemic highlighted the potentially discriminatory nature of these exclusionary practices (Kelly & Cordell, 1996). Between 1992 and 1993, 15% of all new AIDS cases reported were in women, and almost 75% of these women were either Black or Hispanic (Allen, 1994). In 1986, NIH drafted its first policy promoting the inclusion of women in clinical trials (LaRosa, 1994). Since the implementation of this policy, women of childbearing potential have been allowed to participate in phase 1 clinical trials if they are not pregnant. However, they must be advised of the potential for fetal damage if they become pregnant and must agree to use effective contraception while participating in a study (Merkatz & Junod, 1994).

In 1990, NCI established the Office of Research on Women's Health to promote research on women's health issues and increase the participation of women in clinical trials. The NIH Revitalization Act, passed by Congress in 1993, mandated the inclusion of women and minorities in all NIH-sponsored clinical trials (Pinn, 1994). Women and minorities were frequently excluded or marginalized in clinical research, including oncology trials, because of societal norms, ethical dilemmas, and discriminatory practices. Some researchers have defended these exclusions by citing misconceptions about physiologic differences or treatment responses (Jenei et al., 2021; Vidal et al., 2024), whereas others have shed light on participation barriers, including healthcare access disparities, institutional mistrust, and cultural and language obstacles (Daitch et al., 2022). As a result of the NIH Revitalization Act, the participation of women in clinical trials is growing. Study data show women comprised 49% of NCI cooperative study enrollments between 1996 and 2002 for cancer treatment (Murthy et al., 2004). However, an analysis of NCI clinical trials from 2005–2020 revealed a decline, with women representing 41.7% of participants compared to their 49.5% prevalence in the U.S. cancer population (Choradia et al., 2024).

American science author Rebecca Skloot's *The Immortal Life of Henrietta Lacks* (2010) brought attention to the ethical, racial, and medical issues surrounding the use of Henrietta Lacks' cells, known as HeLa, which were taken without her consent in 1951. The book highlighted the significant scientific breakthroughs made possible by HeLa cells while raising awareness about the lack of informed consent, racial disparities in health care, and the exploitation of marginalized communities in medical research (Skloot, 2010). Cells were retrieved to diagnose her cancer; however, additional cells were taken without her knowledge or consent to contribute to research and are still being used in research today. Her family was aware of the use of their mother's cells but was unaware of the full impact those cells had made in laboratories worldwide until Skloot started communicating with them. With the use of Henrietta Lacks' cells and the publication of Skloot's book, bioethics began evolving, and the public became aware of the triumphs and tribulations of research (Nisbet & Fahy, 2013).

The history of minorities and women in oncology clinical trials underscores the imperative for ongoing efforts to promote diversity, equity, and inclusion in research. By mitigating systemic obstacles and emphasizing community involvement, researchers can strive for more inclusive and equitable oncology trials that benefit all patients (Vidal et al., 2024).

Children and Older Adults in Clinical Trials

The treatment of children and older adults in the history and background of oncology clinical trials has undergone significant evolution over time. Initially, clinical trials focused on adult populations, with limited attention given to special populations, including children and older adults. With the advancement of the understanding of cancer biology and treatment methods, there has been an increasing recognition of the need for tailored approaches for different age groups (O'Hanlon, 2025). Pediatric oncology has faced unique challenges because of the rarity of childhood cancers and the ethical complexities of enrolling children in clinical trials (Benedetti & Marron, 2021). Early clinical trials in pediatric oncology often involved small cohorts and were primarily conducted in academic medical centers. Legislative milestones in the United States, such as the Pediatric Research Equity Act and the Best Pharmaceuticals for Children Act, have significantly influenced and mandated the incorporation of children into drug clinical trials anticipated for pediatric use (FDA, 2024; National Institute of Child Health and Human Development, n.d.; Schwartz & Feudtner, 2019). A heightened presence of pediatric oncology clinical trials exists, facilitated by specialized cooperative groups and consortia. These endeavors often target distinct pediatric malignancies.

Moreover, the participation of children in cancer clinical trials has far exceeded that of adults. This is, in part, because childhood cancers are rare, and most children with cancer are treated at major academic institutions with access to clinical trials (NCI, 2025). However, because children represent a vulnerable population, special protections have been implemented to safeguard their treatment. In 1983, laws to protect children in clinical trials were added to the Code of Federal Regulations (Burns, 2003; Hirtz & Fitzsimmons, 2002; Sparks, 2002). Concerns have been raised that drugs used to treat adults were being administered without adequate testing in children (Hutchins et al., 1999; NCI, 2025).

In 1998, NIH issued a policy mandating the inclusion of children in clinical trials unless scientifically or ethically contraindicated (NIH, 2015). Then, in 2002, the Best Pharmaceuticals for Children Act was passed, amending the Federal Food, Drug, and Cosmetic Act to improve drug safety and efficacy testing prior to use in children (Burns, 2003). Historically, parental consent alone was sufficient for children under 18 years old to participate in clinical trials. Now this population is asked for their assent, indicating that they are mature enough to understand the trial and the expectations of the study. Although assent, unlike informed consent, is not required by law, many institutional review boards require it (NCI, n.d.-b) (see Chapter 12).

Older adults have historically been underrepresented in clinical trials because of concerns related to comorbidities, potential toxicity, and limited life expectancy. Consequently, there exists a scarcity of evidence-based guidelines for treating cancer in this population. However, given the aging population and the increasing incidence of cancer among older adults, there is a growing recognition of the necessity to include this demographic in clinical research to ensure that treatment recommendations are both evidence based and relevant (Martin et al., 2024; Rosenzweig et al., 2024). Efforts have been initiated to develop geriatric oncology programs and incorporate geriatric assessments into clinical trial protocols to address this disparity. These assessments evaluate factors such as functional status, comorbidities, cognitive function, and social support to better tailor treatment plans to the individual needs of older adult patients with cancer (Lian et al., 2024).

In 1989, FDA published recommended guidelines for the inclusion of older adults in clinical trials. However, older adults continue to be proportionally underrepresented in clinical trials despite cancer incidence and mortality rates being the highest in this population. Suggested reasons for underrepresentation include concerns about toxicities, the presence of comorbid conditions, perceived lack of benefit, advanced stage of disease at diagnosis, lack of awareness, quality-of-life concerns, and a variety of socioeconomic barriers (Hutchins et al., 1999; Lewis et al., 2003; Talarico et al., 2004).

The lack of participation by older adults in clinical trials may not only limit the generalizability of results to this population but also result in less aggressive treatment approaches due to misconceptions about tolerability, thereby compromising survival outcomes (Hutchins et al., 1999; Talarico et al., 2004). Excluding the older adult population is problematic because this group incurs the highest burden of healthcare costs in the United States. Herrera et al. (2010) noted that 36% of personal healthcare dollars are spent on older adults, accounting for 42% of all prescription drug expenditures. Therefore, increased representation of older adults in clinical trials is critically important. To support this, cooperative group trials, such as those involving treatment (e.g., chemotherapy), quality-of-life trials, and registries, are specifically designed to include older adults.

Evolution of National Healthcare Reform

In 2007, the Centers for Medicare and Medicaid Services revised its Clinical Trial Policy to expand coverage for Medicare patients participating in clinical trials. This revision helped to cover expenses accrued during participation in qualified clinical trials. Although many states have adopted various state-specific agreements to cover different aspects of clinical trial participation, there is a lack of consistency among insurance carriers nationwide. In March 2010, the enactment of the Patient Protection and Affordable Care Act introduced requirements for insurance companies to provide coverage for routine costs associated with participating in clinical trials (Mackay et al., 2015). With this in place, patients can choose the best treatment option without worrying that specific tests or procedures will not be covered due to their participation in a clinical trial (Park et al., 2025). The new requirements went into full effect in 2014. The federal law covers all 50 states and the District of Columbia. It includes Employee Retirement Income Security Act plans, as well as self-insured plans that are not mandated by state regulations (Gainotti & Petrini, 2010).

Patient-Centered Care

Patient-centered care in oncology clinical trials has undergone significant evolution, shifting from researcher-focused to patient-centric approaches. Historically, trials assessed treatment efficacy and safety with minimal patient input. However, the rise of patient advocacy groups in the 1970s and 1980s, such as the National Coalition for Cancer Survivorship and the American Cancer Society, underscored the necessity of incorporating patient perspectives. This advocacy incorporated patient-reported outcomes and patient preferences into study designs, reflecting a broader movement toward patient-centered care in the late 20th and early 21st centuries (FDA, 2020). Regulatory agencies, such as FDA and the European Medicines Agency (2023), have further promoted patient engagement through guidance and initiatives aimed at enhancing patient involvement throughout the drug development process.

Oncology trials now emphasize personalized treatment approaches, innovative trial designs, and strategies to improve patient recruitment and retention, ensuring that the needs and perspectives of patients are prioritized through collaborative efforts among all stakeholders (American Cancer Society, n.d.).

The core principles of patient-centered care in oncology clinical trials encompass several key elements:

- Respecting patients' values, preferences, and needs is paramount, ensuring that their perspectives are acknowledged and integrated into their care (Edgman-Levitan & Schoenbaum, 2021; Tseng & Hicks, 2016).
- Comprehensive communication and informed consent are crucial, as they provide patients with clear and understandable information about the trial, enabling them to make informed decisions (Kass et al., 2025; MediPharm Solutions, 2023).
- Coordination and integration of oncology care ensure seamless transitions and collaboration among healthcare providers, enhancing the overall treatment experience (Hall, 2024).
- There is a necessity to address the mental health needs of patients for emotional and psychological support, which is essential in managing the stress associated with cancer treatment (POLA, 2025).
- Involving family and caregivers is key, as it acknowledges their critical role in the patient's support system and actively engages them in the care process to enhance patient outcomes (Adejoh et al., 2020).
- Continuity of care and follow-up are vital, ensuring ongoing support and monitoring that promote sustained

well-being and adherence to treatment plans (Hudon et al., 2012).

- The accessibility and convenience of trial participation are critical, as they minimize barriers to participation and ensure that trials are patient-friendly and accessible to diverse populations (Ford et al., 2008).

Despite these stated principles, there is still notable resistance to patient-centered care.

Institutional resistance to patient-centered approaches persists because of various factors. Financial constraints and resource allocation often pose significant hurdles, limiting institutions' ability to fully implement patient-centered strategies, as highlighted in analyses of healthcare budgeting (Owolabi et al., 2024). Moreover, variability in patient needs and preferences complicates standardization efforts, leading to hesitance in adopting uniform patient-centric approaches across healthcare settings (Chibuike et al., 2024). Ethical considerations and regulatory requirements further exacerbate institutional resistance as institutions struggle to balance patient autonomy with compliance with stringent guidelines (Ahmed, 2024). According to Cruz Rivera et al. (2022), the challenge of measuring and evaluating patient-centered outcomes adds another layer of complexity, with institutions struggling to find suitable metrics and methodologies. Overcoming institutional resistance demands a concerted effort to address these multifaceted challenges, implementing strategies for patient-centered care, and prioritizing patient needs and preferences within healthcare systems.

The role of nursing in clinical trials has evolved significantly, particularly with oncology clinical research nurses, who have become integral to trial implementation and patient care (Hackshaw, 2024; Johnson & Marsh, 2023). Initially, nurses primarily supported patient management by administering treatments and monitoring side effects (Bledsaw, 2023). However, with the growing complexity of clinical trials, oncology clinical research nurses now play a more comprehensive role (Johnson & Marsh, 2023). They act as clinical trial coordinators, ensuring that protocols are adhered to, informed consent is obtained, and patients are fully educated about their treatment options (Zumstein-Shaha & Grace, 2023). These nurses are also involved in data collection, patient advocacy, and the ethical considerations of patient care within trials. Their ability to communicate effectively among physicians, researchers, and patients enhances the quality of care and ensures that trials are conducted ethically. As key research team members, oncology clinical research nurses must remain aware of advancements in clinical trial methodologies and regulatory requirements to continue contributing to the successful execution and integrity of clinical research (Paul & Mahdiani, 2023). This expanded role highlights the importance of ongoing education and awareness among nurses regarding their significant function in clinical trials.

Summary

The evolution of clinical trials has led to significant improvements in the prevention and treatment of numerous diseases, including cancer. Advances in medicine, improved surgical techniques, the development of new drugs and devices, the application of statistical techniques to research studies, the recognition of the need for regulation, and the development of ethical codes have all influenced how clinical trials are now conducted, both in the United States and internationally. The focus is not only on the treatment and prevention of cancer but also on patient-centered management and quality of life. Developments have been made to include more diverse populations and increase outreach activities within communities. Patients are increasingly educated about their diagnosis and potential clinical trials, and they frequently seek out opportunities to participate in research activities.

Key Points

- The progress made in clinical trials has had a positive impact on the prevention and treatment of many diseases, including cancer.
- Factors that have influenced the way clinical trials are conducted include medical and surgical advances, the development of new drugs and devices, the application of statistical techniques to research studies, the recognition of the need for regulation, and the development of ethical codes.
- The focus today is on the treatment and prevention of cancer, symptom management, quality of life, genomics, personalized medicine, patient-centered care, and the use of biospecimens.

The author would like to acknowledge Karri Donahue, MSN, RN, CCRP, and Heather Benzel, BSN, RN, CCRP, for their contribution to this chapter that remains unchanged from the previous edition of this book.

References

Adejoh, S.O., Olorunlana, A., & Adejayan, A. (2020). Patients' experiences of family members' reactions to diagnosis of breast cancer and support in the management of breast cancer in Lagos, Nigeria. *Palliative and Supportive Care, 19*(5), 592–597. https://doi.org/10.1017/S147895152000070X

Ahmed, I. (2024). Autonomous systems in healthcare: Revolutionizing patient care. *Frontiers in Robotics and Automation, 1*(2), 111–130. https://sprcopen.org/index.php/FRA/article/view/133

Allen, M. (1994). The dilemma for women of color in clinical trials. *Journal of the American Medical Women's Association, 49*(4), 105–109.

Alliance for Clinical Trials in Oncology. (n.d.). *History of the Alliance.* https://www.allianceforclinicaltrialsinoncology.org/main/public/standard.xhtml?path=%2FPublic%2FHistory

American Association for Cancer Research. (2023). *AACR cancer progress report 2023.* https://www.aacr.org/wp-content/uploads/2023/11/AACR_CPR_2023_OSPGASummary.pdf

American Cancer Society. (n.d.). *Clinical trials.* https://www.cancer.org/cancer/managing-cancer/making-treatment-decisions/clinical-trials.html

American Cancer Society. (2014). *History of cancer treatments: Chemotherapy.* https://www.cancer.org/cancer/understanding-cancer/history-of-cancer/cancer-treatment-chemo.html

Benedetti, D.J., & Marron, J.M. (2021). Ethical challenges in pediatric oncology care and clinical trials. In A.W. Bauer, R.D. Hofheinz, & J.S. Utikal (Eds.), *Ethical challenges in cancer diagnosis and therapy* (Vol. 218, pp. 149–173). Springer. https://doi.org/10.1007/978-3-030-63749-1_11

Bledsaw, K.R. (2023). *The role of a clinical research nurse: The impact of working remotely* [Doctoral dissertation, The University of Texas Medical Branch].

Burns, J.P. (2003). Research in children. *Critical Care Medicine, 31*(3), S131–S136. https://doi.org/10.1097/01.CCM.0000054905.39382.58

Bush, J.K. (1994). The industry perspective on the inclusion of women in clinical trials. *Academic Medicine, 69*(9), 708–715. https://doi.org/10.1097/00001888-199409000-00005

Centers for Medicare and Medicaid Services. (2007). *Medicare clinical trial policy (CTP): Routine costs in clinical trials.* https://www.cms.gov/regulations-and-guidance/guidance/transmittals/downloads/r74ncd.pdf

Cheson, B.D. (1991). Clinical trials programs. *Seminars in Oncology Nursing, 7*(4), 235–242. https://doi.org/10.1016/0749-2081(91)90061-S

Chibuike, M.C., Grobbelaar, S.S., & Botha, A. (2024). Overcoming challenges for improved patient-centric care: A scoping review of platform ecosystems in healthcare. *IEEE Access, 12,* 14298–14313. https://doi.org/10.1109/ACCESS.2024.3356860

Children's Oncology Group. (n.d.). *Our history.* https://childrensoncologygroup.org/history

Choradia, N., Karzai, F., Nipp, R., Naqash, A.R., Gulley, J.L., & Floudas, C.S. (2024). Increasing diversity in clinical trials: Demographic trends at the National Cancer Institute, 2005–2020. *Journal of the National Cancer Institute, 116*(7), 1063–1071. https://doi.org/10.1093/jnci/djae018

Cooner, F., Ye, J., & Reaman, G. (2023). Clinical trial considerations for pediatric cancer drug development. *Journal of Biopharmaceutical Statistics, 33*(6), 859–874. https://doi.org/10.1080/10543406.2023.2172424

Cruz Rivera, S., Aiyegbusi, O.L., Ives, J., Draper, H., Mercieca-Bebber, R., Ells, C., ... Calvert, M.J. (2022). Ethical considerations for the inclusion of patient-reported outcomes in clinical research: The PRO Ethics Guidelines. *JAMA, 327*(19), 1910–1919. https://doi.org/10.1001/jama.2022.6421

Daitch, V., Turjeman, A., Poran, I., Tau, N., Ayalon-Dangur, I., Nashashibi, J., ... Leibovici, L. (2022). Underrepresentation of women in randomized controlled trials: A systematic review and meta-analysis. *Trials, 23*(1), 1038. https://doi.org/10.1186/s13063-022-07004-2

Del Paggio, J.C., Berry, J.S., Hopman, W.M., Eisenhauer, E.A., Prasad, V., Gyawali, B., & Booth, C.M. (2021). Evolution of the randomized clinical trial in the era of precision oncology. *JAMA Oncology, 7*(5), 728–734. https://doi.org/10.1001/jamaoncol.2021.0379

DeVita, V.T., Jr., & Rosenberg, S.A. (2012). Two hundred years of cancer research. *New England Journal of Medicine, 366*(23), 2207–2214. https://doi.org/10.1056/NEJMra1204479

Dixon, J.R., Jr. (1998). The International Conference on Harmonization Good Clinical Practice guideline. *Quality Assurance, 6*(2), 65–74. https://doi.org/10.1080/105294199277860

Doroshow, J.H. (2023, December 6). What comes after NCI-MATCH? NCI's new precision medicine cancer trials. *National Cancer Institute Cancer Currents Blog.* https://www.cancer.gov/news-events/cancer-currents-blog/2023/new-nci-precision-medicine-trials

Edgman-Levitan, S., & Schoenbaum, S.C. (2021). Patient-centered care: Achieving higher quality by designing care through the patient's eyes. *Israel Journal of Health Policy Research, 10*(1), 21. https://doi.org/10.1186/s13584-021-00459-9

European Medicines Agency. (2023). *Patient engagement: From a patient-centric drug development to authorisation.* https://www.ema.europa.eu/en/documents/presentation/presentation-patient-engagement-patient-centric-drug-development-authorisation-m-mavris-ema_en.pdf

Falzone, L., Salomone, S., & Libra, M. (2018). Evolution of cancer pharmacological treatments at the turn of the third millennium. *Frontiers in Pharmacology, 9,* 1300. https://doi.org/10.3389/fphar.2018.01300

Farah, E., Kenney, M., Kica, A., Haddad, P., Stewart, D.J., & Bradford, J.P. (2023). Beyond participation: Evaluating the role of patients in designing oncology clinical trials. *Current Oncology, 30*(9), 8310–8327. https://doi.org/10.3390/curroncol30090603

Ford, J.G., Howerton, M.W., Lai, G.Y., Gary, T.L., Bolen, S., Gibbons, M.C., ... Bass, E.B. (2008). Barriers to recruiting underrepresented populations to cancer clinical trials: A systematic review. *Cancer, 112*(2), 228–242. https://doi.org/10.1002/cncr.23157

Gainotti, S., & Petrini, C. (2010). Insurance policies for clinical trials in the United States and in some European countries. *Journal of Clinical Research and Bioethics, 1*(1), 1–8. https://doi.org/10.4172/2155-9627.1000001

George, S., Duran, N., & Norris, K. (2014). A systematic review of barriers and facilitators to minority research participation among African Americans, Latinos, Asian Americans, and Pacific Islanders. *American Journal of Public Health, 104*(2), e16–e31. https://doi.org/10.2105/AJPH.2013.301706

Good, M., Castro, K., Denicoff, A., Finnigan, S., Parreco, L., & Germain, D.S. (2020). National Cancer Institute: Restructuring to support the clinical trials of the future. *Seminars in Oncology Nursing, 36*(2), 1501003. https://doi.org.10.1016/j.soncn.2020.151003

Grimes, D.A., Hubacher, D., Nanda, K., Schulz, K.F., Moher, D., & Altman, D.G. (2005). The Good Clinical Practice guideline: A bronze standard for clinical research. *Lancet, 366*(9480), 172–174. https://doi.org/10.1016/s0140-6736(05)66875-4

Hackshaw, A. (2024). *A concise guide to clinical trials.* Wiley. https://doi.org/10.1002/9781119502678

Hall, K. (2024). Incorporating upstream oncology nurse navigation to improve timeliness to treatment in lung cancer: A quality improvement project. *Journal of Oncology Navigation and Survivorship, 15*(2). https://www.jons-online.com/issues/2024/february-2024-vol-15-no-2/5031

Harden, V.A. (1987). A short history of the National Institutes of Health. *National Institutes of Health Office of NIH History and Stetten Museum.* https://history.nih.gov/illustrated-histories/a-short-history-of-nih-1887-1987

Haynes, M.A., & Smedley, B.D. (Eds.). (1999). *The unequal burden of cancer: An assessment of NIH research and programs for ethnic minorities and the medically underserved.* National Academies Press.

Herrera, A.P., Snipes, S.A., King, D.W., Torres-Vigil, I., Goldberg, D.S., & Weinberg, A.D. (2010). Disparate inclusion of older adults in clinical trials: Priorities and opportunities for policy and practice changes. *American Journal of Public Health, 100*(Suppl. 1), S105–S112. https://doi.org/10.2105/AJPH.2009.162982

Hirtz, D.G., & Fitzsimmons, L.G. (2002). Regulatory and ethical issues in the conduct of clinical research involving children. *Current Opinion in Pediatrics, 14*(6), 669–675. https://doi.org/10.1097/00008480-200212000-00003

Hudon, C., Fortin, M., Haggerty, J., Loignon, C., Lambert, M., & Poitras, M.-E. (2012). Patient-centered care in chronic disease management: A thematic analysis of the literature in family medicine. *Patient Education and Counseling, 88*(2), 170–176. https://doi.org/10.1016/j.pec.2012.01.009

Hutchins, L.F., Unger, J.M., Crowley, J.J., Coltman, C.A., & Albain, K.S. (1999). Underrepresentation of patients 65 years of age or older in cancer-treatment trials. *New England Journal of Medicine, 341*(27), 2061–2067. https://doi.org/10.1056/NEJM199912303412706

International Council for Harmonisation of Technical Requirements for Pharmaceuticals for Human Use. (1996a). *Guidance for industry E6 good clinical practice: Consolidated guidance.* https://www.govinfo.gov/content/pkg/GOVPUB-HE20-PURL-LPS113971/pdf/GOVPUB-HE20-PURL-LPS113971.pdf

International Council for Harmonisation of Technical Requirements for Pharmaceuticals for Human Use. (1996b). *ICH Harmonized Tripartite Guideline: Guideline for good clinical practice E6(R1).* https://media.tghn.org/medialibrary/2011/10/ICH_GCP_1996_Guidelines.pdf

Jenei, K., Meyers, D.E., & Prasad, V. (2021). The inclusion of women in global oncology drug trials over the past 20 years. *JAMA Oncology, 7*(10), 1569–1570. https://doi.org/10.1001/jamaoncol.2021.3686

Jenkins, J., & Hubbard, S. (1991). History of clinical trials. *Seminars in Oncology Nursing, 7*(4), 228–234. https://doi.org/10.1016/0749-2081(91)90060-3

Johnson, E., & Marsh, L. (2023). Clinical research nurse utilisation and role in the conduct of decentralised clinical trials: A literature review. *Journal of Research in Nursing, 28*(3), 214–226. https://doi.org/10.1177/17449871231162497

Kaitlin, K.I., & DiMasi, J.A. (2011). Pharmaceutical innovation in the 21st century: New drug approvals in the first decade, 2000–2009. *Clinical Pharmacology and Therapeutics, 89*(2), 183–188. https://doi.org/10.1038/clpt.2010.286

Kandi, V., Suvvari, T.K., Vadakedath, S., & Godishala, V. (2021). Microbes, clinical trials, drug discovery, and vaccine development: The current perspectives. *Borneo Journal of Pharmacy, 4*(4), 311–323. https://doi.org/10.33084/bjop.v4i4.2571

Karrasch, N. (2025). Modern medical research benefits from the diverse history of clinical trials. *Trialfacts.* https://trialfacts.com/articles/history-of-clinical-trials

Kass, N.E., Meeker-O'Connell, A., Morain, S.R., & Crane, M.A. (2025). Optimizing informed consent—A call to action. *JAMA Health Forum, 6*(5), e250824. https://doi.org/10.1001/jamahealthforum.2025.0824

Kelly, P.J., & Cordell, J.R. (1996). Recruitment of women into research studies: A nursing perspective. *Clinical Nurse Specialist, 10*(1), 25–28. https://doi.org/10.1097/00002800-199601000-00009

Kimmelman, J. (2020). What is human research for? Reflections on the omission of scientific integrity from the Belmont Report. *Perspectives in Biology and Medicine, 63*(2), 251–261. https://doi.org/10.1353/pbm.2020.0017

LaRosa, J.H. (1994). Office of Research on Women's Health: National Institutes of Health and the women's health agenda. *Annals of the New York Academy of Sciences, 736,* 196–204. https://doi.org/10.1111/j.1749-6632.1994.tb12832.x

Lee, S.J.C. (2009). Science, surveillance, and the politics of redress in health disparities research. *Race/Ethnicity: Multidisciplinary Global Contexts, 3*(1), 51–74. http://www.jstor.org/stable/25595024

Lewis, J.H., Kilgore, M.L., Goldman, D.P., Trimble, E.L., Kaplan, R., Montello, M.J., ... Escarce, J.J. (2003). Participation of patients 65 years of age or older in cancer clinical trials. *Journal of Clinical Oncology, 21*(7), 1383 1389. https://doi.org/10.1200/JCO.2003.08.010

Lian, S., Hou, X., Liu, W., Li, M., Chen, G., & Ling, Y. (2024). Supportive care needs, quality of life and social support among elderly colorectal cancer patients undergoing chemotherapy: A longitudinal study. *Frontiers in Oncology, 14,* 1437888. https://doi.org/10.3389/fonc.2024.1437888

Lilienfeld, A.M. (1982, Spring). The Fielding H. Garrison Lecture: Ceteris paribus: the evolution of the clinical trial. *Bulletin of the History of Medicine, 56*(1), 1–18.

Lipsick, J. (2023). A history of cancer research: Retroviral insertional mutagenesis. *Cold Spring Harbor Perspectives in Biology, 15*(7), a035873. https://doi.org/10.1101/cshperspect.a035873

Mackay, C.B., Gurley-Calvez, T., Erickson, K.D., & Jensen, R.A. (2015). Clinical trial insurance coverage for cancer patients under the Affordable Care Act. *Contemporary Clinical Trials Communications, 2,* 69–74. https://doi.org/10.1016/j.conctc.2015.12.002

Martin, F.C., Quinn, T.J., Straus, S.E., Anand, S., van der Velde, N., & Harwood, R.H. (2024). New horizons in clinical practice guidelines for use with older people. *Age and Ageing, 53*(7), afae158. https://doi.org/10.1093/ageing/afae158

Maurya, R. (2024). Biomedical ethics in research and clinical practice. In P.K. Prabhakar (Ed.), *Reshaping healthcare with cutting-edge biomedical advancements* (pp. 1–15). https://doi.org/10.4018/979-8-3693-4439-2.ch001

McCaskill-Stevens, W., McKinney, M.M., Whitman, C.G., & Minasian, L.M. (2005). Increasing minority participation in cancer clinical trials: The minority-based community clinical oncology program experience. *Journal of Clinical Oncology, 23*(22), 5247–5254. https://doi.org/10.1200/JCO.2005.22.236

MediPharm Solutions. (2023). *Informed consent and its importance in clinical trials.* https://medipharmsolutions.com/blog/informed-consent-and-its-importance-in-clinical-trials

Merkatz, R.B., & Junod, S.W. (1994). Historical background of changes in FDA policy on the study and evaluation of drugs in women. *Academic Medicine, 69*(9), 703–707. https://doi.org/10.1097/00001888-199409000-00004

Millon-Underwood, S., Sanders, E., & Davis, M. (1993). Determinants of participation in state-of-the-art cancer prevention, early detection/screening, and treatment trials among African-Americans. *Cancer Nursing, 16*(1), 25–33. http://journals.lww.com/cancernursingonline/Citation/1993/02000/Determinants_of_participation_in_state_of_the_art.2.aspx

Mishra, P. (2019). Cancer is not a single disease, but a collection of several diseases. *International Journal of Advanced Research, 7,* 231–248. https://doi.org/10.21474/IJAR01/9217

Mitchell, E., Alese, O.B., Yates, C., Rivers, B.M., Blackstock, W., Newman, L., ... Harris, A.E. (2022). Cancer healthcare disparities among African Americans in the United States. *Journal of the National Medical Association, 114*(3), 236–250. https://doi.org/10.1016/j.jnma.2022.01.004

Murthy, V.H., Krumholz, H.M., & Gross, C.P. (2004). Participation in cancer clinical trials: Race-, sex-, and age-based disparities. *JAMA, 291*(22), 2720–2726. https://doi.org/10.1001/jama.291.22.2720

National Cancer Institute. (n.d.-a). *Cancer clinical trial information for patients and caregivers.* https://www.cancer.gov/research/participate/clinical-trials

National Cancer Institute. (n.d.-b). *Children's assent.* https://www.cancer.gov/research/participate/clinical-trials/safety#childrens-assent

National Cancer Institute. (n.d.-c). *Structure of NCI Cooperative Groups program prior to NCTN.* https://www.cancer.gov/research/infrastructure/clinical-trials/NCTN/structure-NCTN-cooperative-groups

National Cancer Institute. (2003). *National Cancer Institute fact sheet: Community clinical oncology program: Questions and answers.* https://www.govinfo.gov/content/pkg/GOVPUB-HE20-PURL-LPS100240/pdf/GOVPUB-HE20-PURL-LPS100240.pdf

National Cancer Institute. (2005). *Restructuring the national cancer clinical trials enterprise: Report of the Clinical Trials Working Group of the National Cancer Advisory Board.* https://www.cancer.gov/about-nci/organization/ccct/about/ctwg-report.pdf

National Cancer Institute. (2014). *NCI Community Cancer Centers program pilot: 2007–2010.* https://www.nih.gov/news-events/news-releases/nci-launches-pilot-its-community-cancer-centers-program-bring-quality-cancer-care-all

National Cancer Institute. (2015). *Enhancing drug discovery and development.* https://www.cancer.gov/research/areas/treatment/enhancing-drug-discovery

National Cancer Institute. (2019). *NCI Community Oncology Research Program (NCORP).* https://www.cancer.gov/research/infrastructure/clinical-trials/ncorp

National Cancer Institute. (2022). *History of the National Cancer Institute.* https://www.cancer.gov/about-nci/overview/history

National Cancer Institute. (2024). *NCI's clinical trials programs and initiatives.* https://www.cancer.gov/research/infrastructure/clinical-trials

National Cancer Institute. (2025). *Research on childhood cancers.* https://www.cancer.gov/research/areas/childhood

National Commission for the Protection of Human Subjects of Biomedical and Behavioral Research. (1979). *The Belmont Report: Ethical principles and guidelines for the protection of human subject of research.* https://www.hhs.gov/ohrp/regulations-and-policy/belmont-report/read-the-belmont-report/index.html

National Institute of Child Health and Human Development. (n.d.). *Best Pharmaceuticals for Children Act (BPCA).* https://www.nichd.nih.gov/research/supported/bpca

National Institutes of Health. (2004). *Clinical research and the HIPAA Privacy Rule* [NIH Publication No. 04-5495]. https://privacyruleandresearch.nih.gov/pdf/clin_research.pdf

National Institutes of Health. (2015). *Inclusion of children in clinical research: Change in NIH definition.* https://grants.nih.gov/grants/guide/notice-files/NOT-98-024.html

Nisbet, M.C., & Fahy, D. (2013). Bioethics in popular science: Evaluating the media impact of *The Immortal Life of Henrietta Lacks* on the biobank debate. *BMC Medical Ethics, 14,* 10. https://doi.org/10.1186/1472-6939-14-10

Nuremberg Code. (1949). Permissible medical experiments. In *Trials of war criminals before the Nuremberg Military Tribunals under Control Council Law No. 10. Nuremberg, October 1946–April 1949* (Vol. 2, pp. 181–182). https://archive.org/embed/TrialsOfWarCriminalsBeforeTheNurembergMilitaryTribunalsUnderControlCouncil

Office for Human Research Protections. (2016). *Federalwide assurances* (FWAs). https://www.hhs.gov/ohrp/assurances/assurances/index.html

Office for Human Research Protections. (2024). *Federal policy for the protection of human subjects ('Common Rule').* https://www.hhs.gov/ohrp/humansubjects/commonrule/index.html

O'Hanlon, S. (2025). Cancer and older people: A research collection and commentary on the theme. *Age and Ageing, 54*(5), afaf113. https://doi.org/10.1093/ageing/afaf113

Ong, M.B.H. (2020). Participation by minority racial, ethnic groups in NCI-funded trials nearly doubles in 20 years. *Cancer Letter, 46*(26), 6–12. https://cancerletter.com/the-cancer-letter/20200626_1

Orphanopoulos, C.M. (2025). *An interdisciplinary approach to vulnerability: Towards a humane ethics.* Springer Nature.

Owolabi, O.R., Olatoye, F.O., Elufioye, O.A., & Okunade, B. (2024). Reviewing healthcare financial management: Strategies for cost-effective care. *World Journal of Advanced Research and Reviews, 21*(2), 958–966. https://doi.org/10.30574/wjarr.2024.21.2.0523

Park, E.R., Kirchhoff, A.C., Mitchell, C.O., Durieux, N., Foor, A., Kuhlthau, K., ... Donelan, K. (2025). Assessing the effect of virtual navigation interventions to improve health insurance literacy and decrease financial burden in cancer survivors: The HINT II study protocol. *Contemporary Clinical Trials,* 107952. https://doi.org/10.1016/j.cct.2025.107952

Paul, N.W., & Mahdiani, H. (2023). Ethical challenges in clinical studies with adaptive design in oncology. *Clinical Ethics, 18*(2), 148–154. https://doi.org/10.1177/14777509221133974

Piantadosi, S. (2024). *Clinical trials: A methodologic perspective* (4th ed.). Wiley.

Pinn, V.W. (1994). The role of the NIH's Office of Research on Women's Health. *Academic Medicine, 69*(9), 698–702. https://doi.org/10.1097/00001888-199409000-00003

Pohl, S.A., Nelson, B.A., Patwary, T.R., Amanuel, S., Benz E.J., Jr., & Lathan, C.S. (2024). Evolution of community outreach and engagement at National Cancer Institute–designated cancer centers, an evolving journey. *CA: A Cancer Journal for Clinicians, 74*(4), 383396. https://doi.org/10.3322/caac.21841

POLA. (2025, March 11). Mental health support for cancer patients: Boost emotional well-being during treatment. *BeatCancer.* https://beatcancer.eu/resources/mental-health/article/mental-health-support-for-cancer-patients

Protection of Human Subjects, 45 C.F.R. § 46 (2017). https://www.ecfr.gov/current/title-45/subtitle-A/subchapter-A/part-46

Purna Singh, A., Shahapur, P.R., Vadakedath, S., Bharadwaj, V.G., Kumar, D.P., Pinnelli, V.B., ... Kandi, V. (2022). Research question, objectives, and endpoints in clinical and oncological research: A comprehensive review. *Cureus, 14*(9), e29575. https://doi.org/10.7759/cureus.29575

Rosenzweig, M., Belcher, S.M., Braithwaite, L.E., Cuaron, L., Fischer-Cartlidge, E., Lally, R.M., ... Anderson, A. (2024). Research priorities of the Oncology Nursing Society: 2024–2027. *Oncology Nursing Forum, 51*(6), 502–515. https://doi.org/10.1188/24.ONF.502-515

Schwartz, L.A., & Feudtner, C. (2019). Providing integrated behavioral health services to patients with serious pediatric illness. *JAMA Pediatrics, 173*(9), 817–818. https://doi.org/10.1001/jamapediatrics.2019.1683

Sharma, I., Sharma, A., Tomer, R., Negi, N., & Sobti, R.C. (2023). History, evolution, milestones in cancer research and treatment. In R.C. Sobti, N.K. Ganguly, & R. Kumar (Eds.), *Handbook of oncobiology: From basic to clinical sciences.* Springer Nature. https://doi.org/10.1007/978-981-99-2196-6_2-1

Shiely, F., O'Shea, N., Murphy, E., & Eustace, J. (2024). Registry-based randomised controlled trials: Conduct, advantages and challenges—A systematic review. *Trials, 25*(1), 375. https://doi.org/10.1186/s13063-024-08209-3

Şimşek, G.O. (2024). Immunotherapy in the treatment of cancer: Today and tomorrow. *Current Molecular Biology Reports, 10,* 54–64. https://doi.org/10.1007/s40610-024-00161-0

Singh, J. (2015). International conference on harmonization of technical requirements for registration of pharmaceuticals for human use. *Journal of Pharmacology and Pharmacotherapeutics, 6*(3), 185–187. https://doi.org/10.4103/0976-500X.162004

Skloot, R. (2010). *The immortal life of Henrietta Lacks.* Crown.

Sparks, J. (2002). Timeline of laws related to the protection of human subjects. *US National Institute,* 1.

Swann, J.P. (1998). The Food and Drug Administration. In G.T. Kurian (Ed.), *A historical guide to the U.S. government* (pp. 248–254). Oxford University Press.

Talarico, L., Chen, G., & Pazdur, R. (2004). Enrollment of elderly patients in clinical trials for cancer drug registration: A 7-year experience by the U.S. Food and Drug Administration. *Journal of Clinical Oncology, 22*(22), 4626–4631. https://doi.org/10.1200/JCO.2004.02.175

Thota, R., Hurley, P.A., Miller, T.M., Bruinooge, S.S., Lipset, C., Harvey, R.D., ... Nowakowski, G.S. (2024). Improving access to patient-focused, decentralized clinical trials requires streamlined regulatory requirements: An ASCO research statement. *Journal of Clinical Oncology, 42*(33), 3986–3995. https://doi.org/10.1200/JCO.24.00961

Tseng, E.K., & Hicks, L.K. (2016). Value-based care and patient-centered care: Divergent or complementary? *Current Hematologic Malignancy Reports, 11*(4), 303–310. https://doi.org/10.1007/s11899-016-0333-2

Tucker, T.C., Charlton, M.E., Schroeder, M.C., Jacob, J., Tolle, C.L., Evers, B.M., & Mullett, T.W. (2021). Improving the quality of cancer care in community hospitals. *Annals of Surgical Oncology, 28*(2), 632–638. https://doi.org/10.1245/s10434-020-08867-y

Turner, B.E., Steinberg, J.R., Weeks, B.T., Rodriguez, F., & Cullen, M.R. (2022). Race/ethnicity reporting and representation in US clinical trials: A cohort study. *Lancet Regional Health, Americas, 11,* 100252. https://doi.org/10.1016/j.lana.2022.100252

U.S. Food and Drug Administration. (2020). *Patient-focused drug development: Collecting comprehensive and representative input—Guidance for industry, Food and Drug Administration staff, and other stakeholders.* https://resource.nlm.nih.gov/9918230998606676

U.S. Food and Drug Administration. (2024). *Pediatric Research Equity Act (PREA).* https://www.fda.gov/drugs/development-resources/pediatric-research-equity-act-prea

Unger, J.M., Nghiem, V.T., Hershman, D.L., Vaidya, R., LeBlanc, M., & Blanke, C.D. (2019). Association of National Cancer Institute–sponsored Clinical Trial Network group studies with guideline care and new drug indications. *JAMA Network Open, 2*(9), e1910593. https://doi.org/10.1001./jamanetworkopen.2019.1059

Unger, J.M., Shulman, L.N., Facktor, M.A., Nelson, H., & Fleury, M.E. (2024). National estimates of the participation of patients with cancer in clinical research studies based on Commission on Cancer accreditation data. *Journal of Clinical Oncology, 42*(18), 2139–2148. https://doi.org/10.1200/JCO.23.01030

Valdes, K. (2019). Understanding and overcoming barriers to adoption for precision medicine. *Proceedings: DIA 2019 Global Annual Meeting.* https://globalforum.diaglobal.org/issue/august-2019/understanding-and-overcoming-barriers-to-adoption-for-precision-medicine

Vidal, L., Dlamini, Z., Qian, S., Rishi, P., Karmo, M., Joglekar, N., ... Saini, K.S. (2024). Equitable inclusion of diverse populations in oncology clinical trials: Deterrents and drivers. *ESMO Open, 9*(5), 103373. https://doi.org/10.1016/j.esmoop.2024.103373

World Health Organization. (2024). *Guidance for best practices for clinical trials.* https://www.who.int/our-work/science-division/research-for-health/implementation-of-the-resolution-on-clinical-trials/guidance-for-best-practices-for-clinical-trials

World Medical Association. (1996). Declaration of Helsinki. *BMJ, 313,* 1448–1449. https://doi.org/10.1136/bmj.313.7070.1448a

World Medical Association. (2013). World Medical Association Declaration of Helsinki: Ethical principles for medical research involving human subjects. *JAMA, 310*(20), 2191–2194. https://doi.org/10.1001/jama.2013.281053

Zumstein-Shaha, M., & Grace, P.J. (2023). Competency frameworks, nursing perspectives, and interdisciplinary collaborations for good patient care: Delineating boundaries. *Nursing Philosophy, 24*(1), e12402. https://doi.org/10.1111/nup.12402

CHAPTER 2

Drug Development

Victoria Szenes, DNP, RN, CPNP

Introduction

The journey from a promising compound to U.S. Food and Drug Administration (FDA) approval encapsulates centuries of scientific evolution, notably since French chemist and microbiologist Louis Pasteur's germ theory in the 1800s (Gallin, 2018). The medical field, specifically oncology, is propelled by advancements in precision medicine, immunotherapies, and the incorporation of artificial intelligence in drug discovery.

Drugs and biologics are pivotal to therapeutic interventions and follow distinct development and application pathways. Drugs include small molecules and are typically created through chemical synthesis, yielding products with defined structures (FDA, 2018c). Conversely, biologics are derived from living organisms and encompass a range of complex molecules, often produced via recombinant DNA technology. Advances such as biologic therapies and cell and gene therapies highlight the potential for targeted cancer therapy, demonstrating the evolving landscape of therapeutic options.

Understanding the nuances, including the regulatory pathways and manufacturing considerations, is crucial for healthcare professionals. This knowledge ensures they can navigate the complexities of medication management, including the use of biosimilars and interchangeable biologics, which have no clinically meaningful differences in safety and effectiveness and offer more treatment choices and potentially lower-cost options for patients (FDA, 2023b, 2024).

Central to oncology drug development in the United States are the sponsoring entities, typically pharmaceutical or biotechnology companies, and FDA. The Oncology Center of Excellence (OCE) initiatives have been instrumental in providing guidance and support for cancer therapy development (FDA, 2023a). Examples include Project Catalyst, which focuses on guiding and supporting small pharmaceutical companies and academic life science incubators in developing novel cancer therapies, and the Real-Time Oncology Review, which allows for faster review of clinical trial data to expedite approval. These programs are designed to accelerate the review process while ensuring the safety and efficacy of new therapies.

This chapter will detail the drug development process, including history, New Drug Applications (NDAs), the application review process, and drug naming.

Where Does It All Begin?

The path from a promising compound to FDA approval is complex and rigorous, encompassing preclinical and clinical evaluations. Regulatory guidelines in oncology drug development have emphasized the use of adaptive trial designs, which allow trial modifications based on accumulating data, signaling a shift toward more flexible and less costly approaches (FDA, 2018a).

Understanding the disease to be addressed is fundamental to drug development. Researchers delve into the disease's etiology—everything from genetic alterations and their impact on proteins to cellular interactions and the overall effects on patients. This comprehensive understanding is essential for guiding the selection of molecular targets for potential therapeutic interventions.

Following the identification of a disease target, basic research unfolds in two critical phases: lead compound generation and optimization. The initial phase involves identifying a molecule with the potential to alter a disease pathway. This lead generation could be from plant, animal, mineral, microbiology, or semisynthetic/synthetic or recombinant DNA sources (Hughes et al., 2011).

Lead optimization then refines these candidates through rigorous preclinical and animal testing in the laboratory. The testing at this stage is in vitro, which is performed in the laboratory in test tubes and beakers. The other type of testing is in vivo, which is performed in living cell cultures and animal models. During this series of tests, researchers conduct an early assessment of safety, including absorption, distribution, metabolism, excretion, and toxicology (Hughes et al., 2011).

During the rigorous testing in the preclinical phase, a drug is considered successful if it is (a) absorbed into the bloodstream, (b) distributed to the proper site of action in the body, (c) metabolized efficiently and effectively, (d) successfully excreted from the body, and (e) demonstrated to be nontoxic. A compound that demonstrates a favorable profile in preclinical tests can advance to human trials, beginning with an Investigational New Drug (IND) application to FDA. This phase is vital for establishing the compound's safety and efficacy within clinical settings (Hughes et al., 2011).

The Investigational New Drug Application

The IND process is a critical step that facilitates the transition of a promising drug candidate to human clinical trials. Under federal regulations, any drug shipped across a state line must have an approved marketing application (FDA, 2014). The IND is the legally authorized exemption by FDA that allows the drug sponsor to ship within the United States for clinical trial purposes (FDA, 2022).

In the initial stages of preclinical development, the sponsor aims to verify the drug's preliminary safety for human use and to ascertain whether it demonstrates sufficient pharmacologic activity to warrant further development. Once a drug is deemed a promising candidate, the focus shifts toward gathering the requisite data and documentation to demonstrate that early-phase clinical trials can be conducted without subjecting humans to undue risk (FDA, 2022).

The FDA's role in the development of a new drug commences when an IND is submitted. It then begins a review of the drug with the goal of protecting the safety and rights of human participants and ensuring the scientific quality of the clinical investigation.

The following three types of INDs can be submitted to FDA (2022):

- **Investigator IND:** When an investigator is interested in exploring either a compound in development or a new indication for an approved drug, they apply for an IND. Typically, they will request the investigational drug from the manufacturer, but the physician retains responsibility for the trial development and conduct. Often called investigator-initiated trials, these studies are commonly conducted in the oncology therapeutic arena and can bring significant value to the understanding of a compound and potential indications for further research.
- **Emergency use IND:** When there is not enough time to follow the regulated submission pathway for an IND, this mechanism allows for the use of an investigational drug in an emergency. Participants may not meet the requirements for inclusion into the protocol being conducted, or the investigational drug may be indicated when an approved study protocol is not in place. The FDA website (www.fda.gov/drugs/types-applications/investigational-new-drug-ind-application) has tools that will support the physician while ensuring the participant meets the established criteria for an emergency use IND. The IND is obtained via a phone call to FDA.
- **Treatment IND:** This IND can be submitted when an investigational compound is at the end of its promising late-stage testing and is under review by FDA for a serious or immediately life-threatening condition. This would allow for restricted use of the investigational compound per the scope of the IND.

U.S. Food and Drug Administration Review of the Application

The scope of the IND must include information that supports the FDA's understanding of the potential safety of the compound in question for human use. The application must address the following key components (FDA, 2015):

- First, it must include nonclinical pharmacology, pharmacokinetic, and toxicology studies. These studies provide details on the pharmacologic effects and mechanisms of action of the drug in animals and information on the absorption, distribution, metabolism, and excretion of the drug. An integrated summary of the toxicologic effects, drawn from both in vivo animal studies and in vitro experiments, is also required. The specific studies needed depend on the type of drug and the phase of human investigation. If the applicant has any additional data related to use in humans, such as from international clinical trials, these must also be submitted.
- Second, manufacturing information is reviewed and assessed for the chemical composition of the compound, manufacturer location, stability data for the drugs, and information regarding good manufacturing practices.
- Third, the IND must include clinical protocols and investigator information to ensure the development plan is scientifically rigorous and aligned with regulatory standards for participant safety. Investigator qualifications are provided to ensure that research will be sound and follow regulations and Good Clinical Practice. This information is also documented via Form FDA 1572, which is signed by the principal investigator. The application must also include documentation confirming the commitment to obtain informed consent and the review from the institutional review board (FDA, 2010).
- Finally, once submitted, FDA reviews the IND within a 30-day window. There is no formal approval, but it is understood that the agency uses the 30 days to review the submission details to consider the safety and applicability of the protocol from a medical, chemical, pharmaco-

logic, and statistical perspective. If the reviewers feel that not enough evidence demonstrates that the compound is safe to administer in humans, they will institute a clinical hold, and the trial will not move forward until additional data are submitted (FDA, 2018b).

Maintaining and Amending an Investigational New Drug Application

Once an IND is filed, the clinical trial investigation can begin as indicated. The trial is expected to be governed by Good Clinical Practice and applicable regulations. Modifications to an active IND are described under 21 Code of Federal Regulations 312.D. The main categories include the following (IND Application, 1987; FDA, 2021):

- **Information amendments:** Any modifications to ongoing studies, including changes to the study protocol, initiation of new studies under the same indication, or changes in the investigator team, require submission of an IND amendment.
- **Safety reporting**: Sponsors are obliged to report any suspected or actual adverse reaction to study treatment that is serious or unexpected. FDA mandates that these reports be submitted within 15 calendar days following the discovery of any serious adverse events that suggest a significant risk to participants. Unanticipated fatal or life-threatening suspected adverse reactions must be reported to FDA as soon as possible, but no later than seven calendar days following the sponsor's awareness of the event. Any relevant additional information that pertains to the previous IND safety report must be submitted as a follow-up report as soon as possible, but no later than 15 calendar days after the sponsor receives the information (FDA, 2021).
- **Annual reporting:** Even in the absence of active studies, an annual report summarizing the IND's progress and any significant findings must be submitted within 60 days of the IND's anniversary date.

If the drug shows efficacy with acceptable safety in adequate and well-controlled studies, it can be considered for market approval. Data may be submitted to FDA as an NDA for small molecules or a biologic license application (BLA) for biologics. Figure 2-1 illustrates an overview of the drug development process.

Upon approval of the NDA/BLA, a company may begin marketing the drug to consumers. Additional drug testing may continue after the NDA/BLA is approved to gain more data regarding participant quality of life, the cost-effectiveness of treatments, and other epidemiologic parameters. Further clinical trial work may continue after NDA/BLA approval to support new dosages and forms or routes of administration (e.g., patch, IV, oral tablets, oral suspension).

Naming of Drugs

As the investigational agent progresses through drug development, it is typically assigned multiple names. Initially, all compounds (except cell therapies) require a Chemical Abstract Services (CAS) registry number (RN) and chemical name. As the drug moves through clinical development, a generic (nonproprietary) name must be approved by the U.S. Adopted Names Council and the International Nonproprietary Names Committee. These organizations aim for global standardization of drug nomenclature to reduce the risk of prescription drug errors and improve patient safety (Abioye, 2021). The generic name references the mechanism of action, target, or structure in the stem portion of the name. Scientific accuracy and patient safety are the key focuses. It is not promotional or owned by any company. In contrast, the brand name is created and owned by the company that patents the drug. Marketability and patient safety are key focuses. Before any drug reaches the market, it is thor-

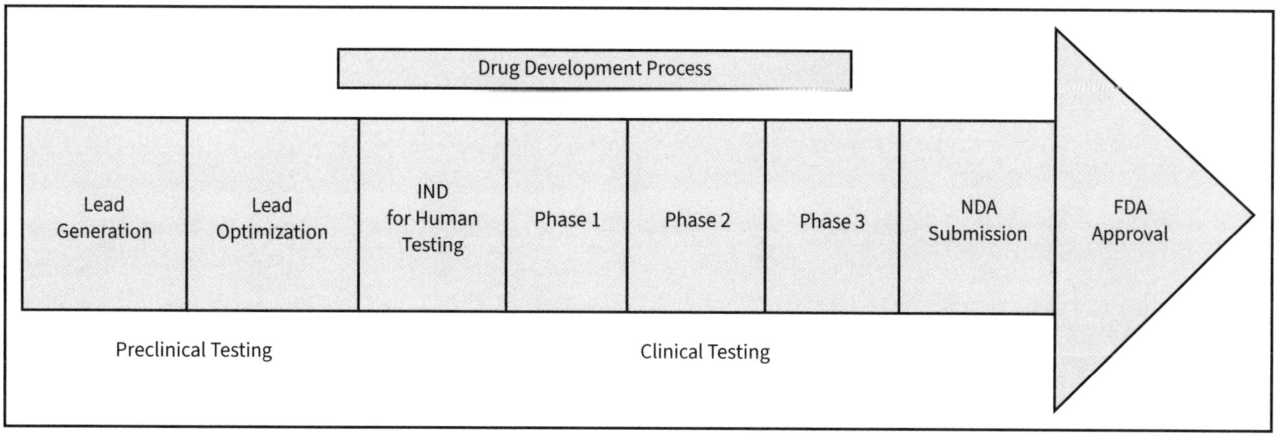

FIGURE 2-1 | Drug Development Process

FDA—U.S. Food and Drug Administration; IND—Investigational New Drug; NDA—New Drug Application oughly examined to identify misleading or potentially confusing messaging (FDA, 2016).

Summary

The landscape of oncology drug development is dynamic, characterized by continuous innovation and stringent regulatory oversight. As the field advances, the integration of new technologies and therapeutic modalities promises to revolutionize cancer treatment. However, the journey from a promising compound to an FDA-approved drug remains a complex and challenging endeavor, underscored by the commitment to enhancing patient outcomes and advancing public health.

Key Points

- FDA and the sponsor have essential roles in U.S. drug development.
- Drug development requires basic science and research.
- In vitro and in vivo experiments are essential prior to administering a new molecule to humans and form the basis of an IND.
- An IND application is a request for authorization from FDA to administer an investigational drug or biological product to humans for clinical trial purposes.

The author would like to acknowledge David Gillogly, MBA, BS, Pamela Perry, MS, and Joan G. Westendorp, MSN, RN, OCN®, CCRP, CIM, for their contribution to this chapter that remains unchanged from the previous edition of this book.

References

Abioye, A.O. (2021). Integrated approach to drug nomenclature. In A. Adejare (Ed.), *Remington* (23rd ed., pp. 23–41). Elsevier Academic Press. https://doi.org/10.1016/B978-0-12-820007-0.00002-7

Gallin, J.I. (2018). A historical perspective on clinical research. In J.I. Gallin, F.P. Ognibene, & L.L. Johnson (Eds.), *Principles and practice of clinical research* (4th ed., pp. 1–15). Elsevier Academic Press. https://doi.org/10.1016/B978-0-12-849905-4.00001-0

Hughes, J.P., Rees, S., Kalindjian, S.B., & Philpott, K.L. (2011). Principles of early drug discovery. *British Journal of Pharmacology, 162*(6), 1239–1249. https://doi.org/10.1111/j.1476-5381.2010.01127.x

Investigational New Drug Application, 21 C.F.R. § 312.D (1987). https://www.ecfr.gov/current/title-21/chapter-I/subchapter-D/part-312

U.S. Food and Drug Administration. (2010, May). *Information sheet guidance for sponsors, clinical investigators, and IRBs: Frequently asked questions – Statement of investigator (Form FDA 1572).* https://www.fda.gov/media/78830/download

U.S. Food and Drug Administration. (2014). *How drugs are developed and approved.* https://www.fda.gov/drugs/developmentapprovalprocess/howdrugsaredevelopedandapproved

U.S. Food and Drug Administration. (2015). *Drug development and review definitions.* https://www.fda.gov/drugs/investigational-new-drug-ind-application/drug-development-and-review-definitions

U.S. Food and Drug Administration. (2016). *Drug name review.* https://www.fda.gov/drugs/fda-drug-info-rounds-video/drug-name-review

U.S. Food and Drug Administration. (2018a). *FDA in brief: FDA modernizes clinical trial designs and approaches for drug development, proposing new guidance on the use of adaptive designs and master protocols.* https://www.fda.gov/news-events/fda-brief/fda-brief-fda-modernizes-clinical-trial-designs-and-approaches-drug-development-proposing-new

U.S. Food and Drug Administration. (2018b). *IND clinical holds* (MAPP 6030.1 Rev. 3). https://www.fda.gov/media/72751/download

U.S. Food and Drug Administration. (2018c). *What are "biologics" questions and answers.* https://www.fda.gov/about-fda/center-biologics-evaluation-and-research-cber/what-are-biologics-questions-and-answers

U.S. Food and Drug Administration. (2021). *IND application reporting: Safety reports.* https://www.fda.gov/drugs/investigational-new-drug-ind-application/ind-application-reporting-safety-reports

U.S. Food and Drug Administration. (2022). *Investigational New Drug application.* https://www.fda.gov/drugs/types-applications/investigational-new-drug-ind-application

U.S. Food and Drug Administration. (2023a). *Biosimilar and interchangeable biologics: More treatment choices.* https://www.fda.gov/consumers/consumer-updates/biosimilar-and-interchangeable-biologics-more-treatment-choices

U.S. Food and Drug Administration. (2023b). *Real-time oncology review.* https://www.fda.gov/about-fda/oncology-center-excellence/real-time-oncology-review

U.S. Food and Drug Administration. (2024). *OCE programs and projects overview.* https://www.fda.gov/about-fda/oncology-center-excellence/oce-programs-and-projects-overview

CHAPTER 3

Types of Clinical Research: Background

Donglan Xia, PhD, RN, OCN®

Introduction

Clinical research is evolving. Although the time-honored designs of experimental and observational studies continue to provide the foundation for clinical research, this field recognizes that the rapid translation of scientific advances to the clinical setting is increasingly important. Medical and scientific experts agree that clinical research methods and designs must progress to meet the growing demand for faster and more efficient translation of scientific discoveries into patient care. This is especially important for treating serious illnesses such as cancer, where advancing therapies can lead to improved outcomes and better quality of life. During the past decade, there has been an exponential increase in the number of registered clinical trials. In 2010, there were 82,859 registered trials, and by 2025, this number had surged to 520,886 (ClinicalTrials.gov, n.d.).

Clinical trials are a vital process for evaluating the safety and efficacy of new treatments, diagnostic methods, and preventive strategies. They provide valuable data to guide clinical practice, inform regulatory decisions, and advance scientific understanding of cancer biology. As the clinical trial industry continues to expand, there is an increasing focus on improving access, enhancing the welfare of study participants, and promoting greater inclusivity. The technological advancements driven by the COVID-19 pandemic have accelerated the development and use of virtual healthcare platforms, even for complex oncology care, which has significantly influenced how clinical trials are conducted (Li & Bergan, 2020).

In response to the unprecedented need for faster development of cancer treatments, the U.S. Food and Drug Administration (FDA) has developed four expedited pathways—Priority Review, Breakthrough Therapy Designation, Accelerated Approval, and Fast Track Designation—so that it can bring drugs for serious diseases to market, offering significant advancements over existing treatments or fill unmet medical needs. Priority Review ensures a quicker evaluation process for drugs with substantial benefits, whereas Breakthrough Therapy Designation provides intensive guidance and faster review for treatments showing significant improvement over current options. Accelerated Approval allows early market access based on surrogate end points, contingent on further confirmation of clinical benefit. Fast Track Designation facilitates rapid development and review for drugs addressing unmet medical needs. These approaches collectively aim to expedite access to vital therapies for patients in need (Kwok et al., 2015; Shahzad et al., 2023).

This chapter will discuss the background and continuing evolution of clinical research design.

Traditional Clinical Research Design

Experimental Versus Observational Clinical Research

Today's clinical research serves as the blueprint for future standard care. Experimental clinical research, also known as clinical trials or interventional or therapeutic research, involves testing various interventions, such as drugs, medical devices, procedures, or behavioral modifications. Before treatment can transition into standard care, research interventions must undergo rigorous testing within a small population of volunteer participants to evaluate their safety, effectiveness, and risk-to-benefit ratio compared to standard treatments. Regulatory agencies, particularly considering advancements in genetically modified cellular therapies, also require long-term safety assessments. The gold standard of an experimental design is the randomized controlled trial, which provides the highest level of evidence-based medicine, particularly in the development of new drugs.

A second type of traditional clinical research is observational. Although this type of research involves voluntary human participants, it does not include planned research alterations or interventions. Participants may be receiving standard medical care or routine procedures, but no experimental interventions or agents are assigned to them. Observational studies provide data related to health outcomes, allowing researchers to define these outcomes in specific groups of participants (Kiani et al., 2022).

The Four Phases of a Clinical Trial

Phase 1 clinical trials are designed to assess the safety of an investigational new drug to human participants, particularly after it has demonstrated efficacy in laboratory and animal studies (phase 0 or preclinical studies). These trials aim to identify the maximum tolerated dose of a drug, ensure a reasonable safety and side effect profile, and detect dose-limiting toxicities. The number of participants enrolled in phase 1 studies is limited to 10–20 patients. The determined maximum tolerated dose can be expanded to more patients in phase 2 trials, where early treatment efficacy is further evaluated.

Phase 2 trials are conducted to assess whether the selected investigational new drug or treatment intervention demonstrates efficacy or clinical response at the specified dose determined by the phase 1 trial. At this stage, more patients will be enrolled and treated. Safety data are continuously monitored throughout treatment. Upon observing promising results in the phase 2 trial, a randomized phase 3 trial will then be necessary to compare the study intervention to the current standard of care (routine care).

Phase 3 trials generally enroll hundreds of patients across multiple locations (multicenter or globally) to ensure statistical reliability and detect less common side effects, except for rare disease indication trials.

A phase 4 clinical trial takes place after a drug or treatment has been approved for public use by regulatory authorities. These trials gather additional information on the drug's long-term safety, efficacy, and optimal use in a broader population. Whereas earlier phases focus on assessing safety and effectiveness in controlled environments, phase 4 trials monitor the drug's performance in real-world settings. See Table 3-1 for a summary of the four phases of clinical trials.

Evolving Clinical Trial Designs in Oncology: Adaptive Trial Designs

Adaptive design in clinical trials allows for optimization of trial procedures (e.g., dosing, sample size, patient population, treatment regimen) based on patient response or interim analysis of the clinical trial. This approach contrasts with traditional fixed designs, where the protocol is set at the beginning and remains unchanged throughout the trial. Adaptive designs allow continued data collection and analysis during the trial. There is a growing trend to integrate different response outcomes and phases into a single clinical trial to accelerate the drug development process and reduce associated time and costs. Adaptive designs align with the FDA's guidance to enhance patient safety and optimize resources by allowing real-time, data-driven adjustments during the trial (Zang & Lee, 2014). With meticulous design and planning, adaptive designs use accumulated data to modify the ongoing trial without compromising its integrity and validity. The designs have potential advantages, including improving study power, reducing sample size and total cost, treating more patients with more effective treatments, identifying efficacious drugs for specific subgroups of patients based on their biomarker profiles, and shortening the time for drug development (Zang & Lee, 2014).

Adaptive designs in clinical trials offer several flexible features. Some protocols allow for sample size reassessment to include more patients and generate statistically stronger results. If the interim analysis indicates an inferior treatment arm, it can be discontinued in the middle of the trial. Additionally, patients in the control arm may be allowed to move to a more promising treatment. Adaptive enrichment enables the enrollment of more patients in favorable treatment arms.

Furthermore, separate cohorts can be created to ensure the accessibility and adequate participation of minority groups. Adaptive and seamless designs can be incorporated to enhance the efficiency of clinical trials. Seamless designs facilitate a continuous transition from one phase to the next, such as from phase 1 to 2 (often referred to as phase 1a and 1b, or dose escalation and expansion) or from phase 2 to 3. These approaches reduce the time and resources required for protocol development, allowing promising therapies to advance more quickly through the clinical trial pipeline. For example, in a seamless phase 2 to 3 trial, data from the phase 2 trial can be used to determine key factors, such as the allocation ratio, planned total sample size, and a potentially enriched population for the subsequent phase 3. Data from phase 2 can also be incorporated for data analysis for FDA approval (Buxton et al., 2020).

Master Protocol Designs

In the past 15 years, cancer clinical trials have experienced critical paradigm shifts to fit the need for precision oncology as defined by various biomarkers. Although randomized controlled trials remain the gold standard in oncology, molecular and genomic profiling has been driving changes in oncology clinical research trials, leading to the era of personalized medicine.

New trial designs, such as master protocols encompassing umbrella, basket, and platform trials, have emerged to

TABLE 3-1 | The Four Phases of a Clinical Trial

Phase	Primary Focus	Participants	Key Objectives	Outcomes
Phase 1	Safety and dosage	10–20	Identify the maximum tolerated dose. Detect dose-limiting toxicity.	Assess safe dosage levels and preliminary safety profile.
Phase 2	Efficacy and safety	50–100s	Assess drug efficacy. Monitor ongoing safety.	Determine if the drug works as intended and its safety.
Phase 3	Comparison of the standard of care	100s–1,000s, multicenter	Compare new treatment with standard treatments. Detect less common side effects.	Provide evidence for regulatory approval based on efficacy and safety.
Phase 4	Post-approval safety and long-term efficacy	Thousands, real-world setting	Monitor long-term safety and effectiveness. Detect rare or long-term side effects.	Ensure optimal drug use in the general population.

address the challenges posed by targeted therapies. These designs are widely used in protocols and are set to become the future standard in clinical trial methodology.

A master protocol design allows for the simultaneous evaluation of multiple treatments or interventions within the same protocol framework. It enables the investigation of several research questions or hypotheses under a single protocol, often involving multiple substudies or arms (cohorts) (Di Liello et al., 2021). In this type of trial, patients are typically screened for eligibility based on specific criteria defined in the master protocol. However, upon successful screening, patients are assigned to different substudies or arms based on specific characteristics or biomarkers for treatment. Separate screening procedures might be needed to enroll for specific treatment arms. Each substudy or arm may evaluate a different treatment or intervention, allowing for the simultaneous evaluation of multiple therapies. This type of protocol design offers several advantages, including efficient use of resources, accelerated drug development, and increased flexibility in adapting to new scientific discoveries or changing treatment paradigms. Additionally, it allows for the evaluation of targeted therapies in biomarker-defined patient populations, facilitating the advancement of precision medicine (Di Liello et al., 2021).

A master protocol design refers to a strategy where patient selection and treatment allocation are guided by specific biomarkers, such as genetic variants, protein expressions, or other molecular characteristics. These trials aim to identify subgroups of patients more likely to respond to a particular treatment based on biomarker profile, enabling a more personalized approach to therapy. By targeting treatments to patients with specific biomarkers, these trials increase the likelihood of demonstrating efficacy and optimizing patient outcomes.

Biomarker-driven designs include enrichment, stratified, adaptive, umbrella, and basket trials—each tailored to address different research questions and patient populations. These innovative designs represent a shift toward precision medicine in clinical research, offering the potential to improve treatment outcomes and accelerate drug development (Janiaud et al., 2019).

Decentralized Clinical Research

Clinical trial participation may pose time, cost, and logistical burdens on patients, who may be required to travel to their study centers for treatment administration, additional monitoring, biospecimen collection, or survey completion. This imposes a significant barrier for patients, especially for minority and underserved communities, as they generally lack social support (Fu et al., 2023).

Decentralized clinical trials (DCTs) involve conducting one or more procedures related to clinical trials at locations other than the main trial sites, including local physicians' clinics or participants' homes. The aim is to provide greater convenience for participants, making it easier for them to enroll in clinical trials and reducing the number of visits they need to make to the primary trial sites listed in FDA documents (Park et al., 2024). Although the complexity of oncology research trials makes it hard to conduct them entirely remotely, with careful protocol designs and technologies, the number of on-site assessments can be significantly reduced to ease the burden on clinical research participants. Compared with traditional clinical trials, DCTs represent a paradigm shift from site centered to patient centered. These trials have been gaining significant traction, revolutionizing traditional trial practices (Park et al., 2024).

In DCTs, participants are also more willing to participate when the number of in-person clinic visits is significantly reduced and the trials fit their lifestyles. Therefore, DCTs enable the recruitment of participants from a more diverse geographic location, including rural and underserved settings. In addition, by leveraging telemedicine and remote monitoring, researchers can significantly widen the pool of eligible participants from different geographic locations. Most importantly, because DCT participants have a greater sense of control in terms of scheduling location, time of assessment, and retention, patient engagement is significantly improved (Park et al., 2024).

In 2024, FDA issued *Decentralized Clinical Trials for Drugs and Biologics Guidance for Industry, Investigators, and Other Interested Parties*, which provides recommendations to sponsors on conducting DCTs, including considerations for protocol design, electronic informed consent, remote monitoring, and data collection methods. The COVID-19 pandemic significantly accelerated the adoption of DCTs, as sponsors and researchers embraced newer models to maintain clinical trial continuity while ensuring patient safety and convenience. According to reports, a threefold increase in remote patient interactions is expected to persist, driven by the adoption of telemedicine, direct-to-patient drug shipments, and home healthcare services (Adesoye et al., 2023).

Overall, DCTs offer a patient-centric, technology-enabled approach to clinical research, leveraging digital health innovations to enhance efficiency, inclusivity, and data quality in drug development. As technology continues to evolve and regulatory frameworks adapt, decentralized trial methodologies are poised to become increasingly prominent in the clinical trial landscape (Fu et al., 2023).

Patient-Reported Outcomes and Measures in Oncology Clinical Trials

A patient-reported outcome (PRO) is a measurement of any aspect of health status that comes directly from a patient without the interpretation from a physician or other healthcare professional. In clinical trials, PROs are valuable to assess the impact of a treatment intervention on one or more aspects of patients' subjective health status (Lipscomb et al., 2007). PROs assessments range from the purely symptomatic, such as the response to a headache, to more complex concepts, such as the ability to perform activities of daily living. Data generated by a PRO instrument can provide evidence of a treatment benefit from the patient perspective (Coles et al., 2024). Patient-reported outcome measures (PROMs) are the tools or instruments used to measure PROs. These tools are often self-completed questionnaires, either in a traditional paper format or digital (e.g., electronic tablets, smartphone devices) (Malandrini et al., 2023).

PRO assessment has been increasingly incorporated in oncology clinical trials as a secondary study end point, offering valuable insight regarding patient experience, treatment efficacy, and overall impact on quality of life. Integrating PRO assessments into clinical trials allows researchers to capture the perspective of patients directly, going beyond the traditional clinical end points, such as progression-free and overall survival. This inclusion enables a more comprehensive assessment of treatment benefits and adverse effects, enhancing the overall validity of a trial (Mercieca-Bebber et al., 2018). Incorporating PROs in the clinical trial design facilitates the selection of appropriate outcome measures tailored to specific patient populations and therapeutic objectives. By identifying key interests, such as symptom severity, physical functioning, emotional well-being, and treatment satisfaction, researchers can develop more comprehensive tools that capture the multidimensional impact of their new oncology intervention. Moreover, the inclusion of PROs as a patient-centric approach fosters greater engagement and compliance throughout trials, leading to improved data quality and retention rates. Additionally, PRO data can support regulatory decision-making by offering valuable insights into treatment benefits and risks from the patient's perspective. Overall, integrating PROs into clinical trial design enhances the relevance, validity, and patient-centeredness of research efforts, ultimately leading to more robust and informative trial outcomes (Mercieca-Bebber et al., 2018).

Regulators, clinicians, and patients increasingly recognize PROs in clinical trials as valuable tools to collect patient-centered data. FDA has emphasized PROs in the evaluation of medical investigational product efficacy and safety. Although there may not be specific requirements, it continues to encourage the use of PROs to capture the patient perspective. FDA's *Guidance for Industry: Patient-Reported Outcome Measures: Use in Medical Product Development to Support Labeling Claims* provides recommendations on the selection, development, and validation of PRO measures for use in clinical trials (U.S. Department of Health and Human Services et al., 2006).

Additionally, FDA's Patient-Focused Drug Development initiative involves gathering patient input for regulatory decision-making, including the selection of relevant end points and outcome measures, such as PROs (Kluetz & Bhatnagar, 2021). Although specific requirements may not have drastically changed, sponsors are encouraged to consider PROs in trial designs and engage with FDA early in the development process to ensure that PRO end points are appropriately selected, validated, and analyzed to support labeling claims.

Promoting Clinical Trial Access to Minority and Underserved Communities

Although clinical trials offer significant benefits for patients and the healthcare industry, recruitment and enrollment often face challenges, particularly among minority and underserved communities. Persistent barriers continue to hinder participation from these groups, leading to a lack of diversity in trials (Farb et al., 2023). This underrepresentation can deepen existing disparities, as the participant pool should ideally reflect the demographics of the broader patient population. The barriers to participation are often multifaceted, including limited access to healthcare services, lack of awareness, historical mistrust of the medical system, socioeconomic disparities, lack of health insurance, cultural and language barriers, stigma, structural inequalities, and insufficient diversity among research staff.

Without diversity, there is no clarity as to how trial results apply to underrepresented groups. Diverse trial populations can provide valuable insights into the benefits and risks of health products across demographics. This makes addressing the lack of diversity in clinical trials crucial for ensuring equitable access to safe and effective treatments and improving public health outcomes for all (Farb et al., 2023).

Clinical trial databases serve as repositories of information for clinical studies, offering a centralized platform for researchers, healthcare professionals, patients, and the public to access details about ongoing and completed trials (Paunic et al., 2023). These databases, which also serve as clinical trial search engines, play a crucial role in improving awareness of clinical trials by providing accessibility for users, including physicians, patients, and navigators, to discover relevant research opportunities. Multiple clinical trial databases and repositories have been established worldwide to increase awareness of clinical trials. ClinicalTrials.gov, maintained by the U.S. National Library of Medicine at the National Institutes of Health, is widely regarded as one of the most comprehensive clinical trial databases globally. It covers a vast array of clinical trials conducted worldwide, including both publicly and privately funded studies.

Although multiple clinical trial search engines are available, they may be challenging for individuals with low health and computer literacy to navigate (Paunic et al., 2023). To bridge the gap and ensure that patients have access to available trial information, clinical trial navigating teams can offer additional education and support to prescreened, eligible patients. Institutions have employed culturally sensitive, multilingual professionals to better serve Hispanic and Black patients. These patient navigating teams maintain ongoing communication with enrolled participants to address and overcome barriers that may arise, reducing early trial dropout rates. Additionally, financial resources are allocated to assist with transportation and other expenses, further facilitating participation in clinical trials (Nipp et al., 2019).

Overall, increasing clinical trial access to minorities and underserved communities is essential for promoting health equity, advancing scientific knowledge, and improving healthcare outcomes. By prioritizing diversity and inclusivity in clinical research, researchers can develop more effective and equitable treatments that meet the needs of diverse patient populations.

Artificial Intelligence in Clinical Research

Given the complexity, labor-intensive nature, high cost, and susceptibility to unexpected errors and biases (e.g., gender, race, socioeconomic status) in clinical trials, researchers are increasingly turning to machine learning and artificial intelligence (AI) to optimize clinical trial conduct. Machine learning models can use real-world patient data and provide evidence to loosen clinical trial eligibility criteria and increase enrollment without compromising trial validity (Zhang et al., 2023).

AI can also improve patient enrollment or reduce sample sizes. Researchers have developed clinical trial matching systems or services using natural language processing tools that can extract key information to help determine patient eligibility (Chopra et al., 2023). For example, machine learning has been used to automatically match patients with clinical trials based on specific eligibility criteria. By analyzing patient data against these criteria, the technology narrows down the list of clinical trials for which a patient is most qualified. This saves time for healthcare providers and patients and ensures that patients are matched with trials that best suit their eligibility and medical needs. Studies have shown that AI-based clinical trial matching systems have demonstrated their ability to efficiently and accurately screen patients with cancer for suitable clinical trials (Chopra et al., 2023).

Digital twins (DTs) in drug development and clinical trials are computer-generated models that act as virtual copies of real biologic or physical systems (Bordukova et al., 2024). These digital models, created with the help of AI, allow researchers to run virtual experiments and tests in a digital environment. By using these simulations, researchers can study how drugs might work in the body and predict outcomes before testing them on actual patients, making the process faster and safer. Although available DTs only include a fraction of generative AI's full capabilities, they have already improved the understanding of diseases, aided in discovering biomarkers, and accelerated drug development. These advancements are helping to shape the future of precision medicine. However, overcoming technical and regulatory challenges is essential to unlocking the full transformative potential of DTs in revolutionizing drug discovery and clinical trials (Bordukova et al., 2024).

With its fast-growing capability, AI will revolutionize clinical trials by making them faster, more efficient, and more reliable. From patient recruitment to data analysis and regulatory compliance, AI applications are enhancing every stage of the clinical trial process. As these technologies continue to evolve, their integration into clinical trials will likely become even more sophisticated, further accelerating the development of new treatments and therapies.

Minimal Residual Disease Testing in Clinical Trials

Minimal residual disease (MRD) testing is a highly sensitive method used to detect the presence of cancer cells that remain in the body after treatment, even when these cells are undetectable by traditional diagnostic tools, such as imaging or standard blood or biopsy tests. MRD is detected using advanced techniques, such as next-generation sequencing, flow cytometry, and polymerase chain reaction (Derman et al., 2021; Ye et al., 2019). These techniques offer high sensitivity in identifying even small amounts of residual cancer cells. Early detection of MRD allows clinicians to intervene sooner if a relapse is likely, improving patient outcomes. Continuous MRD monitoring enables timely adjustments in therapy, allowing for early treatment of residual disease and potentially enhancing long-term outcomes.

Integrating MRD assessment into clinical trials offers valuable insights into treatment responses and patient outcomes, improving the efficiency and effectiveness of cancer therapies. For example, in multiple myeloma trials, MRD monitoring was incorporated into an adaptive design. In these trials, participants who achieved MRD negativity were assigned to lower-intensity maintenance treatment, whereas participants who failed to achieve MRD negativity after induction were assigned to additional consolidation or autologous stem cell transplant (Derman et al., 2021; Ye et al., 2019). The importance of using MRD negativity as a primary end point in clinical trial design lies in its ability to provide early and precise indications of treatment efficacy. Differences in the rate of MRD negativity between treatment arms can be assessed within a relatively short time frame of 9–15 months, depending on the treatment duration. This rapid assessment enables the quicker evaluation of the effectiveness of novel therapies, potentially accelerating the regulatory approval process. By providing an early and reliable biomarker for treatment response, MRD negativity helps streamline the development of new treatments, making effective therapies available to patients sooner and improving overall clinical outcomes (Thompson, 2018).

To enhance the monitoring and management of patients with certain types of blood cancers, such as multiple myeloma and acute lymphoblastic leukemia, FDA authorized a highly sensitive next-generation sequencing–based test for MRD detection. This authorization is a significant advancement in the ability to monitor and manage these diseases, as this test offers a high level of sensitivity and accuracy in detecting residual cancer cells that remain after treatment. This could potentially improve patient outcomes through timely interventions and personalized therapy adjustments (FDA Issues Draft Guidance on MRD Testing, 2018).

Optimization of Clinical Trials After the COVID-19 Pandemic

The COVID-19 pandemic has significantly affected clinical trial operations and prompted innovations and optimizations to ensure that clinical research can continue efficiently and safely. During the pandemic, clinical trials encountered considerable disruptions, including delays in launching new studies, challenges in patient enrollment, and difficulties in updating case report forms because of the limited availability of clinical trial staff during lockdown. To address these challenges, the rapid adoption of digital tools and methodologies has been successful. Healthcare facilities quickly adopted videoconferencing platforms, such as Zoom and Microsoft Teams, for conducting remote clinical visits, allowing patients to self-report vital signs, and discussing conditions with physicians from the safety of their homes. Consent and reconsent processes were also conducted remotely through video and phone calls, and signatures were able to be obtained with digital signature platforms.

Data monitoring, meetings, and audits—typically demanding activities for sponsors and researchers—were also effectively transitioned to remote formats without compromising the integrity and quality of clinical research (Castelo-Branco et al., 2021). Hospitals provided secure access to trial documents, enabling remote study monitoring and auditing. The digitization of source documents accelerated data integration into electronic data capture systems. The shift to remote operations, driven by the pandemic, demonstrated that administrative activities in clinical trials can maintain high research standards and should be considered for continued use in the future. Remote meetings, data verification, and monitoring through phone calls, video visits, and emails can be permitted in well-defined settings after establishing validated standard operating procedures. In addition, AI tools and text-mining technologies for data collection, review, and monitoring, when adequately validated, can be used to reduce the workload of clinical research staff (Castelo-Branco et al., 2021).

Beyond clinical trial administrative activities, investigational product management also adapted swiftly during the pandemic to ensure continuity while maintaining patient safety. A key operational change was the direct-to-patient delivery of investigational drugs, which enabled study participants to take part in trials remotely, reducing the need for in-person visits and facilitating ongoing participation (Flet et al., 2020).

The Role of Oncology Clinical Research Nurses

Oncology clinical research nurses (OCRNs) are registered nurses trained to support the comprehensive operations of clinical trials and manage participant care. They are responsible for ensuring protocol adherence, screening, and enrollment, and coordinating all patient care activities for research participants while they are on clinical trials. OCRNs collaborate with the interprofessional research team, including principal investigators, physicians, clinical research coordinators, and study sponsors, to ensure the safe and ethical conduct of the trial (Legor et al., 2021).

The clinical trials industry has experienced remarkable growth, especially in the oncology field, leading to an increased demand for qualified OCRNs. As more clinical trials adopt decentralized or remote models, the need for experienced OCRNs is growing at an unprecedented pace. These nurses are crucial for managing participant care, ensuring protocol adherence, and facilitating communication among interprofessional teams in both hospital and sponsor settings. However, the 2020 National Nursing Workforce Survey reported a consecutive decline in the number of practicing OCRNs in the United States between the 2017 and 2020 surveys, compared to earlier reports in 2013 and 2015 (Johnson, 2022).

This workforce contraction coincides with a surge in clinical trial activity, marking one of the highest volumes of trial starts in modern history and amplifying concerns about adequate OCRN staffing (Flet et al., 2020). The increasing complexity of investigative products, evolving safety profiles, and a growing emphasis on community participant enrollment necessitate OCRN involvement for enhanced safety monitoring and effective interprofessional communication among clinical providers and research collaborators.

In an era of historically high clinical trial activities and increased utilization of remote and decentralized trial models, the need exists for OCRNs with advanced trial management skills to handle complex safety reporting and changes in participant status in these new trial models. Within this scope, OCRNs administer investigational products with unknown safety profiles, requiring a specialized skill set to monitor for subtle health changes that could indicate serious issues. This contrasts with research coordinators, who lack complex medical training and credentials in nursing skills and assessments. OCRNs are also trained to identify and predict safety issues, leveraging their nursing assessment skills to prevent potential injuries to participants. This skill gap underscores the critical role of OCRNs in ensuring participant safety and effective trial management in the evolving landscape of clinical research (Johnson, 2022).

Summary

Clinical trials are rapidly evolving, driven by technological advancements and the need for greater efficiency. These developments have created more efficient, representative, and patient-focused clinical research paradigms while maintaining robust scientific standards. OCRNs serve a key role in the advancement of techniques and trial designs that drive a new age of cancer research.

Key Points

- Adaptive trial designs balance scientific rigor with patient-centric flexibility.
- Inclusive recruitment strategies target underrepresented populations to enhance diversity.
- Remote operational capabilities include digital monitoring and secure data access, which became essential during the COVID-19 pandemic.
- AI-powered solutions have provided intelligent patient matching and workload reductions.
- Precision medicine approaches incorporate genetic and lifestyle factors for targeted therapies.
- The systematic collection of PROs allows for more comprehensive analysis of the real-world impact of treatments.

The author would like to acknowledge Teresa Knoop, MSN, RN, AOCN®, Pamela Carney, MSN, RN, OCN®, and Joan G. Westendorp, MSN, RN, OCN®, CCRP, CIM, for their contribution to this chapter that remains unchanged from the previous edition of this book.

References

Adesoye, T., Katz, M.H.G., & Offodile, A.C., 2nd. (2023). Meeting trial participants where they are: Decentralized clinical trials as a patient-centered paradigm for enhancing accrual and diversity in surgical and multidisciplinary trials in oncology. *JCO Oncology Practice, 19*(6), 317–321. https://doi.org/10.1200/OP.22.00702

Bordukova, M., Makarov, N., Rodriguez-Esteban, R., Schmich, F., & Menden, M.P. (2024). Generative artificial intelligence empowers digital twins in drug discovery and clinical trials. *Expert Opinion on Drug Discovery, 19*(1), 33–42. https://doi.org/10.1080/17460441.2023.2273839

Buxton, M.B., Alexander, B.M., Berry, D.A., Cavenee, W.K., Colman, H., De Groot, J.F., ... Cloughesy, T.F. (2020). GBM AGILE: A global, phase II/III adaptive platform trial to evaluate multiple regimens in newly diagnosed and recurrent glioblastoma. *Journal of Clinical Oncology, 38*(15, Suppl.). https://doi.org/10.1200/JCO.2020.38.15_suppl.TPS2579

Castelo-Branco, L., Awada, A., Pentheroudakis, G., Perez-Gracia, J.L., Mateo, J., Curigliano, G., ... Peters, S. (2021). Beyond the lessons learned from the COVID-19 pandemic: Opportunities to optimize clinical trial implementation in oncology. *ESMO Open, 6*(5), 100237. https://doi.org/10.1016/j.esmoop.2021.100237

Chopra, H., Annu, Shin, D.K., Munjal, K., Priyanka, Dhama, K., & Emran, T.B. (2023). Revolutionizing clinical trials: The role of AI in accelerating medical breakthroughs. *International Journal of Surgery, 109*(12), 4211–4220. https://doi.org/10.1097/Js9.0000000000000705

ClinicalTrials.gov. (n.d.). *Trends and charts on registered studies.* https://clinicaltrials.gov/about-site/trends-charts

Coles, T., Fillipo, R., Plyler, K., Hernandez, A., Henke, D.M., Arizmendi, C., ... Weinfurt, K. (2024). Facets of physical function assessed by patient-reported outcome measures in oncology research. *Quality of Life Research, 33*(7), 1819–1828. https://doi.org/10.1007/s11136-024-03640-0

Derman, B.A., Zonder, J.A., Kansagra, A.J., Grinblatt, D.L., Narula, S., Rayani, S., ... Jakubowiak, A.J. (2021). Interim analysis of a phase 2 minimal residual disease (MRD)-adaptive trial of elotuzumab, carfilzomib, lenalidomide, and dexamethasone (Elo-KRd) for newly diagnosed multiple myeloma (MM). *Journal of Clinical Oncology, 39*(15, Suppl.). https://doi.org/10.1200/JCO.2021.39.15_suppl.8011

Di Liello, R., Piccirillo, M.C., Arenare, L., Gargiulo, P., Schettino, C., Gravina, A., & Perrone, F. (2021). Master protocols for precision medicine in oncology: Overcoming methodology of randomized clinical trials. *Life, 11*(11), 1253. https://doi.org/10.3390/life11111253

Farb, A., Viviano, C.J., & Tarver, M.E. (2023). Diversity in clinical trial enrollment and reporting—Where we are and the road ahead. *JAMA Cardiology, 8*(9), 803–805. https://doi.org/10.1001/jamacardio.2023.2106

FDA issues draft guidance on MRD testing. (2018). *Cancer Discovery, 8*(12), 1502. https://doi.org/10.1158/2159-8290.CD-NB2018-145

Flet, L., Tching-Sin, M., Chanat, A., Gendre, P., & Tibi, A. (2020). Clinical trials: Management of investigational products during the COVID-19 pandemic. *American Journal of Health-System Pharmacy, 77*(16), 1277–1278. https://doi.org/10.1093/ajhp/zxaa146

Fu, S., Gerber, D.E., & Beg, M.S. (2023). Decentralized clinical trials in oncology: Are we ready for a virtual-first paradigm? *Journal of Clinical Oncology, 41*(2), 181–185. https://doi.org/10.1200/JCO.22.00358

Janiaud, P., Serghiou, S., & Ioannidis, J.P.A. (2019). New clinical trial designs in the era of precision medicine: An overview of definitions, strengths, weaknesses, and current use in oncology. *Cancer Treatment Reviews, 73*, 20–30. https://doi.org/10.1016/j.ctrv.2018.12.003

Johnson, E. (2022). Trouble for trials - The worrying state of the research nurse workforce. *Contemporary Clinical Trials, 120*, 106878. https://doi.org/10.1016/j.cct.2022.106878

Kiani, A.K., Naureen, Z., Pheby, D., Henehan, G., Brown, R., Sieving, P., ... Beretelli, M. (2022). Methodology for clinical research. *Journal of Preventive Medicine and Hygiene, 63*(2, Suppl. 3), E267–E278. https://doi.org/10.15167/2421-4248/jpmh2022.63.2S3.2769

Kluetz, P.G., & Bhatnagar, V. (2021). The FDA's patient-focused drug development initiative. *Clinical Advances in Hematology and Oncology, 19*(2), 70–72.

Kwok, M., Foster, T., & Steinberg, M. (2015). Expedited programs for serious conditions: An update on breakthrough therapy designation. *Clinical Therapeutics, 37*(9), 2104–2120. https://doi.org/10.1016/j.clinthera.2015.07.011

Legor, K.A., Hayman, L.L., Foust, J.B., & Blazey, M.L. (2021). The role of clinical research nurses in minority recruitment to cancer clinical trials. *Contemporary Clinical Trials, 110*. https://doi.org/10.1016/j.cct.2021.106590

Li, A.L., & Bergan, R.C. (2020). Clinical trial design: Past, present, and future in the context of big data and precision medicine. *Cancer, 126*(22), 4838–4846. https://doi.org/10.1002/cncr.33205

Lipscomb, J., Gotay, C.C., & Snyder, C.F. (2007). Patient-reported outcomes in cancer: A review of recent research and policy initiatives. *CA: A Cancer Journal for Clinicians, 57*(5), 278–300. https://doi.org/10.3322/CA.57.5.278

Malandrini, F.B., Meregaglia, M., Pinto, C., Di Maio, M., & Ciani, O. (2023). The development of a comprehensive archive of patient-reported outcome measures (PROMs) for clinical research and clinical practice in oncology [Abstract]. *Value in Health, 26*(12, Suppl.), S451.

Mercieca-Bebber, R., King, M.T., Calvert, M.J., Stockler, M.R., & Friedlander, M. (2018). The importance of patient-reported outcomes in clinical trials and strategies for future optimization. *Patient Related Outcome Measures, 9*, 353–367. https://doi.org/10.2147/PROM.S156279

Nipp, R.D., Hong, K., & Paskett, E.D. (2019). Overcoming barriers to clinical trial enrollment. *American Society of Clinical Oncology Educational Book, 39*, 105–114. https://doi.org/10.1200/EDBK_243729

Park, J., Huh, K.Y., Chung, W.K., & Yu, K.S. (2024). The landscape of decentralized clinical trials (DCTs): Focusing on the FDA and EMA guidance. *Translational and Clinical Pharmacology, 32*(1), 41–51. https://doi.org/10.12793/tcp.2024.32.e2

Paunic, M., Rim, C., Hilal, O., Nassar, R., Zaib, F., Touma, K., ... Hamm, C.M. (2023). Engine failures: A critical analysis of current clinical trial websites' search engines. *Journal of Clinical Oncology, 41*(16). https://doi.org/10.1200/JCO.2023.41.16_suppl.e18537

Shahzad, M., Naci, H., & Wagner, A.K. (2023). Association between preapproval confirmatory trial initiation and conversion to traditional approval or withdrawal in the FDA accelerated approval pathway. *JAMA, 329*(9), 760–761. https://doi.org/10.1001/jama.2023.0625

Thompson, P.A. (2018). MRD negativity as a surrogate for PFS in CLL? *Blood, 131*(9), 943–944. https://doi.org/10.1182/blood-2018-01-824177

U.S. Department of Health and Human Services, Food and Drug Administration, Center for Drug Evaluation and Research, Center for Biologics Evaluation and Research, & Center for Devices and Radiological Health. (2006). Guidance for industry: Patient-reported outcome measures: Use in medical product development to support labeling claims (Draft guidance). *Health and Quality of Life Outcomes, 4*, Article 79. https://doi.org/10.1186/1477-7525-4-79

U.S. Food and Drug Administration. (2024). *Decentralized clinical trials for drugs and biologics: Guidance for industry, investigators, and other interested parties.* https://www.fda.gov/media/167696/download

Ye, J.C., Boonstra, P.S., Boyer, D.F., Anderson, L.D., Lipe, B.C., Kin, A., ... Talpaz, M. (2019). A phase 2 study with minimal residual disease (MRD) driven adaptive strategy in treatment for newly diagnosed multiple myeloma with upfront daratumumab-based therapy. *Blood, 134*(1). https://doi.org/10.1182/blood-2019-132204

Zang, Y., & Lee, J.J. (2014). Adaptive clinical trial designs in oncology. *Chinese Clinical Oncology, 3*(4), 49. https://doi.org/10.3978/j.issn.2304-3865.2014.06.04

Zhang, B., Zhang, L., Chen, Q., Jin, Z., Liu, S., & Zhang, S. (2023). Harnessing artificial intelligence to improve clinical trial design. *Communications Medicine, 3*(1). https://doi.org/10.1038/s43856-023-00425-3

CHAPTER 4

Types of Clinical Research: Experimental

Christopher Graham, BSN, RN, OCN®

Introduction

Clinical research is conducted on humans to understand the effects of an intervention on a disease. These interventions could be medical, surgical, or behavioral (National Institute on Aging, 2023). Clinical research studies can be experimental or observational. This chapter will focus on experimental studies. An experimental or interventional study differs from an observational study because patients are assigned to an intervention (National Library of Medicine, 2023). Observational studies monitor patients and compile data without applying an intervention. Researchers may also analyze data that has already been collected (National Institute on Aging, 2023).

For oncology clinical research nurses (OCRNs) to best care for patients participating in a clinical trial and ensure that the clinical trial is being followed appropriately, there are many key concepts to understand. This chapter will present important terms and ideas that explain the various phases and types of experimental clinical trials, as well as key takeaways for OCRNs. A list of important terms used in this chapter can be referenced in Table 4-1.

Terminology Related to Experimental Clinical Research

Randomization

Randomization is an experimental design where patients are assigned to an intervention by chance rather than intentionally being selected (National Institutes of Health [NIH], 2022). Each intervention group, which may also be referred to as an *arm*, is defined in the protocol and could be an experimental, a control, or a placebo arm (National Cancer Institute [NCI], 2024). Randomized controlled trials (RCTs) provide the strongest level of evidence in clinical research and have many benefits, including the following:

- Limiting the differences between each group to ensure that outcomes are due to the treatment and not other variables (Zabor et al., 2020)
- Preventing selection bias when allocating patients to treatment groups (Phillips et al., 2021)
- Blinding the type of treatment a patient is receiving

Patients can be randomized on a clinical trial through various methods, including using a computer, sealed envelopes, or randomly generated numbers (Nair, 2019). To help balance different characteristics in each group, a stratified or block randomization approach may be used. Although the methods are similar, key differences exist (Msaouel et al., 2023). Block randomization is a way to limit certain variables in each group to ensure that they are balanced. This helps equalize variables that may affect study end points. The variables are specified in advance of randomization and consider the baseline characteristics of the patients and the characteristics of patients who have already been assigned treatment (Msaouel et al., 2023). Stratified randomization is a way to group patients based on specific characteristics when interpreting results. Patients with certain characteristics, such as age or performance status, are stratified, and then each group is randomly sampled to ensure a representative population (Msaouel et al., 2023).

OCRNs should understand the randomization process for each clinical trial. Patients should be educated on the process and provided with re-education to ensure initial and ongoing informed decision-making.

Blinding

Blinding in clinical trials is when the treatment assignment for the patient is unknown. When the patient does not

TABLE 4-1 | Important Terms for the Oncology Clinical Research Nurse

Term	Definition
Arm	A group of patients receiving an intervention; each arm could be a control or investigational treatment (National Cancer Institute [NCI], 2024).
Backfilling	Assigning patients to established dose levels that have previously not met the dose-limiting toxicity criteria (Dehbi et al., 2021)
Blinded study	A trial in which patients, and sometimes the treatment team, are not informed of which drug the patient is receiving; blinding helps limit bias (U.S. Department of Health and Human Services, 2022).
Control group	The group, or arm, that receives the standard treatment, not the investigational treatment being studied; it is used as a comparison to the investigational arms (NCI, n.d.).
Disease-free survival	Calculated by determining the length of time from when a patient completes their primary treatment through the time that they survive without signs or symptoms of cancer (NCI, n.d.)
Dose-limiting toxicity	The toxicity of a treatment that is severe enough that it prevents a higher dose from being tested (NCI, n.d.)
End points	An objective measurement in a clinical trial to determine if the intervention is beneficial; each phase of a clinical trial may have different end points. Examples of end points are overall survival, overall response rate, or progression-free survival (NCI, n.d.).
Futility	Analysis before the trial is complete to assess if the trial should be stopped before completion (Ciolino, 2023)
Maximum tolerated dose	The maximum dose of a drug that does not cause unacceptable toxicity (NCI, n.d)
Overall response rate	Calculated by determining the percentage of people within a treatment group who have achieved a partial or complete response to the study treatment over a defined period (NCI, n.d.)
Overall survival	Determined by measuring the time from which a patient is either diagnosed with or starts treatment for a disease to the time at which they are still alive (NCI, n.d.)
Pharmacodynamic	The effects of a drug in the body, including its mechanism of action (Ernstmeyer & Christman, 2023)
Pharmacokinetic	The absorption, distribution, metabolism, and excretion of a drug in the body—often measured in a clinical trial by obtaining blood, urine, or tissue samples (NCI, n.d.)
Phase	The stage of the clinical trial, starting at phase 1 (or less commonly phase 0) and continuing until phase 3. A phase 4 trial is sometimes conducted once U.S. Food and Drug Administration approval has been obtained (U.S. Department of Health and Human Services, 2022).
Placebo	An inactive substance that looks and is administered the same as the investigational drug being studied; it is used to compare to the investigational drug. A control group may contain a placebo alone or in combination with the standard treatment (NCI, n.d.).
Progression-free survival	Measures the time during which a patient lives with a disease that has not worsened and remains stable (NCI, n.d.)
Randomization	An experimental design where patients are assigned to an intervention by chance rather than intentionally being selected for that intervention; phase 3 trials are conducted as randomized controlled trials (U.S. Department of Health and Human Services, 2022).

know which intervention they are receiving, but the provider is informed of the treatment allocation, it is known as a single-blind study (Zabor et al., 2020). When neither patients nor providers know the treatment assignment, it is considered a double-blind study. Blinding helps ensure that outcomes (whether self-reported or provider-assessed) remain unbiased (Zabor et al., 2020). As with randomization, OCRNs should educate patients on the blinding process. Initial and ongoing informed decision-making can be facilitated by re-education.

Control Groups

Depending on the disease being studied, control groups may include a treatment, a placebo, or no treatment at all.

The goal of a control group is to provide an arm of the study to which the experimental arms can be compared (Zabor et al., 2020). OCRNs must understand and educate patients on the type of control being used.

A control group may be an active control, which is an established standard of care treatment by National Comprehensive Cancer Network (n.d.) guidelines and based on updated evidence. The efficacy of experimental arms is compared against an active control (Zabor et al., 2020).

If there is no established standard of care treatment, then the control arm could be a placebo. This is called a placebo-controlled trial, with the goal of showing that an experimental treatment is superior to a placebo (Zabor et al., 2020).

Placebos

A placebo is an inactive substance made to appear like an investigational drug. This helps prevent bias from the treatment team in how patients are cared for and how outcomes are assessed. Placebos are uncommonly used in cancer research but may be used if there are no standard treatments available or in combination with a standard treatment (NCI, 2024). OCRNs must ensure that patients are informed and thoroughly understand if a placebo is being used in the clinical trial and how it will be used. Patients must be aware there is a chance they could receive a placebo, its randomization ratio, and that participating could potentially mean they do not receive an active drug (in trials that are using placebo only and not in combination with standard-of-care treatment). Patients should also be able to explain, or teach back, important concepts, such as the use of placebos and randomization.

Pharmacokinetics

Pharmacokinetic sampling is an important part of clinical trials and is often performed during phase 1 studies, although samples can be tested in all phases. This branch of pharmacology analyzes how the body processes drugs (NCI, n.d.). By measuring drug levels in the body, usually by analyzing blood and urine samples, researchers can determine how a drug is being absorbed, distributed, metabolized, and excreted (National Institute on Aging, 2023). These data are significant because even slight differences in the level of a drug in the body can change the therapeutic effect or cause dose-limiting toxicities (DLTs). Because of this, careful titration and frequent monitoring are necessary (Habet, 2021). Pharmacokinetic samples may require multiple collections at different points during a study, making patient education from OCRNs on these procedures essential.

End Points

End points are objective measures of an outcome used in a clinical trial to help determine if a drug being tested shows benefit (NCI, n.d.). Each phase has different goals and end points to assess. End points can be broken down into the following categories (U.S. Department of Health and Human Services, 2022):

- Primary end points answer the main question being asked in the clinical trial.
- Secondary end points answer other research questions but can provide additional evidence of drug effects.
- Exploratory end points help to answer additional questions but will not aid in answering the main research question. They may provide evidence for a new hypothesis.

Phases of Clinical Trials

Clinical trials are conducted in different stages, referred to as phases. Each phase has a different goal and can vary in design (NIH, 2022). Phases range from 0 to 4, each with an increasing number of participants and with distinct goals.

Phase 0

Phase 0 clinical trials are uncommon and are usually performed in a very small number of patients, generally fewer than 15. They involve giving small doses of the investigational drug to patients to assess how it acts on the body and the cancer (American Cancer Society, 2020). They are not required as part of the drug approval process but may help speed up approval or help investigators determine if testing the drug in a later phase is appropriate.

Phase 1

Phase 1 clinical trials are typically the first time a drug is being tested in humans. The goal of these trials is to determine the safety and maximum tolerated dose (MTD) of study drugs. MTD refers to the highest dose of a study drug that can be given to a human before unacceptable side effects occur. To determine MTD, protocols have predefined toxicities deemed unacceptable, known as DLTs (NCI, n.d.). A DLT is usually a grade 3 or higher non-hematologic toxicity or grade 4 or higher hematologic toxicity and is possibly related to treatment. The toxicity must have occurred during the predetermined window (often the first cycle of treatment) to be considered a DLT (Lee et al., 2021).

Phase 1 trials are conducted on a relatively small number of people, with usually fewer than 100 participants (Torres-Saavedra & Winter, 2022). These trials have been historically performed using a dose escalation method with a 3+3 design to prevent administering subtherapeutic doses of study drugs to patients, maintain safety, and avoid slowing down accrual (Pantoja et al., 2022). In the 3+3 design, three patients are enrolled at one time into a group with a specific dose. If no DLTs are seen, then the trial will enroll three more patients at the next higher dose level. If there is a DLT found in one patient, then three more patients will be enrolled at the same dose. If another DLT occurs in the second set of three patients, then the MTD has been reached, and no more escalation will ensue (Pantoja et al., 2022). OCRNs must be familiar with the MTD and DLT definitions in each phase 1 trial, as they may differ depending on the type of drug under investigation.

The goal of a phase 1 clinical trial has expanded to determine more than just the MTD. In addition to dose and safety, phase 1 trials have begun to evaluate efficacy concurrently (Dehbi et al., 2021). For example, more recent designs may allow for backfilling, or assigning patients to established dose levels that have previously not met DLT criteria. This helps gather more information, such as pharmacodynamics and pharmacokinetics, and is especially useful in the evaluation of immunotherapy or targeted agents where increasing dose levels may not show an increase in efficacy (Dehbi et al., 2021).

Phase 1 trials may involve extra risks and burdens for patients. Extra visits to the clinic or extended clinic visits are often required for research tests and examinations. These tests, such as serial biopsies and pharmacodynamic and pharmacokinetic sampling, may not benefit patients directly and can be burdensome. Phase 1 trials are also more often conducted at large academic institutions, which may mean extended travel for some patients (Bittlinger et al., 2022). For patients to make informed decisions when consenting to a phase 1 trial, OCRNs must educate them on the study schedule, including what extra tests, procedures, or visits are involved and how they may or may not benefit them.

Phase 2

Phase 2 trials aim to continue monitoring the safety of an investigational treatment and evaluate if the treatment is effective against the cancer being studied. These studies include more patients than a phase 1 trial but are still conducted in a relatively small number of individuals, usually hundreds. The efficacy of a drug in a phase 2 trial will help determine if it should be tested in a randomized phase 3 trial with a larger population (Torres-Saavedra & Winter, 2022). Phase 2 trials can be conducted in different designs, such as single-arm trials, non-comparative randomized trials, and comparative randomized trials (Torres-Saavedra & Winter, 2022).

Single-Arm Trials

In single-arm trials, all patients receive the investigational drug. Although this limits the ability to test and analyze efficacy, it helps lessen the number of patients who could receive treatment with an ineffective agent. Just as importantly, it helps limit the number of patients receiving a treatment that may be excessively toxic (Torres-Saavedra & Winter, 2022).

Non-Comparative Randomized Trials

In non-comparative randomized trials, patients are randomized into one of at least two experimental treatment arms. This design does not contain a control arm as a comparator; instead, the investigational arms are compared against a historical control. The arm with the highest response rate is typically selected for further investigation in a future RCT (Torres-Saavedra & Winter, 2022).

Comparative Randomized Trials

Comparative randomized trials in the phase 2 setting, which can be performed as a comparative efficacy trial, help investigators establish evidence to guide a larger phase 3 comparative randomized trial. Comparative efficacy trials seek to determine if the investigational treatment offers improved efficacy as compared to the standard of care (Li & Bergan, 2020). This is often evaluated using a futility analysis or futility stopping rule (Torres-Saavedra & Winter, 2022). A futility stopping rule requires that results be analyzed during an ongoing clinical trial to determine if the trial should be stopped before completion. This approach helps to more promptly stop trials that would have otherwise not shown a statistically significant benefit. The rule also allows for and helps prevent trials that are showing a treatment effect from being stopped early (Ciolino et al., 2023).

Because the goal of a phase 2 trial is usually focused on determining if the drug has activity in the cancer being studied, end points such as overall response rate and disease-free survival are often primary (Torres-Saavedra & Winter, 2022). The overall response rate is calculated by determining the percentage of patients within a treatment group who have achieved a partial or complete response to the study treatment over a defined period (NCI, n.d.). Disease-free survival is calculated by determining the length of time from when a patient completes their primary treatment through the period that they survive without signs or symptoms of cancer (NCI, n.d.). In the phase 2 setting, non-inferiority trials seek to determine if the treatment being studied is not worse than the standard of care and if it may offer benefits such as less toxicity (Li & Bergan, 2020). To assess this, these studies often use quality of life as the primary end point (Torres-Saavedra & Winter, 2022). Quality-of-life assessments measure a patient's subjective determination of their well-being and ability to manage activities of daily living (NCI, n.d.).

Phase 3

Phase 3 clinical trials are conducted as RCTs to compare new treatments to the current standard treatment. They involve hundreds to thousands of patients (National Library of Medicine, n.d.). Phase 3 trials help determine if an investigational treatment exhibits benefit compared to the standard of care in either a comparative efficacy trial or a non-inferiority trial.

Phase 3 trials may be conducted as a double-blind study when feasible. Blinding both patients and providers limits biased observations of efficacy and outcomes (Dawei et al., 2022). Blinding can also help reduce patient dropout because, besides the treatment, patients in all arms are cared for identically (Higgins & Levin, 2023). However, blinding in oncology clinical trials is not always possible, as the side effects of certain drugs may unintentionally unblind patients and providers (Dawei et al., 2022). Also, in situations where a standard-of-care treatment is available, it is not ethical to conduct a placebo-controlled, blinded study. Placebo-controlled trials are often conducted when there is no standard of care option, or the standard of care is not a treatment but is best supportive care or surveillance (Dawei et al., 2022).

The end points of overall survival and progression-free survival in a phase 3 trial are used to help determine clinical benefit (Zhang et al., 2020). Overall survival is determined by measuring the time from when a patient is diagnosed with or starts treatment for a disease to the time at which they are still alive (NCI, n.d.). Progression-free survival measures the time during which a patient lives with a disease that has not worsened and remains stable (NCI, n.d.).

Phase 4

Phase 4 clinical trials are initiated to study drugs that have already received U.S. Food and Drug Administration (FDA) approval and can be helpful in answering questions that went unanswered in earlier phases (Zabor et al., 2020). The main goal of a phase 4 trial, also called a post-marketing study, is to study the safety and effectiveness of a drug over a longer time and among more patients than were able to be studied previously. Because the eligibility criteria are less strict than in phase 3 studies, these trials can help identify rarer toxicities and study effectiveness in real-world situations rather than in the controlled environment of a phase 3 RCT (Henry et al., 2023).

Types of Clinical Trials

Adaptive Trials

Adaptive trials allow changes to occur to the design of a trial when planned prospectively in response to data that have been gathered while the trial is ongoing. The main advantage of an adaptive trial is that it allows adjustments based on information learned during the trial (FDA, 2019). Different types of adaptations may occur, including planned interim analyses, adjustments to sample size or population, and adding or terminating treatment arms (FDA, 2019). A platform trial is an example of an adaptive trial.

Basket Trials

Basket trials (see Figure 4-1) study a targeted intervention among cancers with differing histology but similar characteristics, such as a variant (Park, Hsu, et al., 2020). Usually, these trials will have a single intervention, as it may be challenging to have a control arm among multiple histologies (Park, Hsu, et al., 2020). The goal of a basket trial is to determine if a molecular target is responsive to therapy regardless of the tumor type (Li & Bergan, 2020). Often, basket trials are conducted in the phase 1 or 2 setting (Kasim et al., 2023).

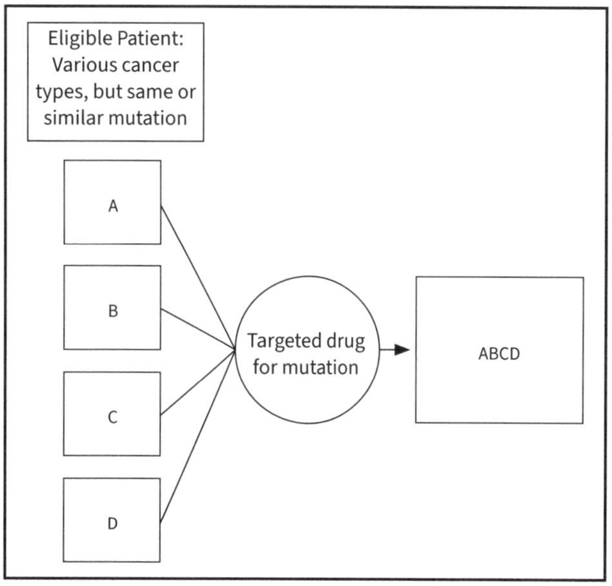

FIGURE 4-1 | Basket Trial Design

Note. Based on information from Park, Hsu, et al., 2020.

Crossover Trials

Crossover trials (see Figure 4-2) are commonly used in oncology and typically allow a patient who had been assigned to the standard of care treatment (in some cases a placebo) to cross over to the investigational treatment at the time of progression. This is known as unidirectional crossover (Hilal et al., 2020). Controversy exists related to conducting crossover trials; although this trial design can be attractive to patients, it may lead to difficulty in assessing trial end points, such as overall survival (Jönsson et al., 2024). Also, crossover trials may expose patients to drugs that have not been proven to show efficacy (Hilal et al., 2020). However, they are often used in situations in which an already FDA-approved treatment is being investigated as a treatment in an earlier line (Haslam & Prasad, 2018).

Parallel Trials

Parallel trials (see Figure 4-3) are the most commonly used design for RCTs (Nair, 2019).

They involve at least two groups of patients receiving different treatments simultaneously (NCI, 2024). Patients remain in whichever arm they were assigned until the study's completion.

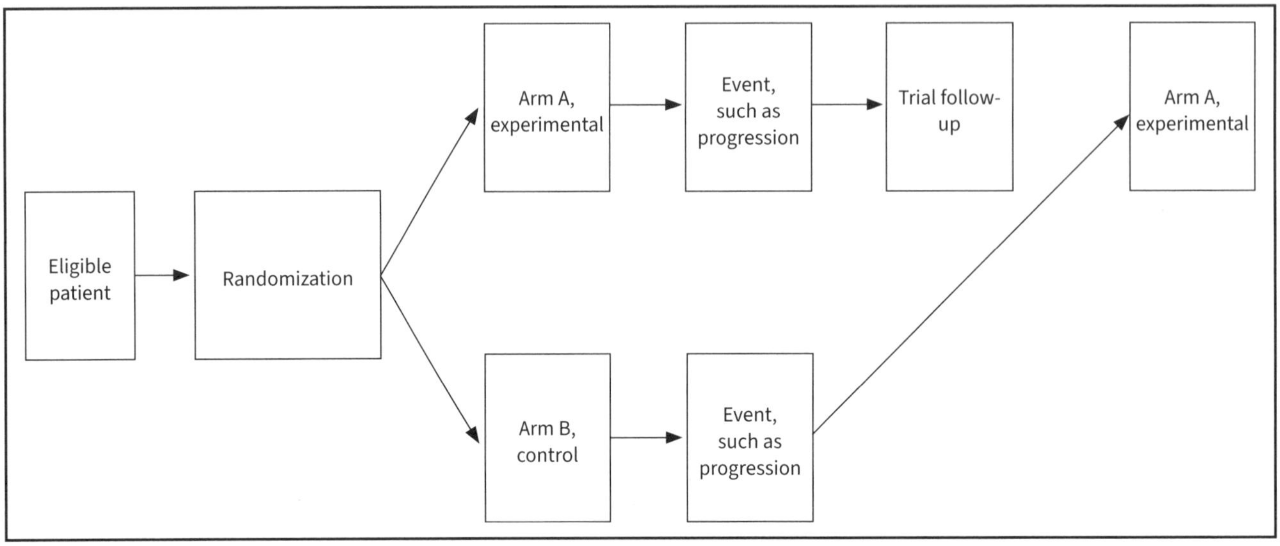

FIGURE 4-2 | Unidirectional Trial Crossover Design

Note. Based on information from Hilal et al., 2020; Nair, 2019.

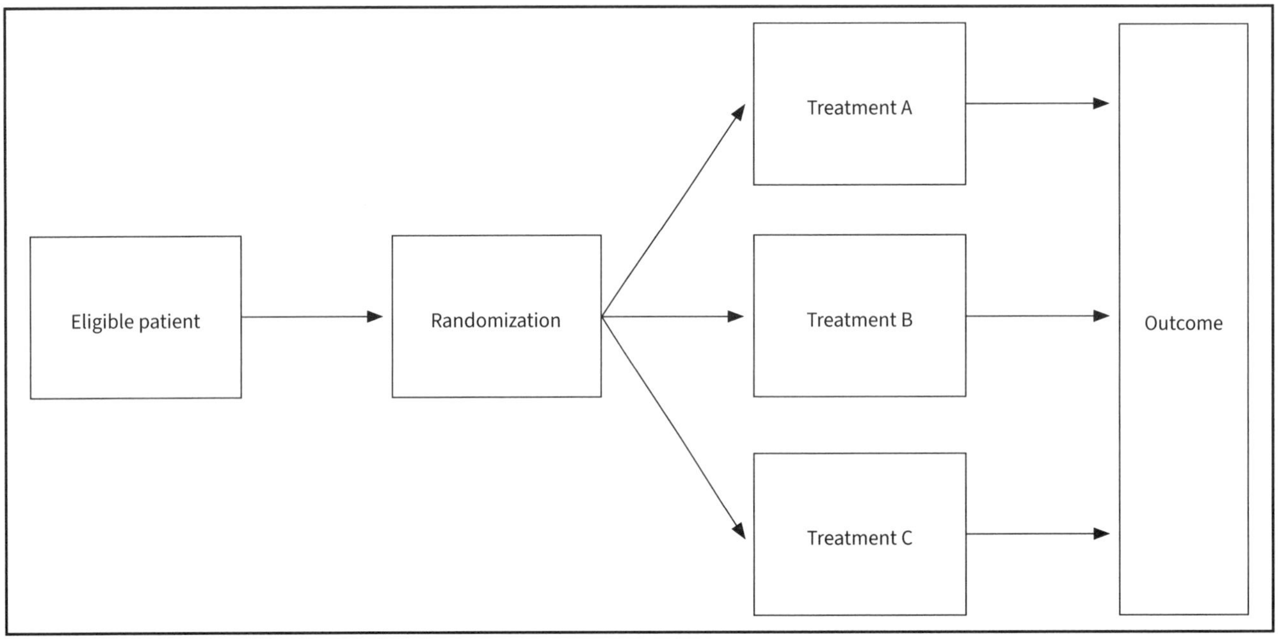

FIGURE 4-3 | Parallel Trial Design

Note. Based on information from Nair, 2019.

Platform Trials

Platform trials (see Figure 4-4) are a type of adaptive trial. They are also known as multiarm multistage trials, and they compare many interventions against a single control group. They allow new investigational arms to be added, and enrollment may be stopped on existing arms that show futility after an interim analysis (Li & Bergan, 2020). The goal of a platform trial is to answer multiple research questions quickly and with lower enrollment than typical RCTs (Noor et al., 2022). Umbrella trials are often conducted using a platform design (Li & Bergan, 2020).

Umbrella

Umbrella trials (see Figure 4-5) are comparable to basket trials, as they study a targeted intervention but differ in that they are conducted on a single disease that is separated into subgroups. An example of these subgroups is multiple variants that are present in a single cancer type

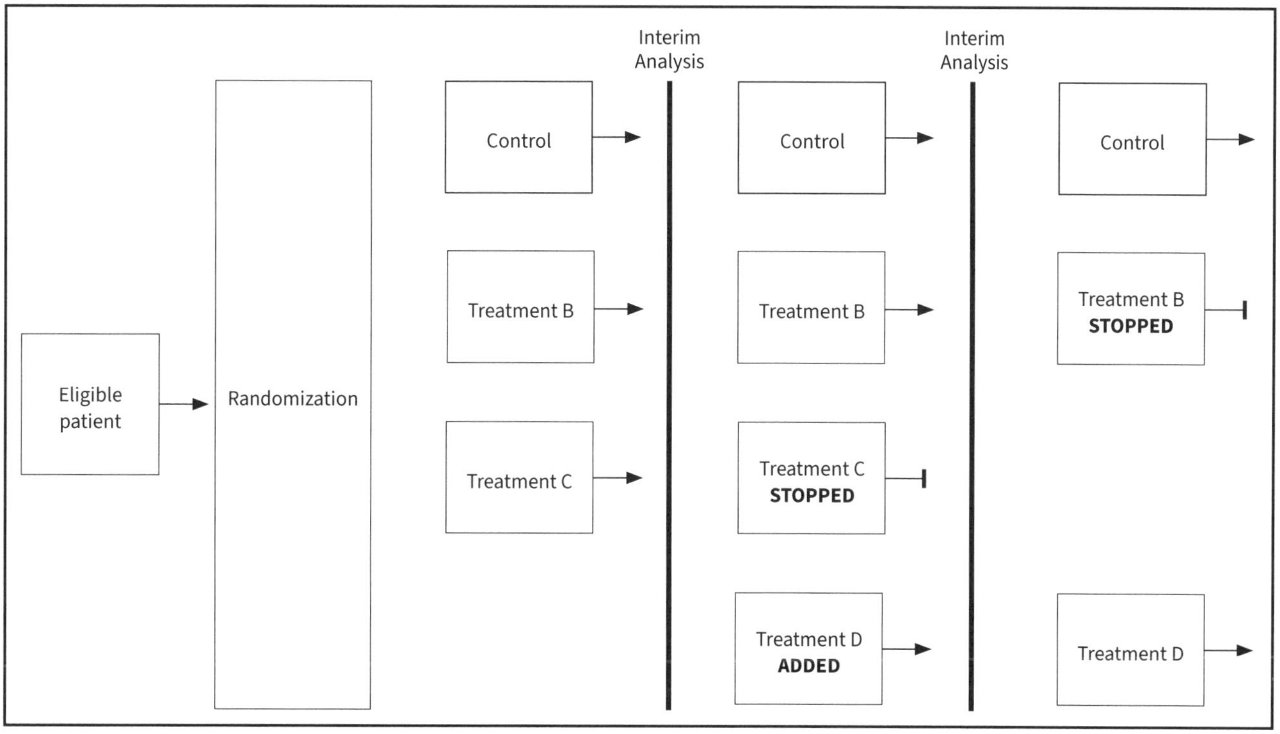

FIGURE 4-4 | Platform Trial Design

Note. Based on information from Li & Bergan, 2020; Park, Harari, et al., 2020.

(Park, Hsu et al., 2020). The goal of an umbrella trial is to determine if different treatments should be used among cancers with the same histology but different molecular profiles (Li & Bergan, 2020). They are often performed in phase 1 or 2 settings, although they may be conducted as a phase 3 trial and are more likely to use randomization and include a control group than basket trials (Park, Hsu et al., 2020).

Implications for Oncology Clinical Research Nurses

Blinding

OCRNs must inform patients if a clinical trial is blinded and explain what a blinded study is, how it is conducted, and whether a placebo is involved. It is also important to review with patients whether they will be unblinded at any time in the future (either during the study, at progression, or after the study has been completed).

Phase 1 Trials

Although OCRNs must ensure that patients are educated on the requirements for any trial being considered, patients must also be informed of the potential extra burden they may be required to undergo during a phase 1 trial. These trials may require additional visits to the treatment center, including on nontreatment days. Correlative studies, such as biopsies and pharmacokinetic sampling, add extra risk and burden without necessarily providing benefit to patients. All study requirements should be reviewed with patients at the time of consent so they are able to make an informed decision on participation.

Placebos

OCRNs must ensure that patients are informed when a placebo is included in a clinical trial. They should educate patients on why a placebo is being used and their chance of receiving one. If the placebo is being used in a crossover trial, OCRNs should be able to educate patients on when they can potentially crossover to the investigational therapy arm. It is critically important that patients can demonstrate their understanding of a placebo-controlled trial in order for them to participate.

Randomization

OCRNs should understand the randomization process, including the ratio to which patients are randomized to the investigational arm (i.e., 1:1 or 2:1 randomization) and the differences between each arm. Patients should be educated on their chances of receiving the investigational drug at the time of consent, which includes the investigational drug, the randomization process, and when randomization occurs. Hence, they are able to make an informed decision on participation.

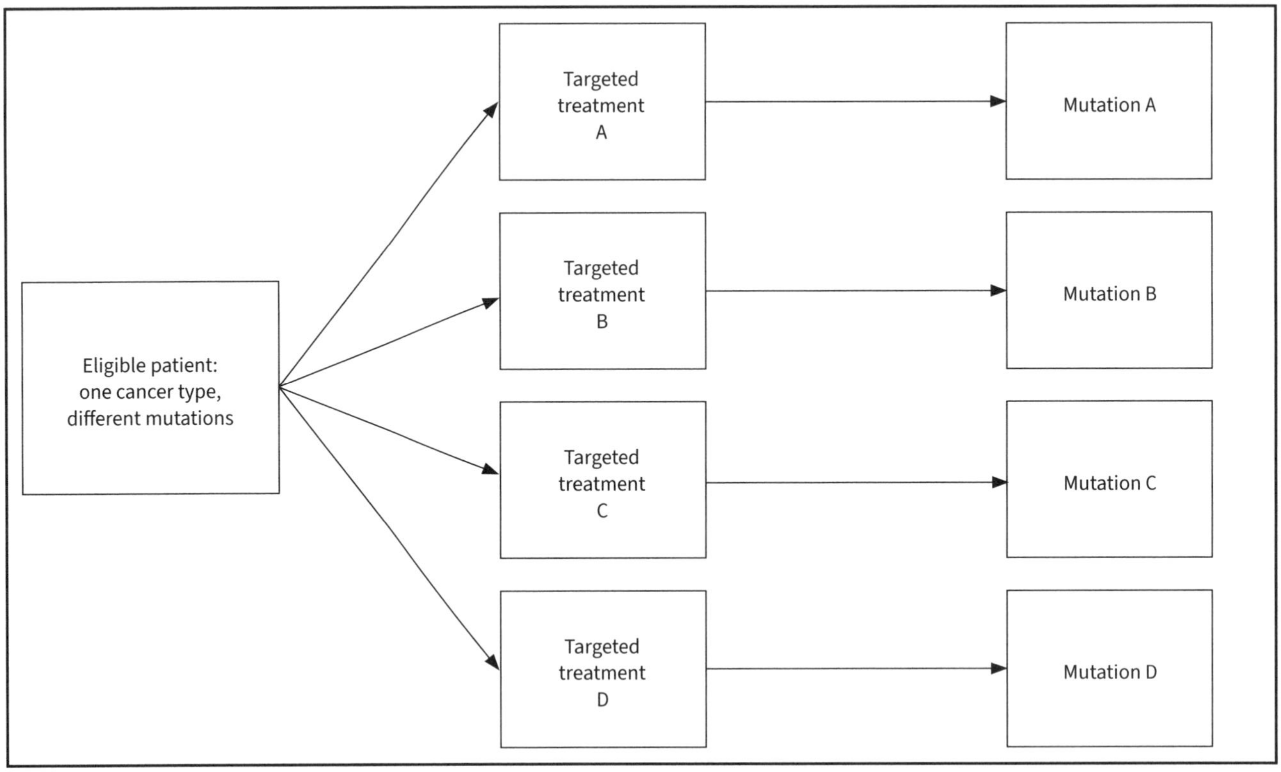

FIGURE 4-5 | Umbrella Trial Design

Note. Based on information from Park, Hsu, et al., 2020.

Summary

For OCRNs to best care for patients and understand clinical trial requirements, many concepts and important terms must be known. Understanding the different designs, phases, and processes in which experimental trials are conducted will allow for more streamlined patient care while enabling nurses to follow the protocol requirements as part of the research team. Just as important, understanding these concepts will allow nurses to appropriately educate patients so they can demonstrate their understanding of essential concepts required for informed consent.

Key Points

- Experimental clinical trials can be complex and vary significantly among phases and designs. OCRNs must understand key concepts to care for and educate patients appropriately.
- Randomization provides the strongest level of evidence in clinical research by preventing biases and limiting the differences between each group to ensure that outcomes are due to the treatment and not other variables.
- Research participants should be informed if randomization is being used, what the groups and treatment arms are, and their chances of being randomly assigned to each group.
- Although uncommon in cancer research, placebos are sometimes used in clinical trials. OCRNs must ensure that participants are informed if a placebo is being used and what the chances are that they could receive it.

The author would like to acknowledge Elizabeth Ness, MS, RN, and Georgia Cusack, MS, RN, AOCNS®, for their contribution to this chapter that remains unchanged from the previous edition of this book.

References

American Cancer Society. (2020, August 18). *Types and phases of clinical trials.* https://www.cancer.org/cancer/managing-cancer/making-treatment-decisions/clinical-trials/what-you-need-to-know/phases-of-clinical-trials.html

Bittlinger, M., Bicer, S., Peppercorn, J., & Kimmelman, J. (2022). Ethical considerations for phase I trials in oncology. *Journal of Clinical Oncology, 40*(30), 3474–3488. https://doi.org/10.1200/JCO.21.02125

Ciolino, J.D., Kaizer, A.M., & Bonner, L.B. (2023). Guidance on interim analysis methods in clinical trials. *Journal of Clinical and Translational Science, 7*(1), e124. https://doi.org/10.1017/cts.2023.552

Dawei, W., Shuangman, M., Huiyao, H., Dandan, C., Yu, T., & Ning, L. (2022). Unblinding at disease progression in double-blinded randomized controlled cancer drug clinical trials: A controversy requires more attention. *Frontiers in Medicine, 9*, 1082445. https://doi.org/10.3389/fmed.2022.1082445

Dehbi, H.M., O'Quigley, J., & Iasonos, A. (2021). Controlled backfill in oncology dose-finding trials. *Contemporary Clinical Trials, 111*, 106605. https://doi.org/10.1016/j.cct.2021.106605

Ernstmeyer, K., & Christman, E. (Eds.). (2023). *Nursing pharmacology* (2nd ed.). Chippewa Valley Technical College.

Habet, S. (2021). Narrow Therapeutic Index drugs: Clinical pharmacology perspective. *Journal of Pharmacy and Pharmacology, 73*(10), 1285–1291. https://doi.org/10.1093/jpp/rgab102

Haslam, A., & Prasad, V. (2018). When is crossover desirable in cancer drug trials and when is it problematic? *European Society for Medical Oncology, 29*(5), 1079–1081. https://doi.org/10.1093/annonc/mdy116

Henry, B.M., Lippi, G., Nasser, A., & Ostrowski, P. (2023). Characteristics of phase IV clinical trials in oncology: An analysis using the ClinicalTrials.gov registry data. *Current Oncology, 30*(6), 5932–5945. https://doi.org/10.3390/curroncol30060443

Higgins, K., & Levin, G. (2023, May 30). *Considerations for open-label clinical trials: Design, conduct, and analysis.* https://www.fda.gov/science-research/fda-science-forum/considerations-open-label-clinical-trials-design-conduct-and-analysis

Hilal, T., Gonzalez-Velez, M., & Prasad, V. (2020). Limitations in clinical trials leading to anticancer drug approvals by the U.S. Food and Drug Administration. *JAMA Internal Medicine, 180*(8), 1108–1115. https://doi.org/10.1001/jamainternmed.2020.2250

Jönsson, L., Sandin, R., Ekman, M., Ramsberg, J., Charbonneau, C., Huang, X., ... Drummond, M. (2014). Analyzing overall survival in randomized controlled trials with crossover and implications for economic evaluation. *Value Health, 17*(6), 707–713. https://doi.org/10.1016/j.jval.2014.06.006

Kasim, A., Bean, N., Hendriksen, S.J., Chen, T.T., Zhou, H., & Psioda, M.A. (2023). Basket trials in oncology: A systematic review of practices and methods, comparative analysis of innovative methods, and an appraisal of a missed opportunity. *Frontiers in Oncology, 13*, 1266286. https://doi.org/10.3389/fonc.2023.1266286

Lee, S.M., Wages, N.A., Goodman, K.A., & Lockhart, A.C. (2021). Designing dose-finding phase I clinical trials: Top 10 questions that should be discussed with your statistician. *JCO Precision Oncology, 5*, 317–324. https://doi.org/10.1200/PO.20.00379

Li, A., & Bergan, R.C. (2020). Clinical trial design: Past, present, and future in the context of big data and precision medicine. *Cancer, 126*(22), 4838–4846. https://doi.org/10.1002/cncr.33205

Msaouel, P., Lee, J., & Thall, P.F. (2023). Interpreting randomized controlled trials. *Cancers, 15*(19), 4674. https://doi.org/10.3390/cancers15194674

Nair, B. (2019). Clinical trial designs. *Indian Dermatology Online Journal, 10*(2), 193–201. https://doi.org/10.4103/idoj.IDOJ_475_18

National Cancer Institute. (n.d.). *NCI dictionary of cancer terms.* https://www.cancer.gov/publications/dictionaries/cancer-terms

National Cancer Institute. (2024). *How do clinical trials work?* https://www.cancer.gov/research/participate/clinical-trials/how-trials-work

National Comprehensive Cancer Network. (n.d.). *About clinical practice guidelines.* https://www.nccn.org/guidelines/guidelines-process/about-nccn-clinical-practice-guidelines

National Institute on Aging. (2023). *What are clinical trials and studies?* https://www.nia.nih.gov/health/clinical-trials-and-studies/what-are-clinical-trials-and-studies

National Institutes of Health. (2022). *NIH clinical research trials and you: The basics.* https://www.nih.gov/health-information/nih-clinical-research-trials-you/basics

National Library of Medicine. (n.d.). *ClinicalTrials.gov glossary terms.* https://clinicaltrials.gov/study-basics/glossary

National Library of Medicine. (2023). *Learn about studies.* https://clinicaltrials.gov/study-basics/learn-about-studies

Noor, N.M., Love, S.B., Isaacs, T., Kaplan, R., Parmar, M.K.B., & Sydes, M.R. (2022). Uptake of the multi-arm multistage (MAMS) adaptive platform approach: A trial-registry review of late-phase randomised clinical trials. *BMJ Open, 12*(3), e055615. https://doi.org/10.1136/bmjopen-2021-055615

Pantoja, K., Lanke, S., Munafo, A., Victor, A., Habermehl, C., Schueler, A., ... Goteti, K. (2022). Designing phase I oncology dose escalation using dose–exposure–toxicity models as a complementary approach to model-based dose–toxicity models. *Pharmacometrics and Systems Pharmacology, 11*(10), 1371–1381. https://doi.org/10.1002/psp4.12851

Park, J.J.H., Harari, O., Dron, L., Lester, R.T., Thorlund, K., & Mills, E.J. (2020). An overview of platform trials with a checklist for clinical readers. *Journal of Clinical Epidemiology, 125*, 1–8. https://doi.org/10.1016/j.jclinepi.2020.04.025

Park, J.J.H., Hsu, G., Siden, E.G., Thorlund, K., & Mills, E.J. (2020). An overview of precision oncology basket and umbrella trials for clinicians. *CA: A Cancer Journal for Clinicians, 70*(2), 125–137. https://doi.org/10.3322/caac.21600

Phillips, M.R., Kaiser, P., Thabane, L., Bhandari, M., Chaudhary, V., Wykoff, C.C., ... Wong, T.Y. (2021). Risk of bias: Why measure IT, and how? *Eye, 36*(2), 346–348. https://doi.org/10.1038/s41433-021-01759-9

Torres-Saavedra, P.A., & Winter, K.A. (2022). An overview of phase 2 clinical trial designs. *International Journal of Radiation Oncology, Biology, Physics, 112*(1), 22–29. https://doi.org/10.1016/j.ijrobp.2021.07.1700

U.S. Department of Health and Human Services. (2022). *Multiple endpoints in clinical trials: Guidance for industry.* https://www.fda.gov/media/162416/download

U.S. Food and Drug Administration. (2019). *Adaptive designs for clinical trials of drugs and biologics: Guidance for industry.* https://www.fda.gov/media/78495/download

Zabor, E.C., Kaizer, A.M., & Hobbs, B.P. (2020). Randomized controlled trials. *Chest, 158*(1, Suppl.), S79–S87. https://doi.org/10.1016/j.chest.2020.03.013

Zhang, J., Pilar, M.R., Wang, X., Liu, J., Pang, H., Brownson, R.C., ... He, J. (2020). Endpoint surrogacy in oncology phase 3 randomised controlled trials. *British Journal of Cancer, 123*(3), 333–334. https://doi.org/10.1038/s41416-020-0896-5

CHAPTER 5

Types of Clinical Research: Observational

Yelena Shames, MSN, ACNP-BC, CNRN

Introduction

Clinical research protocols are generally subdivided into interventional and observational studies (Aggarwal & Ranganathan, 2019). The distinct characteristics of interventional protocols are randomization and the ability of an investigator to manipulate the study interventions. This helps researchers to better understand the causality between exposures and outcomes and adds to data validity. In contrast, in observational studies, researchers merely observe an intervention without influencing the outcomes and examine probable associations between exposures and outcomes (Ramji, 2022). The lack of randomization and control in observational research is confounding and introduces potential biases (see Table 5-1 for information on these biases and related terms). Thus, evidence derived from randomized controlled trials is ranked superior to that derived from observational research (Collins et al., 2020). Despite these limitations, well-designed and adequately powered observational studies can contribute valuable data in patients with rare diseases and those experiencing rare treatment outcomes.

Additionally, observational research plays a role when conducting a randomized controlled trial is unethical, not feasible, or too expensive (Ramji, 2022). Observational epidemiologic studies include broader patient representation and may supplement data extracted from interventional research with real-world data (Collins et al., 2020). Observational research is crucial to generating new hypotheses for future interventional studies (Metelli & Chaimani, 2020).

Observational studies come in various prospective and retrospective designs and can be analytic or descriptive. Patient populations can vary from a single patient to hundreds or thousands of patients, and in most cases, samples are extracted from the available databases. In retrospective studies, the outcome of interest occurs prior to the start of the study. The study population is selected based on a specific outcome. Data that have been previously collected are analyzed to determine risk factors and exposures that led to a specific result (Ramji, 2022). In a prospective study design, researchers select a target population based on risks or exposures. Cases are followed chronologically until the outcome of interest occurs (Wang & Cheng, 2020).

In descriptive studies, researchers observe a selected patient population for the occurrence of health-related events, assess the prevalence of the disease, and evaluate the association between variables or exposures (Gail et al., 2019; Ramji, 2022). Examples of descriptive studies include the following (Aggarwal & Ranganathan, 2019; Bosdriesz et al., 2020):

- Case reports and case series
- Cross-sectional studies
- Ecologic studies
- Qualitative surveys or interviews

In analytical studies, researchers evaluate the incidence of the disease, the association between exposures and outcomes, and identify possible risk factors leading to outcomes (Haley & Huber, 2023). Examples of analytical study designs include the following (Bosdriesz et al., 2020; Ramji, 2022):

- Case-control studies
- Cohort studies
- Some cross-sectional studies

Characteristics and comparison of different observational study designs are provided in Table 5-2.

This chapter will detail the types of observational study designs and their implication on oncology clinical research.

Types of Observational Study Designs

Case Reports and Case Series

Case reports and case series are observational studies that allow clinician investigators to share their experi-

TABLE 5-1 | Glossary of Clinical Research Terminology

Term	Definition
Absolute risk	The probability of the outcome of interest occurring (Gail et al., 2019)
Bias	A systematic error that leads to misinterpretation of study results and false conclusions. It occurs when some variables or outcomes are unintentionally encouraged over others (Wang & Cheng, 2020).
Confidence interval	The range of estimated values (mean value plus and minus variation). It is important to understand when calculating odds ratios (Haley & Huber, 2023).
Confounding	In Merriam-Webster's dictionary, it is defined as confusion or perplexity. In research, confounding variables occur when exposures are influenced by other factors (Miroshnychenko et al., 2022). This can lead to deceptive associations and misinterpretation of the results.
Epidemiology	Studies the association between risks and exposures to health outcomes and evaluates the incidence and prevalence of health outcomes in a specific population (Ahlbom, 2021; Munnangi & Boktor, 2023)
Incidence	New cases of a disease or an outcome of interest that occurred within a specified time interval (Sueyoshi & Huber, 2023)
Internal validity	Describes how well the evidence derived from a specific study supports causal relationships between variables (Gail et al., 2019)
Mean	Represents an average value measured by the sum of all values divided by the total number of values (Fleischmann et al., 2024)
Measurement error bias	Occurs when measurements are either overstated or understated based on statistical methods used for the study (Innes et al., 2021)
Median	Represents the middle value that separates the higher half from the lower half of a data sample (Fleischmann et al., 2024)
Mode	The most frequently occurring value within the data sample (Fleischmann et al., 2024)
Multivariable regression	Regression analysis is a statistical process used to estimate the relationship between dependent and independent variables. The value of a dependent variable can be predicted given the known value of an independent variable. The estimated effect is adjusted for confounders (Bosdriesz et al., 2020). Different forms of regression analysis can be used. To measure the outputs for independent variables, an estimated regression coefficient, confidence interval, and P values can be used (Bzovsky et al., 2022).
Odds ratio	Reflects the proportion of study participants who developed a disease or an outcome of interest compared to those who did not (Sueyoshi & Huber, 2023)
Prevalence	Refers to the proportion of a patient population that developed a disease or an outcome of interest within a specific time frame (National Institute of Mental Health, n.d.)
Recall bias	Occurs when the study participants are unable to recall the information being studied accurately (Khare & Vedel, 2019)
Relative risk	The ratio of the absolute risk of a disease or an outcome of interest occurring in an exposed patient population to the absolute risk of it occurring in an unexposed patient population (Gail et al., 2019)
Selection bias	Occurs when selected study participants do not represent the intended patient population (Wang & Cheng, 2020)
Stratification	The strategy used to mitigate measured confounding variables. All study participants are separated into strata based on the probability of the outcome. Within each stratum, mean outcomes are compared, and a weighted average of the association between exposures and outcomes is computed (Bosdriesz et al., 2020).

ences about unusual health conditions or treatment outcomes (Meade et al., 2024). These studies are descriptive and focus on evaluating the prevalence of common trends among participants who have developed a particular outcome (Fleischmann et al., 2024). In case series, participants are selected based on the presence of common characteristics or a specific outcome. In case reports, the patient population is less than four cases, whereas in case series, it can range from a few cases to hundreds or thousands (Fleischmann et al., 2024). There is no control group, and participants can be followed over time (Munn et al., 2020). The outcomes are reported as a measure of central tendency as mean, median, and mode values (Fleischmann et al., 2024). Case reports and case series can supplement evidence derived from randomized controlled trials or be the only source of evidence in patients with rare diseases. In many instances, case series generate a hypothesis and provide recommendations for future research (Aggarwal & Ranganathan, 2019).

Cross-Sectional Study Design

A cross-sectional study design is often referred to as a *snapshot*, as it allows researchers to simultaneously examine multiple variables, exposures, and outcomes at a single timepoint (Maier et al., 2023). Cross-sectional studies can be analytical or descriptive. A descriptive study design helps to evaluate the prevalence of health outcomes and assess the healthcare needs of a population (Kalantari & Cooper, 2023). In analytical studies, researchers examine an association between exposures and outcomes (Aggarwal & Ranganathan, 2019). Common modalities of cross-sectional study design are qualitative questionnaires and interviews. Cross-sectional studies are cost-effective and time-efficient; researchers can evaluate multiple

TABLE 5-2 | Characteristics of Observational Study Designs

Study Design	Timeline	Main Characteristics	Limitations
Case reports and case series	Retrospective	Provide initial reports on exposures and rare outcomes; helpful for studying rare diseases Provide data on the prevalence of the exposure among study participants who experienced the outcome of interest Help to generate future research hypotheses Data reported by measures of central tendency Inexpensive and time efficient	Do not include a comparison group Unable to determine a causal relationship Susceptible to selection bias
Cross-sectional studies	Single timepoint	Can be descriptive or analytic Allow for the evaluation of multiple variables or outcomes at the same time Evaluate an association between exposures and outcomes Provide information on the prevalence of disease and risks of exposure; helpful in assessing healthcare needs Inexpensive and easy to conduct	Lack of prospective or retrospective follow-up Causality difficult to establish Unable to measure incidence Not used in studying rare diseases Susceptible to confounding and bias
Case-control studies	Retrospective	Compare cases and controls to identify risks Appropriate to study rare diseases and rare outcomes Can focus on a smaller population size Provides data on prevalence and incidence Time- and cost-efficient Association between exposures and outcomes measured as an odds ratio	Causality difficult to establish Difficulty selecting an adequate control sample Susceptible to confounding and bias
Cohort studies	Prospective or retrospective	Evaluate incidence rates Estimate risk of an exposure Suitable design to study rare exposures Can study multiple exposures and outcomes and evaluate an association between exposures and outcomes over time Prospective design to add to internal validity	Causality difficult to establish Longitudinal design makes susceptible to loss to follow-up Susceptible to confounding and bias Require cost and resource availability

Note. Based on information from Aggarwal & Ranganathan, 2019; Fleischmann et al., 2024; Gail et al., 2019; Haley & Huber, 2023; Meade et al., 2023; Munn et al., 2020; Wang & Cheng 2020; Wang & Kattan, 2020.

variables and outcomes simultaneously (Wallace et al., 2022). However, the lack of prospective or retrospective follow-up makes it difficult to evaluate the incidence of a disease or determine direct causal relationships between exposures and outcomes.

A heterogeneous sampling in a cross-sectional study makes it vulnerable to selection bias, as it is often based on prevalent cases and is not representative of the general population (Wang & Cheng, 2020). Incorporating a stratification technique into the study design helps to ensure that the selected sample properly represents the intended target population. In this method, all study participants are subdivided into different groups or strata. Mean values from each stratum are compared, and a weighted average is computed (Bosdriesz et al., 2020). Other limitations of a cross-sectional study design include the risk of confounding, measurement, and recall biases (Aggarwal & Ranganathan, 2019). Implementing multivariable regression analysis helps to reduce confounding and measurement error further. Different forms of regression analysis may be used to predict an association between dependent and independent variables and estimate how the confounding variables may affect the variable of interest (Bzovsky et al., 2022).

Case-Control Studies

Case-control studies are a type of retrospective analytic observational study design that compares a population that developed an outcome of interest to a control group free of that outcome (Haley & Huber, 2023). In case-control studies, researchers determine an association between the exposures and outcomes measured as odds ratios and confidence intervals (Haley & Huber, 2023; Munnangi & Boktor, 2023). An odds ratio is defined as the percentage of patients who have developed an outcome compared to those who have not (Sueyoshi & Huber, 2023). The confidence interval measures the likelihood of an independent variable falling closer to the mean value. Lower confidence interval is associated with higher precision (Bzovsky et al., 2022). Case-control studies are inexpensive, able to assess multiple exposures at a time, and relatively easy to conduct as the patient population can be selected from available databases. A nested case-control study is a subset of case-control studies where the study population is derived from a preexisting cohort study (Ramji, 2022). Similar to cross-sectional studies, case-controlled studies cannot determine incidence rates and are prone to selection and recall biases (Wallace et al., 2022). A properly formulated study question and an adequately selected control group can help mitigate these potential biases (Ramji, 2022).

Cohort Studies

In the hierarchy of evidence, cohort studies provide better internal validity than observational studies. The internal validity demonstrates how well data derived from the study support an association or causal relationship between exposures and outcomes. In contrast, the external validity indicates to what extent the findings described in the study can be generalized to a broader population (Teut et al., 2020). A cohort is defined as a sample population that shares common characteristics (Barrett & Noble, 2019). In these studies, both cases and controls are free of the outcome of interest at the entry into the study. A distinct feature of cohort studies is a longitudinal study design that allows researchers to evaluate exposures at multiple timepoints (Wang & Kattan, 2020). This sequential follow-up provides an opportunity to estimate an association between exposures and outcomes better. Cohort studies can be prospective or retrospective. In cohort studies, outcomes are reported as relative or absolute risks, incidence ratios, and relative odds ratios. An absolute risk is defined as the probability of the outcome of interest occurring (Gail et al., 2019). Cohort studies offer a lot of advantages compared to other observational study designs. They provide information on the incidence of a disease and rare exposures, as well as enable the researcher to measure multiple outcomes at once (Wallace et al., 2022). Cohort studies are less prone to confounding and selection and recall biases. However, the longevity of the study design and broad patient population make cohort studies susceptible to loss to follow-up (Gail et al., 2019).

Implications for Oncology Clinical Research Nurses

In the expanding field of epidemiologic research, studying the occurrence and etiology of health-related events and determining their impact on specific patient populations is of utmost importance (Metelli & Chaimani, 2020). Understanding the incidence and prevalence of such events, along with identifying environmental, nutritional, and genetic factors, aids in better managing the issue and efficiently allocating resources. Insights from the COVID-19 pandemic have prompted researchers to reevaluate how real-world evidence from observational studies can inform clinical decisions and patient treatment strategies. Consequently, the contribution of oncology clinical research nurses in conducting observational studies, gathering qualitative data, and applying real-world evidence in clinical practice is invaluable. With patient advocacy at the forefront, oncology clinical research nurses swiftly establish rapport with patients, aiding in protocol enrollment, record examination, interviews with patients and caregivers, completion of patient-reported outcomes, and both prospective and retrospective data collection. Moreover, the use of qualitative, descriptive design in observational research presents numerous opportunities for oncology clinical research nurses to pursue their own studies, focusing on patient-centered outcomes (Siedlecki, 2020).

Summary

Well-designed observational studies are an essential part of epidemiologic research. They offer valuable insight into the incidence and prevalence of a disease and the risks of exposures and provide an association between exposures and outcomes. Data derived from observational studies help healthcare professionals to understand public health needs better and appropriately allocate necessary resources.

The COVID-19 pandemic highlighted that real-world data acquired from observational studies can efficiently supplement evidence collected from randomized controlled trials (Fox et al., 2022). Observational studies are inexpensive, time-efficient, and easy to conduct. In the field of modern epidemiology, these studies answer important questions about disease and associated risks and exposures (Teut et al., 2020). For patients with rare diseases and those who experienced rare outcomes, observational studies may offer the only available evidence (Wallace et al., 2022). Real-world data extracted from observational research may be generalizable to a broad patient population and can efficiently supplement data derived from experimental studies (Metelli & Chaimani, 2020).

Lack of randomization in observational research precludes it from establishing causal relationships and makes it susceptible to confounding and bias (Gail, 2019). To reduce potential pitfalls of observational study designs, the STROBE (STrengthening the Reporting of OBservational studies in Epidemiology) initiative provides recommendations for the reporting of observational studies (Ghaferi et al., 2021). The guidelines offer a 22-item checklist that outlines criteria for reporting observational research. By requiring standardized reporting, the guidelines aim to improve the reproducibility of data in future studies (Skrivankova et al., 2021). Ultimately, this approach helps to highlight the study limitations and improve the internal validity of the study and the generalizability of the findings. Although not mandatory, most peer-reviewed journals require authors to follow STROBE guidelines (Sharp et al., 2020). Well-defined research questions, a properly selected target population, and the incorporation of contemporary statistical methods can help to mitigate bias and confounding and improve the internal validity of observational studies (Bajwa et al., 2021).

Key Points

- Observational studies come in various retrospective and prospective designs. They are inexpensive, time-efficient, and easy to conduct.
- Observational studies provide valuable insight into the incidence and prevalence of the disease, risk of exposures, and the association between exposures and outcomes.
- Lack of randomization and control in observational studies makes them susceptible to confounding and bias.
- Well-designed and adequately powered observational studies can efficiently supplement data derived from randomized controlled trials and help generate hypotheses for future studies.

The author would like to acknowledge Geri L. Schmotzer, PhD, MSN, MPH, RN, for her contribution to this chapter that remains unchanged from the previous edition of this book.

References

Aggarwal, R., & Ranganathan, P. (2019). Study designs: Part 2 – Descriptive studies. *Perspectives in Clinical Research, 10*(1), 34–36. https://doi.org/10.4103/picr.PICR_154_18

Ahlbom, A. (2021). *Modern epidemiology* (4th ed.) [Book review]. *European Journal of Epidemiology, 36*, 767–768. https://doi.org/10.1007/s10654-021-00778-w

Bajwa, S.J.S., Theerth, K.A., & Gupta, A. (2021). The increasing trend of observational studies in clinical research: Have we forgotten and started defying the hierarchy? *Indian Journal of Anaesthesia, 65*(3), 186–190. https://doi.org/10.4103/ija.IJA_176_21

Barrett, D., & Noble, H. (2019). What are cohort studies? *Evidence-Based Nursing, 22*(4), 95–96. https://doi.org/10.1136/ebnurs-2019-103183

Bosdriesz, J.R., Stel, V.S., van Diepen, M., Meuleman, Y., Dekker, F.W., Zoccali, C., & Jager, K.J. (2020). Evidence-based medicine—When observational studies are better than randomized controlled trials. *Nephrology, 25*(10), 737–743. https://doi.org/10.1111/nep.13742

Bzovsky, S., Phillips, M.R., Guymer, R.H., Wykoff, C.C., Thabane, L., Bhandari, M., & Chaudhary, V. (2022). The clinician's guide to interpreting a regression analysis. *Eye, 36*(9), 1715–1717. https://doi.org/10.1038/s41433-022-01949-z

Collins, R., Bowman, L., Landray, M., & Peto, R. (2020). The magic of randomization versus the myth of real-world evidence. *New England Journal of Medicine, 382*(7), 674–678. https://doi.org/10.1056/NEJMsb1901642

Fleischmann, M., McLaughlin, P., Vaughan, B., & Hayes, A. (2024). A clinician's guide to performing a case series study. *Journal of Bodywork and Movement Therapies, 40*, 211–216. https://doi.org/10.1016/j.jbmt.2024.04.001

Fox, M.P., Murray, E.J., Lesko, C.R., & Sealy-Jefferson, S. (2022). On the need to revitalize descriptive epidemiology. *American Journal of Epidemiology, 191*(7), 1174–1179. https://doi.org/10.1093/aje/kwac056

Gail, M.H., Altman, D.G., Cadarette, S.M., Collins, G., Evans, S.J., Sekula, P., ... Woodward, M. (2019). Design choices for observational studies of the effect of exposure on disease incidence. *BMJ Open, 9*(12), e031031. https://doi.org/10.1136/bmjopen-2019-031031

Ghaferi, A.A., Schwartz, T.A., & Pawlik, T.M. (2021). STROBE reporting guidelines for observational studies. *JAMA Surgery, 156*(6), 577–578. https://doi.org/10.1001/jamasurg.2021.0528

Haley, K.E., & Huber, K.E. (2023). Case-control study. In A.E.M. Eltorai, D.W. Kim, J.A. Bakal, & D.E. Wazer. (Eds.), *Translational radiation oncology* (pp. 223–229). Elsevier. https://doi.org/10.1016/B978-0-323-88423-5.00091-1

Innes, G.K., Bhondoekhan, F., Lau, B., Gross, A.L., Ng, D.K., & Abraham, A.G. (2021). The measurement error elephant in the room: Challenges and solutions to measurement error in epidemiology. *Epidemiologic Reviews, 43*(1), 94–105. https://doi.org/10.1093/epirev/mxab011

Kalantari, J., & Cooper, K. (2023). Cross-sectional study: Design, measures, classic examples. In A.E.M. Eltorai, D.W. Kim, J.A. Bakal, & D.E. Wazer. (Eds.), *Translational radiation oncology* (pp. 189–193).

Elsevier Academic Press. https://doi.org/10.1016/B978-0-12-823026-8.00040-7

Khare, S., & Vedel, I. (2019). Recall bias and reduction measures: An example in primary health care utilization. *Family Practice, 36*(5), 672–686. https://doi.org/10.1093/fampra/cmz042

Maier, C., Thatcher, J.B., Grover, V., & Dwivedi, Y.K. (2023). Cross-sectional research: A critical perspective, use cases, and recommendations for IS research. *International Journal of Information Management*, 102625. https://doi.org/10.1016/j.ijinfomgt.2023.102625

Meade, M., Buchan, L., Stark, M., & Woods, B. (2024). Evidence-based medicine and observational studies. *Clinical Spine Surgery, 37*(5), 242–244. https://doi.org/10.1097/bsd.0000000000001550

Merriam-Webster. (n.d.). Confounding. In *Merriam-Webster.com dictionary.* Retrieved September 1, 2025, from https://www.merriam-webster.com/dictionary/confounding

Metelli, S., & Chaimani, A. (2020). Challenges in meta-analyses with observational studies. *Evidence-Based Mental Health, 23*(2), 83–87. https://doi.org/10.1136/ebmental-2019-300129

Miroshnychenko, A., Zeraatkar, D., Phillips, M.R., Bakri, S.J., Thabane, L., Bhandari, M., & Chaudhary, V. (2022). Cohort studies investigating the effects of exposures: Key principles that impact the credibility of the results. *Eye*, 36(5), 905–906. https://doi.org/10.1038/s41433-021-01897-0

Munn, Z., Barker, T.H., Moola, S., Tufanaru, C., Stern, C., McArthur, A., ... Aromataris, E. (2020). Methodological quality of case series studies: An introduction to the JBI critical appraisal tool. *JBI Evidence Synthesis, 18*(10), 2127–2133. https://doi.org/10.11124/JBISRIR-D-19-00099

Munnangi, S., & Boktor, S.W. (2023). Epidemiology of study design. In *StatPearls.* StatPearls Publishing.

National Institute of Mental Health. (n.d.). *Mental health statistics.* https://www.nimh.nih.gov/statistics

Ramji, S. (2022). Study design: Observational studies. *Indian Pediatrics, 59*(6), 493–498.

Sharp, M.K., Glonti, K., & Hren, D. (2020). Online survey about the STROBE statement highlighted diverging views about its content, purpose, and value. *Journal of Clinical Epidemiology, 123,* 100–106. https://doi.org/10.1016/j.jclinepi.2020.03.025

Siedlecki, S.L. (2020). Understanding descriptive research design and methods. *Clinical Nurse Specialist, 34*(1) 8–12. https://doi.org/10.1097/NUR.0000000000000493

Skrivankova, V.W., Richmond, R.C., Woolf, B.A.R., Davies, N.M., Swanson, S.A., VanderWeele, T.J., ... Richards, J.B. (2021). Strengthening the reporting of observational studies in epidemiology using Mendelian randomisation (STROBE-MR): Explanation and elaboration. *BMJ, 375*, n2233. https://doi.org/10.1136/bmj.n2233

Sueyoshi, M., & Huber, K.E. (2023). Cohort studies. In A.E.M. Eltorai, D.W. Kim, J.A. Bakal, & D.E. Wazer. (Eds.), *Translational radiation oncology* (pp. 231–235). Elsevier.

Teut, M., Walach, H., Varanasi, R., Manchanda, R.K., Oberai, P., Thompson, E., & Ulbrich-Zürni, S. (2020). Recommendations for designing, conducting, and reporting observational studies in homeopathy. *Homeopathy, 109*(3), 114–125. https://doi.org/10.1055/s-0040-1708045

Wallace, S.S., Barak, G., Truong, G., & Parker, M.W. (2022). Hierarchy of evidence within the medical literature. *Hospital Pediatrics, 12*(8), 745–750. https://doi.org/10.1542/hpeds.2022-006690

Wang, X., & Cheng, Z. (2020). Cross-sectional studies: Strengths, weaknesses, and recommendations. *Chest, 158*(1, Suppl.), S65–S71. https://doi.org/10.1016/j.chest.2020.03.012

Wang, X., & Kattan, M.W. (2020). Cohort studies: Design, analysis, and reporting. *Chest, 158*(1, Suppl.), S72–S78. https://doi.org/10.1016/j.chest.2020.03.014

CHAPTER 6

Expanded Access to Investigational Drugs

Yelena Shames, MSN, ACNP-BC, CNRN

Introduction

Randomized controlled trials are the gold standard for the clinical evaluation of bringing a new drug to market. The average approval time from the start of a clinical trial to the final review and marketing approval can take up to eight years—a time frame that patients with serious conditions or rare diseases cannot afford (Michaeli et al., 2024). Thus, for patients with terminal illnesses who have exhausted available treatment options and are ineligible to participate in clinical investigations, an expanded access program (EAP) offers an alternative to obtaining unapproved drugs outside of clinical trials.

The U.S. Food and Drug Administration (FDA) has allowed for the emergency single-patient use of experimental drugs outside of clinical trials since the 1970s (Wasser & Greenblatt, 2023). The compassionate use of investigational drugs was further brought to light by patient advocacy organizations in the 1980s when the HIV/AIDS epidemic necessitated broader access to unapproved therapies (Campbell & Williams, 2021; Polak & Fernandez Lynch, 2023). The FDA Modernization Act of 1997 introduced new standards for compassionate use requests, expanding single-patient use authorization to a broader patient population (Manley et al., 2022).

In 2009, FDA further revised its regulations on expanded access (EA) to investigational drugs for treatment use under an Investigational New Drug (IND) application (21 Code of Federal Regulations [C.F.R.] § 312(i)) (IND Application, 1987). The implementation of these regulatory requirements raised questions from providers, drug manufacturers, and patient activists. In response, FDA issued *Expanded Access to Investigational Drugs for Treatment Use—Questions and Answers* in 2016 to define the rules and regulations for requesting investigational drugs or biologic products outside of clinical trials. Under the new provisions, EAPs were required to be recorded on ClinicalTrials.gov (42 C.F.R. § 11.28(a)(2)(ii)(H) and (c)) (What Constitutes Clinical Trial Registration Information?, 2016). FDA guidance was further updated in 2017 with clarifications related to institutional review board (IRB) review and informed consent requirements.

Updates included the 21st Century Cures Act, which requires drug manufacturers to formalize EA policies and make them publicly available (FDA, 2017). In September 2023, FDA announced the release of its guidance for IRB review of individual patient EA submissions for investigational drugs and biologic products published in the *Federal Register*. Although, statistically, FDA approves 99% of EA requests (FDA, 2018), Right to Try (RTT) legislation was enacted in 2017 with the intention of reducing barriers to accessing unapproved medications. By 2018, RTT was a law in 41 states, creating another pathway for patients to access unapproved therapies (Chapman et al., 2020).

This chapter will discuss the similarities and differences between the two pathways, along with ethical considerations (see Table 6-1).

Expanded Access Programs

Although the compassionate use of an investigational drug and EAP are often used interchangeably in reference to investigational drug access outside of clinical trials, to avoid confusion, guidance defers to the terminology of *Expanded Access to Investigational Drugs for Treatment Use* (FDA, 2017). The primary purpose of an EAP is to diagnose, treat, and monitor patient diseases—not to collect evidence on the safety and efficacy of the investigational intervention.

TABLE 6-1 | Differences and Similarities Between Expanded Access Programs and Right to Try

	Expanded Access Programs	Right to Try
Patient criteria	Must have an immediately life-threatening disease or condition Must have exhausted all available standard treatment options Must be ineligible to participate in clinical trials Provided written informed consent according to U.S. Food and Drug Administration regulations	Must have a life-threatening disease or condition Must have exhausted all available standard treatment options Must be ineligible to participate in clinical trials Informed consent needed but requirements not specified
Investigational drug criteria	Completion of phase 1 trial not required May approve a biosimilar drug when there is a shortage of an approved drug May approve the drug when availability is limited by REMS (Risk Evaluation and Mitigation Strategy) program	Must have completed phase 1 trial Must not be approved for any indication Drug in development for marketing
Regulatory oversight	U.S. Food and Drug Administration Institutional review board	–
Liability	No legal obligations for a manufacturer to provide the drug No legal obligations for a physician to prescribe the drug Allows manufacturer to charge for a direct cost	No legal obligations for a manufacturer to provide the drug No legal obligations for a physician to prescribe the drug Allows manufacturer to charge for a direct cost Physicians or manufacturers not liable for unforeseen harm to the patient unless reckless or willful misconduct committed

Note. Based on information from Agarwal & Saltz, 2020; Chapman, 2020; Lynch, 2023.

Under regulations, FDA defines three types of EAPs:

- EA for individual patients, including for emergency use (21 C.F.R. § 312.310) (Individual Patients, Including for Emergency Use, 2009): Under this provision, EA is generally limited to a single course of therapy for a specified duration. However, under certain circumstances, FDA may grant an exception and authorize multiple courses of therapy, including access to treat a chronic condition or condition that requires extended treatment.
- EA for intermediate-size patient population: This is used when more than one patient with the same disease or condition will be treated, but the patient population is smaller than what would be treated under the existing IND application (21 C.F.R. § 312.315) (Intermediate-Size Patient Populations, 2009)
- EA for widespread treatment use through a treatment IND or protocol (21 C.F.R. § 312.320) (Treatment IND or Treatment Protocol, 2009): This type of EAP is usually used to bridge the gap between the completion of a clinical investigation and final FDA approval (Rizk, 2021).

To be eligible for an EAP, patients must meet specific criteria:

- Patients must have an immediately life-threatening disease or condition defined as a stage of the disease in which there is a reasonable likelihood that death will occur within months without early treatment (21 C.F.R. § 312.300(b)) (General, 2009).
- Patients must have a serious disease or condition associated with morbidity that has a substantial impact on daily functioning. Morbidity needs to be irreversible, persistent, or recurrent (21 C.F.R. § 312.300(b)) (General, 2009).
- Patients must exhaust all approved treatment options and be ineligible to participate in clinical trials (National Cancer Institute, 2024).
- Sufficient scientific evidence exists that benefits justify the risks involved.
- The EAP must not interfere with the initiation, conduct, or completion of clinical trials (21 C.F.R. § 312.300) (General, 2009).
- EA might be granted when a drug has been withdrawn for safety concerns, but there is a patient population for whom benefits continue to outweigh the risks.
- EA might be granted for a biosimilar drug when there is a shortage of an approved drug.
- EA might be granted when the use of an approved drug is limited by a REMS (Risk Evaluation and Mitigation Strategy) program.

The prescribing physician must hold proper licensure and be competent in managing patients receiving investigational medications. The drug manufacturer must agree to supply the drug and should be willing to provide a letter of authorization or grant FDA access to the available safety and efficacy information under the existing IND (see Figure 6-1). Under EAP and RTT provisions, drug manufacturers are not legally obligated to supply the drug outside of clinical trials and may deny access because of a concern with limited drug supply or how information

PHYSICIAN

- Hold appropriate licensure and training and be willing and able to oversee treatment.
- Identify the investigational product that is likely to provide benefits.
- Contact the drug manufacturer to inquire about the availability of the drug.
- Request a letter of authorization that allows FDA access to safety and efficacy data under the existing IND.
- Request institutional review board approval.
- Determine that the probable risks of the unapproved drug are not more significant than the risk from the disease or condition.
- Ensure the patient is eligible.
- Obtain written informed consent in accordance with FDA requirements (21 C.F.R. § 312.305(c)(4)).
- Complete Form FDA 1571 or Form FDA 3926.
- Submit safety reports, annual reports, and end-of-treatment summaries to FDA.

DRUG MANUFACTURER

- Provide contact information.
- Make company policy on EAPs publicly available when registering a clinical trial on ClinicalTrials.gov.
- Allow FDA access to safety and efficacy data under the current IND.
- Provide a written summary of the results of EAPs, including safety reports, number of doses supplied, and number of patients treated (21 C.F.R. § 312.320(c)).
- Approve the use of investigational drugs under EAPs.

FDA

- Based on potential safety and efficacy reports, determine that the potential benefits justify the risks.
- Determine that the patient has a serious or life-threatening condition and no other treatment options are available (21 C.F.R. § 312.305(a)(1)).
- Determine whether there are no alternative treatment options.
- Determine that the patient is ineligible to obtain the drug under clinical trials (21 C.F.R. § 312.310(a)(2)).
- Determine that providing expanded access would not interfere with the conduct of the clinical investigation (21 C.F.R. § 312.305(a)(3)).
- Determine whether the patient may receive treatment under expanded access and grant approval to proceed with the request.

FIGURE 6-1 | Delineation of Responsibilities

C.F.R.—Code of Federal Regulations; EAP—expanded access program; FDA—U.S. Food and Drug Administration; IND—Investigational New Drug

Note. Based on information from Requirements for All Expanded Access Uses, 2009; Scepura et al., 2021; Smith & Redic, 2022; Treatment IND or Treatment Protocol, 2009; U.S. Food and Drug Administration, 2017; Zettler et al., 2021.

collected through the EAP may affect marketing approval (FDA, 2017).

Common barriers to submitting EAP requests reported by healthcare providers include the time commitment required for writing a protocol and completing FDA-required documentation, unfamiliarity with the submission process, lack of knowledge on the availability of unapproved drugs for an indication, local IRB availability, and the deadlines for the IRB review and approval process (Manley et al., 2022). FDA must review the submission and provide its responses within 30 days of submission. However, emergency requests may be approved within one to three days (Smith & Redic, 2022).

Expanded Access and Emergency Use for Individual Patients

Individual patient requests for unapproved drug use outside of clinical trials can be submitted to FDA either as an EA protocol to an existing IND or as an individual EA under a new IND.

In attempts to reduce the administrative burden experienced by physicians, FDA has amended the submission requirements for individual patient IND submissions, including for emergency use. New provisions allow licensed physicians to submit requests either by completing Form FDA 1571 or by selecting the abbreviated Form FDA 3926, which allows them to request a waiver from a full IRB review and request authorization to obtain approval from the IRB chair or a designated member (FDA, 2017). For each patient protocol submitted to an existing IND by the study sponsor, Form FDA 1571 must be submitted.

Either a licensed physician or the sponsor of an existing IND may request EA for a single patient. For requests submitted under a new IND, unless otherwise stated by FDA, a 30-day waiting period is required before treatment can begin. For protocol submissions under an existing IND, the 30-day waiting period is not required, but IRB approval must be included with the request (21 C.F.R. § 312.305) (Requirements for All Expanded Access Uses, 2009). However, for FDA to authorize a subsequent course of treatment, a full IRB review is required.

In an emergency, when waiting for 30 days is not feasible, a physician may request treatment authorization via telephone. Treatment authorized verbally may start immediately, but a physician or a sponsor must submit a written IND request within 15 business days of the initial authorization, and the IRB must be notified within five business days of treatment (21 C.F.R. § 312.310) (Individual Patients, Including for Emergency Use, 2009). For both submissions, FDA requires sponsors and physician investigators to submit safety reports and annual reports as well as to maintain adequate drug disposition records (21 C.F.R. § 312.300) (General, 2009).

Expanded Access for an Intermediate-Size Patient Population

An intermediate-size treatment IND allows physicians to provide EA to more than one patient with the same disease or condition; however, this is generally to a smaller patient population than is treated under the existing IND in clinical trials. FDA does not impose a numerical limit on the number of patients who can be enrolled (FDA, 2017). Single-patient INDs can be merged into intermediate-size INDs to reduce the administrative burden per FDA request.

Intermediate-size EA requests can be submitted either under a treatment IND or as an amendment to a protocol under an existing IND by completing Form FDA 1571 when an investigational drug is being developed for marketing. For submissions under a new IND, a 30-day waiting period is required. FDA may grant authorization to more than one intermediate-size patient population EA IND or protocol submitted by different providers or sponsors (FDA, 2017).

FDA may also grant its approval when a drug has been withdrawn from the market for safety concerns but some patients continue to derive benefits, when a biosimilar drug is requested due to a shortage of an approved drug, and when the availability of an approved drug is limited due to a risk evaluation and mitigation strategy (REMS) (FDA, 2019).

Expanded Access for a Widespread Patient Population

EA for a widespread patient population is usually used to bridge the gap between the completion of a clinical investigation and marketing approval of the investigational drug. EA requests can be submitted by either a licensed physician or the sponsor of the existing IND by completing Form FDA 1571. For submissions under a new treatment IND or as a protocol amendment to an existing IND, a 30-day waiting period is required before treatment can begin unless otherwise noted by FDA (21 C.F.R. § 312.305 (d)(1)) (Requirements for All Expanded Access Uses, 2009). To approve EA of an investigational drug for a broad patient population, FDA requires significant clinical evidence of its safety and efficacy. Clinical evidence is usually collected from phase 2 and 3 trials.

Importantly, data presented at the 2022 American Society of Clinical Oncology Annual Meeting showed that of 2,901 single-patient INDs granted, 534 were for patients aged younger than 18 years (Duke et al., 2022).

The Emergency Use Authorization Program

Emergency Use Authorization (EUA) of unapproved drugs is a form of marketing authorization issued by FDA during public health emergencies to mitigate infectious, biologic, radiologic, chemical, or nuclear threats (Rizk et al., 2021). The Project BioShield Act of 2004 permits the widespread use of an unapproved drug during a public health emergency declaration (Smith & Redic, 2022). In contrast to EA for a widespread patient population, EUA often lacks robust evidence of efficacy and safety, as clinical investigations for that specific indication may not have been completed. Therefore, FDA requires that patients are fully informed and may place additional restrictions to mitigate risks associated with the administration of an investigational product.

When FDA decides to provide an EUA based on available clinical information, enrollment in the EA program for the same drug stops, and the drug is subsequently provided under the EUA program. Unlike other forms of EA, IRB approval for EUA is not required (Samuels et al., 2022); however, FDA may revoke EUA based on updated safety and efficacy reports. During the COVID-19 pandemic, several medications, including remdesivir, convalescent plasma, and hydroxychloroquine, among others, became available under EUA. However, some EUAs were later rescinded and never achieved full market approval (Rizk et al., 2021).

Ethical and Financial Considerations

The COVID-19 pandemic transformed the landscape of EA and EUA programs by increasing public awareness, introducing a new perspective on real-world data collection beyond basic safety reports, and highlighting several ethical considerations related to access to unapproved medications outside of clinical trials.

Physicians with clinical trial experience and those with greater access to and support from their institutional IRBs are more likely to apply for EAPs. This inadvertently creates an inequity between physicians practicing within academic settings and those in the community. Physicians practicing within the community may not be aware of EAPs and may face additional barriers to completing the required application, establishing drug availability, and obtaining approval from an independent IRB (Gould et al., 2022). For instance, for physicians less familiar with clinical trials, there are no available databases that consolidate information on drugs in development linked to a specific clinical indication. This gap in knowledge, combined with a lack of familiarity with writing a required protocol and the administrative submission process for FDA-required forms and a letter of authorization, inhibits physicians practicing outside of academic settings from proceeding with compassionate use requests (Stout et al., 2021). Further, physicians may experience challenges in navigating between two eligible pathways—EA and RTT (Smith & Redic, 2022).

An ongoing debate exists in the literature regarding whether physicians have a moral obligation to discuss the possibility of an EAP with their patients (Vermeulen et al., 2023). Some may worry this may lead to false hope and set up unrealistic expectations for patients with terminal illnesses. This can negatively affect their quality of life by precluding them from pursuing appropriate palliative measures (Bunnik & Aarts, 2021).

Manufacturers are not legally obligated to participate in an EAP. They might deny access to their drug due to concerns about a limited supply availability or how real-world data collected from EAPs might be interpreted by FDA and impact the marketing and approval process (Rozenberg & Greenbaum, 2020). Patients who have not met the inclusion criteria to participate in the clinical investigation might be more susceptible to developing unforeseen adverse events that could negatively reflect on the drug development and approval process (FDA, 2018). This creates a misconception that although EAP and RTT may allow access to an unapproved therapy, drug availability under either of these pathways is not guaranteed (Bunnik & Aarts, 2021).

Financial considerations raise another concern, as many insurance companies may deny reimbursement for treatment associated with unapproved therapies (Polak et al., 2022). Medicare and Medicaid also do not cover the cost of an unapproved drug or any associated expenses (Agarwal & Saltz, 2020). Although some sponsors may provide the drug free of charge, under FDA and RTT provisions, manufacturers are allowed to collect a direct cost of the investigational product, thus contributing to high out-of-pocket expenses for patients (Zettler et al., 2021).

Future Trajectory

The request to use unapproved therapies under the EAP is an unwieldy process. To properly match the drug to the patient, the physician must be familiar with current clinical investigations. Patient eligibility must be determined, and drug availability must be confirmed with the manufacturer. The manufacturer may or may not be able or willing to provide the drug. For EAPs under the current IND, a letter of authorization must be provided to allow FDA access to existing data. Except for urgent single-patient use applications, a treatment plan must be outlined and approved by the local IRB prior to being submitted to FDA (Joly et al., 2023).

To further increase social awareness, address structural inequities, and facilitate the complex application process, FDA continually improves its public website and established an Expanded Access Coordinating Committee aimed at streamlining EA requests (FDA, 2018).

In 2019, FDA launched the Oncology Center of Excellence Project Facilitate Program, a call center staffed with oncology professionals that helps to centralize communication and expedite application review. This program allows oncologists to navigate multistakeholder coordination and streamlines the application submission process (Smith & Redic, 2022). The Project Facilitate Program complements the Reagan-Udall Foundation's Expanded Access Navigator by providing a directory for drug manufacturers and an independent IRB (Scepura et al., 2021).

Lessons learned from the COVID-19 pandemic may present future opportunities to incorporate better real-world data collected from EAPs into the FDA decision-making and approval process. In certain circumstances, specifically for patients with rare diseases, real-world data collection can complement data obtained from RCTs. By providing additional clarification on how the real-world data might be used, FDA could encourage drug companies to have investigational agents more readily available under the EAP (Polak, 2020).

Implications for Oncology Clinical Research Nurses

Oncology clinical research nurses (OCRNs) offer a wealth of experience in managing patients enrolled in clinical investigations. They are indispensable in selecting eligible study participants, assessing and documenting adverse events, and mitigating toxicities and potential safety concerns. OCRNs' familiarity with trial protocols and regulatory reporting requirements, along with their ability to navigate complex clinical trials, uniquely positions them as patient advocates in EA discussions. Thus, OCRNs are vital to increasing public awareness about EAPs, expanding availability to a broader patient population within the community, and ensuring patient-informed decision-making while setting up realistic expectations and connecting patients with available resources.

By assisting physicians with the selection of patients for whom EA might be beneficial, OCRNs help establish enrollments within the community. Furthermore, OCRNs can support physicians by facilitating the cumbersome application process, including locating information on ClinicalTrials.gov and navigating sponsor communication (see Table 6-2).

OCRNs support patients with cancer seeking access to investigational therapies. They provide resources to patients and families by identifying clinical trial options, encouraging peer-to-peer support, matching patients to trials, and increasing their awareness of EAPs (see https://bloodcancerunited.org/resources/patients/clinical-trial-support-center-ctsc).

By providing EAP education to a larger number of patients within the community, OCRNs can help with the equitable selection of eligible patients. Their familiarity with managing patients enrolled in research protocols

TABLE 6-2 | Available Resources For Expanded Access Requests and Review Processes

Source	Website
U.S. Food and Drug Administration (FDA)	
Primary website	www.fda.gov
Center for Drug Evaluation and Research Division of Drug Information	www.fda.gov/about-fda/cder-offices-and-divisions/office-communications-cder-division-drug-information
ClinicalTrials.gov	https://clinicaltrials.gov
Expanded Access: Information for Patients	www.fda.gov/news-events/expanded-access/expanded-access-information-patients
Expanded Access: Information for Physicians	www.fda.gov/news-events/expanded-access/expanded-access-information-physicians
Expanded Access: Information for Institutional Review Boards	www.fda.gov/news-events/expanded-access/expanded-access-information-institutional-review-boards-irbs
FDA's Expanded Access Contact Information	www.fda.gov/news-events/expanded-access/fdas-expanded-access-contact-information
FDA Website Disclaimer	www.fda.gov/about-fda/website-policies/website-disclaimer
Right to Try FDA Fact Sheet	www.fda.gov/media/133864/download
FDA Emergency Call Center telephone (after hours)	866-300-4374
Contact Information for Review Divisions	www.fda.gov/news-events/expanded-access/fdas-expanded-access-contact-information
Oncology Center for Excellence Project Facilitate	www.fda.gov/about-fda/oncology-center-excellence/project-facilitate
Kids v Cancer	
Primary website	www.kidsvcancer.org
Compassionate Use Navigator	www.kidsvcancer.org/compassionate-use-navigator
Blood Cancer United (formerly Leukemia and Lymphoma Society)	
Primary website	www.bloodcancerunited.org
Clinical Trial Support Center	www.bloodcancerunited.org/resources/patients/clinical-trial-support-center-ctsc
Reagan-Udall Foundation	
Primary website	www.reaganudall.org
Expanded Access Navigator	www.reaganudall.org/expanded-access-navigator

enables them to efficiently facilitate the coordination of patient care and assist with real-world data collection and safety reporting.

Summary

Providing patients with access to unapproved therapies is a multifaceted, complex, and ethically complicated process. Over the past few decades, FDA took several steps toward revising its regulations to provide additional clarifications, standardize and simplify the application process, and expedite reviews for emergent requests. Regulatory changes have required drug manufacturers to make their contact information, procedures for submitting EA requests, criteria, and the time frame for reviewing these requests publicly available.

Despite these efforts, misconceptions still exist among patients, physicians, and drug manufacturers about drug availability, costs, application submission processes, and real-world data use. Having a second federal pathway through RTT that omits FDA and IRB reviews and offers legal protection to physicians and drug manufacturers adds to the confusion and brings another layer of ethical considerations.

Collecting data on the safety and outcomes of EAPs may help to reduce bias (Berlanga et al., 2023). Further standardizing and unifying federal pathways for an EA application process, providing additional education and support to physicians within the community, clarifying data collection and reporting requirements, and promoting public awareness would help patients in need of treatment receive access to potentially life-saving therapies.

Key Points

- For patients afflicted with life-threatening or rare diseases with no available treatment options, EAP and RTT offer an opportunity to access investigational drugs outside of clinical trials.
- Although FDA took several steps to facilitate patient access to compassionate investigational drugs, the application process remains logistically complex and is surrounded by ethical, financial, and regulatory considerations.
- Increasing public awareness, offering additional support to physicians and nurses, and standardizing guidance to manufacturers may help to resolve misconceptions and further facilitate patient access to unapproved therapies.

The author would like to acknowledge Deborah A. (Lindberg) Standafer, MBA, BSN, RN-C, CCRC, for her contribution to this chapter that remains unchanged from the previous edition of this book.

References

Agarwal, R., & Saltz, L.B. (2020). Understanding the right to try act. *Clinical Cancer Research, 26*(2), 340–343. https://doi.org/10.1158/1078-0432.CCR-19-2015

Berlanga, P., Ndounga-Diakou, L.A., Aerts, I., Corradini, N., Ducassou, S., Strullu, M., ... Vassal, G. (2023). Measuring safety and outcomes for the use of compassionate and off-label therapies for children, adolescents, and young adults with cancer in the SACHA-France study. *JAMA Network Open, 6*(7), e2321568. https://doi.org/10.1001/jamanetworkopen.2023.21568

Bunnik, E.M., & Aarts, N. (2021). The role of physicians in the expanded access to investigational drugs: a mixed-methods study of physicians' views and experiences in the Netherlands. *Journal of Bioethical Inquiry, 18*(2), 319–334. https://doi.org/10.1007/s11673-021-10090-7

Campbell, M., & Williams, M. (2021). The ethics of access: An AIDS activist won public access to experimental therapies, and this must now extend psychedelics for mental illness. *Front Psychiatry, 12,* 680626. https://doi.org/10.3389/fpsyt.2021.680626

Chapman, C.R., Eckman, J., & Bateman-House, A.S. (2020). Oversight of right-to-try and expanded access requests for off-trial access to investigational drugs. *Ethics and Human Research, 42*(1), 2–13. https://doi.org/10.1002/eahr.500038

Duke, E., Kormanik, N.L., Barone, A., Singh, H., Beaver, J.A., Pazdur, R., ... Donoghue, M.B. (2022). FDA analysis of expanded access use in pediatric patients from 2015 to 2020. *Journal of Clinical Oncology, 40*(Suppl. 16), 1529. https://doi.org/10.1200/JCO.2022.40.16_suppl.1529

General, 21 C.F.R. § 312.300 (2009). https://www.ecfr.gov/current/title-21/chapter-I/subchapter-D/part-312/subpart-I/section-312.300

Gould, P., Salam, T., Kimberly, L., Bateman-House, A., & Lynch, H.F. (2022). Perspectives of academic oncologists about offering expanded access to investigational drugs. *JAMA Network Open, 5*(11), e2239766. https://doi.org/10.1001/jamanetworkopen.2022.39766

Individual Patients, Including for Emergency Use, 21 C.F.R. § 312.310 (2009). https://www.ecfr.gov/current/title-21/chapter-I/subchapter-D/part-312/subpart-I/section-312.310

Intermediate-Size Patient Populations, 21 C.F.R. § 312.315 (2009). https://www.ecfr.gov/current/title-21/chapter-I/subchapter-D/part-312/subpart-I/section-312.315

Investigational New Drug Application, 21 C.F.R. § 312 (1987). https://www.ecfr.gov/current/title-21/chapter-I/subchapter-D/part-312

Joly, M.M., Edwards, T.L., Jerome, R.N., Mainor, A., Bernard, G.R., & Pulley, J.M. (2023). Taking AIM at serious illness: Implementing an access to investigational medicines expanded access program. *Frontiers in Medicine, 10,* 1287449. https://doi.org/10.3389/fmed.2023.1287449

Lynch, H.F. (2023). Devil in the details: Physician duties and expanded access. *Journal of Law, Medicine, and Ethics, 51*(1), 1–14. https://doi.org/10.1017/jme.2023.54

Manley, H., Sisk, B.A., Master, Z., & Scott, C.T. (2022). Prescribing unproven cancer drugs: Physician perspectives on expanded access and right to try. *Journal of Law and the Biosciences, 9*(2). https://doi.org/10.1093/jlb/lsac031

Michaeli, D.T., Michaeli, T., Albers, S., Boch, T., & Michaeli, J.C. (2024). Special FDA designations for drug development: Orphan, fast track, accelerated approval, priority review, and breakthrough therapy. *European Journal of Health Economics, 25*(6), 979–997. https://doi.org/10.1007/s10198-023-01639-x

National Cancer Institute (2022). *Ways to access experimental cancer drugs.* https://www.cancer.gov/about-cancer/treatment/drugs/access-experimental

Polak, T.B., Cucchi, D.G.J., van Rosmalen, J., Uyl-de Groot, C.A., & Darrow, J.J. (2022). Generating evidence from expanded access use of rare disease medicines: Challenges and recommendations. *Frontiers in Pharmacology, 13,* 913567. https://doi.org/10.3389/fphar.2022.913567

Polak, T.B., & Fernandez Lynch, H. (2023). The ethics of expanded access research. *Journal of the American Medical Association, 329*(13), 1057–1058. https://doi.org/10.1001/jama.2023.2204

Polak, T.B., van Rosmalen, J., & Uyl-de Groot, C.A. (2020). Expanded access as a source of real-world data: An overview of FDA and EMA approvals. *British Journal of Clinical Pharmacology, 86*(9), 1819–1826. https://doi.org/10.1111/bcp.14284

Requirements for All Expanded Access Uses, 21 C.F.R. § 312.305 (2009). https://www.ecfr.gov/current/title-21/chapter-I/subchapter-D/part-312/subpart-I/section-312.305

Rizk, J.G., Forthal, D.N., Kalantar-Zadeh, K., Mehra, M.R., Lavie, C.J., Rizk, Y., ... Lewin, J.C. (2021). Expanded access programs, compassionate drug use, and emergency use authorizations during the COVID-19 pandemic. *Drug Discovery Today, 26*(2), 593–603. https://doi.org/10.1016/j.drudis.2020.11.025

Rozenberg, O., & Greenbaum, D. (2020). Making it count: Extracting real-world data from compassionate use and expanded access programs. *American Journal of Bioethics, 20*(7), 89–92. https://doi.org/10.1080/15265161.2020.1779857

Samuels, E., Champagne, E., Gravelin, M., Racklyeft, J., & Weatherwax, K. (2022). Adapting an expanded access program to enable investigational treatments for COVID-19. *Journal of Clinical and Translational Science, 6*(1), e77. https://doi.org/10.1017/cts.2022.403

Scepura, B., Chan, M., Kim, T., Boehmer, J., Goldberg, K.B., & Pazdur, R. (2021). Oncology expanded access and FDA's Project Facilitate. *Oncologist, 26*(10), e1880–e1882. https://doi.org/10.1002/onco.13910

Smith, A.J.F., & Redic, K.A. (2022). Single-patient expanded access: A primer for pharmacists. *American Journal of Health-System Pharmacy, 79*(23), 2118–2127. https://doi.org/10.1093/ajhp/zxac242

Stout, J., Smith, C., Buckner, J., Adjei, A.A., Wentworth, M., Tilburt, J.C., & Master, Z. (2021). Oncologists' reflections on patient rights and access to compassionate use drugs: A qualitative interview study from an academic cancer center. *PLOS ONE, 16*(12), e0261478. https://doi.org/10.1371/journal.pone.0261478

Treatment IND or Treatment Protocol, 21 C.F.R. § 312.320 (2009). https://www.ecfr.gov/current/title-21/chapter-I/subchapter-D/part-312/subpart-I/section-312.320

U.S. Food and Drug Administration. (2017). *Expanded access to investigational drugs for treatment use – Questions and answers: Guidance for industry.* https://www.fda.gov/media/85675/download

U.S. Food and Drug Administration. (2018). *Expanded access program report.* https://www.fda.gov/media/119971

U.S. Food and Drug Administration. (2019). *FDA's application of statutory factors in determining when a REMS is necessary: Guidance for industry.* https://www.fda.gov/regulatory-information/search-fda-guidance-documents/fdas-application-statutory-factors-determining-when-rems-necessary

What Constitutes Clinical Trial Registration Information?, 42 C.F.R. § 11.28 (2016). https://www.ecfr.gov/current/title-42/chapter-I/subchapter-A/part-11/subpart-B/section-11.28

Vermeulen, S.F., Hordijk, M., Visser, R.J., & Bunnik, E.M. (2023). Do physicians have a duty to discuss expanded access to investigational drugs with their patients? A normative analysis. *Journal of Law, Medicine and Ethics, 51*(1), 172–180. https://doi.org/10.1017/jme.2023.53

Wasser, J.S., & Greenblatt, D.J. (2023). Applying real-world data from expanded-access ("compassionate use") patients to drug development. *Journal of Clinical and Translational Science, 7*(1), e181. https://doi.org/10.1017/cts.2023.606

Zettler, M.E., Jeune-Smith, Y., Feinberg, B.A., Phillips, E.G., Jr., & Gajra, A. (2021). Expanded access and right to try requests: The community oncologist's experience. *JCO Oncology Practice, 17*(11), e1719-e1727. https://doi.org/10.1200/OP.20.00569

SECTION II.
Clinical Trials: Fundamental Information

CHAPTER 7

Legal, Regulatory, and Legislative Issues

Crystal D. Chu, PhD, RN

Introduction

Knowledge, understanding, and application of research-related laws and regulations are expected of all individuals involved in the conduct of clinical research, regardless of role. Past unethical actions in human participant research have led to the development of legal and regulatory processes that guide clinical research. The history of this evolution can be found in peer-reviewed articles, books written about clinical trials, or online regulatory groups. Oncology clinical research nurses (OCRNs) must stay up-to-date as these documents evolve to reflect the advances in ethics and clinical care and ensure the protection of research participants.

This chapter will introduce and familiarize OCRNs with the overarching legal, regulatory, and legislative aspects of conducting clinical research. The elements of clinical research to which these principles and standards apply are presented in depth in other chapters of this publication.

Historical Overview

Historical injustices, abuse, and inequity of research participants have led to the development of laws, regulations, and guidelines that protect research participants and form the foundation for best clinical research practices worldwide. The selected historical events and timelines presented in this chapter are not exhaustive of all injustices, and the protection of research participants continues to evolve.

Nuremberg Code

The beginning of the modern era for protecting human participants can be traced to after World War II (WWII). Prior to WWII, limited rules and protocols for human medical experimentation existed. A protocol that introduced the concept of informed consent was developed in Germany in 1931 in response to a failed vaccination experiment (Sass, 1983). However, none of these carried the force of law or were subjected to advanced legal scrutiny. This changed during the Nuremberg Medical Trial (Weindling, 2022).

During WWII, pseudoscientific experiments were performed on unwilling prisoners in German concentration camps. Nazi doctors performed extraordinarily unethical and malicious acts in the name of medical research. As the details of these acts emerged, the United States and its WWII allies developed the Nuremberg Code (1949), a set of 10 standards used by the Nuremberg Military Tribunal to evaluate experimentation on humans conducted by the Nazis (Weindling, 2022). The Allies held these trials in 1946–1947 to prosecute German war criminals. In the ruling of the tribunal in the case of the United States of America versus Karl Brandt et al., the court outlined a list of six (later expanded to 10) characteristics of legitimate human research. The document went well beyond the existing American Medical Association directives and the German Guidelines on Human Experimentation of 1931 (Sass, 1983), becoming the foundation for the Nuremberg Code (Weindling, 2022). Since its initial publication in 1949, the Nuremberg Code has remained unchanged. However, it has served as a template for subsequent laws, rules, codes, and guidance documents. The principles of the Nuremberg Code, and later the Declaration of Helsinki, have been incorporated into U.S. law in Title 45 of the Code of Federal Regulations (C.F.R.), specifically Part 46, Protection of Human Subjects (2017).

Declaration of Helsinki

The principles of the Nuremberg Code were reinforced when the World Medical Association (WMA) developed and adopted the *Declaration of Helsinki: Recommendations Guiding Medical Doctors in Biomedical Research Involving Human Subjects.* First issued in 1964, it is a statement of ethical principles to serve as guidance in the conduct of medical research. The Declaration of Helsinki builds upon the 10 principles of the Nuremberg Code, stating that identifiable human material and data are considered part of medical research (WMA, 2013). The document provides numerous ethical principles. In 2024, its 11th revision became the official version (WMA, 2024).

National Institutes of Health

In 1953, the National Institutes of Health (NIH) developed a policy to protect human participants by requiring an independent prospective review of clinical research studies on healthy volunteers conducted at the NIH Clinical Center. The initial policy only applied to healthy volunteers; patients enrolled in clinical trials received no additional protection, which was in line with the prevailing medical community opinion at the time. In the 1960s, as federal funding for research increased, interest in protecting the rights and well-being of research participants also grew. In 1966, NIH developed the first Public Health Service policy for the protection of human participants, which applied to all clinical research conducted and funded by the U.S. Department of Health, Education, and Welfare, later renamed the U.S. Department of Health and Human Services (HHS) (Slutsman & Nieman, 2018).

National Research Act

The U.S. Public Health Service's Untreated Syphilis Study at Tuskegee was conducted between 1932 and 1972 (Centers for Disease Control and Prevention [CDC], 2024). The study did not obtain informed consent, and the researchers withheld treatment for syphilis from an underserved population of rural Black men to learn about the natural progress of the untreated disease. In response to the unethical conduct and recognition of the lack of protection for human participants in the United States, an advisory panel ended the study in 1972, and the National Research Act was subsequently developed (CDC, 2024).

The National Research Act required the U.S. Department of Health, Education, and Welfare to codify its human participant protection policy, which occurred on May 30, 1974 (CDC, 2024; Office for Human Research Protections [OHRP], 1993; Slutsman & Nieman, 2018). The Protection of Human Research Subjects regulations outline the role and responsibilities of the institutional review board (IRB), as well as the informed consent process (see Chapter 12). The National Research Act established the National Commission for the Protection of Human Subjects of Biomedical and Behavioral Research, which eventually authored the historic *The Belmont Report* (OHRP, 2009, 2022a).

The Belmont Report

The Belmont Report: Ethical Principles and Guidelines for the Protection of Human Subjects of Research, written by the National Commission in 1978 and published in the *Federal Register* in 1979, is the standard for the ethical conduct of clinical trials. It was named after the Belmont Conference Center in Elkridge, Maryland, where a 12-member commission met to develop the report. These guidelines, along with HHS human participant protection regulations, constitute the basis for existing human participant protection standards in the United States (OHRP, 2022a). *The Belmont Report* outlines the distinction between research and practice and identifies the basic ethical principles for conducting clinical research, including remarks on the application of each principle (National Commission, 1979).

Distinction Between Research and Practice

OCRNs must understand the distinction between clinical practice and research (see Table 7-1). The objective of clinical practice is to diagnose and provide preventive, curative, or palliative treatment to improve the health of individuals. Conversely, the objective of clinical research is to test a hypothesis or hypotheses concerning the use of a clinical intervention, draw conclusions about the hypothesis based on the responses of study participants (captured in the form of data), and then report generalized conclusions from the research, thereby contributing to the knowledge base of healthcare science. Practice and research often happen concurrently, especially in the development of new treatments. It is important to consider what is standard practice; if an activity occurs sig-

TABLE 7-1 | Distinction Between Practice and Research

Concept	Description
Clinical practice	Diagnosis; provision of preventive, curative, or palliative treatment to improve the health of an individual
Clinical research	Testing hypothesis or hypotheses concerning the use of a clinical intervention, drawing conclusions based on responses of study participants, and reporting conclusions, thereby contributing to the knowledge base of healthcare science (to improve the health of other individuals) and allowing for replication of the research
Clinical research of clinical practice interventions	Combines clinical practice and clinical research

Note. Based on information from National Commission for the Protection of Human Subjects of Biomedical and Behavioral Research, 1979.

nificantly outside of that, it should be reviewed for the protection of human participants (National Commission, 1979).

Basic Ethical Principles

The Belmont Report identifies three unifying ethical principles for the conduct of clinical research: respect for persons, beneficence, and justice (see Table 7-2).

Respect for persons acknowledges the autonomy of study participants. It incorporates a requirement to protect those with diminished autonomy, such as children and individuals with mental illness, senility, or dementia. Autonomy refers to an individual's ability to make their own decisions freely and voluntarily based on sound judgment. Respect for the autonomy of study participants includes ensuring that participants have sufficient knowledge of the study to enable them to make an informed decision about participating (i.e., the informed consent process). *The Belmont Report* includes descriptions of the required elements of the informed consent form, as well as consideration of ethical standards undergirding the process of informed consent (National Commission, 1979).

Beneficence is defined by two general principles: not harming study participants and protecting them against potential harm while maximizing the benefits of their participation. Although beneficence is generally understood to apply to individuals, it also applies to society at large and to the institutions in which the research is conducted.

The Belmont Report addresses the nature of risks and benefits as they apply to clinical research and their disclosure in the informed consent document. Risk is defined as the probability of harm to participants and the potential severity of that harm. The report also lists harms other than physical and psychological harm (e.g., legal, social, financial, economic) that should be considered when comparing the risks and benefits of a study. The benefit in clinical research is defined as the positive value related to health or welfare. Benefits should be examined, as they affect not only the study participant but also society in general, in particular, people with the health condition under study (National Commission, 1979). The risk–benefit assessment is conducted as part of the ethical review of a study, typically by an IRB or ethics review committee.

Justice addresses the responsibility of researchers to ensure that the population from which study participants are recruited will benefit from the research. From a historical context, this concept addresses the benefits of the research and critically examines the burden. Examples of injustices (the experimentation in the Nazi concentration camps or the Tuskegee syphilis study) within research have occurred. It is essential to prevent the burden of research on humans, particularly those within vulnerable populations (i.e., socioeconomically disadvantaged or racial and ethnic minorities), and to avoid exploiting vulnerable individuals for the sake of ease in recruitment strategies (National Commission, 1979).

TABLE 7-2 | Application of The Belmont Report

Principle	Application
Respect for persons • Individuals are autonomous agents. • Individuals should be treated with respect. • Persons with diminished autonomy need additional protection.	Informed consent • Participants must be given the opportunity to choose what shall or shall not happen to them. • The consent process must include three elements: – Information sharing – Comprehension – Voluntary participation
Beneficence • Human participants should not be harmed. • Research should aim to maximize potential benefits and minimize potential risks.	Assessment of risks and benefits by the investigator and the institutional review board or ethics review committee
Justice • The benefits and burdens of research must be distributed fairly.	Selection of participants • Procedures and outcomes in the selection of research participants should be fair. • Eligibility criteria should include those who may benefit and exclude those who may be harmed.

Note. Based on information from National Commission for the Protection of Human Subjects of Biomedical and Behavioral Research, 1979.

Regulatory Authority

Several groups with regulatory authority are involved in conducting clinical trials. In the United States, the conduct of clinical trials is governed at the federal level by regulations enacted by HHS and other agencies (e.g., Department of War, Department of Veterans Affairs). HHS is the principal agency responsible for protecting the health of the U.S. population. This agency comprises 12 operating divisions, including NIH, CDC, the Agency for Healthcare Research and Quality, the Centers for Medicare and Medicaid Services, and the U.S. Food and Drug Administration (FDA) (HHS, 2024a). An organizational chart is available online at www.hhs.gov/about/agencies/orgchart.

The two main regulatory groups within HHS with whom OCRNs could interact are OHRP and FDA. The interaction will be either direct or indirect depending upon the type of research, who funds the research, and how the OCRN role is implemented at the research site. Table 7-3 presents various categories of clinical trials, along with the regulatory agency, center, or office providing oversight. The con-

TABLE 7-3 | Regulatory Authority Based on Type of Study and Sponsor

	Federal Agencies With Clinical Trial Oversight					
	FDA **Title 21 C.F.R.**		**OHRP** **Title 45 C.F.R. Part 46**		**DOD** **Title 32 C.F.R. Part 219**	
Type of Study						
Biologic agents conducted under an IND: • Vaccines • Blood and blood products for transfusion and/or manufacturing into other products • Allergenic extracts, which are used for both diagnosis and treatment (e.g., allergy shots) • Human cells and tissues used for transplantation (e.g., tendons, ligaments, bone) • Gene therapies • Cellular therapies • Tests to screen potential blood donors for infectious agents such as HIV	✓	CBER	✓	If HHS funded For gene therapy, OBA oversight	✓	If DOD funded
Devices conducted under an IDE	✓	CDRH	✓	If HHS funded	✓	If DOD funded
Drugs conducted under an IND: • Any article intended for use in the diagnosis, cure, mitigation, treatment, or prevention of disease • Any article, other than food, intended to affect the structure or any function of the body of man or other animals • New indication of an already marketed drug (known as a supplemental IND)	✓	CDER	✓	If HHS funded	✓	If DOD funded
Type of Sponsors for Oncology Clinical Trials						
DOD	✓	CDER, CBER, CDRH if using an IND or IDE		–	✓	–
NIH and NCI, including cooperative group studies	✓	CDER, CBER, CDRH if using an IND or IDE	✓	–		–
Private (e.g., biopharmaceutical industry, foundations)	✓	CDER, CBER, CDRH		–		–

Depending on the study sponsor, two sets of regulations may have to be followed. For example, an NCI study using an IND agent must adhere to both OHRP and FDA regulations.

CBER—Center for Biologics Evaluation and Research; CDER—Center for Drug Evaluation and Research; CDRH—Center for Devices and Radiological Health; C.F.R.—Code of Federal Regulations; DOD—Department of War; FDA—U.S. Food and Drug Administration; HHS—U.S. Department of Health and Human Services; IDE—Investigational Device Exemption; IND—Investigational New Drug Application; NCI—National Cancer Institute; NIH—National Institutes of Health; OBA—Office of Biotechnology Activities; OHRP—Office for Human Research Protections

Note. Based on information from Food and Drugs, 2025; Protection of Human Subjects, 2017, 2018.

tent covered by these regulations is compared in Table 7-4. Although Title 21 and Title 45 (Part 46) regulate different types of research, the human participant protection regulations are similar.

Both OHRP and FDA have regulations and several guidance documents that OCRNs will need to review. By definition, guidance documents are intended to provide a framework for conduct and recommendations for managing an operation, such as conducting clinical trials, but are not legally binding. In many instances, they serve as the foundation for the development of standard operating procedures and may be incorporated into legally binding requirements at a later date. Compliance with guidance documents represents adherence to the current standards of practice. OCRNs must be aware of the guidance documents applicable to the type of research being conducted and the research setting, including international, national, and local documents.

Office for Human Research Protections

OHRP was established in 2000 by HHS to protect the rights, welfare, and well-being of research participants. It is part of the Office of the Assistant Secretary for Health within the Office of the Secretary. Before 2000, human participant protection by HHS was limited to NIH-funded studies, with oversight from the NIH Office for Protection from Research Risks (OHRP, 2024b; Slutsman & Nieman, 2018).

OHRP's focus is on the IRBs and the informed consent process. It is the regulatory authority for 45 C.F.R. § 46, which includes the following (OHRP, 2025):

- **Subpart A:** Basic HHS Policy for Protection of Human Research Subjects (the Common Rule)
- **Subpart B:** Additional Protections for Pregnant Women, Human Fetuses, and Neonates Involved in Research
- **Subpart C:** Additional Protections Pertaining to Biomedical and Behavioral Research Involving Prisoners as Subjects
- **Subpart D:** Additional Protections for Children Involved as Subjects in Research
- **Subpart E:** Registration of Institutional Review Boards

The first codified federal policy for the protection of human research participants was established in 1974. In 1991, this policy, informally known as the Common Rule, was issued by 15 other federal agencies and departments. The Common Rule is 45 C.F.R. § 46 (OHRP, 2025).

As with any law or regulation, the Common Rule requires revision over time. OHRP provides a history of revisions to the Common Rule, and the latest published version, as of June 19, 2018, is referred to as the *2018 Requirements* (OHRP, 2025). OCRNs should be aware that 45 C.F.R. § 46 may change again and should check the OHRP website for current regulations.

OHRP is also responsible for compliance agreements and registration of IRBs. Institutions that conduct federally funded human participant research are required to obtain a Federalwide Assurance (FWA) for compliance with 45 C.F.R. § 46 prior to initiation of any clinical research. All IRBs listed on the FWA and those in the United States who

TABLE 7-4 | Content of Titles 21 and 45 of the U.S. Code of Federal Regulations Related to Clinical Trials

Title	Part	Topic Addressed
Title 21 (U.S. Food and Drug Administration): Food and Drugs	Part 11	Electronic records and signature
	Part 50	Protection of human subjects
	Part 54	Financial disclosure by clinical investigators
	Part 56	Institutional review boards
	Part 312	Investigational New Drug application
	Part 314	Application for U.S. Food and Drug Administration approval to market a new drug
	Part 601	Licensing
	Part 812	Investigational device exemptions
	Part 814	Premarket approval of medical devices
Title 45 (Common Rule): Public Welfare and Human Services	Part 46	Protection of human subjects
	Part 46, subpart A	Basic Health and Human Services policy for the protection of human research subjects
	Part 46, subpart B	Additional protection pertaining to research development and research activities involving fetuses, pregnant women, and human in vitro fertilization
	Part 46, subpart C	Additional protection pertaining to research development and research activities involving prisoners as research subjects
	Part 46, subpart D	Additional protection pertaining to research development and research activities involving children as research subjects

review FDA-regulated clinical trials must register with OHRP (HHS, 2021).

U.S. Food and Drug Administration

Not all clinical research conducted in the United States is funded by HHS. FDA has oversight of the laws for which it has authority (e.g., foods, drugs, biologics, devices, tobacco), regardless of who funds the research. FDA obtains its statutory authority through several acts of U.S. Congress (i.e., sets of laws), including the Federal Food, Drug, and Cosmetic Act; the Prescription Drug User Fee Act; the Prescription Drug Marketing Act; and the FDA Modernization Act of 1997. FDA is composed of centers and offices that ensure all regulations are followed (FDA, 2025b):

- Center for Biologics Evaluation and Research
- Center for Devices and Radiological Health
- Center for Drug Evaluation and Research
- Center for Food Safety and Applied Nutrition
- Center for Tobacco Products
- Center for Veterinary Medicine
- Human Foods Program
- Office of Clinical Policy and Programs
- Office of External Affairs
- Office of Minority Health and Health Equity
- Office of Operations
- Office of Policy, Legislation, and International Affairs
- Office of the Chief Scientist
- Office of Women's Health
- Oncology Center of Excellence

FDA also has regulations related to the protection of human participants: 21 C.F.R. § 50 Protection of Human Subjects and 21 C.F.R. § 56 Institutional Review Boards were codified in 1980 and 1981, respectively (Food and Drugs, 2025). The rules and regulations are developed by government departments and agencies based on laws passed by U.S. Congress. The regulations are published in the Code of Federal Regulations and are cited, for example, as 21 C.F.R. § 50. Each agency then provides nonbinding guidance documents, published in the *Federal Register*, which represent the agency's current stance on a particular subject to provide further direction. The U.S. agencies involved in clinical research provide an overview of their involvement in clinical research, including regulations and various guidance documents, on their respective websites. For more legal terms OCRNs may encounter related to the development of regulations, see Table 7-5.

The FDA regulations that apply to clinical research include electronic records and electronic signatures, informed consent, protection of human participants, financial disclosure by clinical investigators, approval of investigational new drugs, approval of new drugs, investigational device exemptions, and premarket approval of medical devices. In addition to the regulations, FDA (2025d) has several guidance documents.

> Guidance documents represent the agency's current thinking on a particular subject. They do not create or confer any rights for or on any person and do not operate to bind FDA or the public. An alternative approach may be used if such approach satisfies the requirements of the applicable statutes, regulations, or both. (para 1.)

FDA guidance documents may be found by searching the Division of Drug Information Database, available online at www.fda.gov/regulatory-information/search-fda-guidance-documents.

International Council for Harmonisation of Technical Requirements for Pharmaceuticals for Human Use

The International Council for Harmonisation of Technical Requirements for Pharmaceuticals for Human Use (ICH), established in 1990, develops and maintains major international standards for the conduct of research involving human participants (ICH, n.d.-a). It brings together the drug regulatory authorities of the European Union, Japan, and the United States (represented by FDA), along with pharmaceutical trade associations from these three regions, to discuss the scientific and technical aspects of product registration. ICH's mission is to achieve greater harmonization in the interpretation and application of technical guidelines and requirements for product registration, thereby reducing duplication of testing and reporting performed during the research and development of new medicines. This harmonization is to ensure that safe, effective, and high-quality medicines are developed and registered in the most resource-efficient manner (ICH, 2023).

The scope of ICH guidelines covers a broad range of topics related to conducting clinical research. In 2005, ICH divided the guidelines into four categories: quality (Q), efficacy (E), safety (S), and multidisciplinary (M), with numbered revisions to each guideline (e.g., R1, R2). The ICH topics are contained within one of these categories. Examples of guidelines located within the "M" category include the *Medical Dictionary for Regulatory Activities,* the *Common Technical Document,* and *Electronic Standards for the Transfer of Regulatory Information* (ICH, n.d.-b).

The guidelines have been updated over time to ensure clinical research rigor, safety, and quality reporting while incorporating the use of modern technology. In 2025, *ICH Harmonised Guideline: Guideline for Good Clinical Practice E6(R2)* was updated to *E6(R3)*, with updates including increased transparency in clinical trial registration and reporting (ICH, 2025). This guideline is critical for OCRNs to read and incorporate into practice.

International Standards, Laws, and Guidelines

Internationally conducted clinical trials are becoming increasingly more prevalent as the communication and technical capacities for these endeavors increase. OCRNs will have more opportunities to coordinate trials at an international level and must be aware of the legal and regulatory standards of other countries.

Although internationally conducted research offers the potential for tremendous benefit, it compounds the requirements for ensuring accountability and compliance. Annually, OHRP updates a compilation of international human research standards, which can be found at www.hhs.gov/ohrp/international/compilation-human-research-standards/index.html. This serves as a comprehensive reference for international research.

TABLE 7-5 | Glossary of U.S. Legal Terms

Term	Definition
Act	A person performs an action in accordance with their free will (Merriam-Webster, n.d.-a).
Act of Congress	A new law is made by the U.S. Senate and House of Representatives, usually after it has been signed by the President (Cambridge Dictionary, n.d.).
Administrative Agency	A government body authorized to implement legislative directives by developing more precise and technical rules than would be possible in a legislative setting. Many administrative agencies also have law enforcement responsibilities (Cornell Law School, 2025).
Code	A systematic compilation or revision of law or legal principles that is arranged especially by subject; a set of rules or regulations that is promulgated by a body (as a professional organization) and that regulates its industrial or professional practices (Merriam-Webster, n.d.-b)
Code of Federal Regulations	The Code of Federal Regulations (C.F.R.) is the codification of the general and permanent rules published in the *Federal Register* by the executive departments and agencies of the Federal Government (Office of the Federal Registrar, 2023).
Common Rule	The U.S. Department of Health and Human Services regulations for the protection of human participants in research (Title 45 C.F.R., § 46) includes five subparts. Subpart A, also known as the Common Rule, provides a robust set of protections for research participants (Protection of Human Subjects, 2018).
Federal Register	This daily bulletin of administrative and executive rules, regulations, orders, and notices is published by the federal government (Merriam-Webster, n.d.-c).
Guidance Documents	These documents are prepared for the U.S. Food and Drug Administration's (2025c) staff, regulated industry, and the public to describe its interpretation of policy on a regulatory issue.
Guidelines	This documentation indicates or outlines a policy or conduct (Merriam-Webster, n.d.-d). For example, the National Institutes of Health (2024b) guidelines cover practices related to aspects of clinical research.
Law	Definitions include the rule of conduct or action prescribed or formally recognized as binding or enforced by a controlling authority, a body of laws, the control or authority of the law, the whole body of laws and doctrines relating to one subject, and the legal profession (Merriam-Webster, n.d.-e).
Legal	Definitions include relating to law or the processes of law, deriving authority from or founded on law, fulfilling the requirements of law, having a status derived from law, or created by operation of especially statutory law (Merriam-Webster, n.d.-f).
Negligence	This action is the failure to exercise the degree of care expected of a person of ordinary prudence in like circumstances in protecting others from a foreseeable and unreasonable risk of harm in a particular situation (Merriam-Webster, n.d.-g).
Regulation	A rule or order is issued by an executive authority or regulatory agency of a government and has the force of law (Merriam-Webster, n.d.-h).
Rule	A rule is all or part of a statement (as a regulation) by an administrative agency that has general or particular applicability and future effect, and that is designed to implement, interpret, or prescribe law or policy or that describes the organization, procedure, or practice of the agency itself (Merriam-Webster, n.d.-i).
Statute	Definitions include a law enacted by the legislative branch of a government, an act of a corporation or its founder intended as a permanent rule, and an international instrument setting up an agency and regulating its scope or authority (Merriam-Webster, n.d.-j).

Privacy and Confidentiality

Health Insurance Portability and Accountability Act

In response to the public's concern about the potential abuse of health information confidentiality, the U.S. Congress passed the Health Insurance Portability and Accountability Act of 1996. As required by U.S. Congress, HHS was to establish regulations that would determine how health information was to be protected. These regulations, 45 C.F.R. § 160 General Administrative Requirements, 45 C.F.R. § 164, Subpart A Security and Privacy, and 45 C.F.R. § 164, Subpart D Standards for Privacy of Individually Identifiable Health Information, are commonly known as the Privacy Rule. Compliance was required as of April 14, 2003 (HHS, 2024b). The regulations introduced new terminology, including *protected health information* (PHI) and *covered entities*. PHI relates to the individual but also includes relatives, employers, and household members. The data considered PHI include the following (HHS, 2022):

- Names
- Geographic information (e.g., street address, city, county, zip code)
- Dates related to the individual (e.g., date of birth, date of admission or discharge, date of death)
- Telephone numbers (e.g., fax numbers)
- Email addresses and other internet identifiers (e.g., web universal resource locators [URLs], internet protocol [IP] addresses)
- Social Security numbers
- Medical record numbers
- Health plan beneficiary numbers
- Account numbers
- Certificate and license numbers
- Vehicle identifiers (e.g., license plate numbers)
- Device identifiers
- Biometric identifiers (e.g., fingerprints, voice prints)
- Full-face photographic images
- Any other unique identifying numbers, characters, or codes

Covered entities are health plans, healthcare clearinghouses, and healthcare providers that transmit health information electronically in connection with transactions defined by the Health Insurance Portability and Accountability Act. An independent researcher is not considered a covered entity and, therefore, does not have to comply with the Health Insurance Portability and Accountability Act privacy policies. However, very few researchers are totally independent. A researcher is considered part of a covered entity if they are a healthcare provider engaging in covered electronic submissions or are employed by a covered entity.

The Privacy Rule does allow disclosure for research purposes. The rule established conditions for the disclosure or use of PHI, including preparatory review for research, research on decedents' information, and de-identification of PHI. Research involving data, mobile health applications, and biospecimens is subject to this rule. The disclosure of PHI requires authorization either by waiver or participant authorization. The authorization for the disclosure of PHI for research has specific requirements. In some instances, the core elements may be included in the informed consent document (HHS, 2022). OCRNs should refer to the Office for Civil Rights, HHS websites, and their institution's compliance and privacy division for specific information.

Genetic Information Nondiscrimination Act

On May 21, 2008, the Genetic Information Nondiscrimination Act (GINA) was signed into law in the United States, thereby affecting how clinical researchers handle genetic information. GINA prohibits discrimination based on genetic information for health insurance or employment purposes. The Office for Civil Rights collaborated with NIH, the Department of Labor, the Centers for Medicare and Medicaid Services, the Department of the Treasury, and the Equal Employment Opportunity Commission before issuing regulations for the enforcement of GINA. The regulations are found in 29 C.F.R. § 1635 (GINA, 2010).

GINA has two specific areas of implication in research: IRB criteria for approval and requirements for informed consent. IRBs should consider the provisions of GINA when evaluating whether genetic research meets the criteria necessary for approval. In particular, IRBs should consider whether the risks are minimized and reasonable in relation to anticipated benefits and whether adequate provisions are in place to protect the privacy of participants and maintain the confidentiality of the data.

GINA is also relevant to informed consent. When investigators develop and IRBs review the consent processes and documents for genetic research, they should consider whether and how the protections provided by GINA should be reflected in the consent document's description of risks and provisions for ensuring the confidentiality of the data (OHRP, 2009).

Clinical Trial Registration and Patient Open Access

The need for a reliable way for the public to find the status of ongoing clinical trials and the results of completed clinical trials was addressed in the late 1990s. The FDA Modernization Act of 1997 mandated the establishment of a registry for federal and privately funded clinical trials of experimental treatments for serious or life-threatening diseases or conditions. In 2007, the FDA Amendments Act, specifically Section 801, expanded the scope of required trials (e.g., device trials) and required the reporting of clinical trial results (e.g., primary outcome, adverse events, demographics). Additionally, in 2008, U.S. Congress passed the Consolidated Appropriations Act, which directed NIH to create a public access policy for NIH-funded research. The result was PubMed Central, a free full-text archive with more than 2.4 million articles in biomedicine and life sciences (National Library of Medicine, 2008).

Patient open access to clinical trials refers to patients being informed about the outcomes of ongoing and recently completed or analyzed studies. The importance of knowing both negative and positive study outcomes has been identified as an unmet expectation. Although study sponsors, whether private or public, are eager to share the positive outcomes, the publishing of negative results is often delayed or absent in the literature. The Cochrane Collaboration, which publishes widely respected data reviews and meta-analyses of available clinical trials, issued a position statement emphasizing the importance of timely access to data from all clinical trials. Cochrane called for the following strategies to improve access (Cochrane Community, 2013):

- All trials should be registered before recruitment.
- Full trial protocols should become publicly available and free of charge.
- A summary of the results of all outcomes should become available within 12 months of study completion.
- De-identified data sets should become available free of charge.
- A call should occur for government agencies to take action to increase public access to data.

Subsequently, in 2016, HHS issued an update to the FDA Amendments Act Section 801, further expanding the availability of information about clinical trials. This regulation, 42 C.F.R. § 11 Clinical Trials Registration and Results Information Submission, is also known as the Final Rule and has been in effect since 2017 (NIH, 2024c).

In 2022, as an effort to build on progress since 2013, the White House Office of Science and Technology Policy released the memorandum *Ensuring Free, Immediate, and Equitable Access to Federally Funded Research* (Nelson, 2022).

Another form of public access is to information about types of cancer, clinical trials, and eligibility criteria for specific trials. Both the National Cancer Institute's website (www.cancer.gov) and the National Library of Medicine's public registry (www.clinicaltrials.gov) provide the public and healthcare professionals with access to information on clinical trials for a wide range of diseases, conditions, and health problems. The commercial-based website CenterWatch (www.centerwatch.com) has a mission to provide reliable information concerning clinical trials to healthcare professionals and the public. OCRNs should visit these sites to ensure that the information is accurate.

Federal Clinical Trial Legislation

Proposed legislation (bills) concerning clinical trials is submitted to both houses of the U.S. Congress. The submission of a bill does not guarantee that the bill will become law. For example, in 2005, the Fair Access to Clinical Trials Act was introduced but not passed (S. 467, 2007; S. 470, 2005). Although the act failed, subsequent bills have passed, and clinical research continues to evolve.

The Improving Access to Clinical Trials Act of 2009 was signed into law in October 2010 (S. 1674, 2010). In this law, U.S. Congress recognized that to advance medical treatments, increased participation in clinical trials is necessary. The primary focus was improved access for individuals receiving Supplemental Security Income and Medicaid benefits. Before this law, individuals receiving these benefits might not have been allowed to receive any monetary compensation for participating in clinical trials. Although their compensation may be nominal, the additional income could have been sufficient to increase the individual's income above the level required to receive Medicaid or Supplemental Security Income benefits. The Improving Access to Clinical Trials Act permits these individuals to receive payments without the threat of losing benefits (S. 1674, 2010).

Subsequently, the Patient Protection and Affordable Care Act was signed into law in March 2010. The act aimed to enhance access to healthcare insurance, increase consumer protection, improve the quality of care and system performance, increase access to preventive care and screenings, reorganize the healthcare workforce, and address rising healthcare costs. The clinical trials coverage in the act incorporated many points from the Improving Access to Clinical Trials Act. This act expanded the requirements for health insurance plans (e.g., commercial plans, plans through the Federal Employee Health Benefits Program, self-insured employer-sponsored plans, state self-insured plans) to cover certain costs associated with participation in clinical trials. These plans are required to cover routine costs, including all items and services typically covered for a patient not enrolled in a clinical trial, associated with high-quality, phase 1–4 trials for cancer and other life-threatening diseases (American Society of Clinical Oncology, 2014). The coverage must also be available to an individual if the clinical trial is conducted outside their state of residence. The American Cancer Society Cancer Action Network (n.d.) continues to support and advocate for coverage from the Affordable Care Act and works to decrease health disparities.

Determining the status of ongoing national legislation in any aspect of research involving human participants is possible by checking the *Federal Register* (www.federalregister.gov) for recent activity.

State Clinical Trial Legislation

State laws and regulations have a significant impact on clinical trials and may vary in terms of additional informed consent requirements or privacy notifications. OCRNs and clinical research teams need to collaborate with their IRBs to fulfill both federal and state requirements for clinical trials (OHRP, 2022b). The National Conference of State Legislators website (www.ncsl.org) is an additional resource for finding the latest news regarding health policy research and accessing answers to state-specific questions about the state legislature.

Retention of Records

All study-related records must be retained after the study is completed, meaning that all participants have been recruited and have completed the study, and that all data have been collected and analyzed. ICH, OHRP, and FDA have varying requirements. Completion requirements vary by entity (see Figure 7-1). If local record retention policies are stricter than federal requirements, it is necessary to comply with the stricter local policy.

Shipment of Research Specimens

Some clinical studies require that specimens be shipped to laboratories specified by the sponsor for analysis and processing. Specimens containing body fluids or human tissue that may be stored on dry ice or in formalin are considered hazardous materials. The Occupational Safety and Health Administration, the Department of Transportation, and the International Air Transport Association (IATA) regulate the shipment of these materials. The specific regulations for packaging and shipping to prevent spillage during the transport of these specimens are listed in Category B Infectious Substances (IATA, 2023). The Federal Aviation Administration, the Federal Highway Administration, the Federal Railroad Administration, and the U.S. Coast Guard enforce the regulations within the United States.

Although research specimens are exempt from more stringent shipping requirements, the specific packaging and labeling requirements must be followed. IATA provides an exemption for patient specimens from dangerous goods regulations and considers research specimens to be patient specimens. These specimens are designated for shipping as a biologic substance in 3.6.2.2.2.2 Category B, commonly referred to as UN 3373 (IATA, 2023).

Although IATA requires training for anyone packaging and shipping materials that meet the IATA definition of dangerous goods, this requirement does not apply to those packing and shipping Category B specimens (IATA, 2023). The required training involves understanding the specifics of the regulations for packaging and shipping specimens. IATA encourages obtaining an understanding of the dangerous goods regulations for packaging and shipping. Some sponsors will require training specific to a given study.

Compliance Issues

The monitoring of clinical research activities for compliance with regulatory measures is an evolving field that has raised awareness of the importance of protecting research participants. OCRNs must stay updated on the latest regulations and guidelines by checking the OHRP website and signing up for email updates. They can also subscribe to FDA email updates pertaining to human participant protection at www.fda.gov/science-research/science-and-research-special-topics/clinical-trials-and-human-subject-protection.

Noncompliance

Not adhering to regulations or the protocol may be a form of regulatory noncompliance. This may be discovered during a sponsor's monitoring visit, a routine scheduled audit, or by someone involved in the research organization who may later become identified as a whistle-blower. The reporting of the event will initiate a more in-depth investigation conducted by the appropriate government agency, such as FDA or OHRP.

The consequences of noncompliance with federal regulations depend on the severity of noncompliance. Three different classifications of noncompliance exist: noncompliance, continuing noncompliance, and serious noncompliance. The *NIH Policy Manual* (2023, p. 35) defines noncompliance in the following ways:

- Noncompliance is the failure of an investigator to follow the applicable laws, regulations, or institutional policies governing the protection of human participants in research or the requirements or determinations of the IRB, whether the failure is intentional or not.
- Continuing noncompliance is a pattern of recurring noncompliance that either has resulted in, or, if continued, may result in harm to participants or otherwise materially compromise the rights, welfare, or safety of subjects; affect the scientific integrity of the study; or compromise the validity of the results. The pattern may comprise a repetition of the same noncompliant actions or different noncompliant events. Such noncompliance may be unintentional (e.g., due to lack of understanding, knowledge, or commitment) or intentional (e.g., due to deliberate choice to ignore or compromise the requirements of any applicable regulation, organizational policy, or determination of the IRB).
- Serious noncompliance is when noncompliance, whether intentional or not, results in harm or otherwise materially compromises the rights, welfare, or safety of the participant. Noncompliance that materially affects the scientific integrity or validity of the research may be considered serious noncompliance, even if it does not result in direct harm to research subjects

Intent, awareness, and regard for what was performed carry significant weight when determining whether mis-

ICH GCP E6(R3): 3.16.3. Record Keeping and Retention:	45 C.F.R. § 46.115	21 C.F.R.	NIH Policy Statement 8.4.2 Record Retention
• The sponsor (or subsequent owners of the data) should retain the sponsor-specific essential records pertaining to the trial in accordance with the applicable regulatory requirements. • The sponsor should inform the investigators/institutions and service providers, when appropriate, in writing of the requirements for the retention of essential records and should notify the investigators/institutions and service providers, when appropriate, in writing when the trial-related records are no longer needed in accordance with applicable regulatory requirements. • The sponsor should report to the appropriate authorities any transfer of ownership of the essential records as required by the applicable regulatory requirements. The sponsor should also inform the investigator if sponsorship of the trial changes.	• IRB Records: Documentation should be retained 3 years after completion of the study. • All records pertaining to the study include copies of research materials reviewed, minutes of IRB meetings, continuing review activity, statements of significant new findings provided to subjects, and all correspondence between the IRB and investigator.	• Part 56.115: IRB Records: Documentation should be retained at least 3 years after completion of research. • Part 312.62: Sponsor and Investigators: – Documentation should be retained 2 years after a marketing application is approved for the drug; or – If an application is not approved for the drug, documentation should be retained until 2 years after shipment and delivery of the drug for investigational use is discontinued and FDA has been notified.	• 2 C.F.R. § 200.334: Documentation of all NIH-sponsored studies should be retained for at least 3 years after the study ends.

FIGURE 7-1 | Comparison of Duration of Record Retention

C.F.R.—Code of Federal Regulations; FDA—U.S. Food and Drug Administration; ICH GCP—International Council on Harmonisation of Technical Requirements for Registration of Pharmaceuticals for Human Use Good Clinical Practice; IRB—institutional review board; NIH—National Institutes of Heath

Note. Based on information from Food and Drugs, 2025; International Council on Harmonisation of Technical Requirements for Registration of Pharmaceuticals for Human Use, 2025; National Institutes of Health, 2024a; Protection of Human Subjects, 2017.

conduct has occurred. Both OHRP and FDA will enforce consequences against the study sponsor, the institution, or the investigator to ensure compliance. OHRP addresses issues of noncompliance related to IRB procedures and research institutions' human research protection programs. Examples of noncompliance that may generate an investigation from OHRP are research conducted without IRB review or approval, inadequate review of research at IRB meetings related to a lack of expertise of members or insufficient review of materials, poorly maintained records, or inadequate procedures around informed consent (OHRP, 2024a).

FDA may find noncompliance related to clinical trial registration, false or misleading information, or failure to submit required clinical trial information (FDA, 2025a). When FDA finds regulatory noncompliance, it can obtain a court order requiring that the study be stopped at the site, institution, or sponsor level; charge the violator with a crime; seize the goods involved; bar the violator from future participation in a New Drug Application; impose a civil monetary penalty; or issue a written notice or warning. Consequences of noncompliance can include the following (FDA, 2025a):

- Temporary suspension of the investigator
- Lifetime suspension of the investigator
- Names of disqualified or restricted investigators listed in the *Federal Register*
- Names of disqualified or restricted investigators listed on the FDA website indefinitely, even after the restriction has been lifted
- Penalties, including fines or prison sentences
- IRB functions suspended

Research Misconduct

According to the Office of Research Integrity (n.d., para. 1), "research misconduct means fabrication, falsification, or plagiarism in proposing, performing, or reviewing research, or in reporting research results." It does not include "honest error or differences of opinion." Scientific integrity is crucial for maintaining public trust in the research process and is the foundation of the scientific community's reputation (Colbert et al., 2018).

In 1989, in response to growing public concern about research integrity, the Institute of Medicine (now the National Academy of Medicine) released *The Responsible Conduct of Research in the Health Sciences* (Rubenstein et al., 1989). Subsequently, in 2002, it released a second report, *Integrity in Scientific Research: Creating an Environment That Promotes Responsible Conduct* (Rubenstein et al., 2002). Notably, in 2015, NIH updated the requirements of research training to emphasize ethics and integrity (Colbert et al., 2018).

In an effort to increase the visibility of research misconduct, Retraction Watch (www.retractionwatch.com), an online forum, was created in 2010. Some examples of misconduct highlight the use of artificial intelligence programs, such as ChatGPT, for the writing, falsification, or fabrication of results or unreliable data.

The most challenging aspect of determining research misconduct is determining the intention. The Office of Research Integrity and other organizations must assess and approach the process to determine if it was an honest error or if the misconduct was intentional, knowingly or recklessly (Colbert et al., 2017).

Financial Fraud and Abuse

Financial fraud and abuse occur when the management of clinical trial funds is not handled honestly and accurately. For example, more funding is requested for a study than is necessary, or improper billing practices are employed. Clinical research billing and reimbursement may involve multiple departments in the clinical setting. OCRNs must review current laws, regulations, and billing practices to avoid errors, such as billing multiple parties for the same service (double-dipping).

Without meticulous documentation and a clear understanding of the services offered, Medicare or any other insurance party can be billed for services that are intended to be paid by the sponsor of a clinical trial. It is necessary to know which clinical trial activities or procedures are standard of care and which are research related to determine the appropriate payer. Conducting a coverage analysis by collaborating across relevant departments to prevent common billing errors is considered best practice for OCRNs (Jackson, 2020).

Additionally, it is important to understand the financial fraud and abuse laws that apply to physicians. For example, reimbursement fraud can be prosecuted under the False Claims Act and is primarily enforced by the U.S. Department of Justice. This requires knowledge that false or fraudulent claims and false statements were made to the government (Office of Inspector General, n.d.). Financial fraud and abuse in clinical trials may also occur in relation to the Stark Law, which prohibits physicians from providing health service referrals to an entity with which they have a financial relationship. A financial relationship may involve investment, ownership, or a compensation arrangement (Centers for Medicare and Medicaid Services, 2024; Office of Inspector General, n.d.). For example, funds forwarded by an institution to a principal investigator not employed by the hospital would fall under the umbrella of the Stark Law. The fiscal management of clinical trials must be done with knowledge, accuracy, accountability, and integrity.

Negligence

Negligence is defined as a failure to act to meet acceptable standards of nursing competence and scope of practice (Jacoby & Scruth, 2017). Although OCRNs adhere to a written, IRB-approved protocol, the potential exists for malpractice or negligence to occur. As individuals licensed by the state, OCRNs must work within the scope of that state's nurse practice act. This means that they may not assume roles that are not assigned to their level of license.

Implications for Oncology Clinical Research Nurses

OCRNs are required to comply with the nurse practice act for their state and institution and must adhere to the most stringent regulations. Whether acting as study coordinators, site managers, clinical research associates, study monitors, regulatory associates, or project managers, OCRNs must be aware of the current regulatory and compliance standards and informed about any changes being considered. Reading beyond nursing literature and subscribing to professional journals will provide increased exposure to proposed changes in clinical trials involving regulatory and compliance issues. Journals from nursing or clinical trials–related organizations may contain articles of interest to OCRNs.

Although the legal and legislative processes are not common areas of expertise for OCRNs, they should not be ignored and should be taken seriously. One way to obtain the latest information is to read the *Federal Register*. Furthermore, OCRNs can offer a unique perspective and knowledge base to elected officials and their staff. Elected officials are not experts in the field like OCRNs. Involvement in these processes can include submitting comments to officials, visiting their offices, and advocating for a cause. Other ways to become involved include the following:

- Join or establish a government or legislative committee within a local chapter of a professional organization. For example, the Oncology Nursing Society offers various opportunities for members to get involved (www.ons.org/network-advocacy/advocacy-health-policy).
- Make or obtain a list of current federal representatives and senators, state senators and representatives, and local elected officials. The list should include contact information (e.g., address, phone numbers, email addresses, social media handles). A listing of U.S. senators and representatives may be found at www.house.gov/representa-

tives/find-your-representative. State representatives may be found on each state's website.

- Seize the opportunity to express an opinion directly to representatives through action. Examples include:
  - Voting
  - Writing a letter and sending it with a return receipt requested
  - Sending an email
  - Making use of active social media application
  - Attending meetings related to clinical trials and health policy with representatives

Summary

The origin, development, and application of laws, regulations, and guidelines in clinical trials is a constantly evolving and complex subject that has moral, ethical, and legal implications at the state and federal levels. The U.S. government and local healthcare institutions have established several systems to ensure the safety and well-being of research participants and guide the conduct of clinical trials. OCRNs must maintain a steadfast commitment to ensure the protection of individual research participants while advocating for continued advancements that will reinforce the public's trust.

Key Points

- OCRNs need to be knowledgeable and understand research-related laws and regulations. Legal compliance with the most stringent law or regulation is required, whether it is the national or local jurisdiction's standard.
- In the United States, regulations are developed from laws passed by U.S. Congress and are legally binding. All federally conducted or funded research must follow 45 C.F.R. § 46. The authority for this regulation is with OHRP.
- Existing laws and regulations may be amended to address new issues or concerns regarding the well-being of human research participants.
- Guidelines provide direction on how to follow regulations. These are not legally binding in the United States but may be in other countries.
- Laws, regulations, and guidelines for the conduct of clinical research are based on the premise that human research participants are to be protected. Every aspect of the development, conduct, and evaluation of clinical trials is subject to examination for compliance with established ethical and legal standards.

The author would like to acknowledge Sally Brown, MGA, BSN, RN, OCN®, CBCN®, CCRP, Susan Markus, MS, BSN, RN, OCN®, and Carol Anne Bales, MSN, RN, CCRP, for their contribution to this chapter that remains unchanged from the previous edition of this book.

References

American Cancer Society Cancer Action Network. (n.d.). *Access to health insurance.* https://www.fightcancer.org/what-we-do/access-health-insurance

American Society of Clinical Oncology. (2014). *ASCO information guides on Affordable Care Act's clinical trials coverage requirement.* https://connection.asco.org/do/asco-information-guides-affordable-care-acts-clinical-trials-coverage-requirement

Cambridge Dictionary. (n.d.). Act of Congress. In *Cambridge Dictionary.* Retrieved June 26, 2025, from https://dictionary.cambridge.org/us/dictionary/english/act-of-congress

Centers for Disease Control and Prevention. (2024). *About the Untreated Syphilis Study at Tuskegee.* https://www.cdc.gov/tuskegee/index.html

Centers for Medicare and Medicaid Services. (2024). *Physician self-referral.* https://www.cms.gov/medicare/regulations-guidance/physician-self-referral?redirect=/physicianselfreferral

Cochrane Community. (2013). *Access to data from all trials.* https://community.cochrane.org/organizational-info/resources/policies/organizational-position-statements/access-data-all-trials

Colbert, M.C., Nussenblatt, R.B., & Gottesmann, M.M. (2018). Integrity in research: Individual and institutional responsibility. In J.I. Gallin & F.P. Ognibene (Eds.), *Principles and practice of clinical research* (4th ed., pp. 33–46). Elsevier Academic Press.

Cornell Law School. (2025). *Administrative agency.* https://www.law.cornell.edu/wex/administrative_agency

Fair Access to Clinical Trials Act of 2005, S. 470, 109th Cong. (2005). https://www.govtrack.us/congress/bills/109/s470/text

Fair Access to Clinical Trials Act of 2007, S. 467, 110th Cong. (2007). https://www.govtrack.us/congress/bills/110/s467/text

Food and Drugs. (2025). 21 C.F.R. https://www.ecfr.gov/current/title-21

Genetic Information Nondiscrimination Act of 2008, 29 C.F.R. § 1635 (2010). https://www.ecfr.gov/current/title-29/subtitle-B/chapter-XIV/part-1635

Genetic Information Nondiscrimination Act of 2008, Pub. L. No. 110-233, 122 Stat. 881. (2008). https://www.govinfo.gov/content/pkg/PLAW-110publ233/pdf/PLAW-110publ233.pdf

Improving Access to Clinical Trials Act of 2009, S. 1674, 111th Cong. (2010) (enacted). https://www.govtrack.us/congress/bills/111/s1674/text

International Air Transport Association. (2023). *3.6.2 Division 6.2—Infectious substances.* https://www.iata.org/contentassets/b08040a138dc4442a4f066e6fb99fe2a/dgr-64-en-3.6.2.pdf

International Council for Harmonisation of Technical Requirements for Pharmaceuticals for Human Use. (n.d.-a). *History.* https://www.ich.org/page/history

International Council for Harmonisation of Technical Requirements for Pharmaceuticals for Human Use. (n.d.-b). *ICH guidelines.* https://www.ich.org/page/ich-guidelines

International Council for Harmonisation of Technical Requirements for Pharmaceuticals for Human Use. (2023). *Overview of ICH.* https://admin.ich.org/sites/default/files/2023-11/OverviewOfICH_2023_1115_0.pdf

International Council for Harmonisation of Technical Requirements for Pharmaceuticals for Human Use. (2025). *ICH harmonised guideline: Guideline for good clinical practice: E6(R3).* https://database.ich.org/sites/default/files/ICH_E6%28R3%29_Step4_FinalGuideline_2025_0106.pdf

Jackson, M. (2020). Good financial practice and clinical research coordinator responsibilities. *Seminars in Oncology Nursing, 36*(2), 150999. https://doi.org/10.1016/j.soncn.2020.150999

Jacoby, S.R., & Scruth, E.A. (2017). Negligence and the nurse. The value of the code of ethics for nurses. *Clinical Nurse Specialist, 31*(4), 183–185. https://doi.org/10.1097/NUR.0000000000000301

Merriam-Webster. (n.d.-a). Act. In *Merriam-Webster.com dictionary.* Retrieved June 26, 2025, from https://www.merriam-webster.com/dictionary/act#legalDictionary
Merriam-Webster. (n.d.-b). Code. In *Merriam-Webster.com dictionary.* Retrieved June 26, 2025, from https://www.merriam-webster.com/dictionary/code#legalDictionary
Merriam-Webster. (n.d.-c). Federal Register. *Merriam-Webster.com dictionary.* Retrieved June 26, 2025, from https://www.merriam-webster.com/legal/Federal%20Register
Merriam-Webster. (n.d.-d). Guidelines. In *Merriam-Webster.com dictionary.* Retrieved June 26, 2025, from https://www.merriam-webster.com/dictionary/guidelines
Merriam-Webster. (n.d.-e). Law. In *Merriam-Webster.com dictionary.* Retrieved June 26, 2025, from https://www.merriam-webster.com/dictionary/law#legalDictionary
Merriam-Webster. (n.d.-f). Legal. In *Merriam-Webster.com dictionary.* Retrieved June 26, 2025, from https://www.merriam-webster.com/dictionary/legal#legalDictionary
Merriam-Webster. (n.d.-g). Negligence. In *Merriam-Webster.com dictionary.* Retrieved June 26, 2025, from https://www.merriam-webster.com/dictionary/negligence#legalDictionary
Merriam-Webster. (n.d.-h). Regulation. In *Merriam-Webster.com dictionary.* Retrieved June 26, 2025, from https://www.merriam-webster.com/dictionary/regulation#legalDictionary
Merriam-Webster. (n.d.-i). Rule. In *Merriam-Webster.com dictionary.* Retrieved June 26, 2025, from https://www.merriam-webster.com/dictionary/rule#legalDictionary
Merriam-Webster. (n.d.-j). Statute. In *Merriam-Webster.com dictionary.* Retrieved June 26, 2025, from https://www.merriam-webster.com/dictionary/statue
National Commission for the Protection of Human Subjects of Biomedical and Behavioral Research. (1979, April 18). *The Belmont Report: Ethical principles and guidelines for the protection of human subjects of biomedical and behavioral research.* https://www.hhs.gov/ohrp/regulations-and-policy/belmont-report/read-the-belmont-report/index.html
National Institutes of Health. (2023). *NIH policy manual.* https://policymanual.nih.gov
National Institutes of Health. (2024a). *NIH grants policy statement.* https://grants.nih.gov/grants/policy/nihgps/html5/section_8/8.4.2_record_retention_and_access.htm
National Institutes of Health. (2024b). *NIH guidelines.* https://oir.nih.gov/sourcebook/ethical-conduct/research-ethics/nih-guidelines
National Institutes of Health. (2024c). *Policy and regulation on* ClinicalTrials.gov *registration and reporting.* https://grants.nih.gov/policy/clinical-trials/reporting/understanding.htm
National Library of Medicine. (2008). ClinicalTrials.gov *to include basic results.* https://www.nlm.nih.gov/pubs/techbull/so08/so08_clinicaltrials.html
Nelson, A. (2022). *Memorandum for the heads of executive departments and agencies: Ensuring free, immediate, and equitable access to federally funded research.* https://bidenwhitehouse.archives.gov/ostp/news-updates/2022/08/25/breakthroughs-for-alldelivering-equitable-access-to-americas-research
Nuremberg Code. (1949). *Trials of war criminals before the Nuremberg military tribunals under Control Council Law No. 10* (Vol. 2, pp. 181–182). https://www.hhs.gov/ohrp/archive/nurcode.html
Office for Human Research Protections. (1993). *Institutional review board guidebook.* https://wayback.archive-it.org/org-745/20150930181805/http://www.hhs.gov/ohrp/archive/irb/irb_guidebook.htm
Office for Human Research Protections. (2009). *Genetic Information Nondiscrimination Act (GINA): OHRP Guidance (2009).* https://www.hhs.gov/ohrp/regulations-and-policy/guidance/guidance-on-genetic-information-nondiscrimination-act/index.html
Office for Human Research Protections. (2022a). *The Belmont Report.* https://www.hhs.gov/ohrp/regulations-and-policy/belmont-report/index.html
Office for Human Research Protections. (2022b). *Use of a single institutional review board for cooperative research.* https://www.hhs.gov/ohrp/regulations-and-policy/requests-for-comments/draft-guidance-use-single-institutional-review-board-for-cooperative-research/index.html
Office for Human Research Protections. (2024a). *Compliance and reporting.* https://www.hhs.gov/ohrp/compliance-and-reporting/index.html
Office for Human Research Protections. (2024b). *History.* https://www.hhs.gov/ohrp/about-ohrp/history/index.html
Office for Human Research Protections. (2025). *45 CFR 46.* https://www.hhs.gov/ohrp/regulations-and-policy/regulations/45-cfr-46/index.html
Office of Inspector General. (n.d.). *Fraud and abuse laws.* https://oig.hhs.gov/compliance/physician-education/fraud-abuse-laws
Office of Research Integrity. (n.d.). *Definition of research misconduct.* https://ori.hhs.gov/definition-research-misconduct
Office of the Federal Registrar. (2023). *About the Code of Federal Regulations.* https://www.archives.gov/federal-register/cfr/about.html
Protection of Human Subjects, 32 C.F.R. § 219 (2018). https://www.ecfr.gov/current/title-32/subtitle-A/chapter-I/subchapter-M/part-219
Protection of Human Subjects, 45 C.F.R. § 46 (2017). https://www.ecfr.gov/current/title-45/subtitle-A/subchapter-A/part-46
Rubenstein, A.H., Anlyan, W.G., Angell, M.E., Barber, B., Daddario, E.Q., Davie, J.M., ... Weinberg, R.A. (1989). *The responsible conduct of research in the health sciences.* https://www.nap.edu/openbook.php?record_id=1388&page=R1
Rubenstein, A.H., Bebeau, M.J., Bondurant, S., Cox, D.R., Dynes, R.C., Frankel, M.S., ... Zigmond, M.J. (2002). *Integrity in scientific research: Creating an environment that promotes responsible conduct.* https://www.ncbi.nlm.nih.gov/books/NBK208712/pdf/Bookshelf_NBK208712.pdf
Sass, H.-M. (1983). Reichsrundschreiben 1931: Pre-Nuremberg German regulations concerning new therapy and human experimentation. *Journal of Medical Philosophy, 8*(2), 99–111. https://doi.org/10.1093/jmp/8.2.99
Slutsman, J., & Nieman, L. (2018). Institutional review boards. In J.I. Gallin & F.P. Ognibene (Eds.), *Principles and practice of clinical research* (4th ed., pp. 47–61). Elsevier Academic Press. https://doi.org/10.1016/B978-0-12-849905-4.00004-6
U.S. Department of Health and Human Services. (2021). *Register IRBs and obtain FWAs.* https://www.hhs.gov/ohrp/register-irbs-and-obtain-fwas/index.html
U.S. Department of Health and Human Services. (2022). *Guidance regarding methods for de-identification of protected health information in accordance with the Health Insurance Portability and Accountability Act (HIPAA) Privacy Rule.* https://www.hhs.gov/hipaa/for-professionals/privacy/special-topics/de-identification/index.html#coveredentities
U.S. Department of Health and Human Services. (2024a). *HHS agencies and offices.* https://www.hhs.gov/about/agencies/hhs-agencies-and-offices/index.html
U.S. Department of Health and Human Services. (2024b). *HIPAA for professionals.* https://www.hhs.gov/hipaa/for-professionals/index.html
U.S. Food and Drug Administration. (1997). *The FDA Modernization Act of 1997.* https://www.fda.gov/regulatory-information/food-and-drug-administration-modernization-act-fdama-1997/fda-backgrounder-fdama
U.S. Food and Drug Administration. (2007). *FDA Amendments Act, Section 801.* https://www.govinfo.gov/content/pkg/PLAW-110publ85/pdf/PLAW-110publ85.pdf#page=82
U.S. Food and Drug Administration. (2025a). ClinicalTrials.gov *- notices of noncompliance and civil money penalty actions.* https://www.fda.gov/science-research/fdas-role-clinicaltrialsgov-information/clinicaltrialsgov-notices-noncompliance-and-civil-money-penalty-actions
U.S. Food and Drug Administration. (2025b). *FDA overview organization chart.* https://www.fda.gov/about-fda/fda-organization-charts/fda-overview-organization-chart
U.S. Food and Drug Administration. (2025c). *Guidance documents (medical devices and radiation-emitting products).* https://www.fda.

gov/medical-devices/device-advice-comprehensive-regulatory-assistance/guidance-documents-medical-devices-and-radiation-emitting-products

U.S. Food and Drug Administration. (2025d). *Guidances/Drugs.* https://www.fda.gov/drugs/guidance-compliance-regulatory-information/guidances-drugs

Weindling, P.J. (2022). From the Nuremberg "Doctors' Trial" to the "Nuremberg Code." In S. Gallin and I. Bedzow (Eds.), *Bioethics and the Holocaust* (vol. 96, pp. 219–228). International Library of Bioethics. https://doi.org/10.1007/978-3-031-01987-6_12

World Medical Association. (2013). *Public to be consulted over changes to the WMA's Declaration of Helsinki.* https://www.wma.net/news-post/public-to-be-consulted-over-changes-to-the-wmas-declaration-of-helsinki

World Medical Association. (2024). *Declaration of Helsinki—Ethical principles for medical research involving human subjects.* https://www.wma.net/what-we-do/medical-ethics/declaration-of-helsinki

CHAPTER 8

Good Clinical Practice

Anita Moore, MS, BSN, RN

Introduction

How do clinicians know whether the new knowledge reported from a clinical study was based on valid data or whether the research was conducted ethically? Good Clinical Practice (GCP) in conducting research refers to an internationally recognized standard that ensures ethical and scientific quality in human participant research (Committee for Human Medicinal Products, 2016). GCP adherence ensures that the rights, safety, and well-being of human participants involved in research are protected and promotes data integrity and reliability (Committee for Human Medicinal Products, 2016). To enforce GCP as a requirement, governments can transpose these recommended guidelines into regulations to ensure that standards are achieved. Thus, understanding GCP is critical for oncology clinical research nurses (OCRNs) and others who participate in clinical research operations.

This chapter will review the origins of GCP to help readers understand the significance of the GCP guidelines, the evolution of the International Council for Harmonisation of Technical Requirements for Pharmaceuticals for Human Use (ICH) (formerly known as the International Conference on Harmonisation) GCP guidance, application of GCP in practice, and essential recordkeeping as part of GCP.

Origins of Good Clinical Practice

The overarching objectives of GCP are to protect study participants' rights, safety, and well-being and ensure that trial data are credible (Committee for Human Medicinal Products, 2016). These standards are integral to countering past scientific misconduct and advancing ongoing efforts to safeguard the health, well-being, and safety of clinical research participants worldwide (ICH, 2023a). By understanding the historical evolution of GCP, researchers, healthcare workers, and the public will better appreciate the significance and importance of adhering to the overarching principles of the GCP standard. See Figure 8-1 for a timeline of accomplishments in GCP.

Starting with contemporary history, in the aftermath of World War II, the Nuremberg Trials exposed horrific medical experiments performed by doctors on concentration camp victims in Nazi Germany. The Nuremberg Code was the first internationally adopted document outlining a code of ethics and standards to which physicians were expected to conform when performing experiments on human participants (International Military Tribunal, 1949). Later, in 1964, the World Medical Association published the first version of the Declaration of Helsinki, which built upon the Nuremberg Code and emphasized the ethical principle that medical research with therapeutic intent may only be conducted on human participants if the benefits outweigh the risks (World Medical Association, 2025).

Milestones in the U.S. federal regulations governing the protection of human participants include the passage of the Kefauver-Harris Amendments to the Food, Drug, and Cosmetic Act in 1962. This was the result of the discovery of a tragic link between fetal abnormalities and the use of thalidomide (U.S. Food and Drug Administration [FDA], 2018b). The Kefauver-Harris Amendments required that written informed consent be obtained to participate in experimental treatments and that drug manufacturers demonstrate efficacy prior to obtaining market approval (FDA, 2018a). These amendments and the investigational drug regulations of 1963 introduced many new procedures in the United States that strengthened control over investigational new drugs and facilitated the creation of the New Drug Application process (Federal Register, 1963).

In 1979, *The Belmont Report* summarized the basic ethical principles: respect for persons, beneficence, and justice. It also established boundaries between practice and research and served as an essential reference for institutional review boards (IRB) reviewing federally funded

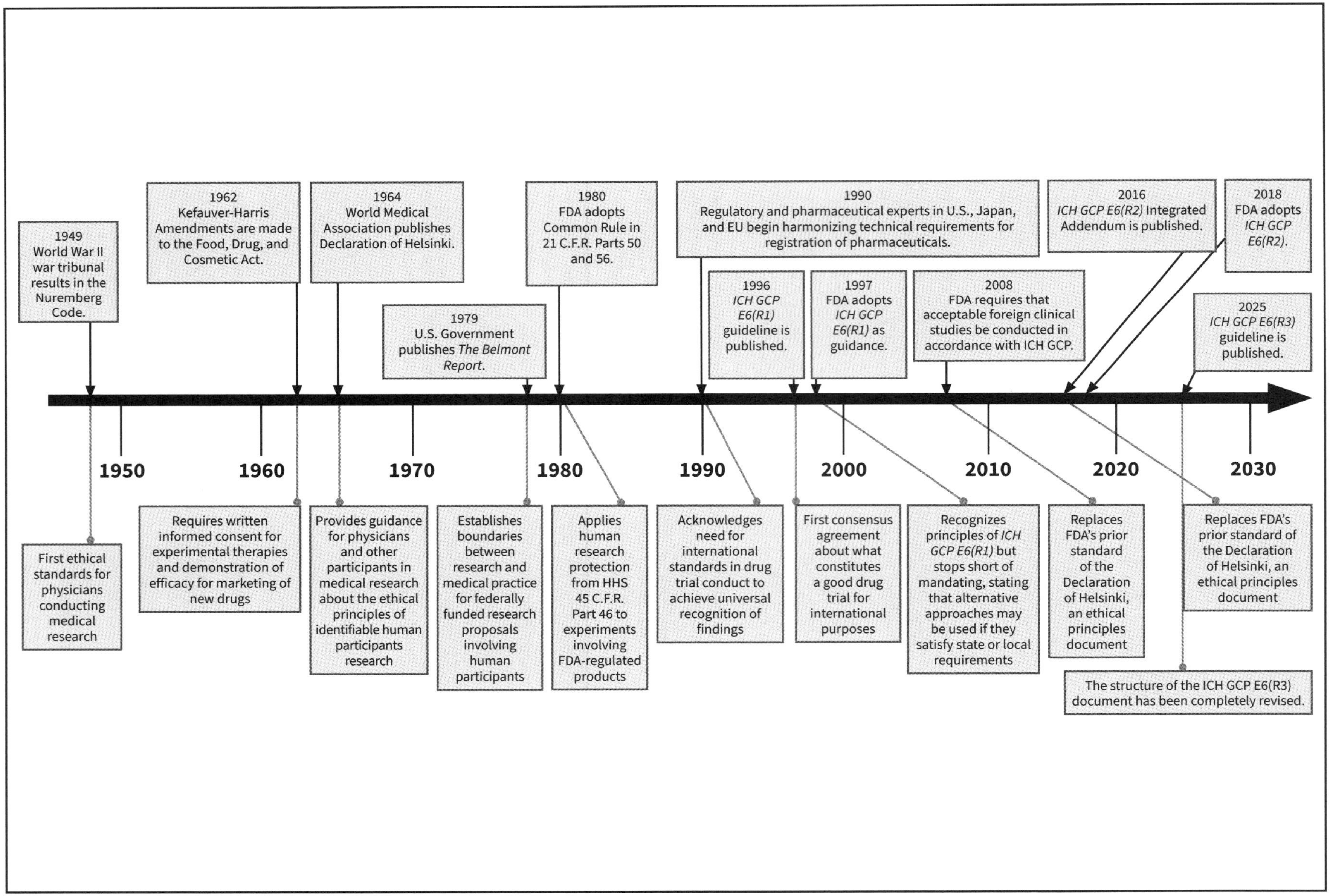

FIGURE 8-1 | Good Clinical Practice Timeline

C.F.R.—Code of Federal Regulations; EU—European Union; FDA—U.S. Food and Drug Administration; GCP—Good Clinical Practice; ICH—International Council on Harmonisation of Technical Requirements for Registration of Pharmaceuticals for Human Use human participant research proposals (National Commission for the Protection of Human Subjects of Biomedical and Behavioral Research, 1979).

The U.S. Department of Health and Human Services (HHS) federal policy for the Protection of Human Research Subjects was revised in 1991, and 15 federal departments and agencies became official signatories with the policy becoming law in their own Code of Federal Regulations (C.F.R.) sections (Office for Human Research Protections [OHRP], 2025). For all participating departments and agencies, these regulations outline the basic provisions for IRBs, informed consent, and assurances of compliance and are governed by the authority of that department or agency. Title 45 C.F.R. Part 46 Subpart A, Protection of Human Subjects (2017), became commonly referred to as the Federal Policy or the Common Rule. The Common Rule protects the rights and the welfare of human participants in federally supported and conducted research and applies to any institution engaged in this research. In addition to HHS regulations, FDA regulates clinical investigations of products under its jurisdiction (e.g., drugs, biological products, and medical devices). FDA is not considered a Common Rule agency because its regulations differ. However, it is required to harmonize with the Common Rule whenever permitted by law (i.e., 21st Century Cures Act of 2016) (OHRP, 2025). The FDA regulations under its jurisdiction are published in Title 21 C.F.R. Chapter 1, Part 50 (Protection of Human Subjects), Part 56 (IRBs), Part 312 (Investigational New Drug Application), and Part 812 (Investigational Device Exemptions) (Food and Drugs, 2025).

The Evolution of the International Council for Harmonisation Good Clinical Practice

The evolution of the ICH GCP ethical and scientific quality standards for clinical research conduct has progressed over time. GCP is viewed as necessary to provide assurances of clinical research participant protection and that credible and reliable evidence exists for making informed decisions about medical practice and public health. Clinical trials are an essential aspect of medical research, and GCP guidelines are critical for validating that trials are conducted ethically and with the highest integrity (ICH, 2023b).

The GCP efficacy guideline document that was initially approved by the ICH Steering Committee in 1996, *ICH Harmonised Tripartite Guideline: Guideline for Good Clinical Practice E6(R1)*, was an expert opinion about what constituted best practices for clinical research conduct. In *E6(R1)*, ICH originally defined *GCP* as "an international ethical and scientific quality standard for designing, conducting, recording and reporting trials that involve the participation of human subjects" (ICH, 1996, p. 1). Within that same year, the three ICH regions (European Union, Japan, and the United States) had adopted similar, but not identical, versions of the guidance document. Despite differences between the versions, the three regions agreed that the underlying principles did not differ by region; most of the differences were without any real impact on users (ICH, n.d.), and adherence to the standard was nevertheless crucial to maintaining the harmonization reached. *E6(R1)* described the responsibilities and expectations for conducting clinical trials. Adherence to this documentation became required for all international submissions that were approved by regulatory agencies in the three regions (ICH, 1996).

ICH GCP guidelines have changed in response to various developments in the medical research landscape. Now in its fourth decade of ongoing work, ICH is focused on expanding the benefits of harmonization beyond its original founding regions. A major milestone was reached in 2015, marked by several transformative changes: enhanced international outreach, a restructured governance model, broader dissemination of information about ICH processes to a wider range of stakeholders, and the formal establishment of ICH as a legal entity to ensure a more stable operational framework (ICH, n.d.).

The resultant ICH association established an overarching governing body with the aim of focusing global pharmaceutical regulatory harmonization efforts within a single forum, enabling pharmaceutical regulatory authorities and relevant industry organizations to participate more actively in the harmonization initiatives (ICH, n.d.). Out of this work, an integrated addendum to the guidance, *ICH Guideline for GCP E6(R2) Integrated Addendum*, was finalized on December 15, 2016, with an effective date of June 14, 2017 (Committee for Human Medicinal Products, 2016). *E6(R2)* was intended to address evolutions in technology and clinical trial practices and to encourage greater efficiency in clinical trials (ICH, 2016). It attempted to align with the modern regulatory landscape, addressing the evolutions in technology and clinical trial practices that occurred since the *E6(R1)* release.

Published on January 6, 2025, ICH Harmonised Guideline for GCP *E6(R3)* aimed to address specific and potentially unique aspects of an individual clinical trial to support efficient approaches to trial design and conduct (ICH, 2025). *E6(R3)* is not an integrated addendum to the previous ICH GCP versions. This guideline has a new structure composed of an introduction, principles, annexes, appendices, and a glossary (ICH, 2025). These extensive revisions are intended to enable easier and faster updates in the future and to provide clarity and better readability that impact all the trial conduct processes from planning to reporting (Bhatt, 2023). Where appropriate, the revisions retain key concepts and guidance from earlier versions. However, as technology, methodologies, and trial designs have advanced, updates have been made to address gaps, resolve inconsistencies, and support a broader range of clinical trial approaches (ICH, 2019). The principles are envisioned to apply across clinical trial settings and are expected to remain relevant as technological and methodologic advances occur (ICH, 2023a). The revisions were made to align more closely with the regulatory environment by clarifying how GCP principles apply to a wider variety of trial types and data sources and by introducing flexibility to support the use of new technologies in clinical trials (ICH, 2023b). The revised guideline supports innovation in clinical trial design and conduct while still providing guidance to protect participants and ensure reliable results. "The principles are interdependent and should be considered in their totality to ensure ethical trial conduct and reliable results" (ICH, 2025, p. 3). A comparison of the three *ICH GCP E6* versions can be found in Figure 8-2.

Modifications in the *ICH GCP E6(R3)* include principles designed to apply across all types of clinical trials and settings and to remain applicable as technology and methods evolve; annexes, including its appendices, intended to provide guidance on applying the principles to clinical trials appropriately; and an updated glossary section with new and replacement terms (ICH, 2025). For example, *trial participant* replaces *subject*, *agreement* replaces *contract*, a *clinical trial* is classified as any *interventional investigation* in human participants, and *source records* replaces *source documents* and *data*. New terms have also been added, such as *assent, data acquisition tool, metadata, reference safety information, signature*, and *suspected unexpected serious adverse reactions* (ICH, 2025).

The structure, principles, definitions, descriptions, and assurance elements of *E6(R3)* have been modified to promote improved, more efficient, and flexible approaches to trial design and conduct while maintaining patient safety and data integrity (TransPerfect Life Sciences, 2023). See Table 8-1 to use as a reference outlining the changes that have been made regarding the transition from *E6(R2)* to *E6(R3)* and how the revisions can be applied in practice.

The Application of Good Clinical Practice

Clinical trials conducted in accordance with ICH GCP ensure that the rights, safety, and well-being of research participants are protected, that conduct is consistent with the principles originating in the Declaration of Helsinki, and that clinical trial results are reliable (ICH, 2025). The overarching principles of GCP provide a flexible framework for clinical trial conduct and are structured to guide all processes from planning to reporting.

ICH GCP provides a unified standard to facilitate the mutual acceptance of clinical trial data by applicable regulatory authorities worldwide. Although ICH GCP guidelines have evolved throughout each version, the foundational themes remain: that research participants are protected and clinical trial results are reliable.

As a practical application example of how one U.S. agency implemented GCP, FDA announced in March 2018 the availability of the guidance, *E6(R2) Good Clinical Prac-*

ICH GCP E6(R1)	ICH GCP E6(R2)	ICH GCP E6(R3)
• Described the responsibilities and expectations of stakeholders, including investigators, monitors, sponsors, and institutional review boards and independent ethics committees in the conduct of clinical trials • Covered the aspects of monitoring, reporting, and archiving of clinical trials • Incorporated appendices for the investigator's brochure and essential documents for the conduct of a clinical trial	• Included an integrated addendum to encourage implementation of improved and more efficient approaches to clinical trial design, conduct, oversight, recording, and reporting given the evolution in technology and risk management processes • Continued to ensure human participant protection and reliability of results • Updated the standards for electronic records and essential documents, intended to increase clinical trial quality and efficiency	• Updated *trial conduct* to include processes from planning, initiating, performing, and recording oversight, evaluation, analysis and reporting activities as appropriate • Aimed to be universally applicable across diverse clinical trial settings and types, ensuring their relevance and applicability in the face of rapid technological and methodological advancement thus providing guidance throughout the life cycle of the clinical trial • Emphasized digital technology, ethics, and quality to subsequently increase the responsibilities of ethics committees, investigators, and sponsors • Constructed so that its principles remain applicable to trials involving human participants • Provided annexes and appendices for appropriate interpretation and application of the principles

FIGURE 8-2 | Comparison of International Council for Harmonisation Good Clinical Practice Guidelines

GCP—Good Clinical Practice; ICH—International Council on Harmonisation of Technical Requirements for Registration of Pharmaceuticals for Human Use

Note. Based on information from International Conference on Harmonisation of Technical Requirements for Registration of Pharmaceuticals for Human Use, 2016; International Council for Harmonisation of Technical Requirements for Pharmaceuticals for Human Use, 2025.

tice: Integrated Addendum to E6(R1). This announcement promoted the *E6(R2)* as guidance with its improved and more efficient approaches to clinical trial design, conduct, oversight, recording, reporting, and updated standards for electronic records and essential documents (Federal Register, 2018). This FDA guidance was intended as recommendations to improve clinical trial quality and efficiency while maintaining human participant protections and reliability of trial results (Federal Register, 2018; FDA, 2018a). Unlike the FDA regulation Title 21, which is legally binding and enforceable, the implementation of ICH GCP has never been mandatory for FDA-regulated research. For FDA, the ICH GCP documents are used as a representative guide. FDA recognizes that an alternative approach to the guidance may be used if such an approach satisfies the local and state requirements, noting that it does require harmonization with the Common Rule whenever permitted by law (i.e., 21st Century Cures Act of 2016) (OHRP, 2025).

Although the regulatory members of the ICH assembly endorsed the final version of the *E6(R3)* on January 6, 2025 (ICH, 2025), the European Medicines Agency announced an effective date of July 23, 2025 (Committee for Human Medicinal Products, 2025). Additional guidance may be added to *E6(R3)* to address GCP considerations that arise (ICH, 2024).

Essential Recordkeeping as Part of Good Clinical Practice

To assist OCRNs, investigators, and study team members in ensuring ethical trial conduct and reliable results, GCP requires essential records to be kept that are gener-

TABLE 8-1 | Good Clinical Practice E6(R3) Key Summary of Changes

Principle	ICH GCP E6(R3)	ICH GCP E6(R2) References	Practice
1	Ethical Principles • Origin in the Declaration of Helsinki, consistent with GCP and applicable regulatory requirements • Ensuring the rights, safety, and well-being of participants	2.1, 2.2, 2.3, 2.7, 2.11 • Combines *ICH E6(R2)* principles 1, 2, 3, 7, and 11	*Revision* • Making sure not to exclude particular participant populations unnecessarily • Permitting a wider range of qualified health professionals *Practice (rights, safety, and well-being of participants)* • Prevail over the interests of science and society • Require periodic review of new safety information • Need to balance risks and benefits to participants and society • Selection of participants representative of the anticipated population • Qualified physician, dentist, or other health professional responsible for medical decisions and care • Protection of the confidentiality of participants' identity Includes promoting representative participant selection and permits a wider range of health professionals to be responsible for medical decisions if this is in accordance with local regulatory requirements
2	Informed Consent	2.9	*Revision* • Taking into consideration relevant aspects of the trial *Practice* • Freely given informed consent before clinical trial participation • Information adequate to make an informed decision about participation • Focus on critical aspects of the trial protocol • Consent obtained as soon as possible in emergency situations Formally P9, the requirement for prior documented consent; *delayed consent/consent to continue* in the emergency setting, and flexible consent provisions in accordance with applicable regulatory requirements and processes approved by the IRB/IEC
3	Institutional Review Board Independent Ethics Committee • IRB/IEC approval • IRB/IEC review and compliance with the protocol	2.6	*Revision* • Periodic review according to applicable regulatory requirements *Practice* • Conduct of trial in compliance with IRB/IEC approved protocol • Periodic review of the trial by the IRB/IEC Formally P6 with an additional statement confirming the requirement for the periodic review of a trial by the IRB/IEC

(Continued on next page)

TABLE 8-1 | Good Clinical Practice E6(R3) Key Summary of Changes *(Continued)*

Principle	ICH GCP E6(R3)	ICH GCP E6(R2) References	Practice
4	Science • Scientific knowledge • Should be scientifically sound and fit for the intended purpose	2.4, 2.5 • Combines former *ICH E6(R2)* P4 and P5	*Revision* • Periodic review of scientific knowledge and approaches to determine whether modifications to the trial are needed *Practice* • Adequate nonclinical and clinical information on investigational product • Scientifically sound clinical trial design based on state of knowledge and experience with the investigational products • Periodic review of current scientific knowledge and approaches Includes a statement that trials should "reflect current scientific knowledge and experience" and the requirement for periodic review of current scientific knowledge and approaches to determine the need for modifications
5	Qualified Individuals • Individuals qualified by education, training, and experience	2.8	*Revision* • Individuals with different expertise and training needed across all phases of a clinical trial *Practice* • Designed and conducted by individuals qualified by education, training, and experience to perform their respective tasks Formally P8, now with examples of individuals who should be qualified; broadens the range of qualified personnel; examples include physicians, nurses, pharmacists, researchers, ethicists, technology experts, trial coordinators, monitors, auditors, and biostatisticians
6	Quality • Quality built into the scientific and operational design and conduct • Building quality into clinical trials	2.13	*Revision* • The quality and amount of the information generated to support good decision-making *Practice* • Quality of a clinical trial is a fitness for purpose, meaning fit for what is intended • Quality by design identified prospectively with focus on factors fundamental to the protection of participants, the reliability and interpretability of the trial results • Strategies implemented to avoid, detect, address, and prevent recurrence of serious noncompliance with GCP, the trial protocol, and applicable regulatory requirements Formally P13, but with a focus on *fitness-for-purpose* and *critical to quality* concepts; strategies to avoid, detect, and prevent serious noncompliance should be implemented.
7	Risk Proportionality • Participant risk, importance of data, and avoid unnecessary burden • Adopting proportionate approaches to trial conduct	–	*New* • Focus on participant's safety and the reliability of results • Risks beyond those associated with standard medical care *Practice* • Trial processes proportionate to the risks to human protection and data reliability • Emphasis on the risks to participants beyond those associated with standard medical care • Prospective management of risks critical to quality factors • Avoiding unnecessary burden New principle on risk proportionality, including clarification that *trial risks* are risks beyond those posed by standard care; critical to quality risks should be managed prospectively and to avoid unnecessary burden.

(Continued on next page)

TABLE 8-1 | Good Clinical Practice E6(R3) Key Summary of Changes *(Continued)*

Principle	ICH GCP E6(R3)	ICH GCP E6(R2) References	Practice
8	Protocol • Described in a clear, concise, scientifically sound, and operationally feasible protocol	2.5	*Revision* • A well-designed trial protocol is fundamental to the protection of participants and for the generation of reliable results. • Scientific objectives should be clear and explicitly stated in the protocol. • The protocol and other documents (e.g., statistical analysis plan, data management plan) for trial execution should be clear, concise, and operationally feasible. *Practice* • Well-designed for human protection and data reliability • Explicit scientific objectives • Clear, concise, feasible protocol, plans, or documents Formally P5; clarifies that scientific objectives be explicitly stated and that trials be operationally feasible
9	Results • Reliable results • Trials should generate reliable results.	2.10	*Revision* • Trial processes should support the key trial objectives. • Clinical trials should incorporate efficient and well-controlled processes for managing records through appropriate management of data integrity. • Clinical trials should be transparent, with registration on publicly accessible databases and the public posting of clinical trial results. *Practice* • Quality and information should be fit for purpose and sufficient to provide confidence in the results generated and supportive for good decision-making. • Systems and processes that aid in data capture, management and analyses, and quality of the information should be fit for purpose and proportionate to the risks and importance of acquired data. • Computerized systems should be fit for purpose, with a focus on factors critical to the quality and integrity of trial data. • Efficient and robust processes should be in place for managing record integrity, traceability, and protected information for accurate reporting, interpretation, and verification. • A secure retention of essential records should be in place for the required period. • Trial registration and results posting should be transparent. New principle including the former P10; requires fit-for-purpose systems; promotes transparency, timely registration, and communication of results
10	Roles and Responsibilities • Roles and responsibilities of the sponsor and the investigator • Roles and responsibilities should be clear and documented.	–	*New* • Clarification of transfer of activities by the sponsor and delegation by the investigator • Maintenance of appropriate oversight *Practice* • Responsible for respective activities: tasks, duties, or functions • Agreements clearly define roles, activities, and responsibilities. Where activities have been delegated to service providers, the trial conduct, quality, and data integrity reside with the sponsor or investigator, respectively. • Responsible for the appropriate oversight of the activities New principle covering delegation of activities, agreements with clarity of roles and responsibilities, and the requirement for sponsors and investigators to have oversight of any trial activities they delegate.

(Continued on next page)

TABLE 8-1 | Good Clinical Practice E6(R3) Key Summary of Changes *(Continued)*

Principle	ICH GCP E6(R3)	ICH GCP E6(R2) References	Practice
11	Investigational Products • Investigational product should be manufactured in accordance with applicable Good Manufacturing Practice standards and managed in accordance with product specifications and the trial protocol.	2.12	*Revision* • Investigational products should be carefully managed to align with treatment assignment and maintain blinding, where applicable. • The investigational product provided to the trial participant should retain its quality. *Practice* • Manufactured in accordance with Good Manufacturing Practice standards • Measures to retain the quality of the investigational product • Use of investigational product in accordance with the protocol and relevant trial documents • Manufacturing, handling, and labeling of investigational product to align with treatment assignment and maintain blinding, where applicable • Labeling of investigational product in compliance with regulatory requirements • Adequate measures to ensure handling, shipping, storage, dispensing, returning, and destroying or alternatively disposing of investigational product Formally P12 with expanded content, including measures to retain the quality of investigational products, labeling, and shipping

GCP—Good Clinical Practice; ICH—International Conference on Harmonisation of Technical Requirements for Registration of Pharmaceuticals for Human Use; IEC—independent ethics committee; IRB—institutional review board

The principles are interdependent and should be considered in their totality to ensure ethical trial conduct and reliable results.

Note. Based on information from International Conference on Harmonisation of Technical Requirements for Registration of Pharmaceuticals for Human Use, 2016; International Council for Harmonisation of Technical Requirements for Pharmaceuticals for Human Use, 2025.

ated before, during, and after the conduct of a clinical trial. These records are collected, maintained, and retained in a way that ensures that they remain complete, readable, readily available, and directly accessible upon request by regulatory authorities.

If trial records are produced, they are considered essential and should be retained (ICH, 2025). For example, when collecting and maintaining essential records, GCP requires the investigator's brochure; the signed protocol and subsequent amendments during the trial; dated documents that are submitted to, issued by, and approved by the IRB or independent ethics committee; completed signed and dated informed consent forms; completed participant identification code list and enrollment log; notifications of serious adverse events and other safety information; source records; data and relevant metadata; the final report; and more (ICH, 2025). This is not all-inclusive of what may be deemed necessary records. Complying with and adhering to the GCP essential recordkeeping requirements provides relevant information about the clinical trial, documents oversight of the safety of research participants, contains data and relevant metadata that would be needed to be able to reconstruct the trial, produces consistency with the conduct of the clinical trials, and provides quality worldwide.

Summary

Clinical trials are the scientific foundation for improving patient and public health outcomes. The ICH GCP guideline was initially established to provide international standardization for the conduct of clinical trials, assure participants that they are properly protected, ensure that trial data are credible, and facilitate the submission and approval of new medical products.

OCRNs, investigators, and study team members must be fully aware of their obligations and responsibilities required by the sponsors, local oversight bodies, and applicable federal regulatory agencies prior to conducting research. OCRNs play an instrumental role in ensuring research participant safety and integrity in studies that lead to improved care. Knowledge of GCP is critical for all those involved in clinical research.

Key Points

- GCP in clinical trial conduct is designed to protect participants' rights, safety, and well-being and ensure the credibility of trial data.

- *E6(R1)* defined GCP as an international ethical and scientific quality standard for the design, conduct, performance, monitoring, auditing, recording, analysis, and reporting of clinical trials.
- *E6(R2)* delineated GCP as a standard for the design, conduct, performance, monitoring, auditing, recording, analysis, and reporting of clinical trials that ensures that the data and reported results are credible and accurate and that the rights, integrity, and confidentiality of research participants are protected.
- *E6(R3)* describes GCP as an international, ethical, scientific, and quality standard for the conduct of trials that involve human participants. Clinical trials conducted in accordance with this standard will help to ensure that the rights, safety, and well-being of research participants are protected, that the conduct is consistent with the principles that have their origin in the Declaration of Helsinki, and that the clinical trial results are reliable. The term *trial conduct* includes planning, initiating, performing, recording, oversight, evaluation, analysis, and reporting activities as appropriate.
- HHS codified the Common Rule in Title 45.
- FDA GCP refers to a collection of regulations, guidance, and recommendations for clinical trials involving drugs, biologic products, and medical devices that are under FDA authority.
- FDA requirements are codified in Title 21.
- Essential records permit and contribute to the evaluation of the ethical conduct of a trial and the reliability of the results produced.
- OCRNs, investigators, and other research team members conducting human participant research are required to know what constitutes proper study conduct as defined by local and federal oversight bodies and study sponsors.

The author would like to acknowledge Patricia C. Woltz, PhD, RN, for her contribution to this chapter that remains unchanged from the previous edition of this book.

References

21st Century Cures Act, Pub. L. No. 114–255, § 1002 (2016).

Bhatt, A. (2023). The revamped Good Clinical Practice E6(R3) guideline: Profound changes in principles and practice! *Perspectives in Clinical Research, 14*(4), 167–171. http://doi.org/10.4103/picr.picr_184_23

Committee for Human Medicinal Products. (2016). *ICH guidelines for good clinical practice E6(R2): Step 5* (Publication No. EMA/CHMP/ICH/135/1995). European Medicines Agency. https://www.ema.europa.eu/en/documents/scientific-guideline/ich-guideline-good-clinical-practice-e6r2-step-5_en.pdf

Committee for Human Medicinal Products. (2025). *ICH E6 (R3) Guideline for good clinical practice (GCP): Step 5* (Publication No. EMA/CHMP/ICH/135/1995). European Medicines Agency. https://www.ema.europa.eu/en/documents/scientific-guideline/ich-e6-r3-guideline-good-clinical-practice-gcp-step-5_en.pdf

Federal Register. (1963, October 11). *Federal Register* (Vol. 28, p. 10972). https://archive.org/details/sim_federal-register-find_1963_28_index/page/72/mode/2up?q=10972

Federal Register. (2018, March 1). *Federal Register* (Vol. 83, No. 41, pp. 8882–8883). https://www.govinfo.gov/content/pkg/FR-2018-03-01/pdf/2018-04154.pdf

Food and Drugs, 21 C.F.R. (2025). https://www.ecfr.gov/current/title-21/chapter-I

International Conference on Harmonisation of Technical Requirements for Registration of Pharmaceuticals for Human Use. (1996, June 10). *Guideline for good clinical practice E6(R1).* https://media.tghn.org/medialibrary/2011/10/ICH_GCP_1996_Guidelines.pdf

International Council for Harmonisation of Technical Requirements for Pharmaceuticals for Human Use. (n.d.). *The evolution of ICH.* https://www.ich.org/page/history

International Council for Harmonisation of Technical Requirements for Pharmaceuticals for Human Use. (2016). *ICH harmonised guideline: Integrated addendum to ICH E6(R1): Guideline for good clinical practice E6(R2).* https://database.ich.org/sites/default/files/E6_R2_Addendum.pdf

International Council for Harmonisation of Technical Requirements for Pharmaceuticals for Human Use. (2019). *ICH E6(R3): Final concept paper.* https://database.ich.org/sites/default/files/E6-R3_FinalConceptPaper_2019_1117.pdf

International Council for Harmonisation of Technical Requirements for Pharmaceuticals for Human Use. (2023a). *ICH E6(R3): Draft guideline.* https://database.ich.org/sites/default/files/ICH_E6%28R3%29_DraftGuideline_2023_0519.pdf

International Council for Harmonisation of Technical Requirements for Pharmaceuticals for Human Use. (2023b). *ICH E6(R3): Step 2 presentation.* https://database.ich.org/sites/default/files/ICH_E6%28R3%29_Step%202_Presentation_2023_0613.pdf

International Council for Harmonisation of Technical Requirements for Pharmaceuticals for Human Use. (2024). *ICH harmonised guideline: Guideline for good clinical practice E6(R3): Annex 2.* https://database.ich.org/sites/default/files/ICH_E6%28R3%29_Annex%202_Step2_DraftGuideline_2024_1024_0.pdf

International Council for Harmonisation of Technical Requirements for Pharmaceuticals for Human Use. (2025). *ICH harmonised guideline: Guideline for good clinical practice: E6(R3).* https://database.ich.org/sites/default/files/ICH_E6%28R3%29_Step4_FinalGuideline_2025_0106.pdf

International Military Tribunal. (1949). *Trials of war criminals before the Nuremberg military tribunals under Control Council Law No. 10* (Vol. 2, pp. 181–182). United States Government Printing Office.

National Commission for the Protection of Human Subjects of Biomedical and Behavioral Research. (1979, April 18). *The Belmont Report: Ethical principles and guidelines for the protection of human subjects of research.* U.S. Department of Health, Education, and Welfare. https://www.hhs.gov/ohrp/regulations-and-policy/belmont-report/read-the-belmont-report/index.html

Office for Human Research Protections. (2025). *Federal policy for the protection of human subjects ('Common Rule').* https://www.hhs.gov/ohrp/humansubjects/commonrule/index.html

Protection of Human Subjects, 45 C.F.R. § 46 (2017). https://www.ecfr.gov/current/title-45/subtitle-A/subchapter-A/part-46

TransPerfect Life Sciences. (2023). *ICH E6(R3): Understanding the updated Good Clinical Practice guidelines (GCP) and their future impact.* https://lifesciences.transperfect.com/blog/ich-e6r3-understanding-updated-good-clinical-practice-guidelines-gcp-and-their-future-impact

U.S. Food and Drug Administration. (2018a). *E6(R2) Good Clinical Practice: Integrated addendum to ICH E6(R1): Guidance for Industry.* https://www.fda.gov/media/93884/download

U.S. Food and Drug Administration. (2018b). *Part III: Drugs and foods under the 1938 act and its amendments.* https://www.fda.gov/about-fda/changes-science-law-and-regulatory-authorities/part-iii-drugs-and-foods-under-1938-act-and-its-amendments

World Medical Association. (2025). *WMA Declaration of Helsinki: Ethical principles for medical research involving human subjects.* https://www.wma.net/policies-post/wma-declaration-of-helsinki

CHAPTER 9

Standard Operating Procedures

Elaine Esler, MSN, RN, OCN®, NE-BC

Introduction

Standard operating procedures (SOPs) are written documents that provide a detailed approach to performing a particular process and delineate the responsible parties for the process. They are used in numerous settings to ensure consistency, transparency, and high-quality workflow adherence (Roje et al., 2023).

Consistent use of an approved SOP provides adherence to organizational practices, reduces work effort and errors, and improves data comparability, credibility, and defensibility (U.S. Environmental Protection Agency [EPA], 2007). The International Council on Harmonisation of Technical Requirements for Registration of Pharmaceuticals for Human Use (ICH, 2016) defines SOPs as "detailed, written instructions to achieve uniformity of the performance of a specific function" (p. 7). ICH's *Guideline for Good Clinical Practice E6(R1)* also states that the sponsor is responsible for implementing and maintaining quality assurance and quality control systems with written SOPs to ensure that trials are conducted and data are generated.

This chapter will help oncology clinical research nurses (OCRNs) understand the value of research site SOPs, describe the relationship between SOPs and quality management, provide an overview of the development and maintenance of SOPs, and recommend topics for SOP development for research sites.

Standard Operating Procedures and Quality Management

A quality management plan describes an organization's quality system. It identifies the organizational structure, policies and procedures, functional responsibilities of management and staff, lines of authority, and processes for planning, implementing, documenting, and assessing all activities conducted under the organization's quality system. Quality assurance includes performing routine self-audits, modifying existing or implementing new SOPs for issues identified during the internal quality assurance process, recording minor and major violations, and applying corrective action plans (Manghani, 2011).

Properly established and managed quality control and quality assurance systems with integral, well-written SOPs provide a systematic and consistent approach to quality and performance improvement at a clinical trial site. These systems ensure that trials are performed as designed, that Good Clinical Practice guidelines are followed, and that participants' rights, welfare, and safety are protected (St Germain & Good, 2018). SOPs provide an infrastructure that confirms that quality controls and quality assurance systems are integrated within overall operations at research sites. They play a crucial role in a quality system, promoting teamwork, providing concise guidance, and empowering staff. This leads to enhanced opportunities for skill development, uniform execution, and minimized potential for errors. The use of quality management plans in combination with SOPs, supportive supervision, and rapid data feedback contribute to high-quality data collection (Bernardi et al., 2023).

Clinical research sites that have quality management plans in place with effective SOPs demonstrate their understanding of research regulations and a commitment to quality research.

Developing Standard Operating Procedures

The development and use of SOPs minimize variation and promote quality through consistently implementing a process or procedure within an organization, even with temporary or permanent personnel changes. "If not written correctly, SOPs are of limited value. In addition, the best written SOPs will fail if they are not followed" (EPA, 2007, p. 1). SOPs should be organization specific and constructed to guarantee ease and efficiency in use. Internal formatting will vary with each organization and the type of SOP written. The level of detail provided in the SOP may differ based on whether the process is critical and the frequency and number of people involved in a specific procedure (EPA, 2007).

The organization should have a procedure in place for determining what needs to be documented. Individuals knowledgeable about the activity and the organization's internal structure should write these SOPs. A team approach can be followed, especially for multitasked processes where the experiences of several individuals are critical; this method promotes adoption by potential end users (EPA, 2007).

It is helpful to organize a site's operations by key business components or core operational functions when determining categories, topics, and resources for SOP development. Several resources have recommendations for specific SOP development for clinical research sites. The U.S. Food and Drug Administration and the Office for Human Research Protections have guidance documents that interpret regulations available on their websites (see Figure 9-1). The American Society of Clinical Oncology recommends topics for SOP development through its position statement on minimum standards and exemplary attributes of clinical trial sites (Zon et al., 2008). Figure 9-2 outlines the key business components and core functions of an organization's clinical trial operations and includes a list of related topics to assist with SOP development.

Developing a set of SOPs can be overwhelming. It is a time-intensive process requiring commitment from all levels of the organization; however, it is well worth the effort in the long run. An organization needs to identify the key areas where SOPs are necessary and determine the standards, regulations, guidelines, and evidence-based/best practices that are applicable to its quality management plan and SOP development (see Figure 9-1). The following steps should be considered when organizing an effort to create SOPs (EPA, 2007):

- Prioritize the list based on risk or need.
- Develop a standard approach to SOP development and writing.
- Follow a team-based approach for SOP development and problem-solving whenever possible. Form a task force or focus group to map the current process, identify gaps and opportunities for improvement, and brainstorm and problem-solve to define the process further.
- Incorporate end-user review to gain consensus that procedures and expectations are appropriate and achievable. Pilot the SOP if possible.
- Establish an evaluation and review system to ensure that SOPs are adhered to and that the steps are correct and appropriate.

Figure 9-3 provides an example of a decision-making and planning matrix for SOP development.

Writing Standard Operating Procedures

SOPs should be created by individuals who are experienced in the topic and reviewed by external parties for clarity, comprehension, and reliability within the context of the organization. In the creation of clinical trial–related SOPs, an interprofessional team will likely be required. OCRNs, investigators, coordinators, and regulatory, budget, pharmacy, and laboratory personnel are some of the groups that may be needed to contribute to SOPs. Team writing for SOPs guarantees that comprehensive knowledge acquired from different perspectives is applied. Writing teams do not have to sit together to write. They can write portions of an SOP and edit individual items independently; then, one person can combine the individual contributions. For example, Hollmann et al. (2020)

International Conference on Harmonisation Guidelines
- www.ich.org/products/guidelines.html

National Cancer Institute (NCI)
- NCI Division of Cancer Treatment and Diagnosis Cancer Therapy Evaluation Program Resources for Clinical Trials in NCI Networks: http://ctep.cancer.gov/investigatorResources/default.htm#guidelines_policies
- NCI Investigator's Handbook: https://dctd.cancer.gov/research/ctep-trials/for-sites/investigator-handbook.pdf

U.S. Department of Health and Human Services Office for Human Research Protections (OHRP)
- OHRP Regulations, Policy, and Guidance: www.hhs.gov/ohrp/policy/index.html
- International Compilation of Human Research Standards: www.hhs.gov/ohrp/international/compilation-human-research-standards/index.html

U.S. Food and Drug Administration (FDA)
- Clinical Trials Guidance Documents: www.fda.gov/science-research/clinical-trials-and-human-subject-protection/clinical-trials-guidance-documents
- FDA Office of Good Clinical Practice (GCP) query email account: gcp.questions@fda.hhs.gov
- Archived replies to GCP queries indexed by topic: www.fda.gov/ScienceResearch/SpecialTopics/RunningClinicalTrials/RepliestoInquiriestoFDAonGoodClinicalPractice/default.htm
- Code of Federal Regulations–Title 21–Food and Drugs: www.fda.gov/medical-devices/medical-device-databases/code-federal-regulations-title-21-food-and-drugs

Other Regulations and Standards
- The Health Insurance Portability and Accountability Act of 1996 Privacy and Security Rules: www.hhs.gov/ocr/privacy
- OHRP: Guidance: www.hhs.gov/ohrp/regulations-and-policy/guidance/index.html
- Association for the Accreditation of Human Research Protection Programs Accreditation Standards: www.aahrpp.org
- U.S Department of Transportation Pipeline and Hazardous Materials Safety Administration guidance: www.phmsa.dot.gov/guidance
- American Society of Clinical Oncology Statement on Minimum Standards and Exemplary Attributes of Clinical Trial Sites: https://doi.org/10.1200/JCO.2007.15.6398

FIGURE 9-1 | Resources for Developing Standard Operating Procedures

Policy #	Categories	Title/Description	Effective Date	Revision Date	Last Literature Review	Associated Documents
	General and Administrative	• Development of Standard Operating Procedures (SOPs) • Site Research Mission, Organization, Scope, and Responsibilities • Research Staff Qualifications and Training • Research Site Communication Plan • Affiliate Institutional Network • Conflict of Interest in Research • Clinical Trial Patient Education and Outreach				Training materials; reference to related SOPs within the institution
	Protocol Management	• Protocol Activation and Implementation Plan • Study Recruitment Plan • Protocol Training • Institutional Review Board (IRB) Submissions • Regulatory Files • Protocol Termination • Archiving Study Files • Investigational Drug Management				Reference to related IRB SOPs
	Patient Management	• Study Recruitment • Informed Consent Process • Study Participant Study File • Study Participant Case Management on a Trial • Investigational Drug Administration and Treatment Plan • Adverse Event Reporting • Specimen Collection and Handling				Related clinical procedures
	Data Management	• Source Documents • Storage and Archiving • Information System Adherence				
	Quality Assurance	• Audits and Inspections • Monitoring Visits • Data Safety and Monitoring Committee • Electronic Health Record Access for External Audits • Quality Management Program				Audit tools
	Protocol Financial Management	• Research Participant Billing Adherence • Financial Review Process • Contractual Review Process • Medicare Coverage Analysis				

FIGURE 9-2 | Example of a Standard Operating Procedures Table of Contents and Document Management

Note. Based on information from U.S. Food and Drug Administration, 2009; Zon et al., 2008.

recommended the use of a shared server or cloud-based document-sharing platform.

Once combined, the draft SOP should be reviewed before editing the final version. Ideally, the writing team should meet at least once to establish the objectives. SOPs should be written with sufficient detail so that employees with limited experience or knowledge of the procedure can successfully reproduce the procedure when unsupervised. For detailed and complex procedures, mapping the process is helpful. *Mapping* involves taking each step in the procedure and making it more efficient and easier to follow. Once the mapping is completed, the team will convert the process to an outline, diagram, flow chart, or another format that will make it easy to understand (EPA, 2007).

Whenever possible, an organization should pilot the SOP prior to broader use, as this will provide an opportunity to evaluate its effectiveness. Subsequent revisions can

Category	Subcategory/ Topics	Current Process	Current Documentation of Process	Process Not Defined and Needs to Be Developed	Regulatory/ Standards/ Guidelines/Best Practice Resources for SOP Development	Content Expert Reviewer	SOP Developer(s) Key Personnel Involved in Process Development	SOP Required? Yes/No Cross-Reference (SOP available through another department)
Research specimen ordering, collecting, processing, storing, and shipping	Staff training and competencies	Yes	Orientation checklist and annual competencies			Biohazard compliance officer	Clinical research associate and clinical research nurse	Yes
			Hazmat training		International Air Transport Association	Compliance officer		No (see system policy for hazardous material shipment)
	Research study laboratory manual and supplies	Yes		Study specific				Yes
	General research laboratory supplies	Yes	Laboratory supply inventory and storage					Yes
		No	Ordering and disposal					
	Laboratory procedures	Yes	General laboratory manual	Study specific	Biohazard precautions	Laboratory manager		Yes
	Research laboratory patient orders and internal coordination	Yes	Electronic health record instructions for ordering research samples		Research billing regulations	Oncology clinical research nurse		Yes
		Yes	Coordination instructions			Clinical manager		
		Yes	Central calendar—group wide					
		Yes	Calendar template					
	Research laboratory processing	No				Laboratory manager		Yes
	Research study laboratory shipping	Yes			Hazmat			Yes
	Laboratory specimen archiving/freezer	No				Laboratory manager		Yes

FIGURE 9-3 | Example of a Decision-Making and Planning Matrix for Standard Operating Procedure Development

SOP—standard operating procedure

Note. Based on information from U.S. Environmental Protection Agency, 2007.

then be made based on the feedback. Supplementing SOPs with checklists, work instructions, guidelines, and workflow charts will assist with adoption and adherence. SOPs should be reviewed prior to release for adequacy and completeness. They should adhere to all applicable legal, ethical, and regulatory requirements (Akyar, 2012). The finalized SOPs should be approved by the organization's line of authority as outlined in the quality management plan (e.g., director of the research office). See Table 9-1 for specific sections and items to include in SOP documentation

Implementing Standard Operating Procedures

When possible, SOPs should be validated by one or more individuals with appropriate training and experience in the process. A standard approach should be developed for the implementation or distribution of SOPs for broader

TABLE 9-1 | Items to Include in a Standard Operating Procedure Document

Item	Description
SOP document information	Policy identifier: SOP identification number and organization Category: If applicable Title: Clearly identifies the activity or procedure Date: Effective date and/or revision date
SOP author or reviewer and approver	Include name, title, and credentials of the person who created, reviewed, or revised the policy, as well as the person who approved the SOP. The determination of the level of signature should be defined for developing SOPs within the organization. The reviewers should be knowledgeable and experienced with the content of the SOP.
References or resources	Policy and procedure should be based on current evidence-based practice or a regulation, law, or accreditation that is mandating the policy. List related SOPs, supporting documentation, applicable regulations, and/or guidelines.
Table of contents	A table of contents may be needed to quickly refer to lengthy SOPs, locate information, and denote changes or revisions made only to certain sections of an SOP.
Purpose	The purpose is the intent of the SOP, or the stated goal or purpose of the policy.
Scope	The scope provides an overview of the process and the range of activities that apply to the SOP, as well as any limitations or exceptions.
Responsibilities	This section outlines the individuals and areas required to comply with the policy. For individuals, titles or roles should be used, and names should be avoided.
Policy	A policy is a position statement that describes the organization's approach to a particular situation. It reflects the rules and is process based.
Definitions	Definitions or terminology may need to be clarified. Explanations of words or phrases unique to the document or topic should be included to add to the readers' understanding of the basic policy.
Procedure	The definitive steps to carry out the policy. Procedures are action-oriented, outlining chronologically the specific steps needed to act. The SOP should be drafted in a flow diagram or outline to assist in making the steps efficient or determining any gaps in the process or need for involving other people in development. Content should be clear, concise, thorough, and comprehensive, using tables, matrices, checklists, diagrams, and examples.
Effectiveness criteria/quality control measures	All appropriate quality assurance and quality control measures or activities should be described to ensure adherence with the procedure.
Policy dissemination	A systematic approach should be developed to confirm SOP implementation and associated training and frequency of SOP review. Minimally, all SOPs should be reviewed during new staff orientation, annually, and at the time SOPs are revised.
Appendices	Additional documents, given the situation, can be used as the best method to accurately convey the necessary information and facilitate the consistent implementation of an SOP, such as examples, documentation tools, checklists, flow charts, diagrams, decision trees, and algorithms.

SOP—standard operating procedure

Note. Based on information from U.S. Environmental Protection Agency, 2007.

use. Implementation should include a process for training current and new staff, and providing documentation of training, as well as metrics to evaluate effectiveness and adherence over time as a quality assurance measure. The training plan should include a regular annual review and staff competency review of SOPs to ensure adherence. It is helpful to use the individuals who were involved in SOP development as facilitators for implementation and ongoing quality assurance (EPA, 2007).

Maintaining Standard Operating Procedures

SOPs need to remain current to be useful; therefore, whenever procedures, standards, regulations, or guidelines are changed, SOPs should be updated and reapproved. SOPs should be reviewed on a regular basis (e.g., annual or biennial) to verify that policies and procedures remain current and appropriate (Hollman et al., 2020).

SOPs should be part of a controlled document system, including document identifiers, version dates, and statuses. SOP distribution must always be documented and controlled, and when obsolete SOPs are required to be retained for any purpose, they should be suitably identified to prevent unintended use. For historical and legal purposes, SOPs should be archived in the event they need to be referenced (Dubinsky & Henry, 2022).

Table 9-1 provides an example of how to manage SOPs and related documents, which can easily be converted into an electronic data management system.

Summary

SOPs are integral to an organization's quality management plan, which ensures that the conduct and results of clinical trials meet regulatory and ethical standards. Effective SOPs provide the framework for quality controls and quality assurance systems integrated within the research site's overall operations. An organizational commitment at all levels and from all individuals at the site is required for a quality system to succeed.

OCRNs need to know their organization's SOPs and quality management plan, and they should become involved in the development and implementation of SOPs. The national clinical research environment is changing rapidly, and a commitment to quality management by all is needed to protect human research participants, data integrity, and quality clinical research.

Key Points

- A quality management program will adhere to Good Clinical Practice guidelines to produce quality study results.
- SOPs are integral to an organization's quality management program.
- A procedure for determining appropriate SOPs should be developed.
- SOP development should include a team approach whenever possible and involve content experts and resources.
- Quality measures should be integrated within individual SOPs.
- SOPs should be reviewed regularly to evaluate credibility and appropriate adherence to regulations, best practices, and standards.
- Investment in the development and maintenance of SOPs will save time and effort and ensure a quality operation.

The author would like to acknowledge Cecilia Petrowsky, MSN, RN, CCRC, OCN®, for her contribution to this chapter that remains unchanged from the previous edition of this book.

References

Akyar, I. (2012). Standard operating procedures (What are they good for?). (2012). In I. Akyar (Ed.), *Latest research into quality control* (pp. 367–391). InTechOpen. https://doi.org/10.5772/50439

Bernardi, F.A., Alves, D., Crepaldi, N., Yamada, D.B., Lima, V.C., & Rijo, R. (2023). Data quality in health research: Integrative literature review. *Journal of Medical Internet Research, 25*, e41446. https://doi.org/10.2196/41446

Dubinsky, P.M., & Henry, K.A. (2022). *The fundamentals of clinical research: A universal guide for implementing good clinical practice.* Wiley.

Hollmann, S., Frohme, M., Endrullat, C., Kremer, A., D'Elia, D., Regierer, B., & Nechyporenko, A. (2020). Ten simple rules on how to write a standard operating procedure. *PLoS Computational Biology, 16*(9), e1008095. https://doi.org/10.1371/journal.pcbi.1008095

International Council for Harmonisation of Technical Requirements for Pharmaceuticals for Human Use. (2016). *ICH harmonised guideline: Integrated addendum to ICH E6(R1): Guideline for good clinical practice E6(R2).* https://database.ich.org/sites/default/files/E6_R2_Addendum.pdf

Manghani, K. (2011). Quality assurance: Importance of system and standard operating procedures. *Perspectives in Clinical Research, 21*(1), 34–37. https://doi.org/10.4103/2229-3485.76288

Roje, R., Tomić, V., Buljan, I., & Marušić, A. (2023). Development and implementation of research integrity guidance documents: Explorative interviews with research integrity experts. *Accountability in Research, 30*(6), 293–330. https://doi.org/10.1080/08989621.2021.1989676

St Germain, D., & Good, M. (2018). Data management in clinical trials. In J.I. Gallin, F.P. Ognibene, & L.L. Johnson (Eds.), *Principles and practice of clinical research* (4th ed., pp. 531–545). Elsevier Academic Press. https://doi.org/10.1016/B978-0-12-849905-4.00030-7

U.S. Environmental Protection Agency. (2007). *Guidance for preparing standard operating procedures.* https://www.epa.gov/sites/default/files/2015-06/documents/g6-final.pdf

U.S. Food and Drug Administration. (2009). *Guidance for industry: Investigator responsibilities—Protecting the rights, safety, and welfare of study subjects.* https://www.fda.gov/downloads/Drugs/Guidances/UCM187772.pdf

Zon, R., Meropol, N.J., Catalano, R.B., & Schilsky, R.L. (2008). American Society of Clinical Oncology statement on minimum standards and exemplary attributes of clinical trial sites. *Journal of Clinical Oncology, 28*(15), 2562–2567. https://doi.org/10.1200/JCO.2007.15.6398

CHAPTER 10

Ethics of Clinical Research

Reneé Kurz, DNP, FNP-BC, AOCNP®, and Victoria Szenes, DNP, RN, CPNP

Introduction

Ethics in clinical research are vital to safeguard the protection, rights, and welfare of human participants while supporting scientific progress. All nurses, especially oncology clinical research nurses (OCRNs), must understand and apply ethical principles in their roles. Clinical research is essential for advancing medical knowledge and developing new treatments to improve health outcomes. However, history has demonstrated that research involving human participants has, at times, been ethically compromised (see Chapter 1). Notable examples include the Jewish Chronic Disease Hospital study, the Willowbrook hepatitis studies, and the U.S. Public Health Service Untreated Syphilis Study at Tuskegee (Arras, 2008; Jones, 2008; Robinson & Unruh, 2008). Pioneering American anesthesiologist and medical ethicist Henry Knowles Beecher's 1966 article in the *New England Journal of Medicine* exposed ethical misconduct occurring within prestigious research institutions in the United States. Beecher identified 22 ethically questionable studies and emphasized that the ethical integrity of research relies not only on external guidelines but also on the personal moral responsibility of investigators (Beecher, 1966). These cases highlighted the need for strict ethical standards and led to the development of essential ethical codes of conduct.

Foundational ethical codes include the Nuremberg Code, enacted after the Nazi war criminal trials (Nuremberg Trials), which emphasized the essential role of participants' voluntary consent in research (Annas & Grodin, 2008; Weindling, 2008). It became the prototype for subsequent ethical frameworks. Other important codes of conduct, such as *The Belmont Report*, outlined three key principles: beneficence, respect for persons, and justice (National Commission, 1979). See Chapter 8 for more information about the Nuremberg Code and *The Belmont Report*. The World Medical Association (1997) developed the Declaration of Helsinki as a statement of ethical principles of medical research involving human participants, including research using identifiable human material or data.

This chapter explores seven main principles of ethics in clinical trial research that OCRNs should be familiar with: social and clinical value, scientific validity, fair participant selection, favorable risk–benefit ratio, independent review, informed consent, and respect for participants.

The Seven Principles

Social and Clinical Value

Clinical trials are designed to answer meaningful questions about preventing, treating, or managing disease. The potential value of these answers must justify asking participants to accept some risk or inconvenience for others. The Institute of Medicine (now the National Academy of Medicine) and other institutions have suggested that limited-value studies (e.g., small, underpowered studies) make little impact on the overall goals of science (Lo & Field, 2009; Saver, 2012). Resources for clinical research are limited, so it is essential to design studies that avoid unnecessarily exposing participants to risk without the potential for individual or societal benefit.

Scientific Validity

Ethical research must be scientifically rigorous. Valid and reliable instruments, an appropriate sample size determined through power analysis, and a well-planned methodology are critical to generating credible results (Waltz et al., 2010). Conducting a power analysis is essential to determine appropriate sample size, minimizing type II errors (indicating that there is no statistical difference when, in fact, there is) and ensuring the ability to detect significant outcomes. Ethically, researchers should avoid exposing participants to risks without the power to determine treatment efficacy. Beecher (1966) concluded, "an experiment is ethical or not at its inception; it does not become ethical post hoc" (p. 372), underscoring the importance of proactive, critical appraisal during study design.

Randomized controlled trials (RCTs) are considered the gold standard for scientific validity. These trials minimize bias by randomly assigning patients to different groups (e.g., treatment versus placebo). Blinding helps further eliminate bias, especially double blinding, when the participant and the investigator are both blinded to the intervention or study drug. RCT results should be included in systematic reviews and inform clinical practice guidelines (Granholm et al., 2022).

As oncology research has evolved, precision medicine and studies driven by biomarkers have become more prominent. These types of studies frequently use basket and umbrella designs. Basket trials evaluate a targeted therapy for multiple diseases that share common molecular alterations or risk factors, whereas umbrella studies look at multiple targeted therapies for a single disease and stratify into subgroups based on different molecular or other predictive risk factors (Park et al., 2020). However, other types of clinical trials (e.g., prevention) and methodologic designs (e.g., epidemiologic, observational, historical) may also shed light on complex problems, thus being considered of scientific and societal value (Emanuel et al., 2000). Examples of potential research questions that add social and scientific value are outlined in Figure 10-1.

Other important research-related terms and processes that OCRNs need to be aware of include *equipoise*, *randomization*, and *placebo*. Often, participants may seek the advice of OCRNs to help explain the specifics of these terms as part of the informed consent process.

Researchers designing an RCT, for example, and proposing to test the safety and efficacy of an intervention must be in a state of equipoise. Equipoise is an important ethics-related term in RCTs because it represents a state of professional uncertainty regarding the superiority of the treatment arms. Ethically, physicians or nurse investigators cannot assign participants to inferior care or treatment because of their professional codes of conduct and their therapeutic obligations to patient care (Miller & Joffe, 2011). The term *clinical equipoise* was proposed to provide an ethical ground to conduct randomized controlled clinical trials.

- What are the benefits and burdens of COVID-19 vaccine research?
- What innovative strategies minimize health disparities in the recruitment and retention of human participants in clinical research?
- What are the personal and societal costs of caregiving now, once an individual is diagnosed with cancer?
- What is the added value of community-based participatory research in meeting the healthcare goals of differing communities?
- What is the role of interprofessional team science in translating research from the bench to the bedside?
- What defines a "good death" from the point of view of individuals, families, and healthcare providers, and how is it different or similar among them?

FIGURE 10-1 | Examples of Research Questions That Add Social and Scientific Value

In RCTs, randomization is a method where study participants are assigned to a treatment group. This process of assigning groups by chance is explained to research participants as similar to flipping a coin. Participants are often concerned about being randomized to a placebo. A Harris Interactive Survey conducted in the United Kingdom reported that of patients who were aware of a clinical trial, 71% of eligible patients opted not to participate. Approximately 37% of these individuals chose not to participate because of the perception that the standard treatment was better, 31% for concern of receiving a placebo, 22% for fear of being treated like guinea pigs, and 21% because of travel distance (Chaudhari et al., 2020).

Researchers might propose a placebo-controlled trial in which the experimental drug is compared to a placebo (inactive substance). Emanuel and Miller (2001) contended that placebo-controlled trials can be ethically justified for the following reasons: (a) there is a compelling methodologic argument to use a placebo, (b) a thorough and stringent ethical review has taken place, and (c) the risk of serious patient harm is null, and the risks of receiving a placebo are minimized to the greatest extent possible. Thus, these important ethics-related terms in RCTs must be outlined in the informed consent document as well as during the informed consent process and in a way that is understandable to participants.

Fair Participant Selection

Recruitment to studies should reflect the diversity of the population affected by the conditions being studied. Under the Code of Federal Regulations (C.F.R.) Title 21 § 56.111, institutional review boards (IRBs) must ensure that participant selection is equitable before approving research (Criteria for IRB Approval of Research, 2023). This includes consideration of the purposes of the research and the setting in which it will be conducted.

Diversity in clinical trial recruitment ensures the generalizability of results and promotes health equity. Neither privilege nor vulnerability should influence inclusion or exclusion without scientific justification. The National Cancer Institute and the American Society of Clinical Oncology have been strong advocates for expanding participation to underrepresented groups, including racial and ethnic minorities, individuals from rural or low-resource areas, and non-English–speaking populations (National Cancer Institute, 2025; Oyer et al., 2022).

To address barriers to participation, decentralized trials and community-based research initiatives can bring studies closer to participants' homes. OCRNs are well-positioned to identify strategies for improving access and ensuring inclusive enrollment practices. They can advocate for thoughtful recruitment strategies and provide input to make trial participation feasible and equitable for diverse communities.

Favorable Risk–Benefit Ratio

Research and clinical practice were defined and differentiated in *The Belmont Report* as both separate and distinct concepts, although they can and sometimes do overlap (see Figure 10-2). In fact, participants may not perceive them differently, primarily when research is conducted at the bedside, where care is traditionally given and received. This is imperative to the understanding of informed consent and requires immediate clarification. Medical or clinical care is meant to benefit an individual; therefore, a provider's primary commitment is to address the patient's immediate health and well-being. Conversely, research can potentially benefit individuals, but its goal is to improve care and treatment for future patients. Research represents a systematic process that is aimed at testing specific hypotheses meant to generalize knowledge.

Appelbaum et al. (1982) first discussed the term *therapeutic misconception*, arguing its existence when patients believe that they will personally benefit or receive therapeutic gain from all aspects of research participation. Building off of this, Appelbaum et al. (1987) stated that "to maintain a therapeutic misconception is to deny the possibility that there may be major disadvantages to participating in clinical research that stem from the nature of the research process itself" (p. 20). Significant empirical research with differing groups of patient populations enrolled in clinical research (e.g., cancer, Parkinson disease, mental health) has highlighted several participant- and study-level factors that may place patient-participants at risk for therapeutic misconception (Appelbaum et al., 2004; Kim et al., 2009). This includes those who are older, less educated, or in poorer health, as well as those with limited options and an increased sense of optimism (Appelbaum et al., 2004).

Horng and Grady (2003) delineated other aspects of participants' misunderstanding beyond the therapeutic misconception, including therapeutic misestimation and therapeutic optimism. An uneven risk–benefit assessment can lead to a therapeutic misestimation, either "underestimating the risks, overestimating the benefits, or both" (Horng & Grady, 2003, p. 13).

Fostering optimism or hope in research participation is central to many patients' ability to cope with their illness and does not necessarily undermine their ability to make autonomous decisions (Horng & Grady, 2003; Jansen, 2006). However, therapeutic optimism can be unrealistic, and more data are needed to better understand the role of hope in the lives of participants and at what point it biases their research-related decisions.

Kim et al. (2009) called on researchers and related professionals to refocus their attention on therapeutic misconception using a different lens. OCRNs should continue to foster hope, but at the same time, statements that reflect a misconception or misestimation should be carefully considered within the overall context of the participant's decision-making process (Kim et al., 2009). They can address this by asking participants to articulate their understanding of the purpose, aims, risks and benefits, and other aspects of the study and how they arrived at a risk–benefit calculus for themselves. Open and consistent dialogue is the key to allaying misunderstandings and improving knowledge associated with the research process. Figure 10-3 provides strategies that OCRNs can use to address misconceptions and therapeutic misestimation.

Research
Research designates an activity designed to test a hypothesis, permit conclusions to be drawn, and thereby to develop or contribute to generalizable knowledge (expressed, for example, in theories, principles, and statements of relationships). Research is usually described in a formal protocol that sets forth an objective and a set of procedures designed to reach that objective.

Practice
Practice refers to interventions that are designed solely to enhance the well-being of an individual patient or client and that have a reasonable expectation of success. The purpose of medical or behavioral practice is to provide diagnosis, preventive treatment, or therapy to particular individuals.

FIGURE 10-2 | Definitions of Research and Clinical Practice Addressed in *The Belmont Report*

Note. From *The Belmont Report: Ethical Principles and Guidelines for the Protection of Human Subjects of Research*, by National Commission for the Protection of Human Subjects of Biomedical and Behavioral Research, 1979. https://www.hhs.gov/ohrp/humansubjects/guidance/belmont.html. In the public domain.

Independent Review

To minimize potential conflicts of interest and to ensure studies are ethically acceptable, IRBs were established to

- Revisit the study's purpose, aims, and research questions to address whether it still reflects participants' goals and preferences.
- Clarify terms such as *randomization*, *placebo*, and *equipoise* or any other misunderstandings as needed.
- Inform participants of any study changes as the protocol progresses.
- Discuss the risks and benefits of the study.
- Call a family and care team meeting to discuss ethical, procedural, or other concerns with the principal investigator and others integral to the protocol.
- Design informational brochures that can be shared with participants to clarify aspects of the clinical trial. These brochures will need to be approved by the institutional review board of record.

FIGURE 10-3 | Strategies to Address Concerns Related to Therapeutic Misestimation in Clinical Research

Note. Based on information from Horng & Grady, 2003.

review and approve research involving human participants and to ensure that all human research is conducted with federal, institutional, and ethical guidelines and regulations. IRBs have the authority to approve, require modifications to, or disapprove research. IRBs ensure that 45 C.F.R. § 46.111 criteria for research are met, including the following (Criteria for IRB Approval of Research, 2023):

- Risks to participants (subjects) are minimized.
- Risks are reasonable in relation to anticipated benefits, if any.
- The selection of participants is equitable.
- Informed consent is sought and appropriately documented.
- Adequate provisions for data monitoring are provided to ensure participant safety.
- Privacy and confidentiality of the data are protected.
- Special provisions for ensuring the protection of vulnerable participants are clearly delineated, where applicable.

The IRB provides investigators and institutions with written documentation of all decisions.

An IRB includes at least five members, preferably from various racial, gender, and cultural backgrounds (Protection of Human Subjects, 2017). The members must consist of at least one researcher, one nonresearcher, and one person who is not affiliated with the institution. Members often are physicians, pharmacologists, clergy, nurses, social workers, and bioethicists. If a study is presented that requires additional expertise, the IRB can invite a particular individual to consult, although they will not have voting privileges (Protection of Human Subjects, 2017). Additionally, no IRB may have a member participate in the initial or continuing review of any project in which the member has a conflicting interest, except to provide information requested by the IRB.

OCRNs who serve on IRBs often provide a broad lens by which to evaluate risks and benefits to the participants from both a clinical and human protection perspective. As knowledgeable care providers, they are often able to easily recognize or forecast procedural irregularities or potential for adverse events. For example, an OCRN may identify burdensome procedures or suggest more explicit consent language. Whether serving as an IRB member or caring for research participants, nurses are responsible for promoting sound science and protecting the rights and welfare of patients enrolled in clinical trials (Grady & Edgerly, 2009).

Informed Consent

Informed consent is a process by which a participant voluntarily confirms their willingness to participate in a protocol. It must occur before any research activity begins, and participants must be provided with ample time to ask questions and make an informed decision. It respects the right of individuals to determine what is in their best interest. In *Schloendorff v. Society of New York Hospital*, 211 N.Y. 125, 105 N.E. 92 (1914), Justice Cardozo wrote the following opinion:

> Every human being of adult years and sound mind has a right to determine what shall be done with his own body; and a surgeon who performs an operation without his patient's consent commits an assault for which he is liable in damages. This is true except in cases of emergency where the patient is unconscious and where it is necessary to operate before consent can be obtained.

Thus, informed consent involves the voluntary consent and autonomous authorization of patients after they understand the purpose, risks, benefits, and other study-related aspects of the treatment or research being proposed. Informed consent consists of (a) disclosure of information, (b) decisional capacity (to understand the information and make a decision), (c) voluntariness on behalf of participants, and (d) comprehension of information (Emanuel et al., 2000; National Commission, 1979). Figure 10-4 describes what should be discussed with patients in research.

A potential gap exists between what participants are ideally expected to understand and what they actually comprehend. Many studies demonstrate that factors such as educational level, serious illness, age, and trust in the researcher influence informed consent (Flory & Emanuel, 2004; Joffe et al., 2001). Moreover, the Office for Human Research Protections regulations designated several groups of participants as vulnerable—those who have a diminished capacity to provide informed consent—and in need of additional safeguards, including (a) adults with diminished capacity, (b) children, (c) pregnant women, neonates, and fetuses, and (d) prisoners (Protection of Human Subjects, 2017). Although informed consent is an essential element for the ethical conduct of research with human participants, it is

- The nature and purpose of the study
- The risks and benefits
- The right to withdraw at any time without penalty
- The alternatives that might be available
- The name of the individual to contact in case of an emergency (generally the principal investigator or other study team members)
- The voluntariness of patients
- The remuneration of patients, if available
- The way that privacy and confidentiality of patient information will be handled (Certificate of Confidentiality), if needed for sensitive research
- The responsibilities of the participant
- Reasons why the trial may be stopped by the principal investigator or sponsor
- Financial responsibilities of the patient for standard-of-care procedures
- Information on whom the participant can contact for ethical concerns

FIGURE 10-4 | What Should Be Discussed With Potential Research Participants?

Note. Based on information from Appelbaum et al., 1987; Faden & Beauchamp, 1986.

not sufficient (Emanuel et al., 2000; Faden & Beauchamp, 1986).

Research involving children (aged 17 years or younger) includes special requirements and protections as per 21 C.F.R. § 50 Subpart D and 45 C.F.R. § 46 Subpart D (Additional Protections for Children Involved as Subjects in Research, 1983; Additional Safeguards for Children in Clinical Investigations, 2001). These regulations emphasize the need for parental permission and child assent, mirroring the procedure for informed consent used for research involving adults. The child's legally authorized representative must be the one providing permission. Determination of this representative is based on state law. Children capable of assent must also express their willingness to participate.

Participants must be informed of updated information about a research study that might affect their willingness to continue participating in the study. Examples include, but are not limited to, new or modified risks, a change in treatment schedule, and the addition or removal of research tests. When a participant consents to an oncology clinical trial, they have multiple interactions throughout the study. Their condition may change, there can be multiple protocol amendments, arms may open or close, or safety concerns may arise with the study (Ervin & Pettit, 2020). OCRNs should maintain an open dialogue with participants throughout a trial to reaffirm their willingness to continue.

Respect for Potential or Enrolled Participants

Participants' confidentiality must be protected throughout a study. OCRNs should de-identify personal information when corresponding with sponsors, uploading scans, and entering information into case report forms. Throughout an oncology clinical research trial, many opportunities exist for personal health information to be disclosed, making it important that research participant identification numbers are used instead of names and dates of birth on tissue and blood specimens or when sending other study-related items.

Throughout the conduct of a study, it is vital to respect participants' right to change their minds and to withdraw at any time without penalty. Participants may determine that continued involvement no longer aligns with their interests, especially as new information becomes available or their clinical condition changes. Interim analyses, safety concerns, or evolving risk–benefit assessments may also necessitate participant withdrawal, either by choice or because of medical necessity

An often-overlooked aspect of ethical research conduct is the communication of study findings to participants. Although OCRNs are typically diligent in monitoring patients during the trial, it is equally essential to ensure that participants understand what happens after the study concludes. Sharing study results with participants once available is not only an ethical obligation but also a requirement for federally funded research. Providing this feedback reinforces respect, transparency, and trust between the research team and the participants who contributed to the advancement of knowledge.

Foundation of Ethical Research

Beyond the role of the IRB in human participant protection, scientific integrity must remain a foundational element of ethical research. Scientific integrity is at the core of ethical research and represents a measure of the public's trust in not only individual researchers but also the broader research enterprise. Integrity in science upholds ethical standards and promotes authenticity, transparency, and honesty in all aspects of the research process, ranging from designing the actual study to disseminating the results.

The Institute of Medicine's *Conflict of Interest in Medical Research, Education, and Practice* acknowledged the significance of intellectual honesty in the ethical conduct of research, including fairness in peer review, collegiality, and adherence to standards of practice as outlined between investigators and their research teams in the protection of human participants (Lo & Field, 2009). However, the public is often afraid to participate in research. For example, although patient enrollment in cancer clinical trials has risen to 7.1% as of 2024, participation remains limited (Unger et al., 2024). In a study by Ulrich et al. (2012), clinical research participants expressed sentiments such as, "I often wonder if [the researcher] is not telling me everything," or "People are scared to death to participate." Ethical missteps by investigators and institutions, especially those amplified by media coverage, have significant consequences for participants, professionals, and public trust alike.

Research Misconduct

The U.S. Office of Science and Technology Policy defines research misconduct as "fabrication, falsification, or plagiarism in proposing, performing, or reviewing research, or in reporting research results" (Steneck, 2007, p. 20) (see Figure 10-5). Research misconduct does not include differences of opinion. Actual reports of misconduct vary in the literature, with Pryor et al. (2007) reporting 18% of research coordinators knowing of integrity violations.

Other areas not formally defined as research misconduct can create ethical concerns, such as protocol violations; inconsistencies in the process of informed consent, data collection, and data management; pressures to recruit and retain patient-participants; failure to report adverse events in a timely fashion; modification of procedures without IRB approval; conflicts of interest; and authorship disputes. OCRNs are a vital link between participants and the principal investigator. In their qualitative work on study coordinators' (or OCRNs') critical role in human partici-

Fabrication
Making up data or results and recording or reporting them

Falsification
Manipulating research materials, equipment, or processes, or changing or omitting data or results, such that the research is not accurately represented in the research record

Plagiarism
The appropriation of another person's ideas, processes, results, or words without giving appropriate credit

FIGURE 10-5 | Definitions Related to Research Misconduct

Note. From *Federal Policy on Research Misconduct*, by U.S. Office of Science and Technology Policy, 2000. https://ori.dhhs.gov/education/products/RCRintro/c02/b1c2.html. In the public domain.

pant protection, Peng et al. (2023) reported that coordinators are responsible for managing participant recruitment and enrollment, consistency of study implementation, data management and integrity, and compliance with regulatory requirements and reporting. A lack of training, insufficient knowledge of healthcare ethics, significant work-related pressure, and frequent changing of coordinators pose substantial risks to participants (Peng et al., 2023).

The Committee on Assessing Integrity in Research Environments (Institute of Medicine & National Research Council, 2002) has also noted that individual researchers are the most unpredictable and influential variable within the research environment and, in some cases, have shifted blame to study coordinators for questionable practices. However, OCRNs' proximal role to both the participant and the protocol lends itself to immediately addressing any discrepancies before misconduct occurs. All OCRNs should (Richmond & Ulrich, 2013):

- Conduct research with transparency, rigor, and truthfulness.
- Ask questions to clarify concerns related to the conduct of research and seek senior mentorship and support to address questionable research practices.
- Consult with an ethics committee as needed.
- Have a basic understanding of the ethical codes of conduct and the ethical principles of research (i.e., beneficence, respect for persons, justice).
- Contact the IRB for any questions or uncertainty regarding reporting requirements, modifications, or amendments to the protocol.

Conflict of Interest

The ability to financially gain from research has been a source of intense discussion among the research community, the university academy, the pharmaceutical industry, and the public. In research, the secondary financial gain of investigators has the potential to undermine the primary protection of human participants and place them at undue risk. Moreover, Saver (2012) stated that "secondary interests can compromise the design, conduct, and reporting of research, while also threatening subject safety and undermining public trust" (p. 468). OCRNs should be familiar with the Promoting Objectivity in Research (2011) regulations. These regulations specifically address financial conflicts of interest related to the conduct of research and address stock ownership and equity, consulting fees, paid authorship, and individual and institutional reporting requirements. "An individual has a conflict of interest when he or she has personal, financial, professional, or political interests that are likely to undermine his or her ability to meet or fulfill his or her primary professional, ethical, or legal obligations" (Shamoo & Resnik, 2009, p. 191).

Although individuals can disclose their financial conflicts of interest and develop sound management plans with institutional advisory oversight, there has been little focus on other types of conflicts, including nonfinancial conflicts of interest. These intellectual or intrinsic conflicts can undermine research because the pressures for success (e.g., promotion, tenure) may potentially bias one's judgment and contribute to hasty research-related decisions. Barrett (2010) developed a four-tiered system to promote the integrity of research, including personal and professional values, research mentorship, peer review, and IRB oversight. Maintaining research integrity requires a multifaceted approach, and the pragmatic abilities along with the scientific and healthcare expertise of OCRNs provide a protective layer that is essential to the ethical conduct of research.

Ethics Consultation

Consultation with bioethicists and other ethics professionals who are not directly involved in a research study or patient care is sometimes warranted to assist staff, patients, and families in addressing and resolving ethical or communication issues that arise during a clinical trial. These consultations offer expert, unbiased guidance on complex issues. OCRNs may request consultations when consent capacity is unclear, participants or families disagree, they want to seek advice on end-of-life disagreements among study team members, they want to better understand genetic risk implications for family members to determine when disclosure of risk to others is appropriate, or they need guidance on vulnerable population groups.

Evidence suggests that nurses fear retaliation for seeking ethics support. However, Danis et al. (2008) did not find an association between fear of retaliation and decreased requests for ethics consultation. The U.S. Sentencing Commission's *Organizational Sentencing Guidelines* and U.S. Department of Justice enforcement expectations require organizations to provide mechanisms for employees to raise concerns without fear of retaliation, further emphasizing the significance of accessible ethics and compliance resources in clinical research (Dunn et al., 2024).

Consultation provides not only a means of clarifying the ethical issues within the study but also an opportunity to hear all relevant stakeholder voices. Danis et al. (2008, p. 7) noted that assisting researchers and others "in the identification and analysis of ethical issues that arise in the course of conducting research—from the conception of a research question, throughout recruitment and enrollment of research participants, data collection, and even beyond a study's completion" is a primary goal of the consultation service.

Since the 1980s, ethics consultation services have been widely available for practicing clinicians within hospital-based institutions (Danis et al., 2012), and more recently, bioethicists have extended their expertise to the research arena. However, not every institution will have a bioethicist or ethics consultation service. Most academic institutions have an office of research, IRB members, or a compliance officer who can provide insight or guidance on ethics in research-related questions. OCRNs who do not have access to an ethics consultation service can reach out to their IRB representative or check with their professional oncology society for guidelines that might assist them in addressing ethical questions.

OCRNs play a pivotal role in providing patients with accurate information about clinical trials and helping them understand the treatment regimen. As Dresser (2012, p. 74) noted, "patients make trial decisions with a limited and sometimes inaccurate grasp of the facts." This is especially true for patients facing cancer diagnoses, who often experience fear and uncertainty while navigating difficult treatment decisions.

OCRNs have an ethical duty to protect patients from harm and advocate on their behalf; this extends to the research environment and sometimes requires an ethics consultation. Understanding the ethical principles of research, the relevant codes of conduct, the complicated terminology of clinical trials, the importance of informed consent with human participants, and the resources available to assist study team members and others with ethical questions enables OCRNs to safeguard human participants effectively. This commitment reflects the relevant words of Beecher (1966): "an ethical approach to experimentation with man [is] safeguarded by the presence of an intelligent, informed, conscientious, compassionate, responsible investigator" (p. 1360). This includes OCRNs who are integral to research teams and foster critical dialogue among patient participants, principal investigators, and other research team members.

Summary

OCRNs are essential to the ethical conduct of clinical research. They bridge clinical care and research integrity, advocating for participants while upholding study protocols. A strong grasp of ethical principles and practical application empowers OCRNs to protect participants and contribute to responsible science. Fear or uncertainty, including fear of the unknown, can become a barrier to advocacy (Thacker, 2008). As advocates, OCRNs need to exercise ethical assertiveness during research team meetings and interprofessional rounds and advocate as active participants in ethical decisions (Norton & Joos, 2005). New knowledge and experience related to the ethical issues surrounding human participant research come with the responsibility and accountability for OCRNs, as caregivers and research advocates, to strive for full informed consent on the part of each research participant (Wallen & Baker, 2012).

Key Points

- OCRNs are integral members of research teams responsible for the ethical conduct of research.
- Ethical principles (beneficence, respect for persons, and justice) and ethical codes of conduct can guide OCRNs in addressing ethical concerns that arise in clinical research.
- The seven principles of ethics in clinical trial research include: social and clinical value, scientific validity, fair participant selection, favorable risk–benefit ratio, independent review, informed consent, and respect for potential and enrolled participants.
- IRBs are part of the ethical oversight of clinical research and are responsible for protocol review.
- Ethics consultation services can provide support and objective counsel on complex ethical issues that arise in clinical research.
- Knowledge of key ethical terms in clinical research (e.g., *placebo*, *randomization*, *equipoise*) can support OCRNs' conversations with research participants.

References

Additional Protections for Children Involved as Subjects in Research, 45 C.F.R. § 46(d) (1983). https://www.ecfr.gov/current/title-45/subtitle-A/subchapter-A/part-46/subpart-D

Additional Safeguards for Children in Clinical Investigations, 21 C.F.R. § 50(d) (2001). https://www.ecfr.gov/current/title-21/chapter-I/subchapter-A/part-50/subpart-D

Annas, G.J., & Grodin, M.A. (2008). The Nuremberg Code. In E.J. Emanuel, C. Grady, R.A. Crouch, R.K. Lie, F.G. Miller, & D. Wendler (Eds.), *Oxford textbook of clinical research ethics* (pp. 136–140). Oxford University Press.

Appelbaum, P.S., Lidz, C., & Grisso, T. (2004). Therapeutic misconception in clinical research: Frequency and risk factors. *IRB: Ethics and Human Research, 26*(2), 1–8. https://doi.org/10.2307/3564231

Appelbaum, P.S., Roth, L.H., & Lidz, C. (1982). The therapeutic misconception: Informed consent in psychiatric research. *International Journal of Law and Psychiatry, 5*(3–4), 319–329. https://doi.org/10.1016/0160-2527(82)90026-7

Appelbaum, P.S., Roth, L.H., Lidz, C.W., Benson, P., & Winslade, W. (1987). False hopes and best data: Consent to research and the therapeutic misconception. *Hastings Center Report, 17*(2), 20–24.

Arras, J.D. (2008). The Jewish Chronic Disease Hospital case. In E.J. Emanuel, C. Grady, R.A. Crouch, R.K. Lie, F.G. Miller, & D. Wendler (Eds.),

Oxford textbook of clinical research ethics (pp. 73–79). Oxford University Press.

Barrett, R. (2010). Strategies for promoting the scientific integrity of nursing research in clinical settings. *Journal for Nurses in Staff Development, 26*(5), 200–205. https://doi.org/10.1097/NND.0b013e31819b55dd

Beecher, H. (1966). Ethics and clinical research. *New England Journal of Medicine, 274*(24), 1350–1360. https://doi.org/10.1056/NEJM196606162742405

Chaudhari, N., Ravi, R., Gogtay, N.J., & Thatte, U.M. (2020). Recruitment and retention of the participants in clinical trials: Challenges and solutions. *Perspectives in Clinical Research 11*(2), 64–69, https://doi.org/10.4103/picr.PICR_206_19

Criteria for IRB Approval of Research, 21 C.F.R. § 56.111 (2023). https://www.accessdata.fda.gov/scripts/cdrh/cfdocs/cfcfr/CFRSearch.cfm?fr=56.111

Danis, M., Farrar, A., Grady, C., Taylor, C., O'Donnell, P., Soeken, K., & Ulrich, C. (2008). Does fear of retaliation deter requests for ethics consultation? *Medicine, Health Care, and Philosophy, 11*(1), 27–34. https://doi.org/10.1007/s11019-007-9105-z

Danis, M., Largent, E., Grady, C., Wendler, D., Hull, S.C., Shah, S., ... Berkman, B. (2012). *Research ethics consultation: A casebook.* Oxford University Press.

Dresser, R. (2012). *Malignant: Medical ethicists confront cancer.* Oxford University Press.

Dunn, A.M., Good, A.M., Junck, R.D., Ridgway, W.E., & Wykowska, Z. (2024, September). Key updates to the DOJ's evaluation of corporate compliance programs. *Skadden.* https://www.skadden.com/insights/publications/2024/09/key-updates-to-the-dojs-evaluation-of-corporate-compliance-programs

Emanuel, E.J., & Miller, F.G. (2001). The ethics of placebo-controlled trials—A middle ground. *New England Journal of Medicine, 345*(12), 915–919. https://doi.org/10.1056/NEJM200109203451211

Emanuel, E.J., Wendler, D., & Grady, C. (2000). What makes clinical research ethical? *JAMA, 283*(20), 2701–2711. https://doi.org/10.1001/jama.283.20.2701

Ervin, A.-M., & Cobb Pettit, J.B. (2020). Consent forms and procedures. In S. Piantadosi & C.L. Meinert (Eds.), *Principles and practice of clinical trials* (pp. 389–410). Springer. https://doi.org/10.1007/978-3-319-52677-5_46-1

Faden, R., & Beauchamp, T. (1986). *A history and theory of informed consent.* Oxford University Press.

Flory, J., & Emanuel, E.J. (2004). Interventions to improve research participants' understanding in informed consent for research: A systematic review. *JAMA, 292*(13), 1593–1601. https://doi.org/10.1001/jama.292.13.1593

Grady, C., & Edgerly, M. (2009). Science, technology, and innovation: Nursing responsibilities in clinical research. *Nursing Clinics of North America, 44*(4), 471–481. https://doi.org/10.1016/j.cnur.2009.07.011

Granholm, A., Alhazzani, W., Derde, L.P.G., Angus, D.C., Zampieri, F.G., Hammond, N.E., ... Møller, M.H. (2022). Randomised clinical trials in critical care: Past, present and future. *Intensive Care Medicine, 48*(2), 164–178. https://doi.org/10.1007/s00134-021-06587-9

Horng, S., & Grady, C. (2003). Misunderstanding in clinical research: Distinguishing therapeutic misconception, therapeutic misestimation, and therapeutic optimism. *IRB: Ethics and Human Research, 25*(1), 11–16. https://doi.org/10.2307/3564408

Institute of Medicine & National Research Council. (2002). *Integrity in scientific research: Creating an environment that promotes responsible conduct.* National Academies Press. https://doi.org/10.17226/10430

Jansen, L.A. (2006). The problem with optimism in clinical trials. *IRB: Ethics and Human Research, 28(*4), 13–19. http://www.jstor.org/stable/30033204

Joffe, S., Cook, E.F., Cleary, P.D., Clark, J.W., & Weeks, J.C. (2001). Quality of informed consent in cancer clinical trials: A cross-sectional survey. *Lancet, 358*(9295), 1772–1777. https://doi.org/10.1016/S0140-6736(01)06805-2

Jones, J.H. (2008). The Tuskegee syphilis experiment. In E.J. Emanuel, C. Grady, R.A. Crouch, R.K. Lie, F.G. Miller, & D. Wendler (Eds.), *Oxford textbook of clinical research ethics* (pp. 86–96). Oxford University Press.

Kim, S.Y.H., Schrock, L., Wilson, R.M., Frank, S.A., Holloway, R.G., Kieburtz, K., & de Vries, R.G. (2009). An approach to evaluating the therapeutic misconception. *IRB: Ethics and Human Research, 31*(5), 7–14. http://www.jstor.org/stable/25594887

Lo, B., & Field, M.J. (Eds.). (2009). *Conflict of interest in medical research, education, and practice.* National Academies Press.

Miller, F., & Joffe, S. (2011). Equipoise and the dilemma of randomized clinical trials. *New England Journal of Medicine, 364*(5), 476–480. https://doi.org/10.1056/NEJMsb1011301

National Cancer Institute. (2025). *Cancer disparities research.* https://www.cancer.gov/research/areas/disparities

National Commission for the Protection of Human Subjects of Biomedical and Behavioral Research. (1979). *The Belmont report: Ethical principles and guidelines for the protection of human subjects of research.* https://www.hhs.gov/ohrp/humansubjects/guidance/belmont.html

Norton, C., & Joos, O. (2005). Caring for Catherine: A cry to support ethical activism. *Journal of Pediatric Oncology, 22*(2), 119–120. https://doi.org/10.1177/1043454204273771

Oyer, R.A., Hurley, P., Boehmer, L., Bruinooge, S.S., Levit, K., Barrett, N., ... Pierce, L.J. (2022). Increasing racial and ethnic diversity in cancer clinical trials: An American Society of Clinical Oncology and Association of Community Cancer Centers joint research statement. *Journal of Clinical Oncology, 40*(9), 1001–1008. https://doi.org/10.1200/JCO.22.00754

Park, J.J.H., Hsu, G., Siden, E.G., Thorlund, K., & Mills, E.J. (2020). An overview of precision oncology basket and umbrella trials for clinicians. *CA: A Cancer Journal for Clinicians, 70*(2), 125–137. https://doi.org/10.3322/caac.21600

Peng, Z., Ma, Y., Wang, J., Xu, X., Wang, C., & Chen, Y. (2023). Awareness of clinical research coordinators toward ethics and protection of clinical trial patients. *Therapeutic Innovation and Regulatory Science, 57*(3), 561–569. https://doi.org/10.1007/s43441-022-00488-9

Promoting Objectivity in Research, 42 C.F.R. §§ 50.601–50.607 (2011). https://www.gpo.gov/fdsys/pkg/CFR-2011-title42-vol1/pdf/CFR-2011-title42-vol1-part50-subpartF.pdf

Protection of Human Subjects, 45 C.F.R. § 46 (2017). https://www.ecfr.gov/current/title-45/subtitle-A/subchapter-A/part-46

Pryor, E.R., Haberman, B., & Broome, M.E. (2007). Scientific misconduct from the perspective of research coordinators: A national survey. *Journal of Medical Ethics, 33*(6), 365–369. https://doi.org/10.1136/jme.2006.016394

Richmond, T.S., & Ulrich, C. (2013). *Ethical foundations for critical care nursing research.* American Association of Critical Care Nurses. https://www.aacn.org/wd/practice/content/research/ethics-in-critical-care-nursing-research.pcms?menu=practice

Robinson, W.M., & Unruh, B.T. (2008). The Hepatitis experiments at Willowbrook State School. In E.J. Emanuel, C. Grady, R.A. Crouch, R.K. Lie, F.G. Miller, & D. Wendler (Eds.), *Oxford textbook of clinical research ethics* (pp. 80–85). Oxford University Press.

Saver, R.S. (2012). Is it really all about the money? Reconsidering nonfinancial interests in medical research. *Journal of Law, Medicine, and Ethics, 40*(3), 467–481. https://doi.org/10.1111/j.1748-720X.2012.00679.x

Schloendorff v. Society of New York Hospital, 211 N.Y. 125, 105 N.E. 92 (1914).

Shamoo, A.E., & Resnik, D.B. (2009). Responsible conduct of research (2nd ed.). Oxford University Press.

Steneck, N.H. (2007). *ORI introduction to the responsible conduct of research.* https://ori.hhs.gov/sites/default/files/rcrintro.pdf

Thacker, K. (2008). Nurses' advocacy behaviors in end-of-life nursing care. *Nursing Ethics, 15*(2), 174–185. https://doi.org/10.1177/0969733007086015

Ulrich, C.M., Knafl, K.A., Ratcliffe, S., Richmond, T., Grady, C., Miller-Davis, C., & Wallen, G. (2012). *Developing a model of the benefits and burdens of research participation in cancer clinical trials. AJOB Primary Research, 3*(2), 10–23. https://doi.org/10.1080/21507716.2011.653472

Unger, J.M., Shulman, L.N., Facktor, M.A., Nelson, H., & Fleury, M.E. (2024). National estimates of the participation of patients with cancer in clinical research studies based on Commission on Cancer accreditation data. *Journal of Clinical Oncology, 42*(18), 2139–2148. https://doi.org/10.1200/JCO.23.01030

Wallen, G.R., & Baker, K. (2012). Ethical challenges in transitioning to end-of-life care: Exploring the meaning of a "good death." In C.M. Ulrich (Ed.), *Nursing ethics in everyday practice* (pp. 151–161). Sigma Theta Tau International.

Waltz, C., Strickland, O., & Lenz, E. (2010). *Measurement in nursing and health research* (4th ed.). Springer.

Weindling, P.J. (2008). The Nazi medical experiments. In E.J. Emanuel, C. Grady, R.A. Crouch, R.K. Lie, F.G. Miller, & D. Wendler (Eds.), *Oxford textbook of clinical research ethics* (pp. 18–30). University Press.

World Medical Association. (1997). Declaration of Helsinki—Recommendations guiding physicians in biomedical research involving human subjects. *JAMA, 277*(11), 925–926. https://doi.org/10.1001/jama.1997.03540350075038

CHAPTER 11

Elements of a Protocol

Kristen Clemens, BSN, RN, OCN®

Introduction

Clinical trials are a fundamental aspect of medical research, and a protocol is the primary source and reference for all requirements, activities, plans, glossaries, and guidance for operating a specific clinical trial. The research protocol is a roadmap recognized and followed by all participating investigators (Jagadeesh & Balakumar, 2023). With the protocol as its backbone, there is assurance that the trial is followed in the same manner, providing objective consistency across all investigators, sites, and study teams and leading to more robust and accurate data to evaluate the outcome of a study. Well-written protocols, organized and timely data collection and statistical evaluation, and safe and efficiently run trials ultimately lead to new therapy developments and access to life-saving treatments for patients.

This chapter will review the most common elements included in the clinical trial protocol document and provide a detailed breakdown of each. Although some elements of a protocol are essential, the sections that are included may vary depending on the intent, scope, phase, or regulating body of the clinical trial.

Essential Elements

Common elements of a protocol include the following (National Cancer Institute Cancer Therapy Evaluation Program [NCI CTEP], 2014):

- Title page
- Schema
- Objective(s)
- Background and rationale
- Patient eligibility criteria
- Pharmaceutical information
- Treatment plan
- Procedures for patient entry into the study
- Adverse events list and reporting requirements
- Dose modification for adverse events
- Criteria for response assessment
- Monitoring of patients
- Off-study criteria
- Statistical considerations
- Records
- Participation
- Multicenter trials

A protocol includes information required by institutional, national, and international regulatory agencies to conduct a specific research study safely. Although the protocol is robust, it does not include all details regarding the legal, ethical, and regulatory adherence of a study.

Title Page

The title page comprises identifying information about the trial and the involved parties, including the following (National Institutes of Health [NIH], 2023):

- Abbreviated title
- Institutional review board (IRB) reference number
- Other relevant assigned numbers (e.g., Investigational New Drug sponsor, institutional biosafety committee) when available
- Version date (updated with all subsequent amendments)
- The date that all editing of the document was completed (or the date editing began) to ensure consistency throughout the protocol document
- Title
  - Clinical trial type (e.g., phase 1, 1/2, 2, 3)
  - Interventions to be used (e.g., drugs, devices, procedures, observation) and disease entity
- Principal investigator
- Study team members
- Affiliation, address, and contact information (i.e., telephone number, email address) for the principal investigator and study team members
- Investigational agents (if applicable)
- For multi-institutional protocols

- Name of the coordinating center
- Name of the responsible safety monitoring committee

Schema

The schema is a diagrammatic layout of the overall study design (see Figures 11-1 and 11-2). It shows the study steps in chronological order, with a breakdown of cohorts, and may include dose escalation levels if applicable to the protocol. If not in diagram format, a summary narrative may be used instead.

Objectives

The objectives of a protocol describe the overall goal of the study and can include primary and secondary classifications. The objectives answer the scientific question being posed. Primary objectives are the top priority, whereas secondary objectives provide additional data of interest; if not obtained during the study run, they will not affect the end point or final results. The specific objectives depend on the study design (noninterventional vs. interventional) and may include clinical end points (e.g., overall survival, progression-free survival, maximum tolerated dose), surrogate end points (laboratory assessments), patient-reported outcomes, or biomarker studies (Cimino & Braun, 2023).

Background and Rationale

The background and rationale explain the importance of the study and why it is necessary. Background includes information about the disease, device, or disorder being treated, prior research on the topic and published data, current treatment options, and limitations to current practices (NIH, 2023). The rationale contextualizes this information, highlighting the current state of treatment, potential improvements, justifications for further research, and the overall benefits of a safely conducted study.

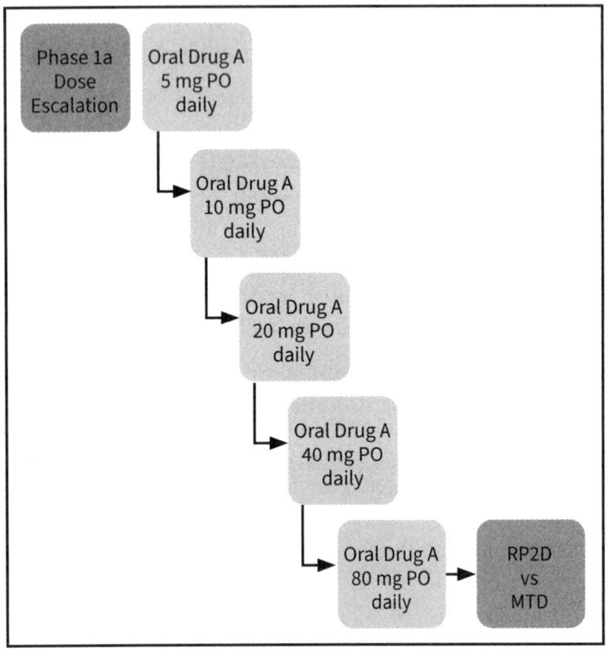

FIGURE 11-1 | Dose Escalation Study Schema

MTD—maximum tolerated dose; RP2D—recommended phase 2 dose

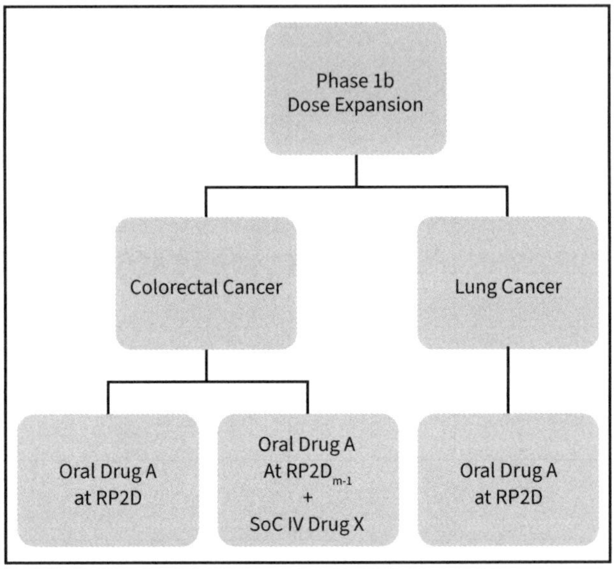

FIGURE 11-2 | Dose Expansion Study Schema

RP2D—recommended phase 2 dose; SoC—standard of care

Patient Eligibility Criteria

Patient eligibility criteria include specific objective characteristics and subjective criteria, based on clinician judgment, that a participant must have (inclusion) or must not have (exclusion) to be eligible for a study (see Figure 11-3). Confirmation that all participants meet the same established criteria is "necessary to ensure the safety of patients participating in a clinical study and to allow for interpretability of the clinical study results" (Spira et al., 2021, p. 2416). The body writing the protocol must balance the level of detail in eligibility criteria with the need to conduct the study safely while achieving accrual goals. "Overly stringent eligibility criteria may unnecessarily limit enrollment, resulting in delayed trial completion, and limiting generalizability of the research results" (Spira et al., 2021, p. 2416). As the study progresses, if the criteria exclude too many participants, the sponsor may need to reevaluate and expand them based on early clinical experience, provided there are no safety concerns. Broadening the eligibility criteria can enhance access, allowing more patients to receive novel therapies during a trial (Spira et al., 2021).

Pharmaceutical Information

Pharmaceutical information details the investigational drug or device being tested. For an oral drug trial, this may include formulations, appearances, dispensing and storage requirements, and dosing guidelines, as well as procedures for receiving shipments, reconciling dispensed drugs, and disposing of unused products.

Inclusion
- Participant must be aged 18 years.
- Participant must have locally confirmed stage IV cancer.
- Participant must have measurable disease based on Response Evaluation Criteria in Solid Tumors (RECIST) definition.
- Participant is willing to follow contraceptive guidance if they have reproductive potential.

Exclusion
- Participant has not recovered from ≥ grade 2 toxicities related to prior anticancer therapy.
- Participant has received anticancer therapy within 21 days or 5 half-lives, whichever is longer, of the start of investigational treatment.
- Participant is on a medication on the Prohibited Medication list, and it cannot be stopped or switched.
- Participant has an uncontrolled or untreated central nervous system disease.

FIGURE 11-3 | Inclusion and Exclusion Criteria

For a medication that must be prepared and administered at a treatment site, guidelines include preparation instructions, safety considerations for the preparer and administrator, expiration timelines, documentation requirements, and any necessary medical equipment or delivery systems required for patient safety.

This section addresses other medications administered during the trial that are not the investigational agent undergoing study, such as standard chemotherapy used in combination with a novel treatment. The protocol will define what medications, therapies, or procedures are allowed, restricted, or used under caution while a participant is on the trial.

If a device is being tested in the study, pharmaceutical information may not apply; however, an alternative section should review the technical and functional details of its operation.

Treatment Plan

The treatment plan describes the investigational intervention and any applicable standard of care or supportive therapies administered in the study, including cycle length, treatment days, duration of administration, instructions for dose adjustment for changes in body weight or body surface area, and total length of treatment (NCI CTEP, 2014).

This information is typically presented in a table titled "Schedule of Assessments," "Schedule of Events," or similar. The table lists all required tests, procedures, assessments, and interventions at all timepoints from prescreening or screening to the end of treatment and long-term follow-up (see Table 11-1). Superscripts or subscripts within the table provide more detailed information on specific laboratory testing, radiologic imaging requirements, and timing of correlatives (e.g., pharmacokinetic and pharmacodynamic draws, biopsies, and electrocardiogram collections) in relation to administration of the investigational agent or device under study.

Procedures for Patient Entry Into the Study

Procedures for patient entry into the study outline requirements for the participant and study team. For the participant, initial testing may be necessary before registration for the study to confirm eligibility and complete any pretreatment or prescreening requirements.

TABLE 11-1 | Schedule of Assessments

Procedure	Screening Day -28 to -1	Cycle 1, Day 1 No Window	Cycle 1, Day 15 +/- 1 Day	Cycle 2+ +/- 3 Days	End of Treatment + 7 Days After Last Dose	Loss to Follow-up +/- 15 Days
Informed consent	X					
Physical examination	X	X		X	X	
Hematology[a]	X	X	X	X	X	
Chemistry[b]	X	X	X	X	X	
Electrocardiogram	X	X		X	X	
Imaging	X			X[c]		X[d]
Drug X infusion		X		X		

[a]White blood cell count, hematocrit, hemoglobin, platelet count, and absolute neutrophil count

[b]Albumin, alkaline phosphatase, total bilirubin, bicarbonate, blood urea nitrogen, calcium, chloride, creatinine, glucose, phosphorus, potassium, aspartate aminotransferase, alanine aminotranferase, and sodium

[c]Imaging should be performed every 4 weeks +/- 7 days until end of treatment.

[d]Imaging continues every 12 weeks +/- 14 days if the participant did not come off the study for disease progression.

For the study team, procedures are primarily administrative, including details on slot allocation and securement, eligibility confirmation, correspondence with the sponsor, and final registration.

Adverse Events List and Reporting Requirements

Adverse events are "any untoward medical occurrence associated with the use of a drug in humans, whether or not considered drug related" (U.S. Food and Drug Administration, 2021, para. 2). This section of the protocol outlines the study's definition of an adverse event, terminology and grading, criteria for a serious adverse events or suspected unexpected serious adverse reactions, or adverse events of special interest. The *Common Terminology Criteria for Adverse Events*, published and updated by NCI, is the most commonly used reference for terminology and grading (NCI CTEP, 2017).

The protocol will specify the information that must be documented (i.e., term, severity, relationship to the study intervention, and expectedness), as well as the timelines for reporting adverse events to the sponsor or the managing regulatory body. It outlines follow-up requirements, including timelines and additional information required for these events (NIH, 2023).

Dose Modifications for Adverse Events

For any therapeutic interventional study, it is essential to specify when and how the dosage of the medications under study can be modified in response to an adverse event, which is crucial for patient safety. The protocol outlines the criteria for dose modification based on the adverse event, as well as its severity, timing, and duration (see Table 11-2). This section provides information on the length of drug hold allowed, rules for restarting or rechallenging, and monitoring and managing treatment-related adverse events.

TABLE 11-2 | Dose Modification Guidelines

Toxicity	Grade	Dose Modification
Hematologic	1–2	No modficiation; continue same dose.
	3	Hold until toxicity resolves to grade 1 or baseline. Reduce by 1 dl.
	4	Discontinue dose.
All other toxicities	1–2	No modficiation; continue same dose.
	3	Hold until toxicity resolves to grade 1 or baseline. Reduce by 1 dl. For second occurrence, reduce by 1 dl.
	4	Discontinue dose.

Note. Based on information from National Cancer Institute Cancer Therapy Evaluation Program, 2017.

For early-phase studies, particularly first-in-human trials, dose modification may be guided by experiences with similar drug classes or from dosing in preclinical animal models. As a study progresses and more data are collected, the protocol may be amended to ensure the safest and most effective treatment for participants, with changes reflected in the protocol version number.

Criteria for Response Assessment

Consistency in data reporting is essential for achieving accurate and reproducible end points in a clinical trial. To evaluate the effectiveness of a therapeutic trial, all investigators must use the same criteria to assess how the disease under study responds to the investigational agent. This section outlines the criteria being used. Examples include the International Working Group response criteria (Kim et al., 2022), Response Assessment in Neuro-Oncology criteria (Qian et al., 2017), World Health Organization criteria, Response Evaluation Criteria in Solid Tumors (RECIST) (Wolchok et al., 2009), and a version of RECIST for immunotherapy trials (iRECIST) (Seymour et al., 2017).

Monitoring of Patients

The monitoring section of the study details the evaluation of participants (e.g., adverse events, adherence) and covers monitoring of study data and safety. This section should identify who will monitor the study, what will be reviewed, and how often by frequency or trial benchmark (Bartrum et al., 2017). Quality assurance monitoring also is performed throughout the study to ensure that all aspects of the trial and applicable regulatory requirements are followed (Bartrum et al., 2017). Regular monitoring and oversight of trial activities improve patient safety, study team adherence, and overall data integrity.

Off-Study Criteria

Off-study criteria outline the reasons a participant should no longer be actively involved in the trial. The decision to come off the study may be based on safety, nonadherence with protocol guidelines, or changes in clinical status.

This section also clarifies the distinction between *off treatment* and *off study*, specifying the data and timepoints the investigator is expected to continue monitoring with the participant. Additionally, it outlines investigator responsibilities regarding participants who withdraw from the study or are considered lost to follow-up (NIH, 2023).

Statistical Considerations

Statistical considerations detail the testing and data analysis methods based on the primary and secondary end points, as well as the timeline for reaching these end points. The timeline to completion accounts for the number of participants (sample size), including those who consent but screen fail and those who begin treatment on the study (NIH, 2023).

Recordkeeping

The protocol specifies the data to be collected, methods of collection, where data are recorded, and duration of storage. Data collection methods include participants' historical medical records, records of adverse events, examinations, imaging, laboratory data, participant questionaries, response criteria assessments, paper records (e.g., investigation medications diaries, pharmacokinetic documents), regulatory documents, and official correspondence with the study sponsor or regulatory bodies. Generally, records should be kept for at least two years from approval of the investigational agent or device for commercial use. If the study concluded without authorization or ended prematurely, records should be kept for two years from when the study was officially discontinued (NIH, 2023).

Participation

Participation refers to the study team members designated to engage in trial activities and their responsibilities in relaying information back to the study sponsor. Led by the principal investigator, the study team is assigned various responsibilities, ranging from entering data for laboratory values to reading radiographic images for response assessment and evaluating and clearing patients on their planned treatment day. Study team members who have met the human research training requirements, along with the locations where participants will engage in required protocol activities, must be designated at the start of the trial and updated throughout the trial when changes occur.

Multicenter Trials

Clinical trials can vary significantly in scope and reach. Some trials may involve multiple centers worldwide and thousands of participants, whereas others may involve a single center with a small number of participants. For trials that are open in multiple institutions, specific guidelines are agreed upon by the study sponsor and participating institutions, including monitoring and auditing agreements, the designation of a coordinating center, and the responsibilities of the protocol chair liaison (NCI CTEP, 2014).

Summary

At first glance, a clinical trial protocol can be intimidating, spanning hundreds of pages. Understanding its key elements can make navigation easier and quicker with continued exposure and review.

Given the specifics of each protocol and the number of studies an oncology clinical research nurse may encounter, it is nearly impossible to know every minute detail. By having a general understanding of the protocol's sections, including what information is included and how to locate it, nurses in this role can quickly navigate and find what is needed, even when working with a protocol for the first time. This expertise highlights the role of the oncology clinical research nurse as a vital and active participant on the research study team.

In the high-stakes world of research involving human participants—especially in developing new treatments for the oncology population—the investigator assumes the responsibility to anticipate, understand, explain, and follow each protocol element. They also serve as educators on the implications of these elements for participants, from the first contact at the time of consent and through their entire time in the study. By adhering to protocol guidelines, investigators and their teams enhance data accuracy, leading to more robust research, continually evolving theories and advancements in cancer treatments.

Key Points

- The protocol is an essential document that acts as the definitive source of information to conduct a clinical trial consistently, safely, and ethically.
- Every interventional protocol will have similar required elements, with some variation based on the type and phase of the trial, scope, and regulatory body overseeing the clinical trial.
- It is imperative for oncology clinical research nurses and all those involved in conducting research to be adept at understanding the elements of a protocol; how to locate, interpret, and apply the information within the protocol; and how to act as a mediator between the study team, principal investigator, and study participants.

The author would like to acknowledge Wendi Mitchell, RN, OCN®, and Zelda Smith, RN, CBCN®, OCN®, for their contribution to this chapter that remains unchanged from the previous edition of this book.

References

Bartrum, E.A., Karp, B.I., & Nussenblatt, R.B. (2017). Writing a protocol. In J.I. Gallin, F.P. Ognibene, & L.L. Johnson (Eds.), *Principles and practice of clinical research* (4th ed., pp. 220–224). Elsevier Academic Press. https://doi.org/10.1016/C2014-0-03999-8

Cimino, J., & Braun, C. (2023). Design a clinical research protocol: Influence of real-world setting. *Healthcare, 11*(16), 2254. http://doi.org/10.3390/healthcare11162254

Jagadeesh, G., Balakumar, P. (2023). Writing research protocols in pharmacological studies. In G. Jagadeesh, P. Balakumar, & F. Senatore (Eds.), *The quintessence of basic and clinical research and scientific publishing* (pp. 45–59). Springer. https://doi.org/10.1007/978-981-99-1284-1_4

Kim, N., Pavletic, S., & Norsworthy, K.J. (2022). Meaningful response criteria for myelodysplastic syndromes. *British Journal of Haematology, 196*(5), 1137–1148. https://doi.org/10.1111/bjh.17838

National Cancer Institute Cancer Therapy Evaluation Program. (2014). *A handbook for clinical investigators conducting therapeutic clinical trials supported by CTEP, DCTD, NCI [v.1.2]*. http://ctep.cancer.gov/investigatorResources/docs/InvestigatorHandbook.pdf.

National Cancer Institute Cancer Therapy Evaluation Program. (2017). *Common terminology criteria for adverse events* [v.5.0]. https://ctep.cancer.gov/protocolDevelopment/electronic_applications/docs/CTCAE_v5_Quick_Reference_5x7.pdf

National Institutes of Health. (2023). *Protocol templates and forms: Interventional drug and device clinical trials protocol template.* https://irbo.nih.gov/confluence/display/ohsrp/Protocol+Templates

Qian, J.M., Mahajan, A., Yu, J.B., Tsiouris, A.J., Goldberg, S.B., Kluger, H.M., & Chiang, V.L.S. (2017). Comparing available criteria for measuring brain metastasis response to immunotherapy. *Journal of Neuro-Oncology, 132*(3), 479–485. https://doi.org/10.1007/s11060-017-2398-8

Seymour, L., Bogaerts, J., Perrone, A., Ford, R., Schwartz, L.H., Mandrekar, S., ... de Vries, E.G.E. (2017). iRECIST: Guidelines for response criteria for use in trials testing immunotherapeutics. *Lancet Oncology, 18*(3), e143–e152. https://doi.org/10.1016/S1470-2045(17)30074-8

Spira, A.I., Stewart, M.D., Jones, S., Chang, E., Fielding, A., Richie, N., ... Gerber, D.E. (2021). Modernizing clinical trial eligibility criteria: Recommendations of the ASCO-Friends of Cancer Research laboratory reference ranges and testing intervals work group. *Clinical Cancer Research, 27*(9), 2416–2423. https://doi.org/10.1158/1078-0432.CCR-20-3853

U.S. Food and Drug Administration. (2021). *IND application reporting: Safety Reports.* https://www.fda.gov/drugs/investigational-new-drug-ind-application/ind-application-reporting-safety-reports

Wolchok, J.D., Hoos, A., O'Day, S., Weber, J.S., Hamid, O., Lebbé, C., ... Hodi, F.S. (2009). Guidelines for the evaluation of immune therapy activity in solid tumors: Immune-related response criteria. *Clinical Cancer Research, 15*(23), 7412–7420. https://doi.org/10.1158/1078-0432.CCR-09-1624

CHAPTER 12

Informed Consent

Cynthia Samborski, MSN, MHA, RN, CCRC

Introduction

Informed consent is a critical step in clinical research, ensuring that participants understand the study's purpose, procedures, risks, benefits, and alternative treatments. Investigators must seek consent under circumstances that allow prospective research participants sufficient opportunity to consider participation and minimize coercion or undue influence. Potential participants should have sufficient opportunity to consider whether to participate (Office of the Commissioner, 2018). This chapter will detail the informed consent process, including information about the consent form, guiding principles and governing bodies, differences between federally funded and non-federally funded research, and protections for special and vulnerable populations. It will also provide a case study on the consent process and hypothetical clinical trial draft guidance.

The Consent Form

The consent form serves a dual purpose: to provide information to the potential participant for their current and future reference and to document the communication between the participant and the investigator (Office for Human Research Participants [OHRP], n.d.-a). The informed consent discussion and form are completed simultaneously to maintain a consistent dialogue and produce a document that confirms the conversation. The oncology clinical research nurse (OCRN), the investigator, and any additional study team members work together to conduct the study. The investigator explains the trial and the consent, and the OCRN assists in the informed consent discussion. Throughout the study, the OCRN plays an integral role in collaborating with the investigator and study team to confirm adherence to the protocol parameters.

According to federal regulations, specifically the Common Rule (45 Code of Federal Regulations [C.F.R.] § 46), informed consent also includes ensuring that recruitment materials are clear, accurate, and not misleading. This includes details about the study's purpose, procedures, risks, benefits, and the voluntary nature of participation (Protection of Human Subjects, 2017). Additionally, recruitment materials must be reviewed and approved by an institutional review board (IRB) to ensure they adhere to these regulations (National Institutes of Health, n.d.).

Guiding Principles and Governing Bodies

According to 21 C.F.R. § 50.20, General Requirements for Informed Consent (1980), except as provided in §§ 50.22, 50.23, and 50.24, investigators must obtain legally effective informed consent from the participant or legally authorized representative (LAR) before involving them in research. Investigators must ask for consent in easy-to-understand language and in such a way that gives individuals enough time to make a decision and avoids any pressure or influence. Consent cannot include language that waives the legal rights to release anyone from liability for negligence.

Several authorities regulate the informed consent process in clinical research. Under the auspices of the U.S. Department of Health and Human Services (HHS), two federal agencies oversee the federal regulations that address informed consent and other aspects of human research protection. OHRP administers the regulations that apply to federally funded research. The U.S. Food and Drug Administration (FDA) administers research funded by non-federal sources, such as pharmaceutical industry trials. Although the regulations overseen by OHRP and FDA were initially developed separately, they both prioritize patient confidentiality and dignity and establish ethical standards that all researchers are expected to follow. The requirements for human research participant safeguards are based on *The Belmont Report* (OHRP, n.d.-a). FDA also requires IRB review and has the authority to approve, require modifications, or disapprove all research activities covered by the IRB regulations (IRB Review of Research, 1981).

The Belmont Report

To prevent the abuse of human research participants, the United States passed the National Research Act (Public Law 93-348) in 1974. Through this, the National Commission for the Protection of Human Subjects of Biomedical and Behavioral Research was created in part to determine the fundamental ethical principles and guidelines for safeguarding human research participants. In 1979, the group issued the landmark *The Belmont Report: Ethical Principles and Guidelines for the Protection of Human Subjects of Research*, which continues to provide the foundation for the conduct of human participant research through three fundamental ethical principles (HHS, n.d.-a):

- **Respect for Persons:** This principle reflects two ethical convictions: individuals should be treated as autonomous agents, and those with diminished autonomy are entitled to protection.
- **Beneficence:** Ethical treatment includes respecting individuals' decisions, protecting them from harm, and making efforts to secure their well-being.
- **Justice:** This principle requires that the benefits and burdens of research be distributed fairly among all participants.

In addition, *The Belmont Report* emphasizes three elements based on respect for individuals: information, comprehension, and voluntariness. *Information* encompasses the following (HHS, 1979):

- The research procedure, its purpose, risks, and anticipated benefits
- Alternative procedures, particularly where therapy is involved
- A statement offering the subject (participant) the opportunity to ask questions
- A statement that permits withdrawal from the research at any time

The element of *comprehension* emphasizes that the way information is presented and the context in which it is presented are just as crucial as the content of the information. A person's capacity to grasp this information depends on their health literacy, reasoning, maturity, and linguistic skills. Therefore, it is essential to tailor the communication of information to align with their comprehension level. According to 45 C.F.R. §§ 46.116 and 46.117, informed consent information must be presented in a language understandable to the participant or their LAR (Documentation of Informed Consent, 2017; General Requirements for Informed Consent, 2017). This includes providing a consent form in the person's native language and, if necessary, using an interpreter to facilitate understanding of both the written document and the consent discussion.

Voluntariness refers to an agreement to participate in research when valid consent is offered and given voluntarily. This element of informed consent requires conditions that are free from coercion and undue influence (HHS, 1979).

Coercion occurs when one person intentionally presents an overt or implicit threat of harm to another to obtain adherence. For example, an investigator might tell a prospective participant that they will lose access to needed health services if they do not participate in the research (HHS, 2023).

Undue influence, by contrast, often occurs through an offer of an excessive or inappropriate reward or other overture to obtain adherence. It arises when one party manipulates another due to a power imbalance, often to the detriment of the weaker party. For instance, an investigator promising psychology students extra credit for research participation may unduly influence them. However, offering non-research alternatives minimizes this risk (HHS, 2023).

U.S. Department of Health and Human Services

HHS enhances the health and well-being of all Americans by providing effective health and human services and by fostering sound, sustained advances in the sciences underlying medicine, public health, and social services (HHS, 2023). OHRP and FDA are responsible for improving the health and welfare of all Americans. These entities play a key role in providing guidance and supervision for clinical research trials. HHS and FDA coordinate efforts to ensure consistent standards and guidelines for human participant research (OHRP, 2023). They oversee the informed consent process to ensure compliance with ethical standards and regulatory requirements (Office of the Commissioner, 2018).

The Code of Federal Regulations

C.F.R. is the codification of the federal government rules and regulations. It contains the final and effective rules of federal agencies, as well as any related official interpretations of the rules. Title 45 of the 50 C.F.R.s is dedicated to Public Welfare. Title 21 is dedicated to Food and Drugs. C.F.R. entries related to clinical research primarily include the following:

- **21 C.F.R. § 50: Protection of Human Subjects** covers informed consent requirements.
- **21 C.F.R. § 56: Institutional Review Boards** outlines the standards for IRBs in clinical investigations.
- **21 C.F.R. § 312: Investigational New Drug Application** governs the use of investigational drugs.
- **45 C.F.R. § 46: The Common Rule** provides the core set of regulations for the protection of human participants in research, including additional protections for vulnerable populations.

U.S. Food and Drug Administration

FDA ensures that medical treatments are safe and effective. It does not create new therapies or conduct clinical trials; it supervises the people who do. FDA staff meet with researchers and inspect clinical trial study sites to safeguard the rights of participants and to confirm the quality and integrity of data (Office of the Commissioner, 2023). Regulation 21 C.F.R. § 50 pertains to the protection of human participants, § 50.20 outlines the general rules for obtaining informed consent, § 50.25 specifies the elements that informed consent should include, and § 50.27 describes the procedures for recording informed consent.

The informed consent requirements in FDA regulations are not intended to preempt any applicable federal, state, or local laws that require additional information to be disclosed for informed consent to be legally effective. If a clinical investigation is conducted or supported by HHS, then the study may additionally be subject to 45 C.F.R. § 46 (Protection of Human Subjects, 2017). When regulations conflict, the ones that provide the highest level of protection to human participants should be followed.

Good Clinical Practice

The International Council for Harmonisation of Technical Requirements for Pharmaceuticals for Human Use (ICH) brings together regulatory agencies and pharmaceutical industry companies worldwide to foster greater alignment of quality standards for drug development and manufacturing. In 2025, it finalized *ICH Harmonised Guideline: Guideline for Good Clinical Practice: E6(R3)*. This is the third revision of ICH's internationally recognized ethical and scientific quality standards for designing, conducting, recording, and reporting trials involving human participants in research. Good Clinical Practice emphasizes informed consent, timely communication of new information, adaptation to participant abilities, protection of participant rights, and scientifically sound research. These guidelines safeguard the interests of participants and maintain the integrity of research.

Institutional Review Boards

In clinical research, protecting human participants is paramount, guided by federal regulations that outline the responsibilities of IRBs. The Common Rule (45 C.F.R. § 46) is the cornerstone of HHS policy, detailing IRB membership requirements, functions, and operations to ensure ethical standards and rigorous review processes. It mandates respect for participants' rights and welfare. Complementing this, FDA regulates clinical investigations through 21 C.F.R. § 56, which sets standards for IRB composition, operation, and responsibilities (Institutional Review Boards, 1981). It outlines criteria for IRB approval, expedited review procedures, and comprehensive recordkeeping to ensure transparency and accountability. Together, these regulations form a robust framework that upholds research integrity and protects human participants, enabling researchers and IRBs to advance science ethically.

The IRB reviews research protocols and informed consent documents to ensure adherence to ethical standards and regulations. It assesses risks, benefits, privacy protections, and consent procedures, ensuring investigators follow approved methods and participants are well-informed. The IRB confirms that the consent process is rigorous and respects participants' autonomy (Office of the Commissioner, 2023). It must also approve all consent forms before any research-related tests are conducted. No research-related tests can be performed until a participant voluntarily agrees to participate in the clinical research study and signs the informed consent document.

Standard of Care Tests

Standard of care testing refers to diagnostic procedures that are widely accepted and used by healthcare professionals for a specific condition. These tests may have been conducted before patients signed a consent form, and the test results are acceptable for use in qualifying patients for a research study. For example, a patient might undergo a computed tomography scan that indicates disease progression or have blood work performed. These tests are classified as standard of care. When assessing eligibility for a study, these test results can be used to qualify the patient, provided they fall within the defined eligibility window. For example, if a computed tomography scan is required within 28 days of signing consent, it is permissible to use a scan conducted within that time frame to determine eligibility.

Differences Between Federally Funded and Non-Federally Funded Research

The Congressional Research Service (2021) defines *federally funded research* as mission driven and often aligned with national priorities and public health goals, such as disease prevention, public health, and national security. It is subject to stringent federal regulations and oversight to ensure ethical standards and public accountability. Federally funded research aims to produce broad, long-term benefits for society, often through basic research that may not have immediate commercial applications.

Non-federally funded research frequently targets specific diseases or conditions and is driven by the interests of private foundations, corporations, or other nongovernmental entities. These entities have greater flexibility in terms of regulatory requirements and can respond more agilely to emerging scientific opportunities. This research is often geared toward developing marketable products or technologies, with a focus on innovation and potential for patents (National Bureau of Economic Research, 2021).

Protections for Special and Vulnerable Populations

Legally Authorized Representatives

Per federal regulations, a LAR is an individual, judicial, or other body authorized under applicable law to consent on behalf of a prospective research participant in a clinical trial. Some states have statutes, regulations, or common laws that specifically address consent by someone other than the research participant (OHRP, n.d.-a). A LAR must be treated the same as a participant in their assessment and understanding of the consent and research requirements.

Children and Adolescents

FDA regulations provide additional safeguards for children enrolled in clinical investigations. Both FDA and the Common Rule rely on 45 C.F.R. § 46 subpart D to protect children as research participants (Additional Protections for Children Involved as Subjects in Research, 1983). If a child is to be enrolled in a clinical investigation, parental or guardian permission must be obtained and documented. When appropriate, a child's assent must also be obtained (FDA, 2023). Definitions related to consent of a child include the following (OHRP, 2025):

- *Children* (younger than age 18 years) are individuals who have not attained the legal age for consent to treatments or procedures involved in research under the applicable law of the jurisdiction in which the study will be conducted.
- *Assent* is a child's affirmative agreement to participate in research.
- *Permission* refers to the agreement of parents or guardians to allow their child or ward to participate in research.
- *Parent* means a child's biologic or adoptive parent.
- A *guardian* is an individual who is authorized under applicable state or local law to consent on behalf of a child to general medical care.

Assent differs from parental or guardian permission for a child's participation in research. IRBs typically mandate seeking a minor child's assent when the child reaches age 7 years unless there is an impairment in decision-making capacity. For children aged 7–11 years, the assent form should be straightforward, enabling the child to comprehend the agreement. Specifically, the form should succinctly convey the following (OHRP, n.d.-b):

- The request for participation in a research study
- The study's purpose
- The approximate duration of participation
- The activities involved upon agreement to participate (e.g., answering questions)
- The immediate foreseeable risks, discomforts, and potential benefits rather than distant or hypothetical outcomes
- The encouragement to ask questions to parents or researchers about the participation
- The voluntary nature of participation, with the option to withdraw at any time
- The awareness of the child's father, mother, or guardian about the invitation to join the study

Investigators should consider the specific characteristics of their study population and decide which elements of informed consent are most relevant for children aged 12–14 years. For adolescents aged 15–17 years, the assent form should be similar to the one used for adult participants (Rochester Institute of Technology, n.d.).

Non-English–Speaking Participants

When prospective participants do not understand English, IRBs and investigators must ensure that the information given to these individuals or their legal LARs is in a language understandable to them (21 C.F.R. § 50.27) (Documentation of Informed Consent, 1981). If consent is not available in a potential participant's native language, they may elect to use a short form. According to 21 C.F.R. § 50.27 and 45 C.F.R. § 46.117, a short form is a written consent document stating that the elements of informed consent required by § 50.25 have been presented orally to the participant or their LAR. When this method is used, a witness must be present for the oral presentation, and the IRB must approve a written summary of what is to be communicated to the participant or their LAR. Only the short form itself is to be signed by the participant or LAR. The witness, the participant (or LAR), and the person giving consent must all sign a summary copy. The participant or LAR will receive a copy of the summary and the short form (21 C.F.R. § 50.27). If the informed consent is translated into the patient's language, a copy of the translated consent should be provided to the participant (Documentation of Informed Consent, 1981).

Older Adults

Studies that include participants with comorbidities will more likely produce results that reflect the clinical realities of older adults in clinical settings (Kuchel, 2019). A 2019 study by Altawalbeh et al. noted that a lack of consistency and repeating questions were the most common obstacles to consent for this population. The authors concluded that ensuring privacy, dedicating more time to the consent process, treating older adults as autonomous individuals, and respecting their cultural beliefs were the most effective strategies. Investigators and OCRNs must be aware of the special needs that some older adults may require during the informed consent discussion (Altawalbeh et al., 2019).

Pregnant Women, Fetuses, and Neonates

Including pregnant patients in research poses unique challenges, but with proper methodologic, ethical, and clinical approaches, it is possible to reduce the knowledge gap and enhance drug safety and availability for this population (Zur, 2023). Pregnancy can intensify or reveal various medical, social, cultural, or psychological vulnerabilities. Nonetheless, pregnant individuals retain their ability to assess risks and benefits and make informed decisions based on their values (Ashcroft, 2016).

According to 45 C.F.R. § 46.204, the government provides the following additional protections for pregnant females and fetuses (Research Involving Pregnant Women or Fetuses, 2001):

- Preclinical studies on pregnant animals and clinical studies on nonpregnant females must provide data on potential risks.
- Risk to the fetus should be minimal or outweighed by direct benefit to the female or important biomedical knowledge.
- If research benefits only the fetus, consent from both parents is needed.
- Researchers must fully inform participants about potential impacts on the fetus or neonate.

As stated in 45 C.F.R. § 46.205, research can include neonates whose viability is uncertain or who are not viable. Consent must cover potential effects on the neonate. Researchers cannot assess neonate viability while a study is ongoing (Research Involving Neonates, 2001).

Prisoners

According to 45 C.F.R. § 46.303, a *prisoner* is any individual involuntarily confined or detained in a penal institution (Definitions, 1978). This includes those sentenced under criminal or civil statutes, detained in other facilities as alternatives to criminal prosecution or incarceration, or pending arraignment, trial, or sentencing.

When conducting research involving prisoners, advocates can be consulted to review protocols and consent forms to prevent exploitation of a population that may not have full access to resources to guarantee their rights. A prisoner advocate in clinical research trials is a voting IRB member who is either a prisoner or a prisoner representative with relevant background and experience. These individuals play a crucial role in ensuring ethical treatment and safeguarding the rights of prisoners involved in research. They can be current or former prisoners, prison chaplains, prison psychologists, social workers, or anyone qualified to represent the rights and welfare of prisoners (OHRP, 2004).

When conducting research involving prisoners, the IRB must make seven specific findings:

- The proposed research falls into one of the permissible categories of research under 45 C.F.R. § 46.306(a)(2) (Permitted Research Involving Prisoners, 1978).
- Risks to prisoners are minimized.
- The research design is sound.
- Adequate provisions are in place for informed consent.
- The research plan includes appropriate safeguards for privacy and confidentiality.
- The research plan provides for equitable participant selection.
- The research plan includes a process for prisoner participation in decision-making regarding research involvement.

According to OHRP (2004), these findings ensure the ethical and responsible conduct of research when working with prisoner populations.

Genetic Testing and Genomic Research

The Genetic Information Nondiscrimination Act (GINA) is a federal law that safeguards against genetic discrimination in employment and health insurance. It makes it illegal for employers and insurance companies to obtain genetic information or use it to discriminate against a research participant. GINA was enacted in 2008 to address concerns related to the misuse of genetic data and ensure equal protection for individuals based on their genetic profile (OHRP, 2009).

Within the informed consent, GINA ensures that participants are informed about their rights and protections against genetic discrimination. This includes recommendations for language that should be included in consent forms to inform participants about their rights under GINA, such as the prohibition of genetic discrimination by health insurers and employers (OHRP, 2009). Additionally, the Equal Employment Opportunity Commission outlines how GINA protects individuals from employment discrimination based on genetic information.

Participant Capacity

Prior to engaging in the consent process, investigators must assess the participant's cognitive capacity and decision-making abilities. Investigators and other research personnel have a legal and ethical obligation to verify that prospective participants possess sufficient knowledge and comprehension of all elements of informed consent. This understanding enables them to make informed decisions about whether to participate in a study. An individual's willingness to sign an informed consent form and the absence of unanswered questions do not necessarily indicate complete comprehension (Association of Clinical Research Professionals, 2013).

Some individuals may have diminished decision-making capacity because of mental disorders, neurologic issues, age, or medication use. Investigators must consider whether a prospective participant's diminished capacity affects their ability to provide informed consent (Mayo Clinic, n.d.).

The presentation of key information at the beginning of the consent process can help facilitate discussions between a prospective participant and an investigator about whether the participant should be involved in a trial (FDA, 2023).

Health Insurance Portability and Accountability Act

A clinical trial Health Insurance Portability and Accountability Act (HIPAA) authorization is a document signed by the research participant that provides permission to allow a covered entity (i.e., clinical research site) to use or disclose protected health information for research (OHRP, 2004), which is also described in the authorization section of the consent form. HIPAA authorization must be written in a manner that is easy to understand for its purposes and to the recipients stated in the authorization. According to HHS

(2018), HIPAA authorization must include the following components:

- A specific description of the information that will be used or disclosed
- The names or specific identification of the individuals authorized to disclose and receive the information
- Identification of the individuals or organizations to whom information will be disclosed
- Description of the use or purpose for disclosure of protected health information
- A time frame for the authorization
- The participant's right to withdraw HIPAA authorization in writing or otherwise, as well as exceptions to withdraw
- A statement that the covered entity may not condition treatment, payment, enrollment, or eligibility for benefits on whether the individual signs the authorization
- The consequences of a refusal to sign the authorization when the covered entity is permitted to condition treatment, enrollment in the health plan, or eligibility for benefits on a failure to obtain authorization

Although federal regulations permit HIPAA authorization to be included in trial-specific informed consent, sponsors and research facilities may opt for a separate document. Participants should receive a copy of this authorization for their records.

The Study Team

Principal Investigator

According to the C.F.R., a principal investigator (PI) is defined as a single individual designated by an organization to lead and direct a research project, possessing an appropriate level of authority and responsibility. The term is often used interchangeably with *investigator* in regulatory documents. However, the PI is typically the lead investigator responsible for the overall conduct of the study at a trial site (Ceh, 2022). Specifically, the investigator is the person under whose immediate direction the drug is administered and dispensed to a participant. The PI is tasked with protecting the rights, safety, and welfare of participants under their care (21 C.F.R. § 50.3) (Definitions, 2025). They are also responsible for educating all research study staff and supervising the processes and procedures.

The PI can assign the task of consenting to a person who has the necessary education, training, and experience. The person obtaining informed consent should be knowledgeable about the clinical investigation and possess the appropriate training and credentials to answer any questions that may arise. These are often referred to as subinvestigators These individuals do not hold the same level of responsibility as the PI, but they are involved in various aspects of the research under the PI's supervision (Ceh, 2022). The PI should have a clear plan for supervising and training staff. The investigator ensures that legally valid, informed consent is obtained (FDA, 2024).

Oncology Clinical Research Nurse

Oncology clinical research nursing is a distinct field that demands a thorough understanding of federal regulations governing clinical research. OCRNs are integral to ensuring clinical oversight and achieving protocol fidelity, all while protecting the safety and autonomy of human research participants. Additionally, they are pivotal in the process of obtaining and maintaining informed consent (Barlow, 2020). The OCRN role is vital to the conduct of clinical trials and is guided by the principle of good ethical practice and ethical codes. C.F.R. provides regulations for the conduct of clinical trials, and the specific roles and responsibilities of OCRNs may be defined by the research institution or the trial protocol (National Institutes of Health Clinical Center, n.d.).

OCRNs' responsibilities can vary widely, including reinforcing the informed consent process by providing patient and caregiver education, advocating for ethical care for research participants, administering investigational drugs, collecting biospecimens, and monitoring for side effects. The Oncology Nursing Society and Oncology Nursing Certification Corporation (2024) identified various skills and abilities often assigned to OCRNs, including navigating barriers to informed consent and collaborating with the PI to ensure that the consent process is performed and documented. They assess the patient's understanding of the information provided during the consent process and ensure comprehension and safety during initial and ongoing clinical trial informed consent discussions.

OCRNs are pivotal in research implementation. They address patient misconceptions, collaborate during the study, and collect data on adverse events. Additionally, they assist with dosing adjustments, reinforce study modifications, and educate patients on amendments or other changes related to the research study.

Case Study: Consent Process

- **Introduction to the trial:** Dr. Smith outlines the trial's purpose, treatment, and potential benefits and risks. Sue, an OCRN, provides a detailed consent document.
- **Assessing understanding:** Sue asks Mr. Bell, the potential research participant, to summarize his understanding of the trial, clarifying any misconceptions.
- **Discussing risks and benefits:** Sue and Dr. Smith discuss side effects and benefits, emphasizing informed decision-making and voluntary participation.

- **Answering questions:** Sue thoroughly answers Mr. Bell's questions about procedures and their impact on daily life; she also addresses his family's concerns.
- **Assessing competency:** Sue ensures that Mr. Bell fully understands the information using a checklist.
- **Obtaining consent:** Sue reviews the consent form with Mr. Bell, who signs it in the presence of the investigator. She provides Mr. Bell with a signed copy for his records.
- **Follow-up**: Sue schedules a follow-up appointment and provides her contact information for any immediate queries.
- **Conclusion:** Sue's compassionate and thorough approach ensures that Mr. Bell is well-informed and comfortable with his decision to participate in the clinical trial, facilitating clear communication and patient support.

A Hypothetical Clinical Trial: Draft Guidance

Key Information Section

Some possible methods to assist people who want to communicate information briefly and clearly include the following:

- Start the discussion by stating the main information about the study. This information can be repeated several times during the consent discussion. Inform potential participants that participation is optional, that they can withdraw at any time, and that their decision will not affect the care they receive.
- Include the purposes of the research, expected duration, and procedures to be followed. This may be a single sentence describing the study and explaining why they are being asked to participate. Given the variability of the study design, details of key information will differ. Discuss the expected duration of their participation, a high-level description of the major procedures, a brief description of medical products and authorization status, and any experimental procedures.
- Provide information on the most common and serious risks and discomforts. Acknowledge that unknown risks can occur.
- Discuss benefits to the participant or prospective participant. If there is no benefit to the participant, this should be clearly stated.
- Clear and concise information should be provided on alternative treatments or procedures.
- Information on compensation and medical treatment for research-related injuries is critical, especially when no compensation is planned.
- Use the teach-back method to validate a patient's understanding of the informed consent. An essential element of this method is using non-shaming language and putting the responsibility for patient understanding on the nurse. Examples of teach-back include the following:
  - "It is my job to explain things clearly. To make sure I did this, please tell me, in your own words, the risks of this trial."
  - "This is important for your safety. I want to make sure you understand. Please tell me how you are going to take the study medications."

Regan (2018) emphasized that the OCRN is ethically and legally required to verbally review and discuss informed consent with patients before they participate in clinical research trials. OCRNs play a crucial role in safeguarding patients' ability to make informed and autonomous decisions during the consent process. Furthermore, OCRNs can offer educational resources and allocate time for patients to ask questions and receive answers throughout the informed consent process.

Documentation of Informed Consent

The IRB must approve a written consent form that documents the informed consent. The participant or the LAR must sign and date the form when they consent. They will receive a copy of the form. A short-form written consent document will state that the elements of informed consent were orally presented to the participant or LAR. There must be a witness for the oral presentation. The IRB will have approved a written summary of the oral presentation, and the participant and LAR will receive copies of the documents (21 C.F.R. § 50.27) (Documentation of Informed Consent, 1981).

Use of Electronic Informed Consent and Consent Waivers

According to OHRP (2021), the research community is increasingly showing interest in using electronic media to supplement or replace paper-based informed consent processes. These electronic processes may enable rapid notification of any amendments to the informed consent that may impact participation in research.

HHS defines *electronic informed consent* as using electronic systems and processes that may include various electronic media, such as text, graphics, audio, video, podcasts, websites, biologic recognition devices, and card readers, to convey study-related information and obtain informed consent. This electronic consent should contain the same essential elements as traditional informed consent and be designed for easy navigation (OHRP, 2021). Hyperlinks can be used to improve accessibility. Additionally, strategies should be implemented to ensure that participants review all consent materials before providing consent. Special attention should be given to participants who may have limited experience with electronic systems, visual impairments, or motor skill challenges (OHRP, 2021).

The process can be done either on-site or remotely. The electronic system must have a way to verify that the person who signs the informed consent electronically is either the participant who will participate in the research study or a LAR (21 C.F.R. § 11.100) (General Requirements, 1997). For remote consenting, the investigator must implement mechanisms for reviewing the consent and allowing sufficient time for participants to ask questions before making a final decision. The OCRN can support this by communicating with the potential participant to ensure their questions are answered and that they feel confident in their decision. Additional strategies include communication through a combination of electronic messages, telephone calls, video conferences, or live chats.

Electronic Signatures

Regulation 21 C.F.R. § 11 establishes standards and guidelines for electronic records and signatures used within the pharmaceutical and healthcare industries, specifically those related to the manufacturing, storage, and distribution of FDA-regulated products (Electronic Records; Electronic Signatures, 1997). It sets forth criteria to ensure authenticity, integrity, and reliability when used (eSignly, 2025). This regulation ensures that electronic records and electronic signatures are considered trustworthy, reliable, and equivalent to paper records and handwritten signatures (General Requirements, 1997).

Waiver of Informed Consent

If an IRB waives the requirement for documentation of informed consent (21 C.F.R. § 56.110), FDA recommends that the elements of the informed consent be reviewed verbally with the participant or LAR (Expedited Review, 1981). Additionally, the IRB may require the investigator to provide participants with a written statement regarding the clinical investigation (OHRP, n.d.-a). The PI and OCRN remain responsible for ensuring that participants comprehend the research, even in cases where formal consent is not obtained for signing.

Protocol Amendments

A sponsor shall submit a protocol amendment describing any change in a protocol that significantly affects the safety of participants, the scope of the investigation, or the scientific quality of the study. Examples include the following (FDA, n.d.):

- A new safety risk
- A change in drug dosage or duration
- Significant change in the design of the protocol
- Addition of new tests or procedures
- A change in investigator
- Amendments reviewed and approved by the IRB before being implemented
- Reconsents or consent addendums

Research is an ongoing process that involves the constant reevaluation of information and procedures. Investigators are ethically obligated to keep participants and LARs apprised of all issues related to participation in the study (University of Virginia, 2024). The participants or LARs should be informed in a timely manner if new information becomes available that may be relevant to their willingness to continue participating in the trial. The communication of this information should be documented (FDA, 2018b). A consent addendum serves as a concise version of study changes. The OCRN and PI must ensure that the patient fully understands these changes before signing to continue participating in the trial.

Summary

OCRNs must grasp the rules, regulations, governing agencies, and historical context that have shaped informed consent regulations. With a focus on patients with cancer, a particularly vulnerable population, the informed consent process is emphasized even more and is often their primary safeguard. OCRNs must collaborate closely with investigators, meticulously review consent forms, actively listen to participant questions, and ensure that participants feel confident in their decisions. A cohesive team of patients, investigators, and OCRNs can help to advance clinical research and elevate medical practice.

Key Points

- Informed consent is crucial in clinical research to ensure that participants understand the study's purpose, procedures, risks, benefits, and alternative treatments. It allows participants to make autonomous and informed decisions about their involvement.
- According to 21 C.F.R. § 50.20, investigators must obtain legally effective informed consent from participants or their LARs before involving them in research. The consent process must provide sufficient time for decision-making and avoid coercion or undue influence.
- The use of electronic systems and processes for informed consent is becoming more prevalent. These systems must convey study-related information clearly and allow for easy navigation. They should also include strategies to ensure that participants review all consent materials and consider the needs of those with limited familiarity with electronic systems.
- OCRNs play a vital role in the informed consent process. They ensure that participants are fully informed and protected, facilitate the consent process, and provide educational opportunities for participants to ask questions and understand the study.
- Special considerations are necessary for obtaining assent from minors and consent from pregnant individuals. Assent forms for children should be straightforward and age-appropriate, and pregnant individuals should be supported in making informed decisions without assuming diminished decision-making capacity.

The author would like to acknowledge Angela D. Klimaszewski, MSN, RN, for her contribution to this chapter that remains unchanged from the previous edition of this book.

References

Additional Protections for Children Involved as Subjects in Research, 45 C.F.R. § 46(d) (1983). https://www.ecfr.gov/current/title-45/subtitle-A/subchapter-A/part-46/subpart-D

Altawalbeh, S.M., Alkhateeb, F.M., & Attarabeen, O.F. (2019). Ethical issues in consenting older adults: Academic researchers and community perspectives. *Journal of Pharmaceutical Health Services Research, 11*(1), 25–32. https://doi.org/10.1111/jphs.12327

Ashcroft, R. (2016). Ethical issues in a trial of maternal gene transfer to improve fetal growth. In F. Baylis & A. Ballantyne (Eds.), *Clinical research involving pregnant women* (pp. 247–263). Springer International.

Association of Clinical Research Professionals. (2013). *The process of informed consent.* https://acrpnet.org/wp-content/uploads/2016/09/ACRPWhitePaperTheProcessofInformedConsent.pdf

Barlow, C. (2020). Human subjects protection and federal regulations of clinical trials. *Seminars in Oncology Nursing, 36*(2), 151001. https://doi.org/10.1016/j.soncn.2020.151001

Ceh, S.E. (2022, February 15). The clinical research investigator: Clarifying the misconceptions. *Clinical Researcher, 36*(1). https://acrpnet.org/2022/02/15/the-clinical-research-investigator-clarifying-the-misconceptions

Congressional Research Service. (2021). *Federally funded research and development centers (FFRDCs): Background and issues for Congress (No. R44629).* https://www.congress.gov/crs-product/R44629

Definitions, 21 C.F.R. § 50.3 (2025). https://www.ecfr.gov/current/title-21/chapter-I/subchapter-A/part-50/subpart-A/section-50.3

Definitions, 45 C.F.R. § 46.303 (1978). https://www.ecfr.gov/current/title-45/subtitle-A/subchapter-A/part-46/subpart-C/section-46.303

Documentation of Informed Consent, 21 C.F.R. § 50.27 (1981). https://www.ecfr.gov/current/title-21/chapter-I/subchapter-A/part-50/subpart-B/section-50.27

Documentation of Informed Consent, 45 C.F.R. § 46.117 (2017). https://www.ecfr.gov/current/title-45/subtitle-A/subchapter-A/part-46/subpart-A/section-46.117

Electronic Records; Electronic Signatures, 21 C.F.R. § 11 (1997). https://www.ecfr.gov/current/title-21/chapter-I/subchapter-A/part-11

eSignly. (2025). *Mastering compliance: The ultimate guide to CFR part 11 and electronic signatures for streamlined operations and increased profits.* https://www.esignly.com/electronic-signature/cfr-part-11-and-electronic-signatures-a-comprehensive-guide.html

Expedited Review Procedures for Certain Kinds of Research Involving No More Than Minimal Risk, and for Minor Changes in Approved Research, 21 C.F.R. § 56.110 (1981). https://www.ecfr.gov/current/title-21/chapter-I/subchapter-A/part-56/subpart-C/section-56.110

General Requirements, 21 C.F.R. § 11.100 (1997). https://www.ecfr.gov/current/title-21/chapter-I/subchapter-A/part-11/subpart-C/section-11.100

General Requirements for Informed Consent, 21 C.F.R. § 50.20 (1980). https://www.ecfr.gov/current/title-21/chapter-I/subchapter-A/part-50/subpart-B/section-50.20

General Requirements for Informed Consent, 45 C.F.R. § 46.116 (2017). https://www.ecfr.gov/current/title-45/subtitle-A/subchapter-A/part-46/subpart-A/section-46.116

International Council for Harmonisation of Technical Requirements for Pharmaceuticals for Human Use. (2025). *ICH harmonised guideline: Guideline for good clinical practice: E6(R3).* https://database.ich.org/sites/default/files/ICH_E6%28R3%29_Step4_FinalGuideline_2025_0106.pdf

Institutional Review Boards, 21 C.F.R. § 56 (1981). https://www.ecfr.gov/current/title-21/chapter-I/subchapter-A/part-56

Investigational New Drug Application, 21 C.F.R. § 312 (1987). https://www.ecfr.gov/current/title-21/chapter-I/subchapter-D/part-312

IRB Review of Research, 21 C.F.R. § 56.109 (1981). https://www.ecfr.gov/current/title-21/chapter-I/subchapter-A/part-56/subpart-C/section-56.109

Kuchel, G.A. (2019). Inclusion of older adults in research: Ensuring relevance, feasibility, and rigor. *Journal of the American Geriatrics Society, 67*(2), 203–204. https://doi.org/10.1111/jgs.15802

Mayo Clinic. (n.d.). *50: Informed consent and assessment of capacity to consent to research.* https://www.mayo.edu/research/documents/50-informed-consent-and-assessment-of-capacity-to-consent-to-research/doc-20180876

National Bureau of Economic Research. (2021). *Are federal and private research funding substitutes?* https://www.nber.org/digest/202103/are-federal-and-private-research-funding-substitutes

National Institutes of Health. (n.d.). *Institutional review boards (IRBs) and protection of human subjects.* https://grants.nih.gov/grants/guide/notice-files/not93-209.html

National Institutes of Health Clinical Center. (n.d.). *Clinical research nursing.* https://www.cc.nih.gov/nursing/crn/2010

Office for Human Research Protections. (n.d.-a). *Informed consent frequently asked questions.* https://www.hhs.gov/ohrp/regulations-and-policy/guidance/faq/informed-consent/index.html

Office for Human Research Protections. (n.d.-b). *Research with children FAQs.* https://www.hhs.gov/ohrp/regulations-and-policy/guidance/faq/children-research/index.html

Office for Human Research Protections. (2004). *Guidance on approving research involving prisoners.* https://www.hhs.gov/ohrp/regulations-and-policy/guidance/prisoner-research-ohrp-guidance-2003/index.html

Office for Human Research Protections. (2009). *Guidance on the Genetic Information Nondiscrimination Act.* Office for Human Research Protections. https://www.hhs.gov/ohrp/regulations-and-policy/guidance/guidance-on-genetic-information-nondiscrimination-act/index.html

Office for Human Research Protections. (2021). *Use of electronic informed consent in clinical investigations: Questions and answers. FDA guidance document.* https://www.fda.gov/regulatory-information/search-fda-guidance-documents/use-electronic-informed-consent-clinical-investigations-questions-and-answers.

Office for Human Research Protections. (2023). *About research participation.* https://www.hhs.gov/ohrp/education-and-outreach/about-research-participation/index.html

Office for Human Research Protections. (2025). *Draft guidance on key information for facilitating understanding in informed consent.* https://www.hhs.gov/ohrp/regulations-and-policy/requests-for-comments/draft-guidance-key-information-facilitating-understanding-informed-consent/index.html#kis-b

Office of the Commissioner. (2018). *Informed consent for clinical trials.* https://www.fda.gov/patients/clinical-trials-what-patients-need-know/informed-consent-clinical-trials

Office of the Commissioner. (2023). *Basics about clinical trials.* U.S. Food and Drug Administration. https://www.fda.gov/patients/clinical-trials-what-patients-need-know/basics-about-clinical-trials

Oncology Nursing Society & Oncology Nursing Certification Corporation. (2024). *Oncology clinical research nurse competencies.* https://www.ons.org/sites/default/files/2025-01/ocrn-competencies-rebrand.pdf

Permitted Research Involving Prisoners, 45 C.F.R. § 46.306 (1978). https://www.ecfr.gov/current/title-45/subtitle-A/subchapter-A/part-46/subpart-C/section-46.306

Protection of Human Subjects, 45 C.F.R. § 46 (2017). https://www.ecfr.gov/current/title-45/subtitle-A/subchapter-A/part-46

Regan, E.M. (2018). Clinical trials informed consent: An educational intervention to improve nurses' knowledge and communication skills. *Clinical Journal of Oncology Nursing, 22*(6), E152–E158. https://doi.org/10.1188/18.CJON.E152-E158

Research Involving Neonates, 45 C.F.R. § 46.205 (2001). https://www.ecfr.gov/current/title-45/subtitle-A/subchapter-A/part-46/subpart-B/section-46.205

Research Involving Pregnant Women or Fetuses, 45 C.F.R. § 46.204 (2001). https://www.ecfr.gov/current/title-45/subtitle-A/subchapter-A/part-46/subpart-B/section-46.204

Rochester Institute of Technology. (n.d.). *Children as research subjects: Assent tips.* https://www.rit.edu/hsro/children-as-research-subjects#assent-tips

U.S. Department of Health and Human Services. (1979). *The Belmont Report: Ethical principles and guidelines for the protection of human subjects of research.* https://www.hhs.gov/ohrp/regulations-and-policy/belmont-report/read-the-belmont-report/index.html

U.S. Department of Health and Human Services. (2018). *Guidance on HIPAA authorizations for future research.* https://www.hhs.gov/guidance/sites/default/files/hhs-guidance-documents/hipaa-future-research-authorization-guidance-06122018%2520v2.pdf

U.S. Department of Health and Human Services. (2023). *About HHS.* https://www.hhs.gov/about/index.html

U.S. Food and Drug Administration. (n.d.). *Protocol amendments (21 CFR 312.30).* https://www.ecfr.gov/current/title-21/chapter-I/subchapter-D/part-312/subpart-B/section-312.30

U.S. Food and Drug Administration. (2018). *ICH E6(R2) Good clinical practice: Integrated addendum to ICH E6(R1).* https://www.fda.gov/media/93884/download

U.S. Food and Drug Administration. (2023). *Informed consent: Guidance for IRBs, clinical investigators, and sponsors. Good clinical practice.* https://www.fda.gov/media/88915/download?trk=public_post_comment-text

U.S. Food and Drug Administration. (2024). *Basics about clinical trials.* https://www.fda.gov/patients/clinical-trials-what-patients-need-know/basics-about-clinical-trials

University of Virginia. (2024). *Re-consenting requirements.* https://research.virginia.edu/irb-hsr/re-consenting-requirements

Zur, R.L. (2023). Protected from harm, harmed by protection: Ethical consequences of the exclusion of pregnant participants from clinical trials. *Research Ethics Review, 19*(4), 536–545. https://doi.org/10.1177/17470161231189843

CHAPTER 13

Protocol Development and Response Assessment

Elizabeth Ness, MS, RN, CRN-BC

Introduction

Careful planning is crucial for the success of a clinical trial. Planning comes before writing the protocol and should include the following aspects:

- Formulating research questions/objectives
- Defining end points and measurement tools
- Determining study design
- Defining study population
- Describing study interventions and required procedures
- Determining sample size and statistical analysis

Planning a clinical trial involves multiple members of the research team, including the principal investigator, statisticians, oncology clinical research nurses (OCRNs), and other providers, investigators, and researchers. OCRNs provide valuable insights into the operationalization of a protocol because of their knowledge of the clinical aspects of patients with the disease under investigation and research regulations.

This chapter will provide information associated with developing an oncology protocol and assessing disease response. See Chapter 11 for additional protocol elements that are not addressed in this chapter.

Objectives and End Points

Formulating a sound research question means it is feasible, interesting, novel, ethical, and relevant. Clear and precise objectives describe how the proposed research question will be accomplished (Jagadeesh et al., 2023). The objectives need to be tied to measurable end points, and a primary objective must be identified. There may also be several secondary or exploratory objectives.

Primary and Secondary Objectives

The primary objective is the most important central question being asked in the protocol and serves as the basis for the study design and sample size. It is a short statement of the purpose of the study that should answer the following questions (Stoney & Johnson, 2017):

- Is this a comparative or descriptive study?
- What are the end points of primary interest?
- What is the research participant population?
- What are the interventions to be used?

Secondary objectives relate to the primary objective and are of secondary importance. These objectives may involve additional aspects of study interest, such as the collection of biospecimens to answer correlative questions or quality-of-life (QoL) measurements.

Direct and Surrogate End Points

End points are selected based on clinical relevance, interpretability, practicality, and affordability to measure. There are direct and surrogate end points. Direct end points are clinically meaningful and directly measure how an individual feels, functions, or survives. They can be objective (e.g., survival, disease exacerbation) or subjective (e.g., patient-reported outcomes [PROs]).

Surrogate, or substitute, end points are alternatives to clinical outcomes and have been used for drug approval under 21 Code of Federal Regulations § 314 Subpart H: Accelerated Approval of New Drugs for Serious or Life-Threatening Illnesses. For example, instead of overall survival, progression-free survival or time to progression could be used as surrogates (Delgado & Guddati, 2021).

OCRNs can play a critical role during protocol development to ensure that the objectives are measurable and have a tool or method for evaluation. They can also review the procedures outlined in the protocol document to ensure that they are related to the objectives and that the institution has the capability to execute the procedures outlined in the study.

OCRNs may consider whether aspects of the study, such as medication adherence, are relevant to nursing practice and should be studied during the trial. They can also consider bringing forward concerns or questions during the protocol development stage to determine if additional objectives can be considered for incorporation into the protocol as a secondary survey or instrument (e.g., QoL) for data collection.

Study Design

The study design is based on the objectives that need to be answered, ethical considerations, as well as the resources that are available within the research organization to be able to implement a clinical trial successfully. The primary objective drives the study design used. The study design should address the following:

- The phase of the study
- The need for early stopping rules
- The number of treatment arms
- How participants are assigned treatment by randomization (i.e., by random choice usually directed by a computer-generated coin toss, by direct assignment, or by other means, such as physician or participant choice)
- How randomization is stratified so that each subgroup of participants, defined by entry characteristics, is balanced between treatment arms

For more information on study designs, including observational designs, see Chapters 3, 4, and 5.

Study Eligibility

Individuals enrolled in a clinical trial will ultimately be those who may benefit from the trial and who are not at a greater risk. Eligibility is written in a format that defines inclusion and exclusion criteria. Inclusion criteria are the elements that must be satisfied before a patient can enter a trial, whereas exclusion criteria identify elements that, if met, will keep the patient from participating in the trial. When writing a protocol, much thought is given to the participant population (Bartrum & Karp, 2017; Stoney & Johnson, 2017). The protocol must specify, through the eligibility criteria, a clearly defined patient group, thereby minimizing any unnecessary or confounding variables in reaching the end points of the study and protecting the patients from a greater risk of harm.

Once determined, eligibility criteria must be strictly followed. For example, if a platelet count of more than $100,000/mm^3$ is required, then patients with a platelet count of $101,000/mm^3$ can be enrolled. Those with a platelet count of $99,000/mm^3$ cannot be enrolled. Similarly, if a hemoglobin level below 10 g/dl is identified in the exclusion criteria, then patients with a hemoglobin level of 9.8 g/dl will not be eligible to participate in the trial. Although it is possible to have an exception granted for minimal variances, it is essential to remember that eligibility criteria were established for the safety of the participant; therefore, exceptions should be rare.

Eligibility criteria should not be too restrictive. Broadening eligibility will enable more patients to participate, making the trial population more representative and the results more generalizable, thereby accelerating accrual. Since 2016, efforts have been made to broaden the eligibility criteria in oncology clinical trials to maximize the generalizability of trial results and increase inclusivity in the study population. Some examples of this include allowing individuals with the following (Kim et al., 2017):

- Patients with previously treated or stable brain metastases are eligible if they meet specific criteria (e.g., not on treatment, off steroids for at least one month prior to enrollment).
- Adolescent and pediatric patients can enroll after safety and toxicity in adults have been established.
- Patients with HIV need to be on effective anti-retroviral therapy with specific criteria identified for cluster of differentiation 4 and T-cell counts.
- Patients with poor kidney function need to have a creatinine clearance of 30 ml/min.

Before proceeding with baseline assessments or study intervention, OCRNs are responsible for confirming that all criteria have been met. This is accomplished by interviewing patients, reviewing the medical record, and obtaining documentation of all required data prior to enrollment. Any concerns about eligibility should be discussed with the principal investigator, who will ultimately be responsible for confirming eligibility.

Pathology

Pathology reports are crucial in determining patient eligibility in oncology clinical trials. Some institutions require a special review if the original pathology was performed at another facility. Clinical trial networks and sponsors sometimes require a centralized review of pathology specimens to ensure consistency. These requirements should be delineated clearly within the protocol.

Stage of Disease

Protocol eligibility criteria identify patients with a specific stage of disease for enrollment. The purpose of staging systems is to classify or describe the extent of disease, providing physicians with sufficient information to determine treatment options and prognostic indicators. The most common system for staging or categorizing the extent of disease for solid tumors is the TNM system. In this system,

T is the primary tumor size, N indicates the regional lymph node involvement, and M represents distant metastasis. It is based on a clinical assessment and workup and has been accepted by the Union for International Cancer Control and the American Joint Committee on Cancer (National Cancer Institute [NCI], 2022). TNM staging is essential for phase 1 and 2 studies, in which the primary goal is to determine the response in a specific stage of a disease. Other staging systems are considered based on the disease. Examples include the following:

- Rai system (used predominantly in the United States) or the Binet system (used widely in the United Kingdom and Europe) for chronic lymphocytic leukemia (Binet et al., 1981; Rai et al., 1975; Shadman, 2023)
- Lugano classification for Hodgkin and non-Hodgkin lymphoma (Cheson et al., 2014)
- International Staging System for multiple myeloma (Palumbo et al., 2015)
- International Neuroblastoma Risk Group staging system for neuroblastoma (Monclair et al., 2009)
- International Retinoblastoma staging system for retinoblastoma (Chantada et al., 2006)

When developing disease-specific inclusion criteria, it may be useful to include the actual staging criteria as an appendix in the protocol with the appendix referenced in the inclusion criteria.

The physician is responsible for assessing the clinical and pathologic stages of a patient's disease. Staging is frequently discussed at tumor board meetings or in consultations with physicians from related disciplines, such as pathology and radiology, and documentation is a requirement of the American College of Surgeons for accreditation. OCRNs typically confirm that staging has been completed and documented in the medical record before enrolling the patients into a study.

Performance Status

In oncology trials, standard scales and criteria are used to quantify a patient's general well-being and objectively assess their ability to perform ordinary tasks (e.g., activities of daily living). These ratings of performance status have been shown to correlate reasonably well with overall survival (Allende-Perez et al., 2022; Assayag et al., 2023; Meyers et al., 2023). Performance status is commonly used in the clinical oncology setting; OCRNs may already be familiar with this concept. When developing a protocol, selecting a performance status scale is typically a component of the inclusion criteria. The two most commonly used performance status scales for adults are the Karnofsky Performance Status Scale (Karnofsky et al., 1948) and the Eastern Cooperative Oncology Group Performance Status Scale (Oken et al., 1982). The Lansky scale (Lansky et al., 1987) is used when a pediatric population is included in a clinical trial. In addition to inclusion criteria, performance status may also be used for stratification in either randomization or data analysis.

Study Interventions and Required Procedures

The protocol should be written to include clear and detailed descriptions of the study interventions (e.g., study drug administration, radiation therapy) and all procedures (e.g., physical examinations, biospecimen collections, radiologic procedures) that will be required for both safety and efficacy assessments. Developing a schedule of events table is beneficial (see Figures 13-1 and 13-2). When determining the frequency of procedures, it is helpful to prioritize what is essential for meeting protocol objectives and assessing participant safety versus what would be valuable but not essential data, as the participant will already be in for a visit. An example would be the value, but not the necessity, of a monthly bone marrow biopsy when disease staging would be routinely needed every two months. It is important to remember that nonessential data, although valuable, may have an invasive or time-intensive component, which can impact accrual or retention.

All procedures should have specified timepoints that delineate when they are to be completed (Bartrum & Karp, 2017; Stoney & Johnson, 2017). It is helpful to build in an allowable range for these periods to accommodate an unforeseen circumstance that might result in deviation from the protocol. For example, if safety laboratory tests are required weekly, the protocol should specify that they must be performed on day 8, plus or minus two days. This assumes the variance will not compromise participant safety.

Biospecimen Collection

Many protocols require the collection of research-specific biospecimens throughout the study. Some of these samples may even be used for eligibility criteria (e.g., vascular endothelial growth factor status), for treatment assignment, or as a stratification variable. It is important that the protocol or a manual of procedures clearly includes the following information (NCI, 2016):

- Types of test tubes or other specimen collection systems to be used
- Timepoint samples to be collected
- Storage of samples until processing (e.g., on ice for no more than 15 minutes, room air)
- Contact person for sample processing
- How samples will be processed (i.e., temperature, speed and duration of time for centrifuge, number of aliquots required)
- Sample storage, including location and freezer temperature
- How and when to ship samples, if applicable
- Identified or de-identified samples
- Description of when, if, and how results will be discussed with the participant

Procedure	Screening	Baseline	Cycle 1					Subsequent Cycles			Off-Treatment Follow-up
			Day X	Day X	Day X	Day X	Day X	Day X	Day X	Day X	
History and physical examination											
Vital signs											
Performance score											
Labs (list specific labs)											
Correlative research samples											
Pharmacokinetics and pharmacodynamics											
Radiologic assessments (list specific studies)											
Other specific assessments (e.g., electrocardiogram, echocardiogram, pulmonary function test)											
Response evaluation											
Adverse events assessment											
Concomitant medications use											

FIGURE 13-1 | Sample Template for Protocol Schedule of Events Table

Off-Treatment Follow-Up

If a study has both off-treatment and off-study criteria, it is essential to specify the study procedures that will be performed once off treatment, including the frequency. Including this information in the schedule-of-events table is helpful to ensure that the data are collected to meet the study objectives.

Protocols with long-term follow-up (e.g., until participant death to measure overall survival) need to identify the following:

- What procedures will be conducted and when
- What data elements will be collected
- Who will be responsible for the continued follow-up
- What measures will secure follow-up for those participants who do not comply with the protocol-specified time (e.g., phone call, return-receipt letter)
- What determines whether a participant is to be deemed "lost to follow-up"

Additionally, the informed consent document should clearly outline the long-term follow-up period and what will be done during this time, such as conducting a phone call or telehealth visit to assess survival.

Oncology Trial End Points and Measurement Tools

The measurement tools used in a protocol need to assess the primary and secondary objectives of the protocol. This typically includes tools to measure safety, response, and QoL, as well as the identification of correlative markers or assays to measure specimens that will be collected on the protocol. In oncology, a standard adverse event measurement tool, the NCI Cancer Therapy Evaluation Program's Common Terminology Criteria for Adverse Events (CTCAE), is used to assess the safety or tolerability of an intervention. The field of oncology also has internationally agreed-upon standards for measuring response for hematologic and solid tumors. These standard tools help to ensure high-quality data that are comparable across studies. When evaluating symptom management end points, numerous QoL surveys or PRO tools are available. Some of these surveys and tools are subject to copyright laws, requiring permission for their use.

Safety End Points

All protocols must address safety. In oncology clinical trials, the standard tool used to measure adverse events is CTCAE. Because of its size, the protocol is often written with the web address for accessing the latest version of the CTCAE. For example, a protocol template could state (NCI CTEP, 2025):

The descriptions and grading scales found in the revised NCI CTEP CTAE version 5.0 will be used for adverse event reporting. All appropriate treatment areas should have access to a copy of CTCAE version 5.0: https://dctd.cancer.gov/research/ctep-trials/for-sites/adverse-events

For more information about CTCAE, see Chapter 22.

	Screening	Baseline	C1 D1	C1 D15	C2 D1	C3+ D1	Q2 Cycles	Off-Treatment Follow-up
Medical history	X							
Concurrent medications	X							
Physical examination	X		X		X	X	X	X
Vital signs	X		X					X
Height	X							
Weight	X				X	X	X	X
Performance status	X		X		X	X		X
Complete blood count with differential, platelets	X		X	X	X	X	X	X
Serum chemistry	X		X		X	X	X	X
Electrocardiogram		X						
B-HCG	X							
Tumor biopsies			X		X			
Radiologic assessment	X					X	X	X
Adverse events assessment		X	X					
Research blood			X		X	X	X	X

FIGURE 13-2 | Example Protocol Schedule of Events Document

C—cycle; D—day; Q—quarter

Disease Response

In the 1970s, the U.S. Food and Drug Administration (FDA) used overall response rate as the primary end point for approving drugs used in oncology. This relied solely on physical and radiologic examination to assess tumor status. However, in the 1980s, FDA began including other end points: disease-free survival, overall survival, improvement in QoL, and relief of tumor-related symptoms (FDA, 2009, 2018; see Table 13-1).

Every protocol must include how disease response will be assessed (i.e., measured). In oncology clinical trials, standards for response criteria have been established, typically through expert consensus, for both solid tumors and hematologic malignancies. Some of the aforementioned staging systems serve as examples. Outside of the research setting, these standards have been used as a guide to help clinicians and patients decide whether to continue therapy.

When using radiologic assessments to evaluate disease response, consistency is crucial to minimize variation between practitioner interpretation and equipment. It is helpful to designate a radiologist to measure tumors at each site while using a consistent methodology (e.g., computed tomography [CT] scan, magnetic resonance imaging, plain films). Ideally, the same scanning equipment should be used, but this may not always be feasible.

TABLE 13-1 | Clinical Trial End Points

End Point	Definition
Overall survival	• Time from randomization until death • Intent-to-treat population
Disease-free survival	• Randomization until recurrence of tumor or death from any cause • Adjuvant setting after definitive surgery or radiation therapy • A large percentage of patients with complete response after chemotherapy
Objective response rate	• The proportion of patients with a reduction of tumor size of a predefined amount and for a minimum time period • Measure from the time of initial response until progression • The sum of partial response patients and complete response patients • Uses standardized criteria when possible
Progression-free survival	• Randomization until objective tumor progression or death • Preferred regulatory end point • Assumes deaths are related to progression
Time to progression	• Randomization until objective tumor progression, excluding deaths
Time to treatment failure	• Randomization to discontinuation of treatment for any reason (e.g., progressive disease, toxicity, death) • Not recommended for regulatory drug approval

Note. Based on information from U.S. Food and Drug Administration, 2018.

Solid Tumor Response Assessment

Best practices for evaluating solid tumors include the following (Eisenhauer et al., 2009):

- Characterizing the overall tumor burden through quantitative evaluation of lesions
- Identifying lesions before initiating therapy
- Using the same method of investigation (e.g., using the same radiographic procedure and equipment) for each assessment timepoint
- Confirming complete and partial responses

Initial attempts to standardize the assessment of solid tumors began as far back as the 1960s with little success. In 1994, an international task force composed of members from the European Organisation for Research and Treatment of Cancer, NCI, and NCI Canada Clinical Trials Group was formed to address this issue. After a retrospective tumor response review of 4,000 patients, the task force made recommendations to simplify response evaluation for solid tumors by using the longest diameter, identifying target and nontarget lesions, and standardizing the assessment of these lesions and new lesions to evaluate overall response. The new criteria, Response Evaluation Criteria in Solid Tumors (RECIST), was intended for solid tumor response assessment in phase 2 clinical trials but was actually used for response assessment in all phases (Therasse et al., 2000). The task force committed to the continual improvement of RECIST, resulting in the 2009 publication of RECIST 1.1 (Eisenhauer et al., 2009).

Understanding how to use RECIST 1.1 involves understanding the measurability of lesions (i.e., whether a disease is measurable or nonmeasurable) and which lesions will be used to determine tumor response (i.e., target or nontarget lesions). Measurable disease is a tumor lesion that is 10 mm or larger, as measured by CT scan (with a slice thickness of 5 mm or less), or twice the slice thickness if the CT scan uses slices thicker than 5 mm. Therefore, when reviewing a CT scan report, it is essential to understand the scanner's slice thickness. When measurements are taken by clinical examination (e.g., using calipers) or via chest x-ray, a measurable lesion is defined as 10 mm or larger and 20 mm or larger, respectively. Nonmeasurable disease encompasses all other lesions, including bone lesions, leptomeningeal disease, ascites, pleural or pericardial effusions, inflammatory breast disease, or cystic lesions (Eisenhauer et al., 2009).

Evaluating tumor response helps in determining the efficacy of study interventions. This evaluation includes lymph nodes. Target and nontarget lesions must be identified at baseline, with the same lesions followed over time. A target lesion is a measurable lesion. There can be a total of five measurable lesions, and all organs with measurable lesions must be represented, with no more than two lesions per organ identified. The selection of target lesions is based on their size and suitability for accurate repeated measurements so that the sum of the diameters becomes the final measurement for target lesions.

Nontarget lesions are any other lesions or sites of disease not classified as a target lesion that are measured as being present at baseline and either present or absent at follow-up. It is acceptable to record multiple nontarget lesions in the same organ or as a single item on a case report form. Lymph nodes are measured using the short axis. To be a target lesion, a lymph node must be 15 mm or larger; a nontarget lesion is a lymph node smaller than 15 mm. If the lymph node is smaller than 10 mm, it is considered normal (Eisenhauer et al., 2009).

To determine the overall response using RECIST 1.1, the individual assessments of both target and nontarget lesions, as well as the assessment of new lesions, are combined. The four response types for target lesions are as follows (Eisenhauer et al., 2009):

- A complete response is characterized by the disappearance of all target lesions, and any pathologic lymph nodes (whether target or nontarget) must exhibit a reduction in the short axis to less than 10 mm.
- A partial response is defined as a 30% or greater decrease in the sum of the diameters of target lesions compared to the baseline sum diameters.
- Progressive disease is at least a 20% increase in the sum of the diameters of target lesions, taking as reference the smallest sum on study (this includes the baseline sum if that is the smallest on study). A relative increase of 20% must have the sum be an absolute increase of at least 5 mm. Progressive disease is also defined as the appearance of one or more new lesions.
- Stable disease is neither a partial response nor progressive disease, as defined by the smallest sum diameters while on study.

Because nontarget lesions have no associated measurements, their response is defined by the presence, absence, or appearance of new lesions. Responses are defined as follows (Eisenhauer et al., 2009).

- A complete response is characterized by the disappearance of all nontarget lesions and normalization of the tumor marker level. All lymph nodes must be nonpathologic in size (less than 10 mm at the short axis). If tumor markers are initially above the upper limit of normal, they must return to normal for a patient to be considered in complete clinical response.
- Noncomplete response/nonprogressive disease is the persistence of one or more nontarget lesions or maintenance of tumor marker levels above the normal limits.
- Progressive disease is the appearance of one or more new lesions or the unequivocal progression of existing nontarget lesions. Unequivocal progression should not typically supersede target lesion status. It must be representative of the overall change in disease status, not just a single lesion increase.

The overall response is best summarized in Table 13-2 for those with measurable disease and in Table 13-3 for those with only nonmeasurable disease. These tables, along with other RECIST information, should be included in the protocol. The NCI Cancer Therapy Evaluation Program (2025) has RECIST language that can be used when writing a protocol.

TABLE 13-2 | Best Overall Response Criteria for Patients With Measurable (Target) Disease

Target Lesions	Nontarget Lesions	New Lesions	Overall Response	Best Overall Response When Confirmation Is Required*
CR	CR	No	CR	≥ 4 weeks confirmation**
CR	Non-CR/ non-PD	No	PR	≥ 4 weeks confirmation**
CR	Not evaluated	No	PR	≥ 4 weeks confirmation**
PR	Non-CR/ non-PD/not evaluated	No	PR	≥ 4 weeks confirmation**
SD	Non-CR/ Non-PD/not evaluated	No	SD	Documented at least once ≥ 4 weeks from baseline**
PD	Any	Yes or no	PD	No prior SD, PR, or CR
Any	PD***	Yes or no	PD	No prior SD, PR, or CR
Any	Any	Yes	PD	No prior SD, PR, or CR

*See RECIST 1.1 manuscript for further details on what is evidence of a new lesion.

**Only for nonrandomized trials with response as primary end point

***In exceptional circumstances, unequivocal progression in nontarget lesions may be accepted as disease progression.

CR—complete response; PD—progressive disease; PR—partial response; SD—stable disease

Note. Patients with a global deterioration of health status requiring discontinuation of treatment without objective evidence of disease progression at that time should be reported as *symptomatic deterioration.* Every effort should be made to document the objective progression even after discontinuation of treatment.

From *CTEP Generic Protocol Template for Cancer Treatment Trial,* by National Cancer Institute Cancer Therapy Evaluation Program, 2025, p. 88 (https://dctd.cancer.gov/research/ctep-trials/trial-development/etctn-protocol-template.docx). In the public domain.

TABLE 13-3 | Best Overall Response Criteria for Patients With Nonmeasurable (Nontarget) Disease

Non-target Lesions	New Lesions	Overall Response
CR	No	CR
Non-CR/non-PD	No	Non-CR/non-PD*
Not all evaluated	No	Not evaluated
Unequivocal PD	Yes or No	PD
Any	Yes	PD

*Non-CR/non-PD is preferred over "stable disease" for nontarget disease since SD is increasingly used as an end point for assessment of efficacy in some trials, so to assign this category when no lesions can be measured is not advised.

CR—complete response; PD—progressive disease

Note. From *CTEP Generic Protocol Template for Cancer Treatment Trial,* by National Cancer Institute Cancer Therapy Evaluation Program, 2025, pp. 88–89 (https://dctd.cancer.gov/research/ctep-trials/trial-development/etctn-protocol-template.docx). In the public domain.

iRECIST

Immunotherapy frequently leads to a response that resembles a tumor flare. Disease response for individuals meeting the criteria for progressive disease per RECIST 1.1 was noted to have a response after being removed from the treatment that was deep and durable. This phenomenon is referred to as *pseudoprogression*, characterized by an increase in lesion size or the visualization of new lesions, followed by a response that may be durable. iRECIST is based on RECIST 1.1 (Seymour et al., 2017). The protocol should specify whether iRECIST will be used to determine the response or if the iRECIST response will be used in conjunction with RECIST. All responses defined using iRECIST criteria are designated with the prefix *i*- (e.g., iCPD is confirmed progressive disease using iRECIST) (Seymour et al., 2017). The iRECIST timepoint and best overall responses are usually recorded separately on a case report form. See Table 13-4 for the iRECIST timepoint response and Table 13-5 for the best overall iRECIST response.

Hematologic Malignancy Response Assessment

Internationally agreed-upon response standards exist for certain hematologic malignancies. Bone marrow assessment is a key component in response assessment (see Table 13-6). This chapter will not review the specific details of each disease response because of the complexity of these standards and the diversity of hematologic malignancies. However, OCRNs should refer to protocol specifics to determine the method for response criteria.

Health-Related Quality of Life

QoL assessment is an additional oncology trial end point of increasing interest. Although the measures of QoL are subjective (i.e., patient reported), their value cannot be overemphasized. With the increasing number of potential treatments available to participants that could prolong life, QoL data as a trial end point can provide information that participants may use for various treatment considerations. FDA has a guidance document to assist in using PRO measures to support a medical product label (FDA, 2009). This may serve as a helpful resource when writing a protocol that has PRO-related objectives.

To determine how to measure a QoL- or PRO-related outcome, the principal investigator needs to select an appropriate QoL or PRO tool. Assessment tools are frequently under copyright, so permission is often required for both the use and analysis of the data. When considering a tool, the developer's website will typically provide both the psychometrics and the population for which the tool has been previously used. Tool development for a specific population's QoL issue requires validation, which is beyond the scope of this publication. However, the tool author or developer can often be contacted and may be able to assist with adapting the application and validating the tool in the proposed study population.

Once the tools have been identified, consideration of when the assessment will be administered is important (e.g., during clinical appointments, at protocol procedure time points), along with the method of delivery (e.g., in person, by mail, electronically). OCRNs can assist in protocol development by ensuring that the protocol incorporates the following:

- Whether the tool can be completed by someone else on behalf of the participant, whether the participant can give verbal responses versus written, or if the response must be written
- Description of when the responses will be reviewed, especially if any items might have immediate clinical implications (e.g., suicidal ideation, harm to others)
- How responses will be returned (e.g., by secure electronic link, via a provided self-addressed, prepaid return envelope)
- Where or how the tools will be stored

Sample Size and Statistical Analysis

It is important to get a statistician involved early in the development process of a clinical trial. They can assist in determining the sample size and selecting the appropriate study design and analysis. Determining the appropriate number of participants needed for a study to answer research questions helps to conserve resources and protect the safety of participants, and allows the study to be completed in a timely manner (International Council for Harmonisation of Technical Requirements for Pharmaceuticals for Human Use [ICH], 2016). The clinical trial results can then be statistically reported with confidence, and those results, either positive or negative, can be disseminated to the scientific community.

TABLE 13-4 | Time Point Response for iRECIST

Target Lesions*	Nontarget Lesions*	New Lesions*	Time Point Response	
			No Prior iUPD**	Prior iUPD**, ***
iCR	iCR	No	iCR	iCR
iCR	Non-iCR/Non- iUPD	No	iPR	iPR
iPR	Non-iCR/Non- iUPD	No	iPR	iPR
iSD	Non-iCR/Non- iUPD	No	iSD	iSD
iUPD with no change OR decrease from last TP	iUPD with no change OR decrease from last TP	Yes	NA	NLs confirms iCPD if NLs were previously identified and increase in size (≥5 mm in SOM for NLT or any increase for NLNT) or number. If no change in NLs (size or number) from last TP, remains iUPD
iSD	iUPD	No	iUPD	Remains iUPD unless iCPD confirmed based in further increase in size of NT disease (need not meet RECIST 1.1 criteria for unequivocal PD)
iUPD	Non-iCR/Non-iUPD	No	iUPD	Remains iUPD unless iCPD confirmed based on further increase in SOM of at least 5 mm, otherwise remains iUPD
iUPD	iUPD	No	iUPD	Remains iUPD unless iCPD confirmed based on further increase in: • Previously identified T lesion iUPD SOM ≥5 mm and/or • NT lesion iUPD (prior assessment - need not be unequivocal PD)
iUPD	iUPD	Yes	iUPD	Remains iUPD unless iCPD confirmed based on further increase in: • Previously identified T lesion iUPD ≥5 mm and/or • Previously identified NT lesion iUPD (need not be unequivocal) and/or • Size or number of new lesions previously identified
Non-iUPD/PD	Non-iUPD/PD	Yes	iUPD	Remains iUPD unless iCPD confirmed based on increase in size or number of new lesions previously identified

*Using RECIST 1.1 principles. If no PsPD occurs, RECIST 1.1 and iRECIST categories for CR, PR, and SD would be the same.

**In any lesion category

***Previously identified in assessment immediately prior to this TP

CR—complete response; iCPD—confirmed progressive disease; NL—new lesion; NLNT—new lesion non-target; NLT—new lesion target; PR—partial response; PsPD—pseudo-progression; RECIST—Response Evaluation Criteria in Solid Tumors; SD—stable disease; SOM—site of metastasis

Note. From *CTEP Generic Protocol Template for Cancer Treatment Trial*, by National Cancer Institute Cancer Therapy Evaluation Program, 2025, pp. 94–95 (https://dctd.cancer.gov/research/ctep-trials/trial-development/etctn-protocol-template.docx). In the public domain.

A clinical trial must be large enough to ensure that the results are statistically valid and can be generalized to the target population. If the study is too small, an important new therapy may be missed, or a toxic or lethal regimen could be accepted for use in a large population. Such a study may also provide incomplete or incorrect information, potentially resulting in a waste of not only time and effort but also limitations on participants and financial resources. Additional considerations when determining the sample size include the phase of the study, strategies for addressing dropouts or withdrawals, and the distinction between medically important and statistically significant differences between interventions (ICH, 1998).

The statistical analysis outlines the methods that will be used to analyze the primary and secondary end points, including any interim or periodic analyses that may be necessary for safety or efficacy. The analysis also focuses on handling stratification, including the selection of participants

TABLE 13-5 | iRECIST Best Overall Response

TPR 1	TPR 2	TPR 3	TPR 4	TPR 5	iBOR
iCR	iCR, iPR, iUPD, NE	iCR, iPR, iUPD, NE	iUPD	iCPD	iCR
iUPD	iPR, iSD, NE	iCR	iCR, iPR, iSD, iUPD, NE	iCR, iPR, iSD, iUPD, iCPD, NE	iCR
iUPD	iPR	iPR, iSD, iUPD, NE	iPR, iSD, iUPD, NE, iCPD	iPR, iSD, iUPD, NE, iCPD	iPR
iUPD	iSD, NE	PR	iPR, iSD, iUPD, NE	iPR, iSD, iUPD, iCPD, NE	iPR
iUPD	iSD	iSD, iUPD, NE	iSD, iUPD, iCPD, NE	iSD, iUPD, iCPD, NE	iSD
iUPD	iCPD	Anything	Anything	Anything	iCPD
iUPD	iUPD	iCPD	Anything	Anything	iCPD
iUPD	NE	NE	NE	NE	iUPD

iCR—immune complete response; iUPD—immune progressive disease; iPR—immune partial response; iSD—immune stable disease; NE—not evaluable that cycle

Note. Table assumes a randomized study where confirmation of CR or PR is not required. Designation "I" for BOR can be used to indicate prior iUPD to aid in data interpretation. For patients with nontarget disease only at baseline, only CR or non-CR/non-PD can be assigned at each TPR but is not shown in the table for ease of presentation.

From *CTEP Generic Protocol Template for Cancer Treatment Trial,* by National Cancer Institute Cancer Therapy Evaluation Program, 2025, p. 96 (https://dctd.cancer.gov/research/ctep-trials/trial-development/etctn-protocol-template.docx). In the public domain.

for the analysis, the approach to handling missing data, and the criteria used to determine study termination (ICH, 1998, 2016). Many statistical issues that arise during data analysis, such as post-randomization dropout or noncompliance with protocol therapy, cannot be foreseen at the time of design. However, every attempt should be made to anticipate data problems that could compromise the analysis.

TABLE 13-6 | Summary of Selected Hematologic Response Assessments

Disease	Methods of Measuring Disease
Malignant lymphomas	Disease response is based on • Nodal masses using fludeoxyglucose (FDG)–positron-emission tomography (PET) or PET/computed tomography (CT) • Spleen and/or liver assessed by CT • Bone marrow biopsy
Acute myeloid leukemia	Disease response is based on • Neutrophils • Platelets • Bone marrow biopsy for blasts • Cytogenetics • Extramedullary disease
Multiple myeloma	Disease response is based on • Serum and urine M protein • Serum free light chain • Bone marrow • Lytic lesion assessment • Calcium level

Note. Based on information from Cheson et al., 2003, 2014; Kumar et al., 2016.

Summary

Interaction among the entire research team is crucial in establishing the objectives, end points, and design for a clinical trial. OCRNs are critical in this interaction, serving as gatekeepers to ensure that the study protocol follows a logical assessment plan and that study procedures and assessments, including disease response and follow-up, are not burdensome on patients (Oncology Nursing Society & Oncology Nursing Certification Corporation, 2024). Each of these considerations must be implemented in an environment that fosters the integrity of the study data.

Key Points

- OCRNs add valuable, clinically applicable knowledge to the design and implementation of a protocol and should be included in the development process.
- OCRNs play a critical role during protocol development to ensure that the objectives are clinically measurable and that a tool or method for evaluating the outcome is included in both baseline and follow-up assessments.
- A critical function of the OCRN role is adherence to study inclusion and exclusion criteria—those elements that define patient eligibility. Inclusion criteria are the elements that must be satisfied before patients can enter into a trial. In contrast, exclusion

criteria identify elements that, if met, will keep patients from participating in the trial.

- When determining the frequency of procedures, it is helpful to delineate between what is essential for meeting protocol objectives and the evaluation of participant safety versus what would be valuable but not essential data when participants return for a study visit.
- RECIST is intended for solid tumor response assessment; determining overall response using RECIST combines the individual assessment for both target and nontarget lesions while assessing for the appearance of new lesions.
- Statistically calculating the appropriate number of participants needed for a study is a critical step to answering the proposed protocol research question while conserving resources and completing the study in a timely manner. Study results can then be statistically reported with confidence, and those results, whether positive or negative, can be disseminated to the scientific community.

The author would like to acknowledge Lydia T. Madsen, PhD, RN, OCN®, AOCNS®, for her contribution to this chapter that remains unchanged from the previous edition of this book.

References

Allende-Pérez, S., Rodríguez-Mayoral, O., Peña-Nieves, A., & Bruera, E. (2022). Performance status and survival in cancer patients undergoing palliative care: Retrospective study. *BMJ Supportive and Palliative Care*. Advance online publication. https://doi.org/10.1136/spcare-2022-003562

Assayag, J., Kim, C., Chu, H., & Webster, J. (2023). The prognostic value of Eastern Cooperative Oncology Group performance status on overall survival among patients with metastatic prostate cancer: A systematic review and meta-analysis. *Frontiers in Oncology, 13,* 1194718. https://doi.org/10.3389/fonc.2023.1194718

Bartrum, E.A., & Karp, B.I. (2017). Writing a protocol. In J.I. Gallin, F.P. Ognibene, & L.L. Johnson (Eds.), *Principles and practice of clinical research* (4th ed., pp. 219–229). Elsevier. https://doi.org/10.1016/B978-0-12-849905-4.00016-2

Binet, J.L., Auquier, A., Dighiero, G., Chastang, C., Piguet, H., Goasguen, J., ... Gremy, F. (1981). A new prognostic classification of chronic lymphocytic leukemia derived from a multivariate survival analysis. *Cancer, 48*(1), 198–206. https://doi.org/10.1002/1097-0142(19810701)48:1<198::aid-cncr2820480131>3.0.co;2-v

Chantada, G., Doz, F., Antoneli, C.B., Grundy, R., Clare Stannard, F.F., Dunkel, I.J., ... Zucker, J.M. (2006). A proposal for an international retinoblastoma staging system. *Pediatric Blood and Cancer, 47*(6), 801–805. https://doi.org/10.1002/pbc.20606

Cheson, B.D., Bennett, J.M., Kopecky, K.J., Büchner, R., Willman, C.L., Estey, E.H., ... Bloomfield, C.D. (2003). Revised recommendations of the International Working Group for diagnosis, standardization of response criteria, treatment outcomes, and reporting standards for therapeutic trials in acute myeloid leukemia. *Journal of Clinical Oncology, 21*(24), 4642–4649. https://doi.org/10.1200/JCO.2003.04.036

Cheson, B.D., Fisher, R.I., Barrington, S.F., Cavalli, F., Schwartz, L.H., Zucca, E., ... Lister, T.A. (2014). Recommendations for initial evaluation, staging, and response assessment of Hodgkin and non-Hodgkin lymphoma: The Lugano classification. *Journal of Clinical Oncology, 32*(27), 3059–3068. https://doi.org/10.1200/JCO.2013.54.8800

Delgado, A., & Guddati, A.K. (2021). Clinical endpoints in oncology - a primer. *American Journal of Cancer Research, 11*(4), 1121–1131.

Eisenhauer, E.A., Therasse, P., Bogaerts, J., Schwartz, L.H., Sargent, D., Ford, R., ... Verweik, J. (2009). New response evaluation criteria in solid tumours: Revised RECIST guideline (version 1.1). *European Journal of Cancer, 45*(2), 228–247. https://doi.org/10.1016/j.ejca.2008.10.026

International Council for Harmonisation of Technical Requirements for Pharmaceuticals for Human Use. (1998). *Statistical principles for clinical trials E9.* https://database.ich.org/sites/default/files/E9_Guideline.pdf

International Council for Harmonisation of Technical Requirements for Registrations of Pharmaceuticals for Human Use. (2016). *Integrated addendum to ICH E6(R1): Guidelines for good clinical practice E6(R2).* https://database.ich.org/sites/default/files/E6_R2_Addendum.pdf

Jagadeesh, G., Balakumar, P., & Senatore, F. (2023). The roadmap to research: Fundamentals of a multifaceted research process. In G. Jagadeesh, P. Balakumar, & F. Senatore (Eds.), *The quintessence of basic and clinical research and scientific publishing* (pp. 3–20). Springer. https://doi.org/10.1007/978-981-99-1284-1_22

Karnofsky, D.A., Abelmann, W.H., Craver, L.F., & Burchenal, J.H. (1948). The use of nitrogen mustard in the palliative treatment of carcinoma. *Cancer, 1*(4), 634–656. https://doi.org/10.1002/1097-0142(194811)1:4<634::AID-CNCR2820010410>3.0.CO;2-L

Kim, E.S., Bruinooge, S.S., Roberts, S., Ison, G., Lin, N.U., Gore, L., ... Schilsky, R.L. (2017). Broadening eligibility criteria to make clinical trials more representative: American Society of Clinical Oncology and Friends of Cancer Research joint research statement. *Journal of Clinical Oncology, 35*(33), 3737–3744. https://doi.org/10.1200/JCO.2017.73.7916

Kumar, S., Paiva, B., Anderson, K.C., Durie, B., Landgren, O., Moreau, P., ... Avet-Loiseau, H. (2016). International Myeloma Working Group consensus criteria for response and minimal residual disease assessment in multiple myeloma. *Lancet Oncology, 17*(8), e328–e346. https://doi.org/10.1016/S1470-2045(16)30206-6

Lansky, S.B., List, M.A., Lansky, L.L., Ritter-Sterr, C., & Miller, D.R. (1987). The measurement of performance in childhood cancer patients. *Cancer, 60*(7), 1651–1656. https://doi.org/10.1002/1097-0142(19871001)60:7<1651::aid-cncr2820600738>3.0.co;2-j

Meyers, D.E., Pasternak, M., Dolter, S., Grosjean, H.A.I., Lim, C.A., Stukalin, I., ... Pabani, A. (2023). Impact of performance status on survival outcomes and health care utilization in patients with advanced NSCLC treated with immune checkpoint inhibitors. *JTO Clinical and Research Reports, 4*(4), 100482. https://doi.org/10.1016/j.jtocrr.2023.100482

Monclair, T., Brodeur, G.M., Ambros, P.F., Brisse, H.J., Cecchetto, G., Holmes, K., ... Pearson, A.D. (2009). The International Neuroblastoma Risk Group (INRG) staging system: An INRG Task Force report. *Journal of Clinical Oncology, 27*(2), 298–303. https://doi.org/10.1200/JCO.2008.16.6876

National Cancer Institute. (2016). *NCI best practices for biospecimen resources.* https://dctd.cancer.gov/data-tools-biospecimens/biospecimens-biobanks/resources/best-practices/best-practices-2016

National Cancer Institute. (2022). *Cancer staging.* https://www.cancer.gov/about-cancer/diagnosis-staging/staging

National Cancer Institute Cancer Therapy Evaluation Program. (2025). *CTEP generic protocol template for cancer treatment trial.* https://dctd.cancer.gov/research/ctep-trials/trial-development/etctn-protocol-template.docx

Oken, M.M., Creech, R.H., Tormey, D.C., Horton, J., Davis, T.E., McFadden, E.T., & Carbone, P.P. (1982). Toxicity and response criteria of the Eastern Cooperative Oncology Group. *American Journal of Clinical Oncology, 5*(6), 649–655. https://doi.org/10.1097/00000421-198212000-00014

Oncology Nursing Society & Oncology Nursing Certification Corporation. (2024). *Oncology clinical research nurse competencies.* https://www.ons.org/sites/default/files/2025-01/ocrn-competencies-rebrand.pdf

Palumbo, A., Avet-Loiseau, H., Oliva, S., Lokhorst, H.M., Goldschmidt, H., Rosinol, L., ... Moreau, P. (2015). Revised International Staging System for multiple myeloma: A report from International Myeloma Working Group. *Journal of Clinical Oncology, 33*(26), 2863–2869. https://doi.org/10.1200/JCO.2015.61.2267

Rai, K.R., Sawitsky, A., Cronkite, E.P., Chanana, A.D., Levy, R.N., & Pasternack, B.S. (1975). Clinical staging of chronic lymphocytic leukemia. *Blood, 46*(2), 219–234. https://doi.org/10.1182/blood-2016-08-737650

Seymour, L., Bogaerts, J., Perrone, A., Ford, R., Schwartz, L.H., Mandrekar, S., ... de Vries, E.G.E. (2017). iRECIST: Guidelines for response criteria for use in trials testing immunotherapeutics. *Lancet Oncology, 18*(3), e143–e152. https://doi.org/10.1016/S1470-2045(17)30074-8

Shadman, M. (2023). Diagnosis and treatment of chronic lymphocytic leukemia: A review. *JAMA, 329*(11), 918–932. https://doi.org/10.1001/jama.2023.1946

Stoney, C.M., & Johnson, L.L. (2017). Development and conduct of studies. In J.I. Gallin, F.P. Ognibene, & L.L. Johnson (Eds.), *Principles and practice of clinical research* (4th ed., pp. 230–218). Elsevier Academic Press. https://doi.org/10.1016/B978-0-12-849905-4.00015-0

Subpart H—Accelerated Approval of New Drugs for Serious or Life-Threatening Illnesses, 21 C.F.R. Part 314 Subpart H (1985). https://www.ecfr.gov/current/title-21/part-314/subpart-H

Therasse, P., Arbuck, S.G., Eisenhauer, E.A., Wanders, J., Kaplan, R.S., Rubinstein, L., ... Gwyther, S. (2000). New guidelines to evaluate the response to treatment in solid tumors. *Journal of the National Cancer Institute, 92*(3), 205–216. https://doi.org/10.1093/jnci/92.3.205

U.S. Food and Drug Administration. (2009). *Guidance for industry: Patient-reported outcome measures: Use in medical product development to support labeling claims.* https://www.fda.gov/media/77832/download

U.S. Food and Drug Administration. (2018). *Clinical trial endpoints for the approval of cancer drugs and biologics: Guidance for industry.* https://www.fda.gov/regulatory-information/search-fda-guidance-documents/clinical-trial-endpoints-approval-cancer-drugs-and-biologics

CHAPTER 14

Virtual Clinical Trials

Elizabeth A. Johnson, PhD, MS-CRM, RN

Introduction

Imagine it is 5 am in the heart of a Montana winter. Clay's mother, weary but resolute, shovels snow from around the car, her breath visible in the bitter cold. With 18 inches of snowfall forecasted by midday, she knows they must leave now, well before sunrise, to make the 240-mile journey to Clay's clinical trial appointment. The earlier they go, the safer the drive. It is not just the storm pushing her to depart at this hour. With overnight lodging near the trial site far beyond her budget, especially after reducing her work hours to care for Clay full time, she has no choice but to make the entire trip in one day. A hotel room means cutting back on the family's groceries or utilities. The clinical trial could be Clay's only chance at slowing his disease, and missing a dose because of the weather or finances is not an option she is willing to consider. Bundling Clay in his favorite blanket, she gently buckles him into the back seat, thanks her parents for watching her other children, and pulls onto the icy road. The sky is still dark, the streets silent—but for Clay's mother, this is what hope looks like.

For many clinical research participants, this scenario is all too familiar. Significant travel burdens and limited resources or supportive services can often strain families or individuals already under considerable stress and pressure from adapting their lives to a schedule of assessments. During the COVID-19 pandemic, clinical trial sponsors and sites faced a flurry of changes to keep research moving, which included the broader adoption of virtual or decentralized participant procedures and visits. Virtual clinical trials, also known as decentralized clinical trials, use technology and local resources to make research participation more accessible. This can include electronic consent and specimen collection at nearby laboratories to reduce the need for participants to travel to a clinical trial site when feasible (Ranganathan et al., 2023; Van Norman, 2021). Although this concept has been actualized through decentralized elements or pieces of clinical research, trials fully remote from the research site became more commonplace during the pandemic, with a 2022 estimation of 81.9% of protocols in one sample having at least one decentralized element of study conduct (de Jong et al., 2022).

This boom in clinical research in community settings has led to an increased need for nursing support, particularly from oncology clinical research nurses (OCRNs) who specialize in oncology clinical trials and can be trained to deliver trial procedures and manage participants in a mobile manner (Beg & Bustos, 2022). In a sample of 85 clinical research executives, nearly half (48%) intended to integrate mobile nursing as a critical element for the success of decentralized trials (Beg & Bustos, 2022). Although listed as a critical element, oncology OCRNs often find themselves managing a multitude of new technologies and an expanding workload of in-person and virtual clinical trial demands, accompanied by variable training and questions related to licensure and scope, which enables decentralized trial conduct.

This chapter will provide an overview of virtual (decentralized) clinical trial concepts, approaches, and conduct considerations. It will also look toward the future trajectory of innovative trial designs that influence how this specialty is used and incorporated, with key stakeholder involvement, to advance opportunity equity and patient centricity in modern research.

What Is in a Name? The Terminology Turmoil

Any search engine inquiry of a *virtual clinical trial* may return several different terminologies, which may either overlap or vary depending on the context of the trial's overall design. A virtual clinical trial lends to a process focus: How do we conduct the trial? The terminology expands to include words that designate trials that are heavily dependent on digital technologies, such as *siteless trials*, *digital trials*, *decentralized trials*, and *remote trials*

(Ranganathan et al., 2023). In these types of trials, the investigative product may be shipped directly to the participant, the consent may be completed via an electronic platform, and participant monitoring may be achieved via electronic questionnaires and wearable devices (Faulkner, 2021). Eligibility criteria will also be virtually evaluated through the use of electronic health record data mining or by having participants self-report their eligibility in an online survey or intake platform. A *siteless trial* may be a misnomer because operations and conduct are still provided at a site level, but the term refers to the absence of in-person visits, which are hallmarks of traditional clinical research (Faulkner, 2021).

Although some approach the use of a term through a focus on process, other stakeholders may use a different term to emphasize the distinguishing characteristics of a study's design or conceptual approach/method. Examples include *decentralized*, *digital*, and *teletrial*.

Decentralized trials are a conceptual approach to conducting research activities at the participant's location rather than on-site. They can be adopted as decentralized elements (a hybrid of on-site and off-site) or fully decentralized, meaning no on-site visits and all activities are conducted in the community or home setting (Faulkner, 2021).

Digital trials can also be viewed through a methodologic lens, specifically in terms of data capture methods that use only technological platforms rather than paper forms (Faulkner, 2021).

A teletrial is a model by which to execute a conceptual design through the process of resource-sharing across research sites and communities (Sabesan, 2023). Through clustered networks of primary and satellite facilities, rural residents, in particular, have the opportunity to access trials closer to home. In contrast, the facilities benefit from a cohesive and standardized approach to trial conduct (Sabesan, 2023). A key example of teletrial success as a model is the Australasian Teletrial Program, which has resulted in not only operational excellence in clinical research but also capacity building and workforce development that enables sustainable growth and outcomes evaluation of the model's use when embedded in decentralized trial designs (Sabesan, 2023; Sabesan et al., 2023).

The terminology and intent may vary, but the overall goal is clear: to make available any element or aspect of clinical research that can be conducted where the participant resides, using technology as a tool to enhance ease of use for both research professionals and participants. This can be achieved by beginning with the end in mind, such as end points or outcomes, which then contextualize the terminology and subsequent paradigm that will steer protocol development and trial execution. As end users and coordinators, OCRNs play an integral role in evaluating virtual clinical trials to match the participant population and local resources, ensuring a safe and ethical clinical trial experience for all involved. Particularly in complex oncology clinical trials, virtual clinical trials have proven to be an opportunity to streamline common pain points, such as ongoing consent and reconsent. Using the appropriate terminology to convey the complexities may enable more effective conversations with local participant groups and sponsors when determining the feasibility and fit-for-purpose of the research in relation to the needs of the population of interest.

Historical Overview of Virtual Clinical Trial Development and Adoption

Although virtual clinical trials have been used for some time in observational or lower-risk trials, their use increased exponentially during the COVID-19 pandemic when access to on-site research resources was constricted. For example, caregivers may have been unable to attend trial visits with their loved ones. OCRNs found themselves working from home, attending certain shifts at their research site, or experiencing a change in duty to clinical service if the research was put on hold. Many sites found themselves in a surge of COVID-19 vaccine trials, and oncology clinical trials faced the constraints of severe drug shortages (e.g., tocilizumab) and material supply shortages (e.g., IV line filters) because of the diversion of resources to clinical units.

From a regulatory perspective, virtual clinical trials were not only pushed to the forefront to keep research moving, but they also exposed the underlying efficiencies that could be actualized if the enterprise pulled together as one to achieve a goal. Common bottlenecks, such as delays in a sponsor's review of informed consent forms or institutional review board (IRB) authorizations, were reduced or eliminated in response to the urgency of the pandemic, which aimed to keep research participants on the study as safely and as long as possible (Maxton et al., 2021).

The U.S. Food and Drug Administration (FDA) issued 84 guidance documents from 2020 to 2022 to harmonize and generate specific guidance related to the conduct of decentralized clinical research. As of May 2025, the Center for Drug Evaluation and Research, a division of FDA, issued draft guidance that garnered 93 separate response submittals from varying organizations during the public comment period (FDA, 2024). One area of significant discussion was the design of decentralized trials, which noted that to facilitate inspection, such as monitoring or audits, a physical location should still be documented as the "site" for Form FDA 1572 and used for participant engagement (FDA, 2024). The selection of the main trial site can influence how training, delegation of responsibilities, and telehealth capabilities are implemented. For example, in its public comment, Advarra highlighted the need for clarification regarding how to document healthcare providers who contribute data for clinical research, particularly when that data also falls under standard-of-care practices (Regulations.gov, 2023b).

Other elements in the draft guidance that sparked animated discussion included how training and delegation of authority are to be managed, given the variance in personnel who may be in contact with participants and support data collection. The International Association of Clinical Research Nurses provided this context in the form of local nursing support when home health, public health, or travel nurses are contracted to extend the outreach of trial activities in remote communities (Regulations.gov, 2023a). Heavy emphasis was applied to the necessary training and infrastructure to ensure consistency in the execution of trial procedures, particularly safety management and reporting of adverse events (Regulations.gov, 2023a). This included recommendations for communication and coordination channels (information exchange) among all stakeholders conducting elements of the clinical trial to support timely data entry, query resolution, and maintain the necessary continuum of care that exists between clinical and research teams.

Progress has been made on other initiatives that affect decentralized or virtual clinical trial conduct, such as the collaboration between sponsors, sites, and FDA on innovative trial design. The Duke-Margolis Institute for Health Policy convened with FDA in a meeting open to the public in March 2024 to engage in open discussion surrounding the conduct of clinical trials in community settings, specifically those that may include decentralized elements, fully virtual design, or hybrid trials that may consist of some traditional site visits (Duke-Margolis Institute for Health Policy, 2024). This convening aimed to open discussion on what modernization of the clinical research enterprise may look like from a stakeholder vantage point, with emphasis on creating the capacity for agility in research-enabled organizations to keep pace with the growth in demand for participant recruitment and retention. The groundwork between the decentralized trial draft guidance and convenings is an example of regulatory and industry collective progress to promote cultural shifts in how trials are perceived, accessed, and designed (see Figure 14-1).

FDA issued final guidance in September 2024, *Conducting Clinical Trials With Decentralized Elements: Guidance for Industry, Investigators, and Other Interested Parties*, which provided expanded detail into key operational considerations for trials outside of the hospital or institution setting. Within the introduction of this guidance, FDA noted that decentralized trials are those best suited for experimental drugs and devices (products) that have "well-characterized safety profiles" and "do not require complex preparation, administration, or medical assessments" (FDA, 2024, p. 3). The guidance continued to note the assumption of using the research site for some activities (thus inclusion of the term *elements* in the title of the guidance) and using elements or sites local to the participant. For those activities or elements local to the participant, FDA clarified that healthcare providers would not be considered subinvestigators or trial personnel, which streamlines the connection between clinical care access and integration of research in local care settings without burdening providers with additional training (FDA, 2024).

Areas of emphasis included in this guidance are the safety of participants, the use of healthcare providers, and how data will be exchanged from local or digital sources of information to research teams (FDA, 2024). FDA encourages clear explanations for participants in the informed consent form of the delineation of procedures and provider use (local and at the research site) to support a comprehensive understanding of the trial's schedule requirements and any associated travel (FDA, 2024).

Example Use Cases
Below is a listing of example decentralized clinical trials (published reports):
- ADAPTABLE study (Schuyler Jones et al., 2021)
- PREDHICT study (Seixas et al., 2023)
- REMOTE study (Orri et al., 2014)
- Trials@Home Consortium (Coyle et al., 2022)

Supplemental Resources for Training and Education
Below is a listing of resources to learn more about decentralized or virtual clinical trials:
- Applied Clinical Trials: *The Past, Present, and Future of Mobile Visits in Decentralized Clinical Trials:* www.appliedclinicaltrialsonline.com/view/the-past-present-and-future-of-mobile-visits-in-decentralized-clinical-trials
- Association of Clinical Research Professionals: Introduction to Decentralized Clinical Trials: https://acrpnet.org/courses/introduction-to-decentralized-clinical-trials-dcts
- Decentralized Trials and Research Alliance: Knowledge Sharing Playbook—Tubestop: www.dtra.org/knowledge-sharing-playbook#tubestop
- Drug Information Association: *Moving Forward With Decentralized Clinical Trials:* www.diaglobal.org/en/course-listing/training/2023/11/moving-forward-with-decentralized-clinical-trials-dcts
- Duke-Margolis Institute for Health Policy: *FDA Convening: Enhancing Adoption of Innovative Clinical Trial Approaches*: https://healthpolicy.duke.edu/events/enhancing-adoption-innovative-clinical-trial-approaches
- Joint Task Force for Clinical Trial Competency: https://mrctcenter.org/clinical-trial-competency

FIGURE 14-1 | Decentralized Clinical Trial Program Exemplars

Core Elements of Virtual Clinical Trial Conduct

Technology

Technology is a pivotal tool used to conduct clinical trials in community and home settings, serving as an extended means of collecting data and connecting with participants. Common instances of technology use include the following (Rosa et al., 2021):

- Electronic patient-reported outcomes
- Wearables
- Remote monitoring devices
- Telehealth platforms
- Mobile applications

Technical support should be verified as available for troubleshooting, either through the vendor's customer service or a centralized contact provided by the trial sponsor or within the research site's information technology department. Training should be made available in multiple forms of media, such as manuals and videos, to aid both clinical research staff and participants, as well as potentially their caregivers (Inan et al., 2020). Evaluation of participant technological acceptance, or the agreeable perception of the technology, is recommended to ensure adherence and engagement (Rosa et al., 2021).

Home or Community Involvement

A significant element of beginning oncology virtual clinical trials is determining the type of engagement in a home or community setting, dependent on what is required per protocol from a resource perspective (Ersek et al., 2019). A first step to this determination is a windshield survey, or community assessment, which categorizes the type of healthcare resources available and population characteristics that may inform the next steps necessary for successful trial conduct. Public health offices and community health needs assessments provided online by local healthcare facilities are great places to begin when first learning about a community. Pragmatic lines of questioning to local insiders should also include resources that support quality of life during cancer treatment or experimental therapy. Such lines of questioning may include the following:

- Where is the nearest grocery store?
- How far is it to the nearest emergency department or urgent care?
- Does this community have consistent internet access?
- Are the roads accessible year-round or seasonally?
- Is there postal service directly to the home or a centralized mail pick-up?
- What options for pharmacies are available locally?
- How does this community define health?
- How many own a smartphone and have access to data plan financial support?

Complementary to community and environmental resources are participant demands on time, effort, and learning that may be requested when wearable devices and online platforms are incorporated (Ersek et al., 2019). Furthermore, how data will be used or shared may be a question asked of potential participants, community leaders, or older adults. The Clinical Trials Transformation Initiative (n.d.) has provided additional questions to ask sponsors upfront to aid in the trust-building process with communities:

- Has a plan been developed for how, when, and what types of health-related information will be returned to participants?
- Can real-time access to individual results be provided in a way that maintains study integrity and participant safety?
- Is the return of data personalized and understandable?
- Have the acceptability, usability, and tolerability of the technology for potential research participants been evaluated?
- Does the informed consent process describe the digital technology, including risks and benefits?
- Are all patient-facing materials as simple as possible and designed to meet the needs of study participants, including those with low health or technical literacy?
- To the extent possible, have measures been taken to protect participant data?
- Is all privacy and confidentiality information clear to potential participants (even if consumer technologies are used in the trial)?

Home-based assessments are important for the safety of participants, OCRNs, and other professionals conducting home visits. Home health services geared explicitly toward clinical research conduct may be contracted by the sponsor or site to perform these home readiness checks as well as trial visits (Tenaerts et al., 2024). The site of record may delegate responsibility for generating nursing orders for home health services based on the study protocol and schedule of assessments. Documentation of these visits may not be integrated into the site's electronic health record and could exist in external systems. Further appraisal may be necessary at the time of contract to ensure the cadence of documentation and visit notes is aligned with data entry expectations.

OCRNs can serve as a point of contact to establish expectations surrounding the anticipated personnel present in the home environment during trial visits to support nurse and patient safety. They may also be in contact with local social services should additional comfort or safety measures be necessary for optimal trial conduct, such as air conditioning, refrigeration if the investigative drug or device is shipped directly and requires temperature control, or language services if translation is needed (Juckett et al., 2023).

Staff Resourcing and Documentation

Although decentralized trials may be conducted with technology or virtual visits, there remains the need to calculate the workload required of OCRNs, similarly to how one may calculate the workload for a traditional, on-site trial. A study of OCRNs and midwives in the United States, United Kingdom, Republic of Ireland, and Australia demonstrated that resource allocation and workload modeling remain a challenge when integrating decentralized trial tasks into the workday of an OCRN who is also supporting on-site activities (Johnson et al., 2024). This includes variations in how staff training is documented and in determining which individuals should be listed on the delegation of authority and training log. For example, the local extension stakeholders, such as public health, local pharmacies, and clinical providers, may collect research-supportive specimens or information (e.g., adverse event safety reporting documentation) within the capacity of their clinical or lay health worker scope. The FDA's final guidance clarifies how documentation practices should vary based on a provider's level of involvement in a participant's research-related care. However, this shift may introduce additional oversight, communication, and training responsibilities for investigators and OCRNs. These considerations must be reflected in the trial budget and in how staff time is allocated across other trials or nonresearch activities (Johnson et al., 2024).

Recruitment and Consent

Consent may be obtained through paper documents sent by mail, in person, or via electronic consent (eConsent). An eConsent may be possible when permitted by a regulatory oversight entity and with a provider platform that enables the audibility and verification of signatures to ensure adherence with trial sponsor requirements, as well as state, federal, and local guidelines and mandates.

Decentralized trial recruitment can occur with the following sources (non-exhaustive):

- Social media
- Databases
- Contract research organization and trial sponsor outreach
- Grassroots organization partnership
- Participant advocate partnerships

Ethical Considerations

The migration of clinical trial activities to locations outside the traditional research site increases the responsibilities of providers, research teams, and the clinical trial network in managing vendors across digital platforms, laboratories, and regulatory systems. Tensions may arise when local providers and research teams lack decision-making authority over vendor selection or operations, especially when these vendors introduce practices that conflict with local norms, cultural expectations, or available resources (Bierer & White, 2023). Additional ethical considerations include but are not limited to the following (Petrini et al., 2022):

- Personal data protection is crucial when a participant's phone is used, for example, to download a research-related mobile application. Participants will need to be supported in their understanding of how to use opt-in, opt-out, and push notifications between research and personal data sources.
- Digital disparity occurs when a research participant may not have the resources to support consistent or solo use of research-provided technologies (e.g., a mobile phone is shared among multiple family members). Changing the technology or not having consistent internet access are additional examples of digital disparities that may affect a community's ability to participate in the trial.
- Regulatory requirements may vary to describe decentralized trial procedures and overall rationale between tribal IRBs, academic or local IRBs, centralized IRBs, and ethics committees. As communities may have varying exposure to decentralized trial concepts or previous trials, OCRNs can support the development or collation of evaluation checklists or source documentation (e.g., vendor manuals, assessment tools) to enable a regulatory board to assess the trial and its potential impact on the local healthcare system and community resources.
- Cold chain custody and investigational product shipment are additional areas of ethical consideration to ensure safe and reliable dispensation. Courier or other mail service access should be evaluated to ensure that the product can be delivered as scheduled across all seasons.
- Privacy and confidentiality are paramount, particularly among small communities or distinct populations. Healthcare providers and community stakeholders may benefit from educational town halls or other meeting styles that emphasize the importance of research and a protected exchange when a participant seeks care or during research visits in community or home settings.

The Role of Oncology Clinical Research Nurses in Virtual Clinical Trials

A specialty since 2016, oncology clinical research nursing has played a crucial role in conducting oncologic decentralized trials, particularly during the COVID-19 pandemic. In one survey of oncologists and patients, patients reported an overwhelming majority as being comfortable with a nurse coming to their home to conduct trial visits and procedures (de Las Heras et al., 2022). Furthermore, patients were less confident in collecting their own specimens or other samples compared to having a nurse collect them (de Las Heras et al., 2022). The licensure permit to conduct nurse visits may vary from state to state and require review prior to proceeding with a decentralized clinical trial (Apostolaros et al., 2020). There may be elements of trial conduct, such as telehealth visits or specific medication administration tasks, that are restricted based on state regulations governing nursing licenses.

OCRNs may be delegated to manage data integrity and data management in decentralized trials actively (Johnson & Marsh, 2023a). This may include recording real-time data at participant homes or validating and transcribing home health (contractor) data collection into a sponsor's electronic data capture platform, as required by the protocol (Johnson & Marsh, 2023a). OCRNs may also need to manage various data sources, including those derived from paper records, electronic transmittal, clinical encounters, or recorded in the electronic health record. Additional vendor platforms may need to be managed by either the OCRN or a delegated staff member, such as electronic patient-reported outcomes, wearable device recordings, and medication adherence trackers.

Participant management practices may vary depending on the research site; however, ensuring that visits are not missed and critical information is not overlooked during remote practices presents new challenges (Johnson & Marsh, 2023a). OCRNs may be contacted by clinical care providers or clinicians should research participants seek care outside of the research site or team. OCRNs can support clinical nurses by conveying contraindicated treatments, side effect profiles, and any dietary restrictions (Johnson & Marsh, 2023b). They may also apprise the study investigators of any change in participant status that may warrant a safety evaluation or need for education or training to support safe clinical care (Johnson & Marsh, 2023b). Figure 14-2 describes actionable steps to support the clinical management of decentralized trial participants as an OCRN.

Future Trends and Practice Considerations

Virtual clinical trials require unique considerations to support operational efficiency because, in practice, they may coincide with traditional trial designs conducted on-site. For example, the nursing coordination of participant visits in a digital domain increases pressure on information technology support with computer and server needs. There also may be changes in workday schedules and the use of a home or remote office, meaning support of outside equipment (e.g., internet, mobile phone). For many sites and healthcare systems or institutions, changes in infrastructure requirements are present across organizational, technological, and physical domains of the clinical research environment.

Organizational

The decision to pursue and conduct a virtual clinical trial comes with cultural shifts at every level of an organization, from leadership to those conducting the clinical trials. OCRNs hold a specialized, expert knowledge of the research protocol in conjunction with their clinical nursing experience. However, OCRNs in the United States have reported challenges with the specialty being visible as a critical, valued component of ensuring trial access to commu-

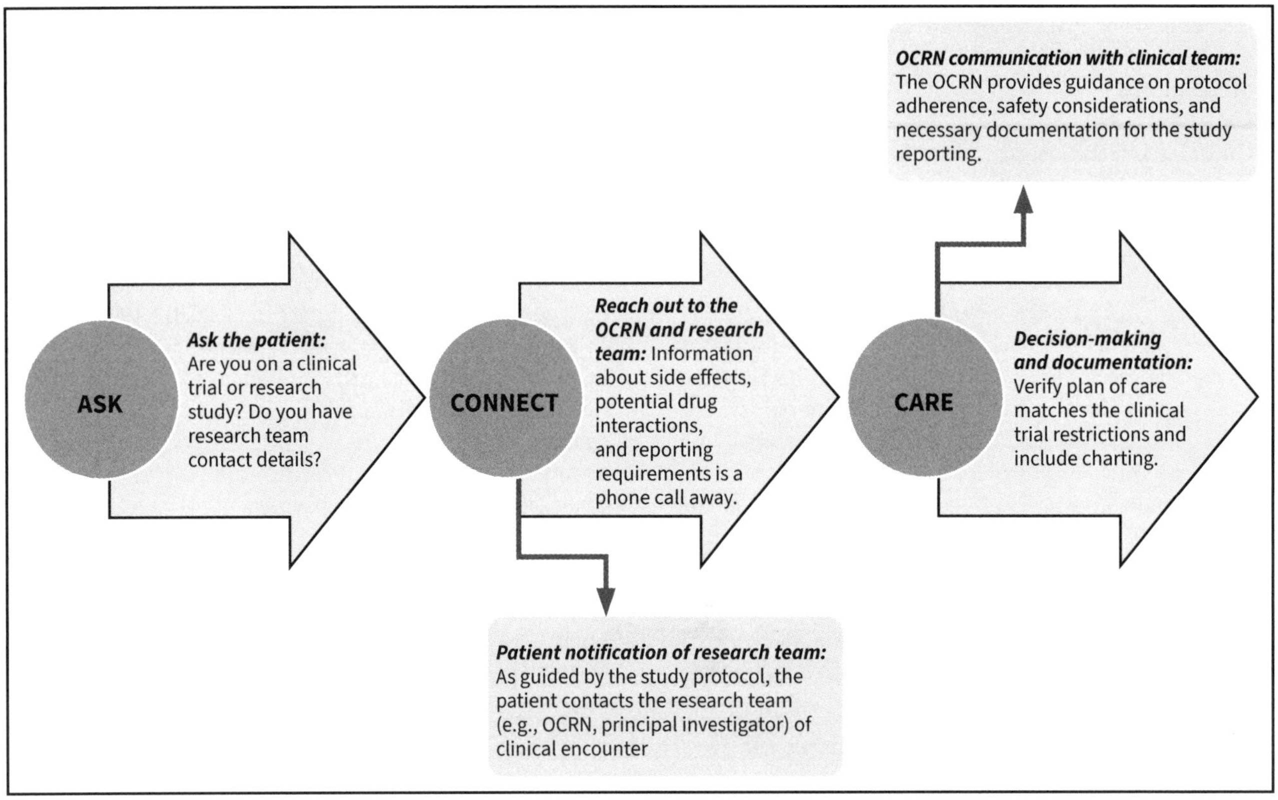

FIGURE 14-2 | Recommended Action Pathway for Clinical Nursing Supportive Care of a Clinical Trial Participant

OCRN—oncology clinical research nurse

Note. Based on information from Johnson & Marsh, 2023b.

nities in the clinical service area. For example, does organizational leadership (i.e., director of nursing, chief nursing officer) include research nursing professionals across coordinator and research unit roles in quality improvement projects or career development opportunities?

Nurses supporting virtual clinical trials may experience a shift from a team-based trial environment to one that may be perceived as professionally isolating if working a remote or hybrid schedule. OCRNs in the United States have reported perceptions of leadership not being aware of the complexities of the research nursing role when the workload is split between traditional and virtual clinical trial conduct, which may cause burnout (Johnson & Rainbow, 2023). During the COVID-19 pandemic, OCRNs in one study felt that they did not experience the same workplace appreciation as clinical nurses, which decreased morale and led to some departing from their organizations (Johnson & Rainbow, 2023). In another study conducted by Showalter et al. (2022), the friction between the needs of the protocol versus the needs of the participant would cause conflict and moral distress among OCRNs, highlighting the importance of providing psychological safety support (particularly those performing new procedures), interacting with new wearable devices, and operating within innovative trial models. Showalter et al. (2022) also noted moral distress among younger aged OCRNs compared to those of advanced age (older than 60 years), which may point to a heightened organizational emphasis on aligning accepted protocols to the values, norms, and roles of those navigating the unknowns associated with experimental drug and device trials.

Education and Mentorship

Educational offerings, supportive mentorship, and resource availability congruent to the workload and tasks associated with virtual clinical trials are interventions protective against burnout and foster resiliency to the variability of modern clinical research (Johnson & Rainbow, 2023). One example of a mentorship program that encompasses education and training is a nurse residency program. These programs, which are traditionally six months in duration, focus on practice-based learning and orient nurses to role-based resources, behaviors, norms, and values through leadership intensives and didactic training (Sutor & Painter, 2020). Although present in more than half of U.S. hospitals and healthcare systems, a lack of standardization exists across residency programs, leaving definitive information sparse on the inclusion of OCRNs (Sutor & Painter, 2020).

Legor et al. (2022) developed and implemented a nurse residency program at the Dana-Farber Cancer Institute that was specific to oncology clinical research for newly licensed nurses and sought ways to improve staff retention, satisfaction, and engagement in preparation to support clinical trials across the organization. This ongoing residency program spans 44 weeks of inpatient, outpatient, and infusion oncology nursing experience. It is guided via a structured curriculum with learning objectives and activities that develop newly licensed nurses into skilled critical thinkers who are adaptive in their approach to supporting trial conduct in the scope of clinical research nursing (Legor et al., 2022).

Per the Society of Clinical Research Associates 2020 Salary Survey, the average age of OCRNs in the sample was 49.1 years compared to the remainder of the overall sample (42.6 years). OCRNs also had the highest rate of retention (average of 7 years at their respective organization) in comparison to 5.2 years with other subgroups (DePaulo, 2020). With many OCRNs approaching retirement, coupled with a contraction in the research nursing workforce, a wealth of organizational and specialty knowledge could be lost if mentorship and buddy programs are not in place to attract nurses to clinical research and be agile for virtual clinical trial delivery (Johnson, 2022). Such programs are also critical to decrease professional isolation and foster familiarity with other research and community team members. They can be formal, such as orientation programs that expose clinical nurses to research as a career opportunity, or informal, such as coffee chats between experienced and novice OCRNs.

Another important avenue involves integrating clinical research nursing into undergraduate nursing curricula to build early awareness of research participants as a distinct patient population. This framing promotes safety-focused care, such as managing adverse events and providing routine support, while also highlighting clinical research nursing as a specialty with diverse opportunities for professional growth and advancement (Capili et al., 2022).

Leadership and Executive Teams

Leadership and executive teams may consider adopting or declining virtual clinical trials based on the degree of risk associated with the system's operations at large. Risk quantifies the potential impact of specific threats on an organi-

STRENGTHS *What is going well or is successful?*	**OPPORTUNITIES** *What are the areas for improvement that improve the likelihood of success or sustained success?*
WEAKNESSES *What are the vulnerabilities to success?*	**THREATS** *What are the internal or external forces that may jeopardize the potential for success?*

FIGURE 14-3 | Strengths, Weaknesses, Opportunities, Threats Analysis

zation's health and may also be compared to actual or estimated benefits. Two tools commonly employed to evaluate risk are the SWOT analysis (Strengths, Weaknesses, Opportunities, Threats) (see Figure 14-3) and Rasmussen's Risk Management Framework.

The SWOT analysis is a popular Lean Six Sigma tool that divides a square into four quadrants, with an element of SWOT represented individually in each quadrant. Brainstorming each SWOT element via bulleted lists enables stakeholders and decision-makers to visually represent the actual or estimated influence a virtual clinical trial may have on clinical research operations. This tool can be used as an ongoing, easy method to appraise the change of risk over time in a high-level manner.

Rasmussen's Risk Management Framework (sometimes referred to as Rasmussen's Ladder) (see Figure 14-4) is a high-level approach to risk evaluation that focuses on the competency or skill level of research professionals compared to different domains of external and internal forces of change that influence the health of the organization or research department. These domains are organized into different system levels, such as the microsystem (the smallest level of system measurement, encompassing the interaction between a patient and a provider), mesosystem (departments or groups of providers), and macrosystem (the organization as a whole or outside influences, including regulation and policy). Risk levels associated with decentralized or virtual clinical trials encompass government (e.g., laws, policies), regulatory (e.g., rules, guidance), company (e.g., standard procedures), management (e.g., operationalization), clinical research team (e.g., translation), and clinical care team (Besel et al., 2023). Together, the system and risk levels can then be compared to the competency or skill set of research professionals to determine the degree or severity of risk associated with the adoption of a virtual clinical trial.

For example, if staff have not been trained on eConsent requirements and best practices but possess strong skill sets in team-based clinical care, leadership may note that the regulatory and management levels of risk are higher than the translational levels associated with clinical care or clinical research teams (Besel et al., 2023).

Technological

The technological connection or integration between all elements of a virtual clinical trial requires close communication and coordination with the site's information technology department and a local assessment of the home or community practice. Some technologies, such as wearable devices and remote monitors, may have the capability to link directly to a vendor platform, data capture system, or the site's electronic health record. These direct connections may require human validation that the information is placed in the correct form fields. Wearable devices and tablets require an internet connection and are thus subject to cybersecurity evaluation to prevent malware or firmware attacks. In home or community practice, appraising internet reliability is common, and many trial sponsors will include an allocation for hotspot devices in the budget. Sites may need to anticipate the need for charging stations or additional ports in research preparation rooms or offices, particularly if multiple wearables or tablets are required. Specific laptops or telehealth workstations may need to be reserved or purchased to support patient visits conducted via videoconferencing.

Physical

A home assessment for the participant is crucial to determine the suitability of performing procedures, such as infusions, in a manner that maintains the safety of both the participant and OCRN or delegate. A third-party contractor, such as a global home health agency, may conduct a home assessment, which typically includes a list of individuals living inside or frequenting the home, availability of heating/cooling and a water source, internet, and candidate regions optimal for procedures (i.e., investigational product preparation, administration, specimen collection, and disposal of waste if not performed with the OCRN or delegate at the end of the visit).

Guidance Updates and Policy

Communications to Healthcare Providers From Firms

As of May 2025, draft revised guidance exists for what is known as "scientific information on unapproved uses of approved/cleared medical products" (SIUU) communications (FDA, 2025). Initially released in 2014, these communications are intended to support healthcare providers in their interpretation of information from firms (e.g., pharmaceutical companies) on the evidence to support off-label use of drugs and devices that have been previously approved or cleared for other intended populations, diseases, or indications (FDA, 2025). In the draft guidance, the onus of interpreting the validity of the evidence, originating from potentially aggregated electronic health record data (real-world evidence) or clinical trials, is now on the healthcare provider (Sah et al., 2023).

As decentralized clinical trials become more commonplace in trial sponsor programs, healthcare providers may see these communications as a means to inform the use of wearables or remote monitoring devices. Healthcare providers will appraise the strengths, weaknesses, validity, and utility of these devices based on the information in the communication. OCRNs have the clinical and research expertise to aid healthcare providers in the local community in interpreting these communications and providing feedback to firms, thus enhancing understanding in regions that may be unfamiliar with clinical research (Sah et al., 2023).

Diversity Action Plans

In April 2022, draft guidance was released that prioritized a focus on adequate representation and enrollment of diverse populations in clinical trials (FDA, 2022). This guidance stems from the overall lack of representation of culturally and linguistically diverse communities in traditional clinical trials. With the advent of decentralized clinical trial designs, there is an opportunity and imperative to recruit and engage community members not only to enhance the validity and generalizability of drug trial findings but also to promote equity in access to novel therapies. For example, rural-dwelling residents are commonly

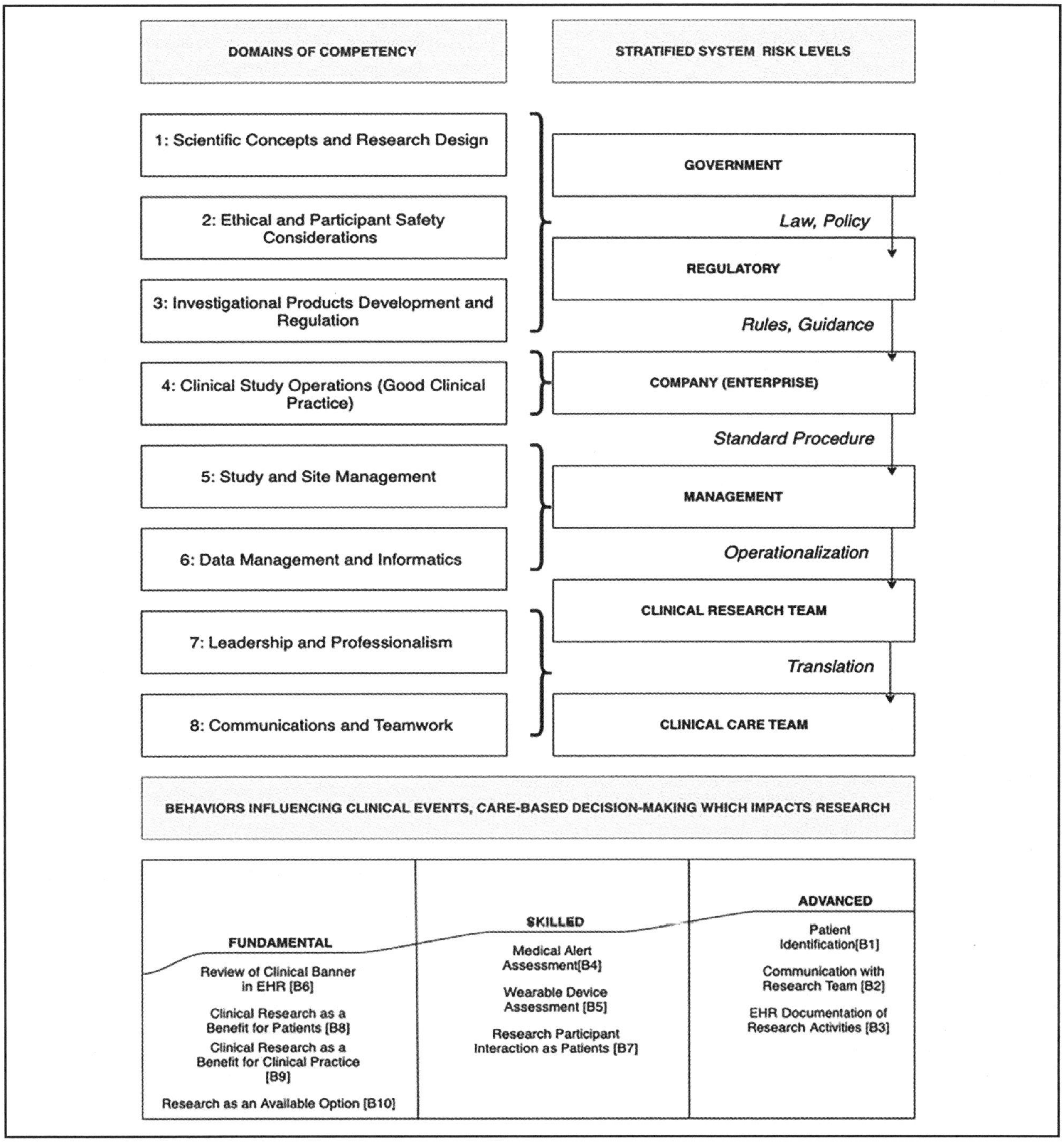

FIGURE 14-4 | Rasmussen Risk Management Framework

EHR—electronic health record

Note. From "Reimagining the Joint Task Force Core Competency Framework for Rural and Frontier Clinical Research Professionals Conducting Hybrid and Decentralized Trials," by J.M. Besel, E.A. Johnson, J. Ma, and B Kiesow, 2023, *Frontiers in Pharmacology, 14,* 1309073 (https://doi.org/10.3389/fphar.2023.1309073). Copyright 2020 by the authors. Licensed under CC BY 4.0 DEED International (https://creativecommons.org/licenses/by/4.0).

under-engaged in oncology clinical trials, with the paucity of National Cancer Institute sites and oncologists operating in these settings (Nelson et al., 2024). As part of diversity action plans, trial sponsors submit to FDA a detailed strategy for recruiting and retaining culturally and linguistically diverse populations in phase 3 and other pivotal clinical trials, ensuring that participants reflect the demographics of the disease, condition, or symptom being studied (FDA, 2022). This policy reflects the growing recognition that a lack of representation in clinical trials contributes to health disparities and reduces the generalizability of trial results, prompting regulators and funders to advocate for inclusive design approaches from the outset of protocol development (Boden-Albala, 2022).

Summary

Virtual clinical trials have demonstrated merit in changing how clinical trial professionals perceive opportunity, equity, and diversity in research data representation. Virtual clinical trials enable OCRNs to advocate for the specialty of oncology clinical research nursing and their participants beyond the bedside or traditional site model. The remote nature extends research careers to include skills in digital management and local liaison roles that facilitate the engagement of underrepresented groups. Although promising to create efficiencies for clinical research nursing workflows, oncology research centers are encouraged to consider physical, technological, and organizational infrastructure capacity needs to accommodate virtual and traditional trial designs to support research nursing well-being and participant satisfaction in their experience. Accepting a new type of trial process or design approach necessitates nursing leadership and advocacy for sponsor-organizational alignment on the role and scope of OCRNs and protocol procedures. The priority attention to virtual clinical trials at the legislative level brings hope and a new promise to progress the clinical research enterprise through expanded stakeholder inclusion and consideration of nursing being at the forefront of advancements in novel oncologic treatments.

Key Points

- Virtual clinical trials are primarily conducted using technology and take place outside of traditional research sites, often in participants' communities or home settings. Although virtual trials may be known by other names, such as decentralized or siteless clinical trials, they share a common element of using technology as a tool to lessen participant burden and increase access to experimental treatments.
- The presence of clinical research participants in community settings introduces ethical, legal, safety, and operational considerations. OCRNs must navigate these challenges to ensure that trials are conducted effectively outside the typical resources available at standard research sites.
- OCRNs play a crucial role in addressing the challenges of virtual clinical trials. They may conduct community assessments, evaluate the digital technologies used in a trial, and serve as navigators for both the sponsor and research team, ensuring that the necessary resources are in place for safe and successful provider assessments and protocol adherence.
- Industry trends and legislative changes reflect a shift toward inclusivity in trial enrollment, an emphasis on continued use of technology to complete trial procedures, and a need for clinical experts (e.g., OCRNs) to build relationships with under-engaged or never-engaged communities. This helps to increase representation in trial data and accelerates recruitment to meet trial end points.

References

Apostolaros, M., Babaian, D., Corneli, A., Forrest, A., Hamre, G., Hewett, J., ... Randall, P. (2020). Legal, regulatory, and practical issues to consider when adopting decentralized clinical trials: Recommendations from the Clinical Trials Transformation Initiative. *Therapeutic Innovation and Regulatory Science, 54*(4), 779–787. https://doi.org/10.1007/s43441-019-00006-4

Beg, S.S., & Bustos, D. (2022). Decentralized and hybrid trials in oncology: Results of a global survey of clinical research executives [Abstract]. *Journal of Clinical Oncology, 40*(28 Suppl.), 102. https://doi.org/10.1200/jco.2022.40.28_suppl.102

Besel, J.M., Johnson, E.A., Ma, J., & Kiesow, B. (2023). Reimagining the joint task force core competency framework for rural and frontier clinical research professionals conducting hybrid and decentralized trials. *Frontiers in Pharmacology, 14,* 1309073. https://doi.org/10.3389/fphar.2023.1309073

Bierer, B.E., & White, S.A. (2023). Ethical considerations in decentralized clinical trials. *Journal of Bioethical Inquiry, 20*(4), 711–718. https://doi.org/10.1007/s11673-024-10341-3

Boden-Albala, B. (2022). Confronting legacies of underrepresentation in clinical trials: The case for greater diversity in research. *Neuron, 110*(5), 746–748. https://doi.org/10.1016/j.neuron.2021.12.008

Capili, B., Baker, L., Thangthaeng, N., Legor, K., Larkin, M.E., & Jones, C.T. (2022). Development and evaluation of a clinical research nursing module for undergraduate nursing schools: Expanding clinical research nurses' outreach. *Journal of Research in Nursing, 27*(1–2), 68–77. https://doi.org/10.1177/17449871211070972

Clinical Trials Transformation Initiative. (n.d.). *Optimizing digital and decentralized clinical trials by engaging patients and sites: Questions to support the implementation of recommendations.* https://ctti-clinicaltrials.org/wp-content/uploads/2021/06/CTTI_DHT_Engaging_Patients_and_Sites_Implementation_Qs.pdf

Coyle, J., Rogers, A., Copland, R., De Paoli, G., MacDonald, T.M., & Mackenzie, I.S. (2021). Learning from remote decentralised clinical trial experiences: A qualitative analysis of interviews with trial personnel, patient representatives and other stakeholders. *British Journal of Clinical Pharmacology, 88*(3), 1031–1042. https://doi.org/10.1111/bcp.15003

de Jong, A.J., Grupstra, R.J., Santa-Ana-Tellez, Y., Zuidgeest, M.G.P., de Boer, A., Gardarsdottir, H., & Trials@Home Consortium. (2022). Which decentralised trial activities are reported in clinical trial protocols of drug trials initiated in 2019–2020? A cross-sectional study in ClinicalTrials.gov. *BMJ Open, 12*(8), e063236. https://doi.org/10.1136/bmjopen-2022-063236

de Las Heras, B., Daehnke, A., Saini, K.S., Harris, M., Morrison, K., Aguilo, A., ... Marcus, R. (2022). Role of decentralized clinical trials in cancer drug development: Results from a survey of oncologists and patients. *Digital Health, 8*. https://doi.org/10.1177/20552076221099997

DePaulo, P.J. (2020). *Subgroup analyses: SOCRA salary survey*. https://www.socra.org/assets/Uploads/SOCRA-Salary-Survey-2020-v2.pdf

Duke-Margolis Institute for Health Policy. (2024, March 18). *Discussion guide: Enhancing adoption of innovative clinical trial approaches*. https://healthpolicy.duke.edu/sites/default/files/2024-03/Discussionguide_Enhancingadoptionofinnovativeclinicaltrialapproaches3.18.2024_0.pdf

Ersek, J.L., Graff, S.L., Arena, F.P., Denduluri, N., & Kim, E.S. (2019). Critical aspects of a sustainable clinical research program in the community-based oncology practice. *American Society of Clinical Oncology Educational Book, 39*, e70–e77. https://doi.org/10.1200/EDBK_238485

Faulkner, K.G. (2021). Decentralized vs digital clinical trials: There is a difference. *Applied Clinical Trials, 30*(12), 12. https://www.appliedclinicaltrialsonline.com/view/decentralized-vs-digital-clinical-trials-there-is-a-difference

Inan, O.T., Tenaerts, P., Prindiville, S.A., Rivera, S.C., Reynolds, H.R., Steinhubl, S.R., & Califf, R.M. (2020). Digitizing clinical trials. *NPJ Digital Medicine, 3*(101). https://doi.org/10.1038/s41746-020-0302-y

Johnson, E. (2022). Trouble for trials—The worrying state of the research nurse workforce. *Contemporary Clinical Trials, 120*, 106878. https://doi.org/10.1016/j.cct.2022.106878

Johnson, E., & Marsh, L. (2023a). Clinical research nurse utilisation and role in the conduct of decentralised clinical trials: A literature review. *Journal of Research in Nursing, 28*(3), 214–226. https://doi.org/10.1177/17449871231162497

Johnson, E., & Marsh, L. (2023b). Unconventional care: When decentralized research models and clinical patient management collide. *Clinical Researcher, 37*(6). https://acrpnet.org/2023/12/unconventional-care-when-decentralized-research-models-and-clinical-patient-management-collide/

Johnson, E., & Rainbow, J. (2023). Exploration of lived experiences and measurement of burnout among US clinical research nurses. *Journal of Nursing Administration, 53*(5), 251–258. https://doi.org/10.1097/NNA.0000000000001280

Johnson, E.A., Hill, G., Smith, H.A., Marsh, L., & Beer, K. (2024). A global pilot comparative, cross-sectional study of clinical research nurses/research midwives: Definition, knowledge base, and communication skills related to the conduct of decentralized clinical trials. *Journal of Clinical and Translational Science, 8*(1), e90. https://doi.org/10.1017/cts.2024.535

Juckett, L.A., Bernard, K.P., & Thomas, K.S. (2023). Partnering with social service staff to implement pragmatic clinical trials: An interim analysis of implementation strategies. *Trials, 24*(1), 739. https://doi.org/10.1186/s13063-023-07757-4

Legor, K.A., Caparrotta, C.M., Sze, C.K., Killion, L.J., & Gross, A.H. (2022). Development and implementation of an oncology clinical research nursing residency program for newly licensed nurses. *Journal of Nursing Administration, 52*(6), 371–376. https://doi.org/10.1097/NNA.0000000000001162

Maxton, F., Darbyshire, P., & Thompson, D.R. (2021). Research nurses rising to the challenges of COVID-19. *Journal of Clinical Nursing, 30*(5–6), e13–e15. https://doi.org/10.1111/jocn.15504

Nelson, J.M., Johnson, E., Kiesow, B., McCrory, B., & Ma, J. (2024). Strengths and opportunities to clinical trial enrollment among BIPOC, rural dwelling patients in the northwest United States: A retrospective study. *Frontiers in Pharmacology, 15*, 1309072. https://doi.org/10.3389/fphar.2024.1309072

Orri, M., Lipset, C.H., Jacobs, B.P., Costello, A.J., & Cummings, C.R. (2014). Web-based trial to evaluate the efficacy and safety of tolterodine ER 4 mg in participants with overactive bladder: REMOTE trial. *Contemporary Clinical Trials, 38*(2), 190–197. https://doi.org/10.1016/j.cct.2014.04.009

Petrini, C., Mannelli, C., Riva, L., Gainotti, S., & Gussoni, G. (2022). Decentralized clinical trials (DCTs): A few ethical considerations. *Frontiers in Public Health, 10*, 1081150. https://doi.org/10.3389/fpubh.2022.1081150

Ranganathan, P., Aggarwal, R., & Pramesh, C.S. (2023). Virtual clinical trials. *Perspectives in Clinical Research, 14*(4), 203–206. https://doi.org/10.4103/picr.picr_184_22

Regulations.gov. (2023a, July 11). *Comment from International Association of Clinical Research Nurses*. https://www.regulations.gov/comment/FDA-2022-D-2870-0016

Regulations.gov. (2023b, July 18). *Comment from Advarra Inc*. https://www.regulations.gov/comment/FDA-2022-D-2870-0017

Rosa, C., Marsch, L.A., Winstanley, E.L., Brunner, M., & Campbell, A.N.C. (2021). Using digital technologies in clinical trials: Current and future applications. *Contemporary Clinical Trials, 100*, 106219. https://doi.org/10.1016/j.cct.2020.106219

Sabesan, S. (2023, July 13). Equitable clinical trial access for regional, rural, and indigenous communities: Leveraging teletrial models as part of decentralized clinical trial systems. *ASCO Daily News*. https://dailynews.ascopubs.org/do/equitable-clinical-trial-access-regional-rural-and-indigenous-communities-leveraging

Sabesan, S., Malica, M., Gebbie, C., Scott, C., Thomas, D., & Zalcberg, J. (2023). Implementation of the Australasian teletrial model: Translating ideas into action using implementation science frameworks. *Journal of Telemedicine and Telecare, 29*(8), 641–647. https://doi.org/10.1177/1357633x211017805

Sah, A., Johnson, E., & Rodriguez-Chavez, I. (2023). *Left to interpretation: Navigating FDA's revised guidance on SIUU communications*. https://globalforum.diaglobal.org/issue/january-2024/left-to-interpretation-navigating-fdas-revised-guidance-on-siuu-communications/

Seixas, A., Richards, S., Moore, J.Q., Izeogu, C., Hollimon, L.A., Jin, P., & Jean-Louis, G. (2023). Precision Recruitment and Engagement of Individuals at Risk for Diabetes and Hypertension in Clinical Trials (PREDHICT): A randomized trial for an E-persuasive mobile application to inform decision making about clinical trials. *International Journal of Environmental Research and Public Health, 20*(23), 7115. https://doi.org/10.3390/ijerph20237115

Schuyler Jones, W., Mulder, H., Wruck, L.S., Pencina, M.J., Kripalani, S., Muñoz, D., ... Hernandez, A.F. (2021). Comparative effectiveness of aspirin dosing in cardiovascular disease. *New England Journal of Medicine, 384*(21), 1981–1990. https://doi.org/10.1056/NEJMoa2102137

Showalter, B.L., Malecha, A., Cesario, S., & Clutter, P. (2022). Moral distress in clinical research nurses. *Nursing Ethics, 29*(7–8), 1697–1708. https://doi.org/10.1177/09697330221090613

Sutor, A., & Painter, J. (2020). Nurse residency programs: Providing organizational value. *Delaware Journal of Public Health, 6*(1), 58–61. https://doi.org/10.32481/djph.2020.04.013

Tenaerts, P., Hernandez, A.F., & Lipset, C. (2024). Clinical trial site readiness for decentralized trials – Fitting trials into today's world. *Journal of Clinical and Translational Science, 8*(1), e43. https://doi.org/10.1017/cts.2024.17

U.S. Food and Drug Administration. (2022). *Diversity plans to improve enrollment of participants from underrepresented racial and ethnic populations in clinical trials: draft guidance for industry*. https://www.fda.gov/regulatory-information/search-fda-guidance-documents/diversity-plans-improve-enrollment-participants-underrepresented-racial-and-ethnic-populations

U.S. Food & Drug Administration. (2024). *Conducting clinical trials with decentralized elements: Guidance for industry, investigators, and other interested parties*. https://www.fda.gov/media/167696/download

U.S. Food & Drug Administration. (2025). *Communications from firms to health care providers regarding scientific information on unapproved uses of approved/cleared medical products: Questions and answers*. https://www.fda.gov/regulatory-information/search-fda-guidance-documents/communications-firms-health-care-providers-regarding-scientific-information-unapproved-uses

Van Norman, G.A. (2021). Decentralized clinical trials: The future of medical product development? *JACC. Basic to Translational Science, 6*(4), 384–387. https://doi.org/10.1016/j.jacbts.2021.01.011

SECTION III.
Recruitment and Retention

CHAPTER 15

Public and Patient Education

Asia S. McCoy, MSN-CRN, RN, OCN®

Introduction

Patients with cancer are faced with many life-altering decisions, including how to best navigate their treatment journey. For many, enrollment in clinical trials can facilitate access to innovative therapeutic interventions with the potential to improve survival outcomes, foster more frequent and comprehensive interactions with interprofessional care teams, and allow patients to play an active role in advancing evidence-based medicine (Shepherd Forbes et al., 2023). What is essential in assisting patients in making informed and educated decisions about their care is health literacy on their part and effective communication on the part of healthcare providers (Holden et al., 2021). Patients and their support systems should be able to understand the information discussed with them and take appropriate action. These are fundamental requirements in the care process. A common trajectory of diagnosis management for patients with cancer will often include an option for participation in a clinical trial.

Healthcare providers have a professional and moral responsibility to provide patients with cancer with complete and comprehensive information regarding their disease and encourage them to be as involved as they wish in decisions regarding their treatment and care (Muscat et al., 2021). However, providing patients with sufficient information to make informed decisions remains a challenge for healthcare providers. Therefore, the ability of oncology clinical research nurses (OCRNs) to identify effective public–patient health education methodologies and promote respective institutional resources can prove instrumental in ensuring the delivery of adequate healthcare services while facilitating participation in clinical trials within their communities. This is of great utility to the overall success of clinical trials. Patient enrollment is the foundation of human participant research, ensuring that trials are adequately powered to detect clinically meaningful differences and enhance the generalizability of trial results across diverse patient populations. Fostering patient participation is both a scientific necessity and a moral imperative in the advancement of oncology care.

OCRNs, along with other healthcare providers, face challenges in providing clinical trial education to patients, staff, and the public, particularly in terms of how and what information is disseminated. Some of the challenges include providing consistent information, involving the collective efforts of many, and securing resources to meet the needs of patients, staff, and the public (Henley et al., 2024).

This chapter will review the literature on methods and resources that OCRNs can use to create awareness about clinical trials among various populations.

The Role of Oncology Clinical Research Nurses in Education

Providing education is a cornerstone of the nurse's role in patient care. The subspecialty of oncology clinical research nursing allows practitioners to apply this core competency in an expanded fashion. Consequently, the role of OCRNs has evolved into a distinct specialty characterized by unique responsibilities and considerations that set it apart from other positions within oncology nursing. The synthesis of these characteristics, combined with the ability to master and coordinate clinical trial–related communication for any audience, is what makes OCRNs a preferred provider for clinical trial education. Providing clinical trial education is a communication-related component of the Oncology Nursing Society (ONS) publication *Oncology Clinical Research Nurse Competencies* (ONS & Oncology Nursing Certification Corporation [ONCC], 2024). These competencies were developed as the framework for the confluent demonstration by OCRNs of critical-thinking skills and implementation of the nursing process to provide leadership in the successful conduct of clinical trials. As such, OCRNs must understand and incorporate into their daily practice a philosophy of continually adding to their knowledge base to further develop their clinical, educational, and cultural competence skills.

The next step in this process is to seek ways to improve lay and, in some cases, professional education on clinical trials. In their pivotal role of overseeing every aspect of the protocol, OCRNs are the key members of the research team most appropriately situated to undertake and achieve this task. Although nurses in this role work in conjunction with other oncology care professionals to provide treatment-related care and information, their primary focus is on educating, treating, and caring for patients through clinical trials. This opportunity enables OCRNs to identify both perceived and actual knowledge gaps in patients, thereby enhancing the effectiveness of research-related education. With this teaching opportunity, OCRNs should ascertain patients' perceived and actual knowledge gaps to improve the adequacy of research information (Chichua et al., 2025).

The Effect of Education on Accrual

Patient education is only the first step toward increasing clinical trial enrollment rates (Asher et al., 2022). Meeting the accrual target is a vital capability that enables the clinical trial to successfully contribute to the development of more effective cancer treatments (Asher et al., 2022). OCRNs are often the de facto members of the clinical trial team for education delivery over the long term. The education OCRNs deliver also has a positive impact on the enrollment of underrepresented populations in clinical trials (Legor et al., 2021). The challenge of this delivery is made increasingly complex by having to analyze a vast array of clinical, technical, and, at times, legal information related to cancer research protocols and distill it into a message that is appropriate and comprehensible to the intended audience. The effectiveness with which this is achieved is a critical yet often underrecognized contributing factor in the overall outcome of clinical trials. The effort can range from providing an individual patient with detailed information on a specific study to an introductory-level presentation for a broader public audience. The intent of the latter approach may be to create awareness of a clinical trial program within the community or to advertise a study better suited to the community at large, such as a prevention study. In either situation, OCRNs must convey certain basic information to aid audiences' understanding of the implications of clinical trial participation.

The literature varies on whether educational efforts have a significant positive impact on accrual outcomes. In some cases, they help to reverse an informational deficit. Doing so may help eliminate distrust or, perhaps, fear that is based on actual or unfounded accounts of research-related misdeeds or the burdens and risks associated with participation in clinical trials. Quinn et al. (2007) found that educational interventions led to increased clinical trial accruals of 8%–33%. Conversely, Black et al. (2022) recognized that a discussion of a clinical trial does not necessarily lead to participation and that many barriers to clinical trial participation exist besides a lack of awareness. Sine et al. (2021) found that educational interventions, while increasing the level of satisfaction attained from the information received, did not demonstrate an increase in subsequent enrollment in clinical trials. Therefore, a recommendation would be to ascertain patients' perceived and actual knowledge and close the gaps to improve the adequacy of research information (Chichua et al., 2025).

In essence, OCRNs are in a unique position because of their constant and consistent contact with patients to guide them through the clinical trial education process by identifying upfront barriers to participation, knowledge deficits, and specific patient–caregiver needs (McKinney et al., 2021).

Individual, Group, and Public Education

OCRNs play a crucial role in educating individuals about clinical trials across three key settings: individual, group, and public. Each of these contexts presents distinct communication challenges and requirements. Effective patient–clinician communication is fundamental in these interactions and should be grounded in strategies that promote clarity, trust, and understanding.

The American Society of Clinical Oncology emphasizes that communication should be patient centered, involving the use of plain language, emotional support, and respect for preferences and values (Gilligan et al., 2017). Additionally, tailoring information to the recipient's needs—including their desired level of detail—and offering content in multiple formats (e.g., written materials, audio, video) can enhance understanding and accessibility. A systematic review by Natale et al. (2021) further underscored that transparency and efforts to build trust and minimize participant burden are essential strategies for increasing recruitment and retention in clinical trials. Ensuring that patients do not feel overwhelmed by information and that their autonomy is respected is crucial for ethical and effective communication. Moreover, Kao et al. (2020) identified essential information elements that support patient decision-making about clinical trial participation. Their findings highlight the importance of providing clear explanations of the trial's purpose, potential risks and benefits, and the logistical commitments required. Encouraging patients to ask questions and providing follow-up discussions to revisit topics and clarify doubts are also integral to the process.

Together, these approaches provide a robust framework for OCRNs to engage in meaningful, supportive, and ethical communication about clinical trials.

Individual Education

A review of the literature highlights ongoing efforts to improve clinical trial education by enhancing patient–provider communication. These interventions are designed to facilitate more meaningful conversations, ultimately promoting a better understanding of clinical trials among patients. Notably, several contemporary studies have explored the use of video-based educational tools as a means to facilitate this process. For example, Yeager et al. (2022) conducted a pilot study using a video intervention to educate patients with breast cancer about clinical trials, reporting that such multimedia tools were both feasible and well-received by patients. Similarly, Vasquez et al. (2023) examined the impact of a novel video intervention designed to prepare patients with blood cancers and their caregivers to discuss clinical trials with their physicians. Their findings suggested that video tools can improve communication readiness and support patient engagement. These studies highlight the potential of tailored multimedia approaches to support patient education. However, variability in patient preferences for information type and decision-making involvement underscores the importance of individualized communication strategies.

Armed with these data, OCRNs should consider the population and circumstances under which any adult educational activities are performed, as well as the variables associated with each. Individually oriented education is perhaps the most common example and typically is based at the bedside for inpatient settings or in the clinic for ambulatory settings. OCRNs must be adept at and comfortable with carrying out this effort in either setting while acknowledging that the information recipient may not be well situated to learn in this manner. They can confidently address potential barriers to education by having supplemental resources (e.g., pamphlets, videos) readily available when delivering clinical trial information.

Timing of Education

Providing clinical trial education to a patient is a process, not a singular event. Although the value of providing such education is not a disputed issue, such as with other essential tasks for oncology OCRNs, it requires planning to achieve its intended purpose. Commonly, the process is initiated early on in the clinician–patient relationship. Conventional wisdom would hold that early intervention would be optimal and even preferred. Fleisher et al. (2020) emphasized the importance of using theory-driven, user-centered design in developing communication tools that support informed decision-making. Their development of the MyChoice digital communication tool demonstrated that patient readiness and contextual factors (e.g., emotional state, treatment phase) must be considered to ensure that educational efforts are effective. This highlights that the period when a patient is being evaluated for anticancer therapy may not always represent the most effective moment for introducing complex information about clinical trials.

Steps that can be taken to educate a patient about a specific clinical trial include an initial assessment of their level of comprehension and emotional receptivity status, especially because the discussion often coincides with the initial disclosure of a cancer diagnosis or treatment failure. The opportunity for a prospective study patient to meet with another patient who is currently on or has completed a particular study offers valuable insight into what the patient might expect in terms of side effects, relayed from the point of experience.

Group and Public Education

Although the literature on group or public education for cancer clinical trials remains scarce, such efforts can generally be presumed to occur in healthcare facilities or non-healthcare settings within the community. Healthcare settings outside of OCRNs' practice areas, such as community clinics and offices, offer a venue to reach study participants closer to where they reside. The group setting can offer the advantage of a greater audience, which can make individuals within that group feel more comfortable among similarly interested participants. Non-healthcare settings, such as places of employment, worship, and other community-based centers, can provide information recipients with the advantages of familiarity, proximity, and convenience. In this situation, a potential sense of trust can occur with what can be interpreted as an implied endorsement from the hosting facility. Conversely, mistrust of the healthcare system remains a significant barrier to research participation, with transparency and trust identified as critical factors in improving recruitment and retention across diverse patient populations (Natale et al., 2021). This concept must be acknowledged as a legitimate concern for certain populations in order to implement a diversity-sensitive approach to community education efforts. Such a nursing-led effort is augmented by a community-derived sense of trust toward nurses, as evidenced by Gallup (2024) poll findings that have consistently found the profession rated at the top in honesty and ethics. In non-healthcare group settings, recipients have the opportunity to be exposed to diverse perceptions and questions beyond their own experiences about the provided information. OCRNs should consider this an opportunity to support an open dialogue and provide information that will dispel any misconceptions related to clinical trial participation. This should lead to a better understanding of the educational message and increase the likelihood of more informed decision-making among recipients.

The choice of setting for an educational session is a factor in the public's receptiveness to the message. Despite some compelling instances, the volume of literature on this issue is scant. For example, community-based settings such as barbershops have emerged as innovative and culturally relevant venues for delivering health promotion and research engagement initiatives. Negrete et al. (2024) demonstrated the effectiveness of barbershop collaborations in engaging Black men in lung cancer research, highlighting the potential of such settings to bridge gaps in participation and trust. Similarly, anecdotal information suggested that traditional community gathering places for men, such as barbershops, can provide an environment conducive to health education.

OCRNs can readily identify patients within their healthcare setting who would benefit from clinical trial education. Identifying appropriate patient groups that typically are outside of one's practice setting is more of a challenge but can be achieved by collecting community demographic information (e.g., census data). This can lead to the identification of residential areas and social gathering locations of groups that may be receptive to clinical trial education among a population consistent with that being targeted by the protocol. From there, the specific requirements and eligibility criteria of the protocol will be the determining factors in whether a patient is eligible to participate in and ultimately provides consent to the study.

Opportunities and Preparation for Speaking to the Public

Opportunities to take clinical trial education to a public audience will vary. One approach involves presenting the information to an audience in a non–protocol-specific manner as a public service. This effort could involve making an educational presentation to a school or vocational audience, a club, a civic organization, or the public at large at health fairs or through the use of radio, television, and, increasingly, social media. Regardless of the venue, a basic approach is to focus on providing the history of clinical trials and an explanation of key concepts in the clinical trial process, as well as the implications of study participation, all with an emphasis on the audience achieving at least a basic understanding. The presenter should allow time for and invite questions from the audience.

Preparation for Public Presentations

In preparation for the event, the presenter should create learning objectives for the presentation and conduct pre- and post-testing to gauge the didactic effect, remembering not to assume that merely providing educational material in an accessible form is sufficient to address patients' information needs. A comprehensive downloadable resource is the U.S. Department of Health and Human Services publication *Making Health Communication Programs Work*, available at www.cancer.gov/publications/health-communication/pink-book.pdf. This book is a revised edition, originally published in 1989. The key to making the most out of this publication is to read all the steps and adapt those relevant to a specific program. The tips and sidebars throughout the book offer suggestions on how to tailor the educational event to meet the learning needs of the audience.

Clinical Trial–Specific Public Presentations

A public presentation on clinical trials can be used to bring attention to a specific protocol. Such opportunities arise when the protocol involves a patient population not typically found within the standard practice setting, such as a cancer prevention study or a study related to the emerging field of proteomics research, wherein prospective study participants are healthy volunteers without a cancer diagnosis. Outside of cancer care settings, the healthy population is most likely to be limited to family members and visitors of patients in most other clinical practice areas. Therefore, one would have to seek speaking venues outside their practice setting to reach the necessary audience in meaningful quantities.

Funding Challenges

Funding typically is an issue for most health-related educational outreach activities. If funding for such activities is limited, several community-centered strategies may still support successful outreach. These include collaborating with local volunteers or healthcare organization staff, initiating efforts through smaller pilot events to assess feasibility and engagement, and partnering with trusted community organizations such as churches or civic groups. Brockman et al. (2023) emphasized the importance of leveraging existing community networks and resources as a key strategy for promoting research participation, particularly among rural and underserved populations.

Community-Grounded Interventions

An et al. (2024) employed a community-engaged process to develop a culturally tailored digital decision-support tool for Black patients with cancer. They convened a Community Advisory Board and conducted interviews with Black patients, family members, and providers to guide development and ensure that the content was relevant and acceptable. The resulting multimedia intervention was found to be feasible, acceptable, and culturally appropriate. In a pilot test, it significantly improved participants' knowledge about precision oncology (targeted therapy) and clinical trials, as well as their confidence in making treatment decisions. These findings suggested that a targeted, community-grounded educational intervention can help overcome barriers by empowering Black patients with the information needed to make informed choices about precision medicine and clinical trial participation.

The Role of Social Media in Clinical Trials Awareness

Evidence highlights the growing use of social media as a powerful tool for raising awareness and facilitating recruitment into clinical research. Through a literature review,

Darko et al. (2022) found that social media platforms can significantly expand the reach of clinical trial recruitment efforts by engaging diverse populations, enhancing message dissemination, and providing cost-effective outreach. Although increased visibility and awareness were consistently reported, the review also emphasized that awareness alone does not always translate into willingness to participate. The authors concluded that, although social media can be effective in promoting public knowledge of clinical research, complementary strategies, such as personalized messaging and trust-building initiatives, are often necessary to support actual enrollment decisions.

Credibility

Potential obstacles that can be encountered when making a public attempt at either protocol-specific or non–protocol-specific education include having a credible message and being a credible messenger. Message credibility can be achieved with various audiences through a straightforward and user-friendly presentation of factual and relevant information. It is when the messenger's credibility is either not already established within the audience (i.e., through the messenger or institution's name recognition) or when the presentation fails to convey a credible message that the overall educational objective is not achieved. A preventive action plan for this situation could include identifying a receptive and appropriate audience for the educational presentation and having the information presented by or mediated through a credible messenger, such as a trusted community member.

Explaining the Importance of Eligibility Criteria

As part of public education efforts, a good approach to explaining the importance of eligibility criteria should include pointing out how and why most clinical trials have specific criteria that define a limited patient population. With the advent and expanded use of new targeted and personalized therapies, this often means that, in some instances, a patient's disease must express specific surface biomarkers or have a particular mutational profile related to that therapy to meet increasingly rigid eligibility criteria. Patients who do not meet the specific requirements of a study, especially if the trial has received publicity that is encouraging, may feel that they have been denied opportunity and, consequently, hope. In settings where patients with similar diagnoses can exchange health histories, such as in treatment waiting areas, the necessity for an individualized treatment approach can be misconstrued. It may contribute to an overall misunderstanding or even negative attitudes among patients or the public toward the process by which clinical trials are conducted. They may not understand how randomized clinical trials are the gold standard for testing new treatment concepts, instead seeing them as arbitrary and favoring scientific principles over patient care due to the necessity for such rigidity to satisfactorily evaluate the protocol's end points. The situation can be exacerbated for patients or the public by disagreement within or between the medical and political communities or those with a vested interest when the response rate of a new treatment is not deemed acceptable for regulatory approval. This could, and has, stemmed from a test agent's marginal disease response that appears to benefit some but not enough study patients to be more widely applicable later on to everyday practice or when the treatment's benefits have not outweighed the risks taken. Beyond these controversies, the principle remains that one must ensure compliance with eligibility criteria as evidence of competent protocol management as outlined in the *Oncology Clinical Research Nurse Competencies* (ONS & ONCC, 2024).

Informational Materials

As limitations in human resources and program infrastructure can often affect the capacity to conduct clinical trial education, it is beneficial to be aware of and take advantage of more straightforward yet readily available resources that will meet educational objectives. Printed materials, such as brochures supplied by the study sponsor, particularly those from the National Cancer Institute and some of the cancer cooperative groups, remain a common approach for delivering protocol-specific information. These materials represent a peer-reviewed and often no-cost communication tool. However, the use of informational brochures has its limitations. An article on decision support tool development for cancer clinical trial participation recommended that expert education materials be written in plain language, making it easy to comprehend information the first time it is heard or read (Langford et al., 2019). Most patients made decisions based on their relationships with members of the clinical team. The research group suggested that patient information sheets are influenced more by the needs of the institution than by the educational needs of the patients.

The use of consumer technology is a common means worldwide for providing and acquiring health information. Online health information seeking has become a common practice among U.S. adults. Finney Rutten et al. (2019) found that a substantial majority of adults use the internet to seek health information, with notable increases observed over time as part of broader efforts to meet Healthy People 2020 objectives. Their findings underscore the importance of digital access in shaping how individuals gather information about health conditions, treatments, and preventive care. The rapid adoption of smart handheld devices has enabled point-of-service informational capabilities. Many patients are using internet-derived health information that they have gathered personally or from family or friends. In a sense, the internet and its enabling devices can help level the healthcare playing field and mitigate the barrier to entry by providing information with the click of a key or the swipe of a screen. Vigilance must be exercised to recognize the strengths and weaknesses that these mediums pose as sources of information for clinical trial education. How to best leverage the internet's potential as a conduit for valid and forthright information about clinical trials, as well as how to address the potential barrage of questions from technology-equipped and savvy patients or members of the public, should motivate OCRNs to sharpen their information technology skills. Challenges aside, this informational medium is widely used and has been recognized as an essential tool in navigating today's clinical research landscape. OCRNs must balance internet opportunities with the negative aspects that come with the plethora of health-related information, some of which is either misleading or outright false, performed in the guise of offering hope.

Most cancer institutions provide internet-based information related to cancer care for the public. A mainstay of these websites is information related to clinical trials in general, as well as those offered through the institution. Although the sites provide viewers with information on clinical trials, the availability is typically limited to that vicinity unless patients are willing to travel to the sponsoring institution for care. To reach a broader geographic audience, several publicly or privately sponsored websites are available that provide accurate and current information on all aspects of clinical trial participation, along with registries for listings of actively accruing clinical trials being conducted nationwide. Table 15-1 includes a list of internet resources that may be relevant to the learning objectives for one-to-one education or a specific group educational program.

Although communication remains challenging, video and animation platforms are emerging as a means to provide education on clinical trials to potential participants. Occa and Morgan (2019) conducted a study to investigate the effect of animated videos compared to brochures with and without visuals, as well as National Institutes of Health materials, on knowledge and attitudes toward clinical trials in patients with cancer and those in survivorship. The researchers found positive results regarding the animations, as they improved participants' knowledge about and attitudes toward clinical trials. These animations were more effective than the National Institutes of Health materials in terms of information presentation for participants categorized as having low motivation and low ability to understand health information (Occa & Morgan, 2019). By offering multiple ways of information delivery, animation was helpful in generalizing what can be deemed as complex information.

Healthcare professionals must continue to investigate and develop alternative methods for delivering information to patients and caregivers in the ever-evolving world of clinical trials, thereby assisting with understanding and informed decision-making.

Underrepresented Populations

Oncology clinical trials represent a vital opportunity to improve cancer treatment and prevention. Although participation remains limited across the general oncology population, a 2024 study published in the *Journal of Clinical Oncology* reported that 21.9% of individuals with cancer participate in some form of clinical research, including treatment trials, biorepository studies, genetic studies, and quality-of-life research (Unger et al., 2024). Specifically, enrollment in cancer treatment trials between 2013 and 2017 was 7.1%, a notable increase from previous estimates of 2%–3%.

Despite this progress, disparities in participation persist. Saphner et al. (2021) demonstrated that clinical trial enrollment continues to be disproportionately low among racial and ethnic minorities, older adults, and individuals from lower socioeconomic backgrounds. These disparities raise concerns about the generalizability of findings, as data derived from more homogeneous populations limit our understanding of therapeutic efficacy and safety across diverse groups.

Improving participation among underrepresented populations requires a multifaceted approach. Patients must be equipped with the skills to understand research and scientific concepts, evaluate health information, and make informed decision-making. Equally important, healthcare providers must deliver health education that is accessible, relevant, and culturally tailored to the communities they serve.

Older Adults

The risk of being diagnosed with cancer increases with age. Approximately 88% of all cancers are diagnosed in people aged 50 years or older, and 59% of cases are diagnosed in individuals aged 65 years or older (American Cancer Society [ACS], 2025). The need to include older adults in clinical trials to ensure that the results are applicable to them is clear. However, the expeditious recruitment of an appropriate number of patients that reflects the reality of the population is a constant challenge. As cancer is generally accepted to be a disease most frequently found in the older adult population, OCRNs will most likely find that their educational efforts will be directed toward this group. Despite the growing number of older adults diagnosed with cancer, they remain significantly underrepresented in clinical trials. The care of older patients is often complicated by comorbidities, age-related physiologic changes, and functional

TABLE 15-1 | Clinical Trial Educational Resources

Resource	Description
AccrualNet https://nimict.com/tools/accrualnet	The National Cancer Institute sponsors this website. The site's focus is on professionals caring for clinical research participants. It offers resources, strategies, and tools and contains descriptions and links to professional and patient education resources about clinical trials.
Center for Information and Study on Clinical Research Participation Educational Brochures www.ciscrp.org	This site includes information for patients considering a clinical trial and for professional use, providing potential research participants with an introduction to clinical trials.
CenterWatch www.centerwatch.com	This site provides information on clinical trials for various diseases and conditions.
National Heart, Lung, and Blood Institute www.nhlbi.nih.gov/research/clinical-trials	This site offers information for patients who have heart, lung, blood, or sleep-related diseases or disorders who are interested in clinical trials and funding opportunities.
National Institutes of Health National Institute on Aging https://www.nia.nih.gov/health/clinical-trials-and-studies/what-are-clinical-trials-and-studies	This site addresses the concerns of older adults regarding participation in a clinical trial. It includes free educational pamphlet downloads.
National Institutes of Health Clinical Research Trials and You www.nih.gov/health/clinicaltrials/index.htm	This site provides basic information, patient stories, and educational materials. Spanish language materials are available.

limitations, which can make it challenging to generalize findings from trials primarily involving younger populations. Hagège et al. (2021) emphasized that improving the inclusion of older adults in oncology trials requires stronger collaboration between oncologists and geriatricians. Their study highlighted how interprofessional cooperation can support more appropriate patient selection, assessment, and management, ultimately leading to better-tailored treatments and improved clinical outcomes for older patients.

Patients With Low Incomes

Studies have shown that socioeconomic status has a significant impact on enrollment in cancer clinical trials. Patients with lower annual household incomes are consistently underrepresented in these studies. For instance, individuals with yearly incomes below $50,000 are less likely to participate in clinical trials compared to those with higher incomes, in part due to concerns about the affordability of care during trial participation (Donzo et al., 2024). Financial barriers, including out-of-pocket expenses and inadequate insurance coverage, are major deterrents. These economic challenges contribute to disparities in clinical trial participation, limiting access to potentially beneficial treatments for underserved populations. Moreover, early-phase clinical research participants frequently experience financial toxicity, which includes significant personal financial burden and distress related to treatment costs (Durbin et al., 2025). Specific educational strategies for these patients, such as how to manage indirect and hidden costs (e.g., unpaid leave from work, increased co-pays for visits, hotel costs), could be learning objectives to help patients with low incomes participate in clinical trials. Implementation of a financial toxicity screening tool (e.g., Comprehensive Score for Financial Toxicity [COST]) can help identify the financial burdens patients may face prior to consenting. The lack of adequate insurance coverage for routine care during clinical trials remains a substantial obstacle, undermining efforts to ensure equitable access and slowing progress in cancer research. However, the Patient Protection and Affordable Care Act requires health insurers to pay for routine costs of care in approved clinical trials for cancer and other life-threatening diseases. Covered clinical trials may include trials for treatment, prevention, and early detection.

Hispanics and Latinos

Data that describe clinical trial participation among Latinos, a population that has poor cancer outcomes, are lacking. Latinos are one of the fastest-growing and largest minority groups in the United States, and cancer is the leading cause of death in this population (ACS, 2024b). According to Espinoza-Gutarra et al. (2022), this group accounts for 2.3%–3.9% of participants in cancer clinical trials, with a decline in participation over time. Byrne et al. (2020) examined how translating an online clinical trial recruitment registry from English to Spanish could increase awareness of and willingness to participate in clinical trials. A multiactivity approach was used to translate the registry, which included using plain language, consulting translation professionals and bilingual community speakers, as well as launching and promoting the initiative. Out of the 162 people who registered as Spanish-speaking and of Hispanic ethnicity, 75% were contacted about possible clinical trial eligibility, and 39% expressed willingness to participate in a trial (Byrne et al., 2020). Other outcomes included registrants signing up to receive new trial notifications in Spanish and a higher rate of reported health conditions. Lessons learned included cultural values, the lack of access to technology (with more participants owning smartphones than computers), and barriers to participation that should be addressed to boost exposure and increase enrollment.

Every opportunity to educate and inform should be taken for this vulnerable population. A study by Weston et al. (2024) evaluated clinical trial awareness and willingness among Latino adults (a significant portion being foreign born). With a sample size of N = 600, only about 21% knew that clinical trials (for COVID-19 treatments or vaccines) were available. Nevertheless, among Latinos, increased awareness and higher trust in information significantly predicted willingness to participate. The study further identified trust in healthcare providers as a key informational source—not necessarily translating to awareness or intent—mirroring findings of missed opportunities to educate this population.

Black Americans

Over time, cancer death rates have steadily decreased for Black men and women, but this population still bears a heavy burden of mortality and low survival. According to Lawrence et al. (2022), there was a 2% decrease in cancer-related deaths from 1999 to 2019 in both genders. Black men experienced a faster decrease, at a rate of 2.6% per year, whereas Black women saw a decrease of 1.5% each year (Lawrence et al., 2022). Despite declines, the Black population had the highest death rate and the shortest survival of any racial or ethnic group with cancer in the United States. ACS (n.d.) also outlined that Black immigrants coming into the United States have lower cancer mortality rates than Black natural-born citizens. Black women are 40% more likely to die from breast cancer than their White counterparts, and Black men continue to have the highest rate of death from prostate cancer (ACS, n.d.).

Overall, Black Americans are 26% more likely to die of cancer than their White counterparts (ACS, 2022). Black Americans continue to have lower overall five-year survival rates than White patients with cancer and for each stage of diagnosis for most cancer sites (ACS, 2022). There have been efforts to decrease these disparities, including improved access to health care, more affordable health care, prevention, screening, behavioral and lifestyle changes, and advancements in treatment. The increase in smoking cessation in the Black community has also been a positive factor.

Much of the difference in survival is believed to be because of barriers that limit access to timely, high-quality medical care. Furthermore, Black Americans are more likely to be diagnosed at a later stage of the disease when treatment choices are more limited and less effective (ACS, 2022). This makes accrual to clinical trials very important for this population. Black patients have had a low enrollment rate in therapeutic trials in which a cancer drug was approved in a five-year period; certain factors are not taken into consideration when creating inclusion and exclusion criteria that are sensitive to this population. Providers may not share information on or gauge the attitude of these particular patients toward clinical trials (Awidi & Al Hadidi, 2021).

Due to these factors, Black patients with cancer continue to participate in clinical trials at lower rates than the general population. Besides mistrust of the medical system, one of the most frequently cited, addressable barriers to participation is a lack of accessible and culturally relevant information. Research has shown that tailored educational approaches are effective in improving awareness and shaping attitudes toward clinical trials. For example, a community–academic partnership study examined the informational needs of Black women to inform recruitment strategies more effectively. The findings emphasized the importance of culturally appropriate education and communication in building trust and increasing engagement in clinical trials (Rivers et al., 2019).

American Indians and Alaska Natives

According to the U.S. Centers for Disease Control and Prevention (2025), American Indians and Alaska Natives have some of the highest cancer-related mortality rates of all U.S. ethnic groups. Liver, colorectal, kidney, and stomach cancer incidence rates for both genders in this group are higher than for Whites. Cervical cancer incidence rates for women in this population are also higher than those of White women.

Interest in participating in cancer clinical trials for this population is disproportionately low for several reasons. Mistrust and fear of the medical system persist, alongside limited access to low-cost, quality health care, as well as the exclusion of American Indian and Alaska Native individuals as a racial and ethnicity category in national datasets, which negatively impacts trial recruitment (Mainous et al., 2023). For this group, it is recommended that recruitment strategies be culturally sensitive to demonstrate inclusiveness, cultural humility, safety, and respect. In the 2023 study by Mainous et al., a "circle of trust" was used as a recruitment tool for the trial. The circle involves the tenets of participant, investigator, trusted entity, and community to educate potential participants about and expose them to clinical trials. Engaging potential research participants can also involve community inclusion in protocol development and review, as well as collaboration with American Indian and Alaska Native trial investigators, addressing disparities and ensuring data ownership (Mainous et al., 2023). The findings from this study could be used as an educational platform for OCRNs in working with American Indians and Alaska Natives.

Asian Americans, Native Hawaiians, and Pacific Islanders

Cancer is a leading cause of death for several groups within the Asian American community, and cancer-related mortality rates are higher for Pacific Islanders and Native Hawaiians than those of Whites (ACS, 2024a). The enrollment of Asian Americans, Native Hawaiians, and Pacific Islanders in cancer clinical trials has historically been underrepresented compared to other racial and ethnic groups. A cross-sectional study by Đoàn et al. (2019) found that studies focused specifically on health disparities affecting this population comprised only 0.17% of the National Institutes of Health's total budget over 26 years. This underrepresentation can be attributed to various factors, including but not limited to recruitment and retention challenges, socioeconomic factors, mistrust of healthcare systems, and cultural and language barriers. Financial burdens and limited access to affordable health insurance can contribute to low enrollment. Also posing a challenge are issues with data aggregation. These communities encompass a diverse group of people with distinct health profiles and concerns. Aggregating data under this broad label can mask specific inequalities and needs within subgroups, further complicating efforts to increase representation.

Summary

Educating patients and the public about their potential role in clinical trials is crucial to advancing progress in cancer treatment. The challenges in meeting this objective are significant, presenting OCRNs with opportunities for professional skills development and improved patient care and public relations. This skill was recognized during the formulation of the *Oncology Clinical Research Nurse Competencies* (ONS & ONCC, 2024) and included as a key function in the competent practice of OCRNs. As highly trusted members of the community, OCRNs honor that trust in their role by assessing and reducing health-related knowledge deficits in diverse patient populations through education and teaching. By recognizing the need to use an evidence-based approach in disseminating information to their patient population, as well as to the public, OCRNs can foster better-informed and, potentially, more engaged healthcare consumers. Patient and public outreach education serves to encourage and reinforce a research-supportive relationship between OCRNs and their nursing colleagues by promoting awareness and providing continuous updates on clinical trials.

OCRNs should expand their role to include devising, implementing, and assessing population-appropriate techniques for effectively presenting accurate and up-to-date information about cancer clinical trials, upon which patients can base their treatment decisions or the public can formulate an informed opinion.

Key Points

- Effective communication skills from OCRNs are an essential prerequisite, enabling patients to make informed decisions about their care.
- Education is a process, not a singular event.
- Message credibility can be achieved through a straightforward, user-friendly presentation of factual, relevant, evidence-based information.
- Healthcare providers have a professional and moral responsibility to provide patients with cancer complete and comprehensive information regarding their disease and clinical trial options.
- OCRNs are key members of the clinical trial team, most appropriately situated and suited to undertake education regarding clinical trials.
- OCRNs should ascertain patients' perceived and actual knowledge and close the gaps to improve the adequacy of research information.
- Educational efforts that increase awareness of clinical trials do not necessarily result in increased enrollment.

The author would like to acknowledge David Leos, MBA, RN, OCN®, and Norma Sheridan-Leos, MSN, RN, AOCN®, CPHQ, CPPS, for their contribution to this chapter that remains unchanged from the previous edition of this book.

References

American Cancer Society. (n.d.). *Cancer disparities in the Black community.* https://www.cancer.org/about-us/what-we-do/health-equity/cancer-disparities-in-the-black-community.html

American Cancer Society. (2022). *Cancer facts and figures for African American/Black People 2022–2024.* https://www.cancer.org/content/dam/cancer-org/research/cancer-facts-and-statistics/cancer-facts-and-figures-for-african-americans/2022-2024-cff-aa.pdf

American Cancer Society. (2024a). *Cancer facts and figures for Asian American, Native Hawaiian, and other Pacific Islander people 2024–2026.* https://www.cancer.org/content/dam/cancer-org/research/cancer-facts-and-statistics/aanhpi-cancer-facts-and-figures/aanhpi-cff.pdf

American Cancer Society. (2024b). *Cancer facts and figures for Hispanic/Latino People 2024–2026.* https://www.cancer.org/content/dam/cancer-org/research/cancer-facts-and-statistics/cancer-facts-and-figures-for-hispanics-and-latinos/2024/2024-2026-cancer-facts-and-figures-for-hispanics-and-latinos.pdf

American Cancer Society. (2025). *Cancer facts and figures 2025.* https://www.cancer.org/content/dam/cancer-org/research/cancer-facts-and-statistics/annual-cancer-facts-and-figures/2025/2025-cancer-facts-and-figures-acs.pdf

An, J., Ferrante, J.M., Macenat, M., Ganesan, S., Hudson, S.V., Omene, C., … Kinney, A.Y. (2024). Promoting informed approaches in precision oncology and clinical trial participation for Black patients with cancer: Community-engaged development and pilot testing of a digital intervention. *Cancer, 130*(Suppl. 20), 3561–3577. https://doi.org/10.1002/cncr.35049

Asher, N., Raphael, A., Wolf, I., Pelles, S., & Geva, R. (2022). Oncologic patients' misconceptions may impede enrollment into clinical trials: A cross-sectional study. *BMC Medical Research Methodology, 22*(1), 5. https://doi.org/10.1186/s12874-021-01478-5

Awidi, M., & Al Hadidi, S. (2021). Participation of Black Americans in cancer clinical trials: Current challenges and proposed solutions. *JCO Oncology Practice, 17*(5), 265–272. https://doi.org/10.1200/OP.21.00001

Black, M.D., Esene, L., McClelland, R., Mayer, H., Welch, S., Bauman, G., & Vandenberg, T. (2022). An electronic information kiosk for enhancing patient accrual for cancer clinical trials: A pilot and feasibility study. *Cureus, 14*(5), e25114. https://doi.org/10.7759/cureus.25114

Brockman, T.A., Shaw, O., Wiepert, L., Nguyen, Q.A., Kelpin, S.S., West, I., ... Patten, C.A. (2023). Community engagement strategies to promote recruitment and participation in clinical research among rural communities: A narrative review. *Journal of Clinical and Translational Science, 7*(1), e84. https://doi.org/10.1017/cts.2023.16

Byrne, L.M., Cook, S.K., Kennedy, N., Russell, M., Jerome, R.N., Tan, J., ... Harris, P.A. (2020). Opening doors to clinical trial participation among Hispanics: Lessons learned from the Spanish translation or ResearchMatch. *Journal of Clinical and Translational Science,* 5(1), e46. https://doi.org/10.1017/cts.2020.539

Chichua, M., Mazzoni, D., Marzorati, C., & Pravettoni, G. (2025). The journey of patients in cancer clinical trials: A qualitative meta-synthesis on experiences and perspectives. *Patient Education and Counseling, 130,* 108469. https://doi.org/10.1016/j.pec.2024.108469

Darko, E.M., Kleib, M., & Olson, J. (2022). Social media use for research participant recruitment: Integrative literature review. *Journal of Medical Internet Research, 24*(8), e38015. https://doi.org/10.2196/38015

Đoàn, L.N., Takata, Y., Sakuma, K.K., & Irvin, V.L. (2019). Trends in clinical research including Asian American, Native Hawaiian, and Pacific Islander participation funded by the US National Institutes of Health, 1992 to 2018. *JAMA Network Open, 2*(7), e197432. https://doi.org/10.1001/jamanetworkopen.2019.7432

Donzo, M.W., Nguyen, G., Nemeth, J.K., Owoc, M.S., Mady, L.J., Chen, A.Y., & Schmitt, N.C. (2024). Effects of socioeconomic status on enrollment in clinical trials for cancer: A systematic review. *Cancer Medicine, 13*(1), e6905. https://doi.org/10.1002/cam4.6905

Durbin, S.M., Lundquist, D., Pelletier, A., Petrillo, L.A., Bame, V., Turbini, V., ... Nipp, R.D. (2025). Financial toxicity in early-phase cancer clinical trial participants. *Cancer, 131*(1), e35586. https://doi.org/10.1002/cncr.35586

Espinoza-Gutarra, M.R., Duma, N., Aristizabal, P., Segarra-Vazquez, B., Borno, H., Halbert, C.H., ... Velazquez, A.I. (2022). The problem of Hispanic/Latinx under-representation in cancer clinical trials. *JCO Oncology Practice, 18*(5) 380–384. https://doi.org/10.1200/OP.22.00214

Finney Rutten, L.J., Blake, K.D., Greenberg-Worisek, A.J., Allen, S.V., Moser, R.P., & Hesse, B.W. (2019). Online health information seeking among US adults: Measuring progress toward a Healthy People 2020 objective. *Public Health Reports, 134*(6), 617–625. https://doi.org/10.1177/0033354919874074

Fleisher, L., Bass, S.B., Shwarz, M., Washington, A., Nicholson, A., Alhajji, M., ... Kenny, C. (2020). Using theory and user-centered design in digital health: The development of the *mychoice* communication tool to prepare patients and improve informed decision making regarding clinical trial participation. *Psycho-Oncology, 29*(1), 114–122. https://doi.org/10.1002/pon.5254

Gallup. (2024). *Honesty/ethics in professions.* http://www.gallup.com/poll/1654/honesty-ethics-professions.aspx

Gilligan, T., Coyle, N., Frankel, R.M., Berry, D.L., Bohlke, K., Epstein, R.M., ... Baile, W.F. (2017). Patient–clinician communication: American Society of Clinical Oncology consensus guideline. *Journal of Clinical Oncology, 35*(31), 3618–3632. https://doi.org/10.1200/JCO.2017.75.2311

Hagège, M., Canouï-Poitrine, F., & Derbez, B. (2021). Including older patients in cancer trials: A qualitative study of collaboration between geriatricians and oncologists. *Journal of Geriatric Oncology, 12*(6), 945–951. https://doi.org/10.1016/j.jgo.2021.03.002

Henley, M., DeCotiis, G., FitzGibbon, H., & Singhi, E.K. (2024). Decoding clinical trial jargon: Helping people understand the efficacy end points used in cancer trials. *Future Oncology, 21*(1), 11–14. https://doi.org/10.1080/14796694.2024.2433411

Holden, C.E., Wheelwright, S., Harle, A., & Wagland, R. (2021). The role of health literacy in cancer care: A mixed studies systematic review. *PLOS ONE, 16*(11), e0259815. https://doi.org/10.1371/journal.pone.0259815.

Kao, C.-Y., Aranda, S., Krishnasamy, M., & Hamilton, B. (2020). Identifying essential information to support patient decision-making regarding participation in cancer clinical trials: A Delphi study. *European Journal of Cancer Care, 29*(2), e13188. https://doi.org/10.1111/ecc.13188

Langford, A.T., Hawley, S.T., Stableford, S., Studts, J.L., & Byrne, M.M. (2019). Development of a plain language decision support tool for cancer clinical trials: Blending health literacy, academic research, and minority patient perspectives. *Journal of Cancer Education, 35*(3), 454–461. https://doi.org/10.1007/s13187-019-1482-5

Lawrence, W.R., McGee-Avila, J.K., Vo, J.B., Luo, Q., Chen, Y., Inoue-Choi, M., ... Shiels, M.S. (2022). Trends in cancer mortality among Black individuals in the US from 1999 to 2019. *JAMA Oncology, 8*(8), 1184–1189. https://doi.org/10.1001/jamaoncol.2022.1472

Legor, K.A., Hayman, L.L., Foust, J.B., & Blazey, M.L. (2021). The role of clinical research nurses in minority recruitment to cancer clinical trials. *Contemporary Clinical Trials, 110,* 106590. https://doi.org/10.1016/j.cct.2021.106590

Mainous, A.G., 3rd, Kelliher, A., & Warne, D. (2023). Recruiting indigenous patients into clinical trials: A Circle of Trust. *Annals of Family Medicine, 2*(1) 54–56. https://doi.org/10.1370/afm.2901

McKinney, M., Bell, R., Samborski, C., Attwood, K., Dean, G., Eakle, K., ... Edge, S. (2021). Clinical trial participation: A pilot study of patient-identified barriers. *Clinical Journal of Oncology Nursing, 25*(6), 647–654. https://doi.org/10.1188/21.CJON.647-654

Muscat, D.M., Shepherd, H.L., Nutbeam, D., Trevena, L., & McCaffery, K.J. (2021). Literacy and shared decision-making: Exploring the relationship to enable meaningful patient engagement in healthcare. *Journal of General Internal Medicine, 36*(2), 521–524. https://doi.org/10.1007/s11606-020-05912-0

Natale, P., Saglimbene, V., Ruospo, M., Gonzalez, A.M., Strippoli, G.F., Scholes-Robertson, N., ... Tong, A. (2021). Transparency, trust and minimizing burden to increase recruitment and retention in trials: A systematic review. *Journal of Clinical Epidemiology, 134,* 35–51. https://doi.org/10.1016/j.jclinepi.2021.01.014

Negrete, M., Ademiluyi, A., Karayeva, E., Eskridge, G., Huggins, M., Eskridge, C.M., ... Kim, S.J. (2024). Bridging the gap: Engaging Black men in lung cancer research through barbershop collaboration. *American Journal of Men's Health, 18*(1). https://doi.org/10.1177/15579883241229417

Occa, A., & Morgan, S.E., (2019). Animations about clinical trial participation for cancer patients and survivors. *Journal of Health Communication, 24*(10), 749–760. https://doi.org/10.1080/10810730.2019.1668089

Oncology Nursing Society & Oncology Nursing Certification Corporation. (2024). *Oncology clinical research nurse competencies.* https://www.ons.org/sites/default/files/2025-01/ocrn-competencies-rebrand.pdf

Quinn, G.P., Bell, B.A., Bell, M.Y., Caraway, V.D., Conforte, D., Graci, L.B., ... Bepler, G. (2007). The guinea pig syndrome: Improving clinical trial participation among thoracic patients. *Journal of Thoracic Oncology, 2*(3), 191–196. https://doi.org/10.1097/JTO.0b013e318031cdb6

Rivers, D.A., Pal, T., Vadaparampil, S.T., Adams, L.A., Dash-Pitts, L., & Quinn, G.P. (2019). A community–academic partnership to explore informational needs of African American women as a primer for cancer clinical trial recruitment. *Ethnicity and Health, 24*(6), 679–693. https://doi.org/10.1080/13557858.2017.1367762

Saphner, T., Marek, A., Homa, J.K., Robinson, L., & Glandt, N. (2021). Clinical trial participation assessed by age, sex, race, ethnicity, and socioeconomic status. *Contemporary Clinical Trials, 103,* 106315. https://doi.org/10.1016/j.cct.2021.106315

Shepherd Forbes, R., Bradford, A., Lieschke, M., Shackleton, K., & Hyatt, A. (2023). Patient communication and experiences in cancer clinical drug trials: A mixed-method study at a specialist clinical trials unit. *Trials, 24*(1), 400. https://doi.org/10.1186/s13063-023-07284-2

Sine, S., de Bruin, A., & Getz, K. (2021). Patient engagement initiatives in clinical trials: Recent trends and implications. *Therapeutic Innovation and Regulatory Science, 55*(5), 1059–1065. https://doi.org/10.1007/s43441-021-00306-8

U.S. Centers for Disease Control and Prevention. (2025). *Cancer and American Indian and Alaska Native people.* https://www.cdc.gov/cancer/health-equity/american-indian-alaska-native.html

Unger, J.M., Shulman, L.N., Facktor, M.A., Nelson, H., & Fleury, M.E. (2024). National estimates of the participation of patients with cancer in clinical research studies based on Commission on Cancer accreditation data. *Journal of Clinical Oncology, 42*(18), 2139–2150. https://doi.org/10.1200/JCO.23.01030

Vasquez, T.S., Eggly, S., Sae-Hau, M., DeMairo, K., Figueroa, L., Gambatese, M., ... Bylund, C.L. (2023). Preparing patients to communicate with their doctors about clinical trials as a treatment option: Impact of a novel video intervention for patients with a blood cancer and their caregivers. *Journal of Cancer Education, 38*(5), 1562–1570. https://doi.org/10.1007/s13187-023-02300-0

Weston, C.M., Andrade, E.L., Olawole, W., Vazquez, M.G., Miller, H., Stevens, S.C., ... Dennison Himmelfarb, C.R. (2024). Predictors of willingness to participate in COVID-19 clinical trials among Black and Latino adults. *Journal of Clinical and Translational Science, 8*(1), e217. https://doi.org/10.1017/cts.2024.654

Yeager, K.A., Bai, J., Gogineni, K., Meisel, J.L., Kweon, J., Bruner, D.W., & Waldrop-Valverde, D. (2022). Pilot feasibility study of a video intervention to educate patients with breast cancer about clinical trials. *Journal of Cancer Education, 37*(2), 387–394. https://doi.org/10.1007/s13187-020-01826-x

CHAPTER 16

Accrual Base, Recruitment, and Promotion Strategies

Jessica Schnase, MSN, RN, OCN®, CCRP

Introduction

Oncology clinical trials are often quite complex because of the ever-changing landscape of treatment options. These trials are crucial in driving cancer research forward, making it essential to understand an institution's accrual base and patient population. Recruitment to these complex trials can be challenging due to the specificity of inclusion and exclusion criteria, the overall health of the patients, and the continued stigma associated with participation in a clinical trial. Promotion strategies are sometimes more complex because of the nature of treating patients with cancer.

This chapter will address these important pillars of a clinical trial program. It will also address the challenges of recruitment and provide strategies to increase the number of participants enrolled in cancer trials.

Clinical Trial Enrollment and Emerging Trends

According to the National Comprehensive Cancer Network Guidelines (n.d.), "the best management for any patient with cancer is in a clinical trial." However, "among the National Cancer Institute (NCI)-sponsored trials, around 40% never reach completion, 20% are closed prematurely, with less than 50% meeting enrollment targets" (Mittal et al., 2024, p. 3739). Failing to enroll the required number of participants in a trial can affect its statistical power, potentially leading to the inaccurate reporting of clinically significant effects as statistically insignificant.

Lengthy recruitment periods increase time and expenses, putting clinical trials at risk of being terminated prematurely. In their review of oncology clinical trial design and conduct of phase 1 clinical trials, Araujo et al. (2023) described the importance of flexibility in trials, as well as having clear end points. Trial design plays an imperative role in the success of a clinical trial. Sites should use a design that closely aligns with the author's intentions and their target patient population to foster the trial's success.

Patient participation is trending in a positive direction. Historically, patients with cancer comprised 3%–5% of clinical research participants; however, 2024 data showed that the estimated patient participation in oncology clinical trials was 7.1% (Unger et al., 2024). In this study, patients with cancer also participated in biorepository (12.9%), registry (7.3%), genetic (3.6%), quality-of-life (2.8%), diagnostic (2.5%), and economic (2.4%) studies (Unger et al., 2024). It is worth noting that 21.9% of participants were involved in one or more cancer clinical research trials. Trial enrollment was divided into 21.6% at NCI-designated comprehensive cancer centers, 5.7% at integrated network cancer programs, 5.4% at academic comprehensive cancer programs, and 4.1% at community programs (Unger et al., 2024).

Recruitment Considerations

The recruitment of appropriate and adequate numbers of research participants is an essential component of successful trial completion and the subsequent generation of results. However, recruiting research participants is often a challenging and multifaceted task. Before trial initiation, every effort should be made to identify potential recruitment barriers and select strategies to mitigate them. Discussions should be held with key stakeholders, including physicians, advanced practice providers (APPs), research staff, and administration, to identify and address institutional barriers, thereby allowing research staff to focus solely on patient-related issues. Collaborating with sponsors and using patient resources can enhance patient participation. These can include patient brochures, websites, cell phone applications, or other institutional review board (IRB)-approved tools to help educate patients about the clinical trial.

Barriers to Recruitment

Having a basic understanding and awareness of the challenges and barriers that affect recruitment is essential before attempting to develop and implement recruitment strategies. Although patient-related barriers are often identified and discussed, it is also necessary to be aware of the institutional and organizational barriers that may exist within a particular location.

Barriers to clinical trial participation often involve multiple levels and may be related to patients, healthcare providers, or institutions (Kumar et al., 2022). For example, patient-related barriers may include a lack of awareness, fear of side effects, additional costs, a desire to select the treatment, and added time required. Provider barriers often include a lack of availability of appropriate trials, associated time and costs, and low interest in the study design. Table 16-1 lists examples of barriers and corresponding codes (Kumar et al., 2022).

Structural or institutional barriers may also negatively affect accrual but are not commonly addressed in the literature. Dilts and Sandler (2006) reported on invisible or administrative barriers that occur outside of the patient–provider interaction. The authors divided administrative barriers into three types: procedural, structural, and infrastructural. Procedural barriers refer to the processes or series of steps required to initiate a clinical trial within an institution or research program. Examples of common approval processes within academic centers were studied, often requiring significant, consecutive approvals before a clinical trial can be opened. The levels of approval may begin with the department or unit where the trial will be conducted. Then, the trial must be submitted to an IRB, a scientific review committee, a contracts and grants office, and other relevant entities before it is approved for activation.

TABLE 16-1 | Themes and Codes Related Barriers to Clinical Trial Enrollment

Level of Barriers	Codes on Specific Barriers
Patient	Beliefs/attitude or mistrust, distance to trial site, health insurance coverage, language, and immigration status
Healthcare providers	Limited awareness/knowledge of ongoing clinical trials, time constraints, and non-cooperation of colleagues
Clinical	Strict eligibility criteria and complex clinical design
Institutional/ structural	Policy, limited logistic support (staff, financial, and institutional review board)

Note. From "Barriers for Cancer Clinical Trial Enrollment: A Qualitative Study of the Perspectives of Healthcare Providers," by G. Kumar, P. Chaudbury, A. Quinn, and D. Su, 2022, *Contemporary Clinical Trials Communications, 28,* 100939 (https://doi.org/10.1016/j.conctc.2022.100939). Copyright 2022 by the authors, licensed under CC BY-NC-ND 4.0 DEED (https://creativecommons.org/licenses/by-nc-nd/4.0).

The layout of an organization often causes structural barriers. Different groups or departments have different steps to follow, which frequently leads to confusion and misunderstandings. One department, such as a grants and contracts office, may require a condition to be met; however, the sponsor cannot agree to the condition unless the radiology department concurs with another condition. Further confusion can arise when offices within an institution fail to distinguish between clinical trials and grant research.

Infrastructural barriers are associated with the design of the core institutional system and its interconnections. An example may be an organization that lacks sufficient resources for regularly scheduled, timely IRB meetings, resulting in a delay in evaluating potential clinical trials. These invisible barriers are very real for many research programs.

Minority and Underserved Populations

For cancers such as stomach, prostate, and uterine, mortality rates are two times higher for Black patients (Siegel et al., 2024). This population has the highest death rate and shortest survival of any racial and ethnic group in the United States for most cancers (American Cancer Society [ACS], 2022). The causes of these inequalities are complex and are thought to reflect social and economic disparities more than biologic differences associated with race (ACS, 2022). Between 1975 and 2019, the death rate for all cancers combined was higher among Blacks than Whites, with a prominent gap also seen for men over women (ACS, 2022). Oncology clinical research nurses (OCRNs) must consider this disparity within their institutions and when recruiting patients. Minority and underserved populations, however, often have increased levels of mistrust or misunderstanding of clinical research in addition to healthcare access issues, such as lack of insurance, transportation issues, and language barriers (Anastasi et al., 2024).

Trial Focus

Recruiting participants to treatment-focused clinical trials may require different recruitment and planning strategies than those used in other types of clinical trials, such as cancer control, symptom management, quality-of-life, prevention, screening, or early-detection trials. Potential participants for treatment trials are primarily patients with cancer who have a compelling motivation to treat their disease and are generally accessible in oncology clinics and physician practices. Patients with cancer often experience an array of disease- or treatment-related symptoms, motivating them to participate in a clinical trial that may alleviate these symptoms. When providers discuss these clinical trial options with patients, they "may struggle to assess the risk–benefit ratio and may over-weigh the probability and severity of various types of adverse outcomes associated with clinical trial participation" (Nipp et al., 2019, p. 107).

Unlike treatment and cancer control trials, potential participants in prevention, screening, or early-detection trials typically include healthy individuals from the general population or a defined high-risk group. Accessing these healthy individuals, who may not be as motivated as patients with a disease to participate in a clinical research study, requires additional recruitment planning, strategizing, and effort. Researchers attempting to recruit from these populations should discuss any questions with potential participants to help alleviate any ambivalence they may have toward participation (Anastasi et al., 2024).

Eligibility screening for clinical trials is often time intensive with associated costs that sponsors typically do not cover. Many trials include ancillary components requiring the submission of specimens for the examination of biomarkers. "Clinical trials have evolved, shifting from tumor type–centered to gene-directed, histology-agnostic, with innovative adaptive design tailored to biomarker profiling with the goal to improve treatment outcomes" (Tsimberidou et al., 2020, p. 1); however, screening for biomarker-focused trials increases time-associated efficacy challenges because many patients may need to be screened before actual enrollment of an eligible patient, particularly if the biomarker used for patient selection is of low prevalence in the tumor type of focus.

Estimating the costs associated with identifying and screening patients is crucial for evaluation. In a prospective review of time spent on screening by research staff using a real-time tracking system, Penberthy et al. (2012) found substantial variation in attributed costs by study type and phase, with the average time spent per patient ranging from 3.4 to 8.8 hours and costs ranging from $129 to $336. This translates to an estimated uncompensated annual screening cost of more than $90,000 for the institution, highlighting the substantial cost of screening. Institutions conducting more phase 1 trials were considered to have substantially higher screening-associated costs (Penberthy et al., 2012).

Physician Involvement in Trial Recruitment

Clinical trial recruitment literature has historically reported that the relationship between patients and their physicians is crucial to the success of recruitment into clinical research; there is no doubt that the relationship between the physician and patient is important for participation in cancer research. Patients trust physicians and other healthcare providers to recommend treatments that are in their best interests (Al et al., 2023). Physician involvement in clinical trial recruitment is imperative; however, as busy clinicians, it is unreasonable to expect them to do this without the help of research staff, including OCRNs.

Making Research a Pillar of the Institution

Interprofessional care is the heart of oncology treatment planning. Vose (2023) discussed how treating and caring for patients with cancer requires a complex team of medical professionals working together toward a common goal. Interprofessional teams often include medical oncology, radiation oncology, pathology, radiology, surgical oncology (and other core specialists), tumor registry, genetic counselors, dietitians, and the clinical research team. Having this team understand the importance of the clinical trial program is imperative for success at an institution.

The core research team may include a variety of personnel, such as OCRNs, research managers and coordinators, clinical research associates, regulatory specialists, and quality assurance personnel, who conduct the day-to-day research activities and are employed by the research program. In addition to the physician investigators, the core team plays a crucial role in ensuring accrual. However, when considering recruitment efforts for cancer clinical trials, the research team should extend beyond these individuals to include institutional administrators, other oncology nurses, APPs, private practice personnel, pharmacists, laboratory and finance personnel, radiology services, and patient navigators and advocates. A 2012 Institute of Medicine (now the National Academy of Medicine) workshop illustrated the various roles of research, as well as the sites and researchers required for associated clinical trials (Weisfeld et al., 2012; see Table 16-2).

The entire research team needs to commit to making research a foundation of its culture—one that brings people together to share responsibility with a sense of ownership for clinical trials. A clinical trial culture needs to be supported from the top down, including institution and practice administration, the research program principal investigator, management, and support staff. Most importantly, it must be a foundational practice for the research team. If the research team does not portray the culture of accrual, no one will. A clear message of expectations and predefined, measurable goals must be communicated to everyone on the team. Collis (2023) stated that teamwork should be an integral part of the "DNA of your company." The importance of recruitment and retention needs to be reflected in all day-to-day operations of the research and oncology staff.

An important aspect of recruitment success is having a research staff that is dedicated and responsible for the research process, including recruitment planning, implementation, and follow-up maintenance. Research programs are most effective when staff is assigned solely to the research program. Tools from the American Society of Clin-

TABLE 16-2 | The Four "Laboratories" of a Transformed Clinical Trials Enterprise

Laboratory	Research Goal	Usual Site	Researchers (Methods)	Participants
Innovation	Develop initial evidence about treatments and biological markers and hypotheses.	Academic health and science centers and acute care settings networked with other facilities	Highly trained, with data management expertise (conduct clinical trials)	Small numbers of volunteers per trial, but many trials
Traditional Clinical Research	Determine treatment efficacy, or risks and benefits in carefully defined populations.	Research centers and clinical settings	Trained researchers (conduct clinical trials and CER)	Larger numbers of volunteers, but fewer studies
Health Care Delivery	Evaluate treatment risks and benefits in the context of health care.	Clinical settings	Physicians, nurses, other health professionals (CER; use of EHRs and randomization in clinical practice)	Most patients
Community Engagement	Assess strategies of disease prevention and wellness (including living with chronic disease).	Communities: voluntary health organizations, schools, churches, etc.	Community-based researchers (use patient-reported outcomes; include cluster randomization)	Ordinary citizens

CER—clinical evaluation report; EHR—electronic health record

Note. From *Envisioning a Transformed Clinical Trials Enterprise in the United States: Establishing an Agenda for 2020,* by N. Weisfeld, R.A. English, and A.B. Claiborne, 2012 (www.ncbi.nlm.nih.gov/books/NBK92275/pdf/Bookshelf_NBK92275.pdf). In the public domain.

ical Oncology (2019) Research Community Forum include clinical trial workload assessment strategies that are helpful in assessing staffing needs and workload. One example is the Ontario Protocol Assessment Level, used to gauge the complexity of clinical trials in terms of staffing resources (Lorduy et al., 2020). In a single-site study, Tyson (2023) concluded that the use of standardized processes for determining coordinator effort helps to understand the complexity of clinical trial projects objectively. Leaders can also use this tool at the programmatic level to assess the overall capacity of the clinical trial department to undertake new projects. This can lead to lower staff burnout and increased overall job satisfaction.

The Role of Oncology Clinical Research Nurses in Clinical Trials

The Oncology Nursing Society and Oncology Nursing Certification Corporation (2024) *Oncology Clinical Research Nurse Competencies* state that OCRNs can provide leadership in the conduct of clinical trials, thereby improving outcomes for patients and enhancing study integrity. As a leader and a vital component of the research team, OCRNs can play a key role in reducing the time and effort required of physicians, a significant barrier to recruitment efforts.

OCRNs, working as team members in tandem with physicians, can reduce physicians' burden by prescreening patient charts and, when a potential participant is identified, having the consent document and study-required information available for discussion with the physicians before their encounter with patients. After physicians introduce the clinical trial to patients, they can rely on OCRNs to provide additional trial- and disease-related information to patients and their families. Physicians could then be free to visit with other scheduled patients while OCRNs provide patient education and consent information. After patients have had time to consider their decision, usually at a follow-up visit, OCRNs can ensure trial eligibility criteria are met and, after obtaining signed consent, order any outstanding research-related tests. The physicians would follow up with patients to answer any further questions and concerns. Physicians, OCRNs, and patients become a team throughout the process of enrollment, treatment, and follow-up.

OCRNs can also consider various strategies to enhance recruitment, such as playing a leadership role in implementing recruitment plans, identifying and developing processes to overcome patient-related barriers, and identifying institutional or community-based resources or groups that can assist in achieving the identified recruitment goals (Oncology Nursing Society & Oncology Nursing Certification Corporation, 2024).

Providing Feedback on Recruitment Efforts

Having a leadership team that focuses on feedback regarding recruitment efforts to improve and evaluate the clinical research program is essential to the success of that institute. Accrual statistics can be updated monthly, allowing accrual goals to be tracked against actual enrollment and shared with research staff, investigators, and support personnel. Reports indicating accrual by investigators may be considered as a means of promoting a competitive spirit. Regular email and correspondence to the entire research team can also promote highly accruing investigators or highlight possible recruitment challenges for certain clinical trials. Regularly held research staff meetings provide an opportunity for the team to collectively assess accrual trends, discuss any barriers or problems encountered, and develop possible options for reducing them, as well as providing an opportunity for team building and collaboration.

When non-research staff members have a clear understanding of clinical trial research, what will be required of them, and how the research could benefit them and their community, recruitment will be less burdensome. Research staff should be aware of the clinic or site environment when they are there for research-related purposes and be sympathetic to the clinic staff's day-to-day workload and activities. Every effort should be made not to place unnecessary additional demands on site staff because of research endeavors. A consistent visibility of the research team helps the clinic staff to become familiar with the research. It also has the potential to promote and nurture a partnership between the teams.

Flocke et al. (2017) noted that oncology nurses, or those nurses in the clinic setting, feel they play a vital role in discussing clinical trials but often do not feel comfortable due to a lack of knowledge and other factors (see Figure 16-1). Possible recognition methods could include handwritten thank-you notes placed in personnel files, certificates of appreciation presented at staff meetings or gatherings, gift certificates to a coffee shop, and recognition in newsletters or interoffice communications. Physician investigators, particularly those with high accrual, can be recognized through mechanisms such as newsletters, tumor board conferences, and other cancer program meetings and events. Furthermore, every effort should be made to share the results of clinical trials with both research and non-research staff as an additional opportunity to provide education and reinforce the importance of clinical research, as well as the role the staff played in contributing to the research efforts. This could also garner institutional support, aiding in recruitment strategies.

Roles in Discussing Clinical Trials

Setting matters
- In settings with a CT nurse on staff, oncology nurses clearly understand who initiates discussion of CTs.
- In other settings, oncologists initiate discussion of CTs.

Primary role
- Provide informational assistance to the patient after an initial discussion has taken place.
- Provide emotional support.
- Serve as a patient advocate in the context of the family and clinical team to support the patient's decision.
- Initiating the discussion of CTs is someone else's role.

Barriers to Discussing Clinical Trials

Lack of information
- Lack information on details, logistics, protocol, nuances of patient's case, and scope of trial
- Lack of self-efficacy in explaining CTs
- Uncertain of appropriate timing of discussion in care trajectory
- No clear norms for process or protocol in these discussions

Managing emotions and expectations of patients and their families
- Patients may feel disempowered, as if they are being experimented on.
- Patients may be in denial of their condition and may be offended by "a last-ditch effort."
- Patients may have a false hope that a CT will cure them.

Conflicting priorities
- May lose business for practice if a patient leaves to participate in a CT elsewhere
- Mitigating conflicts of opinion within the family or between the patient and family
- Discomfort in settings with expectations for CT volume

FIGURE 16-1 | Nurses' Perceived Roles in and Barriers to Discussing Clinical Trials With Patients

CT—clinical trial

Note. From "The Role of Oncology Nurses in Discussing Clinical Trials," by S.A. Flocke, E. Antognoli, B.J. Daly, B. Jackson, S.E. Fulton, T.M. Liu, ... N.J. Meropol, 2017, *Oncology Nursing Forum, 44*(5), p. 551 (https://doi.org/10.1188/17.ONF.547-552). Copyright 2017 by Oncology Nursing Society. Reprinted with permission.

Managing Staff Education and Turnover

The research staff should be adequately and appropriately educated regarding clinical trial research. Staff turnover remains high (Adair, 2021); it is important for institutions to properly onboard their research staff and continue to offer education and mentoring opportunities. Staff must understand both the rationale behind clinical research in general and the trial objectives before discussing the trial with patients or potential participants. Staff should also understand how their work could benefit the community of patients whom they serve, as well as the overall goals of the clinical trial department. The individual initiating contact with patients about a clinical trial must be well-informed about the study, able to address all concerns and questions, and convey a culturally sensitive attitude.

Informed consent is a process, not a singular interaction. In a study that included both research staff and participants, O'Sullivan et al. (2021) stated, "The process of informed consent often involves building rapport and trust with the prospective participant and should respect cultural and societal norms, such as involving family members or friends" (p. 2). Research staff should be comfortable with the clinical trial design and requirements, as well as the institutional informed consent process.

Research staff education is of the utmost importance for a clinical research program. Shiri et al. (2023) noted that workers need to engage in continuing professional development to keep and enhance their professional competence. Offering employees these opportunities is beneficial for both the staff and patients. Numerous opportunities for continuing education exist within the research community, including organized groups for research professionals, such as the Society of Clinical Research Associates. Additionally, in the cancer realm, cooperative group meetings or other national groups often have organized meetings with both in-person and virtual opportunities for participation. Many cooperative groups, including NRG Oncology, Eastern Cooperative Oncology Group, and SWOG (Southwest Oncology Group), host annual or semiannual conferences that provide educational opportunities for OCRNs. National research meetings not only provide education but also an opportunity for networking and sharing experiences with staff from other research programs. This can lead to discussions about best practices.

If attending national meetings is too challenging due to budgetary constraints, another option for furthering educational opportunities and networking is online resources, such as NCI's Clinical Trials Reporting Program (www.cancer.gov/about-nci/organization/ccct). This web-based resource and collaboration tool supports professionals involved in the recruitment and retention of participants in clinical trials. It offers a continually updated collection of resources, training materials, and tools, along with an environment for collaborative work, professional development, and the dissemination of accrual best practices.

APPs can obtain the necessary training and guidance from *The Advanced Practice Provider Clinical Trial Manual* (O'Brien et al., 2024). Educational opportunities for APPs involved in the research process at their institution also exist through cooperative groups, such as SWOG. APPs, in partnership with OCRNs, can aid in the understanding and education of research participants.

The Recruitment Process

Achieving enrollment goals is mandatory for a clinical trial to meet end points and answer its scientific question successfully. OCRNs will first need to assess their patient population to capture potential patient enrollment calculations. Before initiating the process of activating a clinical trial, the research program should verify that sufficient potential patients or participants will be available to justify trial activation and that predefined accrual goals are likely to be met. Cancer registries, programs supported by the Centers for Disease Control and Prevention, and NCI's Surveillance, Epidemiology, and End Results program collect information about diagnoses of and deaths from cancer. According to Hill et al. (2023, p. 80), "For more than 40 years, one of the greatest strengths of cancer registries has been their ability to standardize and aggregate cancer data at the population level." Registries can prove to be a valuable resource for research programs as they assess the feasibility of clinical trials. Using these resources can help to identify clinical trial portfolio needs and the necessity of the community of patients that the institution serves. These tools can also be effective in understanding the patient population of the institution. As evidenced by Liu (2021), overly strict inclusion criteria limit access for patients who could potentially benefit from clinical trial enrollment. If the trial does not fit the needs of the institution or its patients, then it will be a failure for both the sponsor and the study staff.

Recruitment Strategies

Once the decision has been made to proceed with the research, key recruitment strategies will need to be implemented. OCRNs will need to screen patients for potential participation in clinical trials. This typically involves an extensive review of the medical chart. To study recruitment to randomized clinical trials, Sampaio et al. (2020) designed a method to optimize time and staffing for managing the demands of screening potential patients effectively. This is an important consideration for programs that employ OCRNs.

By following their institution's informed consent process and protocol diligently, OCRNs can proceed with the enrollment of clinical research participants. This is often a multistep process, where OCRNs' background in critical thinking can assist in ways to increase patient satisfaction with the process (e.g., scheduling appointments for tests on the same day or placing orders for physicians as allowed by their institution) and promote efficiency for protocol requirements (e.g., obtaining local laboratories versus central, as applicable).

Patients and research sites are heterogeneous, indicating that individual methods and tools may vary in effectiveness; a strategy that works for one research program may not be effective for another.

Jiang and Hong (2021) noted the potential of e-health to increase awareness of clinical trials. Using a site's electronic health record for communication, IRB-approved patient-related materials, and information on clinical trial participation could benefit clinical trial programs.

A survey by Adams et al. (2022) reported that 60%–85% of patients reported being more likely to enroll in trials if the burdens of participation were reduced using remote technology. Using electronic tools provided by sponsors, as well as the institution, should be a consideration for enhancing future recruitment efforts.

Bains et al. (2023) concluded that participants from underrepresented racial and ethnic groups were more likely to enroll if the research staff had racial or ethnic concordance.

All the steps in the recruitment process are important; however, ensuring that potential participants are available for specific clinical trials and considering the strategies for recruitment and enrollment are vital. Oncology clinical trial programs should continually assess their recruitment and enrollment strategies to ensure they are aligned with those of the clinical practice with which they are integrated.

Tumor Boards

In the oncology setting, the patient's journey often begins with their physician's presentation of their case at a multidisciplinary tumor board. Dapper et al. (2023) noted that presenting these patient cases in tumor boards can significantly increase trial participation rates. Discussing a potential clinical trial as part of the patient's journey during tumor board meetings can be a quick and efficient way for OCRNs to gather information and gain a deeper understanding of the diagnosis and plan for the patient. OCRNs can also use clinical trial management systems to effectively track patients who are screened and communicate effectively with other team members. Dapper et al. (2023) suggested that having uniform and central trial management software can be helpful in creating continuity, transparency, and quality assurance during the administration of clinical trials. These processes can be beneficial to patients, helping them better understand how the clinical trial fits into their overall plan of care.

Electronic Screening and Artificial Intelligence

Automated systems for eligibility screening using health information technology tools are becoming increasingly prevalent in the clinical trial landscape. Electronic screening systems not only have the potential to assist in evaluating potential participants but also may have the capability to capture information on all screened patients into an electronic screening log, including important information such as reasons for ineligibility. Artificial intelligence (AI) software is being developed and used by many institutions. Lu et al. (2024) highlighted the benefits and potential drawbacks of implementing AI at a research site. They concluded, "The integration of AI in clinical trials offers a promising solution to address the inherent problems associated with traditional clinical trials methodologies and has demonstrated its practicality in clinical trials" (Lu et al., 2024, p. 5). Similarly, Chopra et al. (2023) investigated the potential of AI in clinical trials; however, there is still much to be explored regarding regulation, transparency, and data quality.

The use of software and AI is on the rise in oncology care and clinical trials. These applications range from early cancer detection, diagnosis, classification and grading, molecular characterization of tumors, prediction of patient outcomes and treatment responses, personalized treatment, automatic radiation therapy workflows, novel anticancer drug discovery, and clinical trials (Bhinder et al., 2021). Over time, these tools will likely be further developed and integrated into oncology practices. Institutions will need to evaluate these systems to determine the best use for their clinical trial needs. Following the COVID-19 pandemic, it has become clear that identifying tools for clinical trial administration to reduce provider and staff burden, as well as electronic tools to facilitate patient access and participation in clinical trials, should be a site's top priority (Durden et al., 2024).

The use of clinical trial management systems can also serve as a valuable tool for tracking recruitment efforts and monitoring patient progress throughout the study, thereby enhancing retention strategies (Chaudhari et al., 2020). These systems remain expensive and would need to be evaluated by the site's key stakeholders.

Clinical Trials as a Business

Viewing clinical trials from a business perspective has been investigated as a method to improve accrual (Longbottom et al., 2012; McDonald et al., 2011). Initially, the idea of applying business models to medicine may seem inappropriate; however, they share common goals: businesses strive to find customers and encourage them to purchase what is being offered, and clinical trials aim to recruit physicians and patients, encouraging them to participate (McDonald et al., 2011).

McDonald et al. (2011) applied a business model developed using insights from marketing theory to improve accrual to a national trial assessing treatment options for trauma patients. Multiple business model components were included, such as developing a brand value, devising strategies to overcome resistance, adopting a marketing plan, engaging champions, creating multiaudience messages, achieving buy-in, providing frequent positive reinforcements, and ensuring that trial procedures are simple and can be incorporated into a participating site's established routine. The model offered a consistent framework for planning and managing recruitment and provided the researchers with valuable information that positively influenced accrual to the trial.

Longbottom et al. (2012) also used marketing strategies within a recruitment plan for a cardiology-focused trial. Using multiple techniques, such as developing a unique study logo, trial-specific recruitment materials (i.e., posters, brochures, pocket cards, and template press releases), funding for patient transportation, and flexible appointment schedules, proved beneficial in completing the trial.

Social Media

Recruitment to cancer clinical trials may be enhanced using new and continuously evolving social media technology. Social media or social networking sites are forms of electronic communication that enable people to create online communities and share information, ideas, and personal messages (Britannica Dictionary, n.d.). People within these virtual communities often share common interests and connect from all over the world to engage in conversations and exchange knowledge. The impact of social media is extensive and has fundamentally changed how professional and personal business is conducted. Within the medical world, nurses can now access educational meetings or podcasts. They can also access educational opportunities via Facebook, Instagram, or X (formerly Twitter). A 2020 study by Darmawan et al. found that Facebook and X platforms were the most frequently cited, comprising nearly half of the studies researched. They reported that further discussion is needed about whether the use of social media for recruitment can decrease an institution's recruitment costs.

The use of social media in the recruitment context has numerous advantages. It is cost-effective, fast, interactive, easily accessible, and convenient. Specific patient populations may be targeted through social networking sites such as Facebook, where a sponsor can establish an account focused on a specific drug or disease and customize it to provide clinical trial–specific information. Social media can be used to provide support and direct compliance efforts for participants during and after the trial, as well as during the follow-up period. It can also serve as a means of communication between participants and research program staff, keeping participants motivated and providing feedback or allowing them to ask questions.

Confidentiality issues related to the use of social networking sites need to be considered. Even with the use of antivirus software, there is a risk that hackers may compromise the website, potentially exposing participants' confidential information to unauthorized access. All potential forms of patient recruitment must be presented to the IRB to ensure patient safety, in accordance with the National Institutes of Health *Guidance Regarding Social Media Tools* (2016).

Patient Navigators

The patient navigator role, especially in cancer care, is crucial. These individuals guide patients and their caregivers through diagnosis, treatment, and beyond (Mayo Clinic, n.d.). Patient navigators essentially help individuals navigate their cancer care, which may involve interactions with multiple doctors' offices, clinics, hospitals, outpatient centers, insurance and payment systems, patient support organizations, and other components of the healthcare system. Initially used to improve poor diagnostic follow-up rates among underserved populations, patient navigation is being widely implemented by many healthcare facilities as a means of enhancing cancer programs. Frequently involved with cancer screening processes, patient navigators may be one of the first institutional contacts a newly-diagnosed patient with cancer encounters.

An essential part of the patient navigation process is introducing participation in a clinical trial as a viable treatment option; however, patient navigators are generally not provided with trial-related training. Cartmell et al. (2020) noted that implementing strategies such as patient navigation, which is designed to guide patients through the healthcare system with education and practical support, may help to overcome obstacles to clinical trial recruitment. In this study, a navigator at an NCI-designated site went through trial-related training. They then used a potential barrier checklist, and data was able to be collected about potential barriers to care, and how the patient navigator could help the patient or caregivers overcome these potential barriers. The most common barriers included fear, communication with providers, insurance, and transportation. This study exhibited not only the impact that a patient navigator could have on patient care but also the impact that the entire care team can have in the discussion of clinical trials.

Summary

Recruitment to cancer clinical trials can be challenging. Several factors must be considered before recruitment, during the study phase, and at follow-up. As history has shown, nurses are often the ones who make a significant difference in patient and family care. OCRNs have that opportunity again when promoting and supporting cancer clinical trials.

Key Points

- Recruitment of an appropriate and adequate number of research participants for cancer clinical trials is an essential component of successful trial completion and the subsequent generation of results.
- Barriers to clinical trial participation are many and often involve several levels and factors. Before trial initiation, every effort should be made to identify potential trial-specific recruitment barriers and implement options to reduce them.
- The entire research team needs to commit to making research a foundation of its culture—one that brings people together to share responsibilities with a sense of ownership for clinical trials.
- OCRNs, vital members of research teams, play a key role in reducing barriers to clinical trial recruitment.
- Multiple recruitment strategies are often needed for successful clinical trial accrual.

The author would like to acknowledge Marjorie J. Good, MPH, BSN, RN, OCN®, for her contribution to this chapter that remains unchanged from the previous edition of this book.

References

Adair, T. (2021, March 10). How to motivate and retain clinical research staff. *Society of Clinical Research Associates.* https://www.socra.org/blog/how-to-motivate-and-retain-clinical-research-staff

Adams, D.V., Long, S., & Fleury, M.E. (2022). Association of remote technology use and other decentralization tools with patient likelihood to enroll in cancer clinical trials. *JAMA Network Open, 5*(7), e2220053. https://doi.org/10.1001/jamanetworkopen.2022.20053

Al, P., Hey, S., Weijer, C., Gillies, K., McCleary, N., Yee, M.-L., ... Brehaut, J. (2023). Changing patient preferences toward better trial recruitment: An ethical analysis. *Trials, 24*(1), 233. https://doi.org/10.1186/s13063-023-07258-4

American Cancer Society. (2022). *Cancer facts and figures for African Americans/Black people 2022–2024.* https://www.cancer.org/research/cancer-facts-statistics/cancer-facts-figures-for-african-americans.html

American Society of Clinical Oncology. (2019). *Clinical trial workload assessment strategies at a glance. ASCO Research Community Forum.* https://www.ons.org/sites/default/files/2019-12/2019ASCORCF-ResourcesResearchSites.pdf

Anastasi, J.K., Capili, B., Norton, M., McMahon, D.J., & Marder, K. (2024). Recruitment and retention of clinical trial participants: Understanding motivations of patients with chronic pain and other populations. *Frontiers in Pain Research, 4,* 1330937. https://doi.org/10.3389/fpain.2023.1330937

Araujo, D.A., Greystoke, S., Bates, A., Bayle, E., Calvo, L., Castelo-Branco, J., ... Seymour, L. (2023). Oncology phase I trial design and conduct: Time for a change - MDICT Guidelines 2022. *Annals of Oncology, 34*(1), 48–60. https://doi.org/10.1016/j.annonc.2022.09.158

Bains, A., Osathanugrah, P., Sanjiv, N., Chiu, C., Fiorello, M.G., Siegel, N.H., ... Subramanian, M.L. (2023). Diverse research teams and underrepresented groups in clinical studies. *JAMA Ophthalmology, 141*(11), 1037–1044. https://doi.org/10.1001/jamaophthalmol.2023.4638

Bhinder, B., Gilvary, C., Madhukar, N.S., & Elemento, O. (2021). Artificial intelligence in cancer research and precision medicine. *Cancer Discovery, 11*(4), 900–915. https://doi.org/10.1158/2159-8290.CD-21-0090

Britannica Dictionary. (n.d.). Social media. In *Britannica.com dictionary.* Retrieved September 5, 2025, from https://www.britannica.com/dictionary/social-media

Cartmell, K.B., Bonilha, H.S., Simpson, K.N., Ford, M.E., Bryant, D.C., & Alberg, A.J. (2020). Patient barriers to cancer clinical trial participation and navigator activities to assist. *Advances in Cancer Research, 146,* 139–166. https://doi.org/10.1016/bs.acr.2020.01.008

Chaudhari, N., Ravi, R., Gogtay, N.J., & Thatte, U.M. (2020). Recruitment and retention of the participants in clinical trials: Challenges and solutions. *Perspectives in Clinical Research, 11*(2), 64–69. https://doi.org/10.4103/picr.PICR_206_19

Chopra, H., Annu, Shin, D.K., Munjal, K., Priyanka, Dhama, K., & Emran, T.B. (2023). Revolutionizing clinical trials: The role of AI in accelerating medical breakthroughs. *International Journal of Surgery, 109*(12), 4211–4220. https://doi.org/10.1097/JS9.0000000000000705

Collis, A. (2023, July 3). The power of a teamwork culture: Maximizing your strengths. *Forbes.* https://www.forbes.com/sites/forbesfinancecouncil/2023/07/03/the-power-of-a-teamwork-culture-maximizing-your-strengths

Dapper, H., Dantes, M., Herschbach, P., Algül, H., & Heinemann, V. (2023). Relevance of tumor boards for the inclusion of patients in oncological clinical trials. *Journal of Cancer Research and Clinical Oncology, 149*(10), 7601–7608. https://doi.org/10.1007/s00432-022-04559-0

Darmawan, I., Bakker, C., Brockman, T., Patten, C., & Eder, M. (2020). The role of social media in enhancing clinical trial recruitment: Scoping review. *Journal of Medical Internet Research, 22*(10), e22810. https://doi.org/10.2196/22810

Dilts, D.M., & Sandler, A.B. (2006). Invisible barriers to clinical trials: The impact of structural, infrastructural, and procedural barriers to opening oncology clinical trials. *Journal of Clinical Oncology, 24*(28), 4545–4552. https://doi.org/10.1200/JCO.2005.05.0104

Durden, K., Hurley, P., Butler, D.L., Farner, A., Shriver, S.P., & Fleury, M.E. (2024). Provider motivations and barriers to cancer clinical trial screening, referral, and operations: Findings from a survey. *Cancer, 130*(1), 68–76. https://doi.org/10.1002/cncr.35044

Flocke, S.A., Antognoli, E., Daly, B.J., Jackson, B., Fulton, S.E., Liu, T.M., ... Meropol, N.J. (2017). The role of oncology nurses in discussing clinical trials. *Oncology Nursing Forum, 44*(5), 547–552. https://doi.org/10.1188/17.ONF.547-552

Hill, S.M., Michels, F.S., Knight, K., Goderre, J.L., Terranova, T., Hayes, T., & Kohler, B. (2023). Harnessing the power of cancer registries to advance our understanding of pediatric cancer. *Journal of Registry Management, 50*(3), 80–81. https://pmc.ncbi.nlm.nih.gov/articles/PMC10629798/pdf/jrm-50-80.pdf

Jiang, S., & Hong, Y.A. (2021) Clinical trial participation in America: The roles of eHealth engagement and patient–provider communication. *Digital Health, 7,* 20552076211067658. https://doi.org/10.1177/20552076211067658

Kumar, G., Chaudhary, P., Quinn, A., & Su, D. (2022). Barriers for cancer clinical trial enrollment: A qualitative study of the perspectives of healthcare providers. *Contemporary Clinical Trials Communications, 28,* 100939. https://doi.org/10.1016/j.conctc.2022.100939

Liu, R., Rizzo, S., Whipple, S., Pal, N., Pineda, A.L., Lu, M., ... Zou, J. (2021). Evaluating eligibility criteria of oncology trials using real-world data and AI. *Nature, 592*(7855), 629–633. https://doi.org/10.1038/s41586-021-03430-5

Longbottom, M.E., Roberts, J.N., Tom, M., Hughes, S.E., Howard, V.J., Sheffet, A.J., ... Brott, T.G. (2012). Interventions to increase enrollment in a large multicenter phase 3 trial of carotid stenting vs. endarterectomy. *International Journal of Stroke, 7*(6), 447–453. https://doi.org/10.1111/j.1747-4949.2012.00833.x

Lorduy, K., Brown, V., & Rose, S.J. (2020). Adapting productivity models to improve efficiency and progress in clinical research practice. *Clinical Researcher, 34*(4). https://acrpnet.org/2020/04/14/adapting-productivity-models-to-improve-efficiency-and-progress-in-clinical-research-practice

Lu, X., Chen, M., Lu, Z., Shi, X., & Liang, L. (2024). Artificial intelligence tools for optimising recruitment and retention in clinical trials: A scoping review protocol. *BMJ Open, 14*(3), e080032. https://doi.org/10.1136/bmjopen-2023-080032

Mayo Clinic. (n.d.). *Patient navigators.* https://www.mayoclinic.org/patient-visitor-guide/education-centers/cancer-education/patient-navigators

McDonald, A.M., Treweek, S., Shakur, H., Free, C., Knight, R., Speed, C., & Campbell, M.K. (2011). Using a business model approach and marketing techniques for recruitment to clinical trials. *Trials, 12,* 74. https://doi.org/10.1186/1745-6215-12-74

Mittal, A., Moore, S., Navani, V., Jiang, D.M., Stewart, D.J., Liu, G., & Wheatley-Price, P. (2024). What is ailing oncology clinical trials? Can we fix them? *Current Oncology, 31*(7), 3738–3751. https://doi.org/10.3390/curroncol31070275

National Comprehensive Cancer Network. (n.d.). *NCCN Guidelines®.* https://www.nccn.org/guidelines/category_1

National Institutes of Health. (2016). *Guidance regarding social media tools.* https://www.nih.gov/health-information/nih-clinical-research-trials-you/guidance-regarding-social-media-tools

Nipp, R.D., Hong, K., & Paskett, E.D. (2019). Overcoming barriers to clinical trial enrollment. *American Society of Clinical Oncology Educational Book, 39,* 105–111. https://doi.org/10.1200/EDBK_243729

O'Brien, B., Braun-Inglis, C., Kottschase, L., & Benson, A. (2024). *The advanced practice provider clinical trials research manual* [Password protected]. https://ecog-acrin.org/resources/training-and-education/app-research-manual

Oncology Nursing Society & Oncology Nursing Certification Corporation. (2024). *Oncology clinical research nurse competencies.* https://www.ons.org/sites/default/files/2025-01/ocrn-competencies-rebrand.pdf

O'Sullivan, L., Feeney, L., Crowley, R.K., Sukumar, P., McAuliffe, E., & Doran, P. (2021). An evaluation of the process of informed consent: Views from research participants and staff. *Trials, 22*(1), 544. https://doi.org/10.1186/s13063-021-05493-1

Penberthy, L.T., Dahman, B.A., Petkov, V.I., & DeShazo, J.P. (2012). Effort required in eligibility screening for clinical trials. *Journal of Oncology Practice, 8*(6), 365–370. https://doi.org/10.1200/JOP.2012.000646

Sampaio, S., Sepideh, S., Knight, A., Chambers, J., & Perin., E. (2020). Using workflow mapping to improve the recruitment process in clinical trials. *Society of Clinical Research Associates.* https://www.socra.org/blog/using-workflow-mapping-to-improve-the-recruitment-process-in-clinical-trials

Shiri, R., El-Metwally, A., Sallinen, M., Pöyry, M., Härmä, M., & Toppinen-Tanner, S. (2023). The role of continuing professional training or development in maintaining current employment: A systematic review. *Healthcare (Basel), 11*(21), 2900. https://doi.org/10.3390/healthcare11212900

Siegel, R.L., Giaquinto, A.N., & Jemal, A. (2024). Cancer statistics, 2024. *CA: A Cancer Journal for Clinicians, 74*(1), 12–49. https://doi.org/10.3322/caac.21820

Tsimberidou, A.M., Fountzilas, E., Nikanjam, M., & Kurzrock, R. (2020). Review of precision cancer medicine: Evolution of the treatment paradigm. *Cancer Treatment Reviews, 86,* 102019. https://doi.org/10.1016/j.ctrv.2020.102019

Tyson, K. (2023). *Mapping the OPAL score for clinical trials to coordinator hours: A single site study* (Publication No. 762) [Doctoral dissertation, Medical University of South Carolina]. https://medica-musc.researchcommonMes.org/theses/762

Unger, J.M., Shulman, L., Facktor, M., Nelson, H., & Fleury, M. (2024). National estimates of the participation of patients with cancer in clinical research studies based on Commission on Cancer accreditation data. *Journal of Clinical Oncology, 42*(18), 2139–2148. https://doi.org/10.1200/JCO.23.01030

Vose, J.M. (2023). Multidisciplinary team approach is integral to oncology care. *Oncology, 37*(10), 407. https://www.cancernetwork.com/view/multidisciplinary-team-approach-is-integral-to-oncology-care

Weisfeld, N., English, R.A., & Claiborne, A.B. (2012). *Envisioning a transformed clinical trials enterprise in the United States: Establishing an agenda for 2020.* National Academies Press. https://www.ncbi.nlm.nih.gov/books/NBK114660

CHAPTER 17

Adherence and Retention in Clinical Trials

Tahani Dweikat, MSN, EMHCA, RN, CCRP, AG-CNS, EBP-C, OCN®

Introduction

The recruitment and retention of participants are critical issues in conducting successful clinical trials. Approximately 80% of clinical trials fail to meet recruitment goals within their initial targeted timelines, highlighting a significant challenge for trial teams worldwide (Chaudhari et al., 2020; Desai, 2020). When trials fail to recruit within the envisioned timescale, costs are increased, and the potential for underpowered studies is significant when participant sample sizes fail to meet a recruitment threshold (Fogel, 2018; Shiely et al., 2023). Retention is equally important, as participant dropout or incomplete data can cause problems in the analysis, interpretation, and external validity of the results (Gillies et al., 2021; Shiely et al., 2023).

The importance of adherence and retention in clinical trials cannot be overstated. Adherence directly affects the validity of study findings, as nonadherence can mask the true efficacy of the treatment being evaluated (Poongothai et al., 2023). Furthermore, high rates of attrition and early discontinuation can jeopardize a trial's statistical power, requiring the enrollment of additional participants and increasing the time and cost of the research (Winter et al., 2022). Maintaining patient engagement and follow-up is also crucial for collecting long-term outcome data, such as survival and quality of life (Winter et al., 2022).

This chapter will explore the critical roles of adherence and retention in the success of clinical trials, emphasizing how these factors influence data validity, patient outcomes, and trial efficiency. It will outline the pivotal responsibilities of oncology clinical research nurses (OCRNs) in promoting adherence, educating patients, and maintaining engagement throughout the study. It will also present a framework for excellence in oncology clinical research nursing, define various forms of nonadherence, and discuss contributing factors—ranging from regimen complexity and patient beliefs to financial and logistical barriers. This chapter will additionally examine the challenges in measuring adherence, introduce interventions and tools to support sustained compliance, and highlight the importance of communication, education, and interprofessional collaboration.

The Role of Oncology Clinical Research Nurses in Patient Adherence and Retention

OCRNs are increasingly recognized as vital members of the clinical trial team, particularly in supporting patient adherence and retention throughout the study (Shiely et al., 2023). However, despite their growing importance, the full scope and formal definition of their role in clinical trials remain underdeveloped. Compounding this, OCRNs are often introduced late in the trial planning process and typically have limited input into protocol development (Shiely et al., 2023).

Prior research has shown that trial managers are generally successful at predicting whether sites will recruit effectively (Bruhn et al., 2019). OCRNs are similarly well-positioned to offer insights into recruitment and retention strategies when given the opportunity to engage early (Shiely et al., 2023). Ultimately, fostering a collaborative environment where both patients and clinical staff contribute meaningfully can improve clinical trial outcomes.

A Framework for Excellence in Clinical Trials

The Oncology Clinical Research Nurse Competency Model Framework presents a comprehensive, patient-centered approach to oncology clinical research nursing. At its core are the patient and caregiver, surrounded by three key layers: abilities, skills, and knowledge. These layers are encompassed by nine essential competency domains, including documentation management, ethical standards, informed consent, protocol compliance, financial stewardship, leadership and professional development, data management, patient management, and recruitment and retention (Oncology Nursing Society & Oncology Nursing Certification Corporation, 2024).

This framework emphasizes patient advocacy, research study integrity, and effective communication across all stakeholders. It aligns with established nursing practice standards from the American Nurses Association (2015) and the National Institutes of Health (2025), providing a structured approach to enhance the effectiveness of OCRNs. The model focuses on developing clinical expertise, patient education skills, adherence to ethical standards, collaborative abilities, patient-centered care practices, and quality improvement initiatives.

By integrating resources such as the Collaborative Institutional Training Initiative Program's Good Clinical Practice training and U.S. Food and Drug Administration guidelines, this model equips nurses to navigate complex oncology research, ensure high-quality patient care, promote adherence and retention in clinical trials, and foster a supportive environment for patient engagement (Oncology Nursing Society & Oncology Nursing Certification Corporation, 2024). The framework acknowledges the crucial role of OCRNs in patient education, emphasizing the importance of strong communication skills, the ability to effectively convey treatment protocols, and the significance of medication adherence.

This holistic approach aims to enhance patient outcomes and overall clinical trial success by ensuring that nurses are adequately prepared to support patients throughout their entire clinical trial experience. It provides a structured methodology for enhancing the skills and effectiveness of OCRNs, enabling them to address the multifaceted challenges of oncology research while maintaining a strong focus on patient care and study integrity.

Definitions of Adherence

Adherence refers to the extent to which a person's behavior (e.g., taking medication, following a diet, making lifestyle changes) aligns with the agreed recommendations from a healthcare provider (Mantila et al., 2022). It is the active, voluntary, and collaborative involvement of the patient in a mutually acceptable course of behavior to produce a desired preventive or therapeutic result (Mishra et al., 2021). Initially, *adherence* and *compliance* were used synonymously until the word *compliance* started to take on a negative undertone, such as with a noncompliant patient. *Compliance* implies the negation of the importance of a collaborative relationship between the patient and the healthcare provider. Therefore, *adherence* is preferred in the literature.

Successful clinical trials require careful attention to participant recruitment, retention, adherence, and burden. The term *recruitment* denotes identifying potential participants who meet eligibility criteria and successfully enrolling them (Chaudhari et al., 2020). In contrast, *retention* refers to keeping participants engaged until study completion (Chaudhari et al., 2020). *Adherence*, in a clinical sense, is the measurement of a participant's commitment to following the intervention protocol (Vrijens & Urquhart, 2014).

Nonadherence refers to a patient who fails to comply with the agreed-upon medical advice in a timely and adequate manner. *Intentional* or *primary nonadherence* refers to a patient's conscious decision not to fill a prescription or skip medication doses, often due to personal beliefs or adverse reactions (Martin et al., 2018; Mishra et al., 2021).

Unintentional nonadherence occurs when a patient wants to comply but is unable to do so, often involving dealing with complicated instructions, forgetting to take medications, or not fully understanding the directions (Vrijens & Urquhart, 2014). Mishra et al. (2021) found that some patients discontinued medication upon feeling that their health had improved, whereas opinions and advice from non-medical staff led to nonadherence in other cases.

Factors Interfering With Adherence

Hamstra et al. (2020) reported that factors interfering with medication adherence included experiencing adverse events, perceiving a lack of improvement, being assigned to a placebo arm, having a fear of study procedures, feeling a lack of social support, viewing negative media publicity, undergoing life changes, and facing poverty-related issues.

Nonadherence can be intentional, such as consciously deciding to skip doses because of beliefs or side effects, or unintentional, such as forgetting doses or misunderstanding complex directions. Many factors, such as perceived health status, outside influences, adverse effects, and life circumstances, can contribute to medication nonadherence (Hamstra et al., 2020; Mishra et al., 2021; Vrijens & Urquhart, 2014).

It is essential to evaluate patients for potential factors that contribute to both intentional and unintentional nonadherence. Although factors such as age, gender, race, education level, socioeconomic status, disease state, and severity of disease have been traditionally considered predictors of nonadherence (Miaskowski et al., 2008), qualitative research has identified a broader range of barriers and facilitators that influence medication adherence in those with chronic conditions (Nakajima et al., 2021; Winter et al., 2022). These can be categorized as patient-specific, illness-specific, medication-related, healthcare-related, system-related, sociocultural, logistical, and financial factors (Kvarnström et al.,

2021). Additionally, patient beliefs and attitudes toward their medicines and illness (Belitsi et al., 2023; Rafhi et al., 2024), the patient–provider relationship and communication (Grayek et al., 2022; Hamstra et al., 2020; Lambert-Kerzner et al., 2015), and the lived experience and medication-related burden have been found to play a significant role in both intentional and unintentional nonadherence (Martin et al., 2018).

Study Site Selection

Selecting appropriate study sites is critical, as poor choices can lead to insufficient enrollment, protocol amendments, and inconsistent patient management. The financial impact on patients, including out-of-pocket medical costs, transportation, and lost wages, is often overlooked but can hinder recruitment and retention. Proactively addressing these factors through thoughtful study design and execution is essential for conducting clinical trials that generate valid, reliable results to inform clinical practice (de Viron et al., 2022; Nipp et al., 2019).

Complexity of Regimen

The complexity of a medication regimen can significantly influence adherence. A medical plan that requires substantial lifestyle changes, such as smoking cessation, dietary modifications for weight loss, diabetes, or hypertension, may lead to intentional nonadherence (Kvarnström et al., 2021). The majority of newer agents are metabolized through the CYP3A4 pathway, which further complicates this process. Patients must understand the potential for interactions and adhere to avoiding other medications that are either inducers or inhibitors of the CYP3A4 pathway, as well as certain foods such as grapefruit (Koziolek et al., 2019; Zhao et al., 2021).

However, contrary to previous studies suggesting that regimen complexity is associated with nonadherence, Kvarnström et al. (2021) found that the majority of participants in their study did not perceive their medication regimen as complex, and it was not a significant barrier to adherence. The study participants reported that they adhered to the prescribed medications despite the regimen's complexity.

Regardless, clinical trials have become increasingly complex, requiring participants to be flexible with scheduling, complete medication and side effect diaries, and adhere to strict time frames for obtaining tumor measurements. Many clinical trial staff members are less willing to accommodate holiday schedules for treatment, making it more challenging for patients to adhere to the medical regimen within the confines of a protocol (Chaudhari et al., 2020).

Perception of Benefit

Patients' perceptions of whether the potential benefits of oral anticancer medications outweigh the negative impacts play a significant role in adherence. When patients do not experience symptoms from their cancer, they may doubt the necessity of treatments and be more likely to discontinue them (e.g., endocrine therapy for breast cancer) (Clancy et al., 2020). Even if patients understand the treatment's importance rationally, they can become nonadherent if they do not subjectively feel it provides sufficient benefits to their health or if they experience side effects that severely diminish their quality of life. In such cases, patients perceive the adverse effects as outweighing any potential therapeutic gains (Verbrugghe et al., 2016).

Inadequate provider counseling and information about managing side effects exacerbate negative perceptions (Clancy et al., 2020). Conversely, adherence is higher when patients believe the oral medication is effective and necessary for controlling their cancer progression based on perceiving subjective improvements in their health after initiating therapy (Verbrugghe et al., 2016). Shaping perceptions through education and open communication between patients and providers about balancing the benefits and side effects of these therapies is crucial for promoting adherence to them.

The adage that patients with a cancer diagnosis will strictly adhere to a prescribed treatment is false. The most robust data to dispel this notion were reported in patients with breast cancer who were prescribed endocrine therapy. A study by Lemij et al. (2022) found that in a cohort of 258 older patients (aged ≥ 70 years) with breast cancer receiving adjuvant endocrine therapy, 36% discontinued therapy within two years after initiation.

In the case of endocrine therapy, patients may not believe the regimen will be helpful if they do not experience immediate benefits. Nonadherence is less likely when the therapeutic benefit is experienced soon after initiation of the therapy. If patients take pain medication and the pain is diminished, adherence is more likely. However, if a treatment regimen such as physical therapy is implemented in lieu of a more invasive procedure, patients may not think this is aggressive enough and may not adhere to an at-home regimen or may miss appointments (Lemij et al., 2022).

Randomization

Randomized controlled trials are the gold standard for comparing two or more treatments (An et al., 2020; Hariton & Locascio, 2018; Houle, 2015). However, neither participants nor healthcare providers have control over the outcome of the randomization process. Participants must understand this randomization process (Beghi, 2016; Gillies et al., 2021). They will undoubtedly have treatment preferences before randomization and will either be satisfied or dissatisfied with the outcome; however, participants need to understand that the treatment obtained on either arm of a randomized trial is considered an acceptable treatment option, and discontinuation from the trial based solely on the randomization outcome is discouraged (Lim & In, 2019).

Participant preferences about treatments should be discussed during the informed consent process before enrolling in a randomized trial. Although they may prefer one treatment over another, they must understand that randomization eliminates bias in treatment assignment and strengthens the scientific validity of the trial (Gillies et al., 2021; Houle, 2015). Providing sufficient education and information about trial designs and results, including potential biases, is crucial for increasing awareness and trust in the trial.

Participants should be informed about the purpose and design of research trials before they participate. Researchers should seek participants' consent based on a thorough understanding of the trial. Patients should be able to make an informed decision based on their preferences and values (Kadam, 2017). Research should respect patient autonomy based on providing sufficient information about the trial.

Associated Costs of Treatment

Participating in clinical trials can incur substantial financial costs, which may pose barriers to enrollment and adherence. Health insurance coverage for clinical trial–related expenses varies widely, with many plans limiting coverage to standard-of-care costs (Mitchell, 2021). Participants often face significant out-of-pocket costs for tests, procedures, and office visits required by the trial protocol, but these are considered noncovered services (Liang et al., 2020). Frequent clinic visits necessitate travel expenses and time away from work, further increasing the economic burden (Haleem et al., 2021). Although the Patient Protection and Affordable Care Act has reduced some financial barriers by mandating insurance coverage for routine costs associated with clinical trial participation, financial burdens persist for many patients. Costs related to travel, time off work, and noncovered services can disproportionately affect underserved populations. OCRNs must remain vigilant about assessing patients' financial constraints—especially before enrollment or randomization—to ensure equitable access and to prevent dropouts due to unanticipated financial strain (National Cancer Institute, 2024; Unger et al., 2016).

Access to trial medications also exacerbates financial toxicity. If a portion of the treatment regimen involves commercially available drugs, participants may be responsible for these out-of-pocket costs if lacking adequate prescription coverage (Shankaran, 2021).

Financial burden deters many from clinical trial participation and adherence (Liang et al., 2020; Shankaran, 2021). Clinicians must proactively discuss anticipated costs with participants, assess financial toxicity risk, and connect those struggling with available support resources (Liang et al., 2020). Addressing economic barriers is crucial to ensure equitable access to clinical trials across socioeconomic groups (Liang et al., 2020; Shankaran, 2021).

Patient Characteristics and Comorbidities

Various factors can contribute to medication nonadherence across different age groups. In older adults, cognitive impairment, sensory deficits (e.g., hearing or vision loss), poor quality of life, ineffective coping strategies, and lack of social support increase the risk of nonadherence (Koni et al., 2023). Comorbidities, financial constraints, and complex medication regimens further compound adherence challenges in this population (Aggarwal et al., 2020). For pediatric patients, barriers may include the inability to swallow pills, refusal to participate because of adverse effects, and developmental factors influencing autonomy, especially in adolescence (Shih & Cohen, 2020).

Proactive monitoring and tailored interventions are crucial to address these age-related adherence barriers. Multicomponent strategies involving education, behavioral support, and practical assistance have shown promise in improving medication adherence across the life span (Torres-Robles et al., 2022). A comprehensive understanding of patients' unique risk factors is essential for developing personalized adherence plans (Lemij et al., 2022).

Effective Communication and Collaboration

Patients' relationships with the clinical trial staff and physicians significantly affect adherence. The ability of OCRNs and physicians to educate patients about their diagnosis, treatment options, and participation in clinical trials is crucial for fostering adherence. Although OCRNs serve as the backbone of the clinical trial team, they should not bear the entire burden of disseminating information. Physicians also have a responsibility to understand the protocols and communicate effectively with patients. This collaborative approach is vital for ensuring that patients make informed decisions regarding their treatment options (Shiely et al., 2023).

The relationship between OCRNs and patients is essential. Interactions should convey knowledge, organization, and compassion, promoting a sense of trust and partnership. However, the narrative may inadvertently place excessive pressure on OCRNs, suggesting that they alone prevent adherence issues. This perspective can be unappealing and may undermine the shared responsibility required for successful patient adherence.

Moreover, several factors can hinder adherence, including lack of communication, disorganization, poor instructions, long wait times for required testing, uncomfortable waiting rooms, and unfriendly staff. These elements do not align with the definition of a collaborative relationship (Sharkiya, 2023). To enhance adherence, both OCRNs and physicians must work together to create a supportive environment where patients feel valued and informed.

Assessment for Adherence Throughout the Clinical Trial

Continual adherence assessment from recruitment through trial completion is crucial for OCRNs. Evaluating prior medication-taking behavior can identify potential nonadherence risks. Patients with a history of missed appointments or suboptimal adherence to prescribed therapy may struggle with protocol adherence (Laba et al., 2020). Key considerations include the ability to attend visits, access to reliable transportation, commitment to the trial, and available support resources (Rigatti et al., 2022). Screening for such barriers early minimizes later adherence challenges.

Adherence monitoring should continue post-enrollment, with prompt follow-up and targeted interventions for missed visits or doses (Samper-Pardo et al., 2023). Motivational interviewing, sending text reminders, and involving caregivers in adherence counseling can enhance medication adherence and attendance (Anastasi et al., 2024). A multicomponent approach tailored to each participant's unique barriers is recommended for optimizing protocol adherence (Rigatti et al., 2022).

The Complexity of Measuring Patient Adherence

Determining patient adherence to oral medication remains a complex challenge, with no well-controlled studies conducted to evaluate effective monitoring methods. Indirect methods for assessing adherence include self-report questionnaires, telephone interviews, prescription refill data, manual counting of unused medication, and electronic pill dispensers (Morrison et al., 2020).

However, self-reporting is often unreliable, as patients may intentionally omit or alter information. Manual pill counts can be manipulated if patients remove pills without ingesting them. Although electronic pill dispensers can confirm that medication was dispensed, they cannot verify ingestion, and these devices are often too costly for use in studies.

The Hawthorne effect, where patients modify their behavior because they are aware of being observed, can skew self-reported adherence data (Goodwin et al., 2017). Collateral reports, which involve documentation of adherence through observations verified by healthcare professionals, family, friends, or caregivers, offer another approach but are similarly imperfect (Panahi et al., 2022).

The most objective method for measuring adherence is through pharmacologic markers, such as serum drug levels or metabolites. This method, although accurate, is seldom used because of its complexity (Anghel et al., 2019). Factors such as medication half-life and the timing of ingestion must be considered, making bioassays costly, time-consuming, and more uncomfortable for patients.

Studies have highlighted innovative methods, including digital health technologies and mobile health (mHealth) applications. Arshed et al. (2023) found that digital interventions, including text messaging reminders, significantly improved medication adherence. Another study examined the use of mobile applications to track medication adherence, yielding promising results in improving adherence rates (Peng et al., 2020).

These findings highlight a flourishing life sciences sector that not only fosters medical advancements to enhance lives but also contributes significantly to local and state economies. Sustaining this ecosystem demands a long-term approach backed by stable and predictable policies.

Combatting Nonadherence During a Clinical Trial

Adherence in clinical trials has been diminishing. Failure to recognize nonadherence in a clinical trial misleads the understanding of the true clinical benefit of a treatment in the study. This is particularly true when an oral agent is being studied (Fogel, 2018).

The average adherence rate for patients with chronic conditions remains suboptimal, estimated at around 50% (Burnier, 2024). Failure to account for nonadherence can distort the understanding of a treatment's true efficacy, especially when evaluating oral therapies (Getz et al., 2020).

The risk of nonadherence persists despite the availability of knowledge and interventions, underscoring the crucial role of OCRNs within the clinical trial framework. OCRNs act as central coordinators, facilitating collaboration among physicians, subinvestigators, principal investigators, research teams, and patients throughout the trial process. All members of the research team must work closely with OCRNs to ensure clear communication regarding the study protocol and requirements.

When patients contact a physician and receive permission to alter their appointment or reduce medication intake, this may signal a breakdown in communication and a lack of adherence to trial guidelines. Educating physicians, subinvestigators, and principal investigators on the protocol and its requirements is vital for fostering adherence and ensuring the successful completion of clinical studies (Sharkiya, 2023). The responsibility of guiding patients through the trial process should not fall solely on OCRNs; all members of the research team must engage in proactive communication to address potential issues.

OCRNs should accompany patients during consultations with physicians and principal investigators to minimize errors and enhance adherence. The complexity of managing multiple patients and protocols can lead to oversights, emphasizing the need for collaborative effort among the research team. To mitigate inadvertent physician nonadherence, patients must be instructed to communicate with their OCRNs regarding any challenges they encounter, including difficulties in scheduling appointments or adhering to prescribed treatments (Gborogen & Polek, 2018). It is essential that the entire research team, including physicians and subinvestigators, is involved in this communication process to ensure a unified approach.

Furthermore, OCRNs are responsible for ensuring that necessary laboratory tests and imaging studies are appropriately ordered. In some institutions, OCRNs may enter orders related to the study into the electronic health record, which is subsequently reviewed and signed by a physician or principal investigator. This double-check mechanism serves to confirm the accuracy of treatment dosages and modifications. Continuous interaction with on-treatment patients is essential to confirm that medications, performance status, and side effects are documented and monitored in accordance with institutional guidelines (Flocke et al., 2017).

Nonadherence to a protocol can also arise from insufficient training and the multifaceted roles that OCRNs often assume, such as staff nurses or nurse navigators. Clinical trials are becoming increasingly complex, often incorporating companion studies and quality-of-life assessments at specified timepoints. All members of the research team, including principal investigators and subinvestigators, must thoroughly review study components before implementation to ensure adherence to protocols. Most trials are initiated based on physician requests, particularly in community settings, necessitating that the entire research team verifies the availability of resources required for effective study conduct.

Ongoing interaction with patients receiving treatment is crucial for ensuring the successful management of clinical trials. Principal investigators, treating physicians, and OCRNs must consistently collaborate to verify that medications are administered correctly. Additionally, they should ensure that patients' performance status and any side effects are thoroughly documented and monitored in accordance with institutional guidelines. This diligent oversight not only facilitates adherence to the study protocol but also significantly enhances patient care by enabling timely interventions for potential issues (Flocke et al., 2017).

Interventions and Organizational Tools for Continued Adherence

The process model of adherence intervention emphasizes the identification of health issues and the implementation of behavioral changes supported through organizational, behavioral, and educational strategies (Torres-Robles et al., 2022).

The informed consent form marks the initiation of patient education, which should persist throughout the clinical trial process. Providing patients with thorough explanations regarding trial requirements, treatment options, and potential side effects is crucial. This can be facilitated through various educational modalities, including verbal discussions, written materials, and video presentations tailored to meet the individual learning preferences of patients.

Using organizational tools can significantly aid patients with memory impairments or those who struggle with organization. For example, prefilled calendars with appointments and tests can assist in tracking essential study timelines. Pillboxes marked with specific dates and times also serve as effective reminders (Moore, 2010). Additionally, reminders for appointments and tests can be sent via various communication methods, including email, phone calls, postcards, or letters. Smartphone applications can further support organizational efforts.

A critical component of enhancing patient adherence is the provision of drug diaries by clinical trial sponsors. These diaries help patients track their medication schedules, dosages, and side effects. Educating patients on the importance of these diaries reinforces the notion that adherence is a team effort that involves patients and the clinical trial team (European Patients' Academy on Therapeutic Innovation, 2016).

OCRNs have a pivotal role in educating both patients and caregivers about the importance of adherence, stressing that oral medications are as critical as IV therapies. Educating patients about expected side effects and encouraging them to communicate any issues promptly can lead to better management and adherence (Flocke et al., 2017). The effectiveness of this education can be assessed by encouraging patients and caregivers to repeat key information, ensuring clarity and comprehension (Aremu et al., 2022).

The quality of the relationship between patients and OCRNs plays a critical role in fostering adherence. Establishing a trusting relationship enhances patient commitment to the study. Each patient should ideally have a consistent OCRN who is present during physician consultations to clarify medical information and answer any questions. Checking in with patients during scheduled tests helps ensure their comfort and addresses any immediate concerns. Demonstrating enthusiasm for the study and gratitude for patients' involvement can strengthen this rapport. Keeping patients informed about study updates also maintains their interest and promotes adherence (Oncology Nursing Society & Oncology Nursing Certification Corporation, 2024).

Patients participating in clinical trials should feel valued and recognized. OCRNs can provide positive reinforcement and facilitate access to perks such as free parking or meal vouchers as expressions of appreciation for their participation. However, these incentives should always be presented as tokens of gratitude rather than coercive measures to enroll in clinical trials.

Pharmaceutical Investment in Patient Adherence and Retention

The Pharmaceutical Research and Manufacturers of America (PhRMA) has outlined significant investments made in research and development by its member companies. Over the past two decades, these companies have invested more than a trillion dollars, including a record of more than $102 billion in 2021. This investment has been crucial in driving innovation and the development of new treatments and cures for various diseases (PhRMA, n.d.).

PhRMA highlights the ongoing efforts to advance more than 8,000 medicines currently in clinical development, with nearly 70% classified as potential first-in-class treatments. These novel therapies represent a crucial component of the effort to improve patient outcomes across a range of conditions (PhRMA, n.d.).

The integration of new scientific methodologies and technologies has transformed the research and development process. For instance, decentralized clinical trials have enhanced recruitment efficiency and streamlined data collection, allowing for faster and more effective trials (Coleman & Dang, 2023). Such innovations not only reduce costs but also improve the overall quality of clinical research.

Response to Global Health Crises

The rapid development of COVID-19 vaccines exemplifies the biopharmaceutical sector's ability to respond to urgent public health needs. Collaborations among pharmaceutical companies, regulatory agencies, and public health organizations resulted in unprecedented timelines for vaccine development, demonstrating the potential of a coordinated approach to healthcare challenges (PhRMA, n.d.; World Health Organization, 2023).

Challenges Facing the Biopharmaceutical Sector

Although achievements in research and development are commendable, several challenges threaten the sustainability of these advancements. Legislative changes regarding drug pricing could significantly impact future investments in research and development. Analysts estimate that more than 100 new treatments may be compromised due to these regulations, which may deter companies from investing in the development of new therapies (PhRMA, n.d.).

Moreover, the integrity of intellectual property protections remains a critical concern. Strong intellectual property rights are essential for encouraging innovation and ensuring that the financial risks associated with research and development are mitigated (Office of Science Policy, 2023). Any erosion of these protections could lead to decreased investments and stifle the development of groundbreaking medicines.

PhRMA's extensive investments underscore the critical role that the biopharmaceutical industry plays in advancing medical science and enhancing public health. However, the future of these investments depends on maintaining a supportive regulatory environment and safeguarding the incentives necessary for continued innovation. As the healthcare landscape evolves, addressing these challenges will be essential to ensure ongoing progress in the development of new treatments and therapies.

The Future Framework for Patient Adherence and Retention

Research has expanded our understanding of patient adherence in healthcare settings, building upon classic models of health behavior. Zullig et al. (2018) proposed a new framework that integrates population health science with precision medicine to improve medication adherence and participant retention further. This model emphasizes several key factors influencing adherence, including the following:

- First, clear and personalized communication remains fundamental. Advancements in remote patient monitoring, particularly in heart failure management, present new opportunities for personalized patient education and real-time feedback (Atreja et al., 2018). These technologies enhance the understanding of treatment regimens and allow for more effective patient engagement.
- Second, the patient–provider relationship has evolved to emphasize patient empowerment. Náfrádi et al. (2017) found that patient empowerment, particularly self-efficacy and health locus of control, is significantly associated with medication adherence. This suggests that when patients feel more in control of their health outcomes, they are more likely to adhere to treatment plans.
- Third, interventional tools play a crucial role in improving adherence. Costa et al. (2015) reviewed various interventions, including educational, behavioral, and integrated care approaches. They found that multifaceted interventions tailored to the individual patient's needs were most effective in improving adherence.
- Fourth, addressing barriers to adherence is essential. Kleinsinger (2018) highlighted that nonadherence remains a significant challenge in health care, influenced by medication costs, side effects, and complex regimens. Understanding and addressing these barriers is crucial for improving adherence rates.
- Finally, integrating population health approaches with personalized medicine presents new opportunities for enhancing adherence. Zullig et al. (2018) proposed that combining insights from population-level data with individual patient characteristics enables healthcare providers to develop more effective and targeted strategies to improve adherence.

Modern approaches to enhancing patient adherence and retention integrate personalized communication, patient empowerment, multifaceted interventions, addressing specific barriers, and leveraging both population health insights and precision medicine. This comprehensive approach acknowledges the intricate interplay of factors influencing adherence in contemporary healthcare settings and provides promising strategies for improvement.

Summary

Ensuring patient adherence to clinical trial protocols is crucial for generating valid and reliable data while controlling costs. Maintaining open communication, addressing adherence challenges promptly, and cultivating an appreciation for patients' trial participation can enhance their commitment to protocol requirements. Although more research is needed on optimizing adherence strategies, OCRNs serve as vital advocates for prioritizing adherence and upholding study integrity and validity. Their attentive adherence monitoring and interventions from start to finish are essential for the timely and successful conduct of clinical trials.

Key Points

- Adherence and retention directly affect the outcome and cost of a clinical trial.
- Failure to recognize nonadherence in a clinical trial misleads understanding of the true clinical benefit of a treatment in the study.
- OCRNs should screen for potential nonadherence risk factors and continue to assess adherence past enrollment and randomization.
- OCRNs are key in enhancing patient adherence with early assessment for adherence-related risk factors, assisting patients to overcome obstacles, and educating and working with physicians and interprofessional team members.

The author would like to acknowledge Lisa Francisco, BSN, RN, OCN®, for her contribution to this chapter that remains unchanged from the previous edition of this book.

References

Aggarwal, P., Woolford, S.J., & Patel, H.P. (2020). Multi-morbidity and polypharmacy in older people: Challenges and opportunities for clinical practice. *Geriatrics, 5*(4), 85. https://doi.org/10.3390/geriatrics5040085

American Nurses Association. (2015). *Code of ethics for nurses with interpretive statements.* https://nursing.rutgers.edu/wp-content/uploads/2019/06/ANA-Code-of-Ethics-for-Nurses.pdf

An, M.-W., Duong, Q., Le-Rademacher, J., & Mandrekar, S.J. (2020). Principles of good clinical trial design. *Journal of Thoracic Oncology, 15*(8), 1277–1280. https://doi.org/10.1016/j.jtho.2020.05.005

Anastasi, J.K., Capili, B., Norton, M., McMahon, D.J., & Marder, K. (2024). Recruitment and retention of clinical trial participants: Understanding motivations of patients with chronic pain and other populations. *Frontiers in Pain Research, 4,* 1330937. https://doi.org/10.3389/fpain.2023.1330937

Anghel, L.A., Farcas, A.M., & Oprean, R.N. (2019). An overview of the common methods used to measure treatment adherence. *Medicine and Pharmacy Reports, 92*(2), 117–122. https://doi.org/10.15386/mpr-1201

Aremu, T.O., Oluwole, O.E., Adeyinka, K.O., & Schommer, J.C. (2022). Medication adherence and compliance: Recipe for improving patient outcomes. *Pharmacy, 10*(5), 106. https://doi.org/10.3390/pharmacy10050106

Arshed, M., Mahmud, A.B., Minhat, H.S., Ying, L.P., & Umer, M.F. (2023). Effectiveness of mHealth interventions in medication adherence among patients with cardiovascular diseases: A systematic review. *Diseases, 11*(1), 41. https://doi.org/10.3390/diseases11010041

Atreja, A., Otobo, E., Ramireddy, K., & Deorocki, A. (2018). Remote patient monitoring in IBD: Current state and future directions. *Current Gastroenterology Reports, 20*(2), 6. https://doi.org/10.1007/s11894-018-0611-3

Beghi, E. (2016). The basic structure of a randomized clinical trial. *Frontiers of Neurology and Neuroscience, 39,* 1–7. https://doi.org/10.1159/000445408

Belitsi, V., Tsiampalis, T., Kouvari, M., Kalantzi, V., Androutsos, O., Bonoti, F., ... Kosti, R.I. (2023). Exploring patient beliefs and medication adherence in the Mediterranean context: A cross-sectional study in patients with cardiovascular diseases and cardiometabolic disorders in Greece—The IACT-Study. *Life, 13*(9), 1880. https://doi.org/10.3390/life13091880

Bruhn, H., Treweek, S., Duncan, A., Shearer, K., Cameron, S., Campbell, K., ... Cotton, S.C. (2019). Estimating Site Performance (ESP): Can trial managers predict recruitment success at trial sites? An exploratory study. *Trials, 20*(1), 192. https://doi.org/10.1186/s13063-019-3287-6

Burnier, M. (2024). The role of adherence in patients with chronic diseases. *European Journal of Internal Medicine, 119,* 1–5. https://doi.org/https://doi.org/10.1016/j.ejim.2023.07.008

Chaudhari, N., Ravi, R., Gogtay, N.J., & Thatte, U.M. (2020). Recruitment and retention of the participants in clinical trials: Challenges and solutions. *Perspectives in Clinical Research, 11*(2), 64–69. https://doi.org/10.4103/picr.PICR_206_19

Clancy, C., Lynch, J., O'Connor, P., & Dowling, M. (2020). Breast cancer patients' experiences of adherence and persistence to oral endocrine therapy: A qualitative evidence synthesis. *European Journal of Oncology Nursing, 44,* 101706. https://doi.org/10.1016/j.ejon.2019.101706

Coleman, K., & Dang, D. (2023, June 13). 37 scientists pioneering the future of biomedical research. *Pew.* https://www.pewtrusts.org/en/research-and-analysis/articles/2023/06/13/37-scientists-pioneering-the-future-of-biomedical-research

Costa, E., Giardini, A., Savin, M., Menditto, E., Lehane, E., Laosa, O., ... Marengoni, A. (2015). Interventional tools to improve medication adherence: Review of literature. *Patient Preference and Adherence, 9,* 1303–1314. https://doi.org/10.2147/PPA.S87551

de Viron, S., Trotta, L., Schumacher, H., Lomp, H.J., Höppner, S., Young, S., & Buyse, M. (2022). Detection of fraud in a clinical trial using unsupervised statistical monitoring. *Therapeutic Innovation and Regulatory Science, 56*(1), 130–136. https://doi.org/10.1007/s43441-021-00341-5

Desai, M. (2020). Recruitment and retention of participants in clinical studies: Critical issues and challenges. *Perspectives in Clinical Research, 11*(2), 51–53. https://doi.org/10.4103/picr.PICR_6_20

European Patients' Academy on Therapeutic Innovation. (2016). *Assessing participant adherence during clinical trials.* https://toolbox.eupati.eu/resources/assessing-participant-adherence-during-clinical-trials

Flocke, S.A., Antognoli, E., Daly, B.J., Jackson, B., Fulton, S.E., Liu, T.M., ... Meropol, N.J. (2017). The role of oncology nurses in discussing clinical trials. *Oncology Nursing Forum, 44*(5), 547–552. https://doi.org/10.1188/17.ONF.547-552

Fogel, D.B. (2018). Factors associated with clinical trials that fail and opportunities for improving the likelihood of success: A review. *Contemporary Clinical Trials Communications, 11,* 156–164. https://doi.org/10.1016/j.conctc.2018.08.001

Gborogen, R., & Polek, C. (2018). Communication and organization are top drivers of oral adherence in clinical trials. *Clinical Journal of Oncology Nursing, 22*(3), 333–339. https://10.1188/18.CJON.333-339

Getz, K., Smith, Z., Shafner, L., & Hanina, A. (2020). Assessing the scope and predictors of intentional dose non-adherence in clinical trials. *Therapeutic Innovation and Regulatory Science, 54*(6), 1330–1338. https://doi.org/10.1007/s43441-020-00155-x

Gillies, K., Kearney, A., Keenan, C., Treweek, S., Hudson, J., Brueton, V.C., ... & Aceves-Martins, M. (2021). Strategies to improve retention in randomised trials. *Cochrane Database of Systematic Reviews, 3*(3), MR000032. https://doi.org/10.1002/14651858.MR000032.pub3

Goodwin, M.A., Stange, K.C., Zyzanski, S.J., Crabtree, B.F., Borawski, E.A., & Flocke, S.A. (2017). The Hawthorne effect in direct observation research with physicians and patients. *Journal of Evaluation in Clinical Practice, 23*(6), 1322–1328. https://doi.org/10.1111/jep.12781

Grayek, E.N., Fischhoff, B., Davis, A.L., & Krishnamurti, T. (2022). The value of adherence information during clinical pharmaceutical trials. *Clinical Trials, 19*(3), 326–336. https://doi.org/10.1177/17407745221084127

Haleem, A., Javaid, M., Singh, R.P., & Suman, R. (2021). Telemedicine for healthcare: Capabilities, features, barriers, and applications. *Sensors International, 2,* 100117. https://doi.org/10.1016/j.sintl.2021.100117

Hamstra, M.S., Pemberton, V.L., Dagincourt, N., Hollenbeck-Pringle, D., Trachtenberg, F.L., Cnota, J.F., ... Lacro, R.V. (2020). Recruitment, retention, and adherence in a clinical trial: The Pediatric Heart Network's Marfan Trial experience. *Clinical Trials, 17*(6), 684–695. https://doi.org/10.1177/1740774520945988

Hariton, E., & Locascio, J.J. (2018). Randomised controlled trials—the gold standard for effectiveness research. *BJOG, 125*(13), 1716. https://doi.org/10.1111/1471-0528.15199

Houle, S. (2015). An introduction to the fundamentals of randomized controlled trials in pharmacy research. *Canadian Journal of Hospital Pharmacy, 68*(1), 28–32. https://doi.org/10.4212/cjhp.v68i1.1422

Kadam, R.A. (2017). Informed consent process: A step further towards making it meaningful! *Perspectives in Clinical Research, 8*(3), 107–112. https://doi.org/10.4103/picr.PICR_147_16

Kleinsinger, F. (2018). The unmet challenge of medication nonadherence. *Permanente Journal, 22*(3), 18–33. https://doi.org/10.7812/TPP/18-033

Koni, A.A., Suwan, B.A., Nazzal, M.A., Sleem, A., Daifallah, A., Allah, M.H., ... Zyoud, S.H. (2023). Adherence to oral anticancer hormonal therapy in breast cancer patients and its relationship with treatment satisfaction: An important insight from a developing country. *BMC Women's Health, 23*(1), 114. https://doi.org/10.1186/s12905-023-02276-5

Koziolek, M., Alcaro, S., Augustijns, P., Basit, A.W., Grimm, M., Hens, B., ... Corsetti, M. (2019). The mechanisms of pharmacokinetic food–drug interactions—A perspective from the UNGAP group. *European Journal of Pharmaceutical Sciences, 134,* 31–59. https://doi.org/10.1016/j.ejps.2019.04.003

Kvarnström, K., Westerholm, A., Airaksinen, M., & Liira, H. (2021). Factors contributing to medication adherence in patients with a chronic condition: A scoping review of qualitative research. *Pharmaceutics, 13*(7), 1100. https://doi.org/10.3390/pharmaceutics13071100

Laba, T.-L., Cheng, L., Kolhatkar, A., & Law, M.R. (2020). Cost-related nonadherence to medicines in people with multiple chronic conditions. *Research in Social and Administrative Pharmacy, 16*(3), 415–421. https://doi.org/10.1016/j.sapharm.2019.06.008

Lambert-Kerzner, A., Havranek, E.P., Plomondon, M.E., Fagan, K.M., McCreight, M.S., Fehling, K.B., ... Ho, P.M. (2015). Perspectives of patients on factors relating to adherence to post-acute coronary syndrome medical regimens. *Patient Preference and Adherence, 9,* 1053–1059. https://doi.org/10.2147/ppa.S84546

Lemij, A.A., de Glas, N.A., Derks, M.G.M., Bastiaannet, E., Merkus, J.W.S., Lans, T.E., ... Portielje, J.E.A. (2022). Discontinuation of adjuvant endocrine therapy and impact on quality of life and functional status in older patients with breast cancer. *Breast Cancer Research and Treatment, 193*(3), 567–577. https://doi.org/10.1007/s10549-022-06583-7

Liang, M.I., Pisu, M., Summerlin, S.S., Boitano, T.K.L., Blanchard, C.T., Bhatia, S., & Huh, W.K. (2020). Extensive financial hardship among gynecologic cancer patients starting a new line of therapy. *Gynecologic Oncology, 156*(2), 271–277. https://doi.org/10.1016/j.ygyno.2019.11.022

Lim, C.Y., & In, J. (2019). Randomization in clinical studies. *Korean Journal of Anesthesiology, 72*(3), 221–232. https://doi.org/10.4097/kja.19049

Mantila, K.M., Pasmooij, A.M.G., Hallgreen, C.E., Mol, P.G.M., & van Boven, J.F.M. (2022). Medication adherence measurement methods in registration trials supporting the approval of new medicines: A cross-sectional analysis of centralized procedures in the European Union 2010–2020. *Clinical Pharmacology and Therapeutics, 112*(5), 1051–1060. https://doi.org/10.1002/cpt.2709

Martin, L.R., Feig, C., Maksoudian, C.R., Wysong, K., & Faasse, K. (2018). A perspective on nonadherence to drug therapy: Psychological barriers and strategies to overcome nonadherence. *Patient Preference and Adherence, 12,* 1527–1535. https://doi.org/10.2147/ppa.S155971

Miaskowski, C., Shockney, L., & Chlebowski, R.T. (2008). Adherence to oral endocrine therapy for breast cancer: A nursing perspective. *Clinical Journal of Oncology Nursing, 12*(2), 213–221. https://doi.org/10.1188/08.CJON.213-221

Mishra, P., Vamadevan, A.S., Roy, A., Bhatia, R., Naik, N., Singh, S., ... Legido-Quigley, H. (2021). Exploring barriers to medication adherence using COM-B model of behaviour among patients with cardiovascular diseases in low- and middle-income countries: A qualitative study. *Patient Preference and Adherence, 15,* 1359–1371. https://doi.org/10.2147/ppa.S285442

Mitchell, A.P. (2021). We should treat financial toxicity with curative, rather than palliative, intent [Editorial]. *JCO Oncology Practice, 18*(2), 95–96. https://doi.org/10.1200/OP.21.00540

Moore, S. (2010). Nonadherence in patients with breast cancer receiving oral therapies. *Clinical Journal of Oncology Nursing, 14*(1), 41–47. https://doi.org/10.1188/10.CJON.41-47

Morrison, T.A., Smith, J.R., & Patel, K. (2020). Challenges in monitoring patient adherence to oral medications: A review of indirect assessment methods. *Journal of Clinical Pharmacology, 60*(5), 688–695. https://doi.org/10.1002/jcph.1334

Náfrádi, L., Nakamoto, K., & Schulz, P.J. (2017). Is patient empowerment the key to promote adherence? A systematic review of the relationship between self-efficacy, health locus of control and medication adherence. *PLOS ONE, 12*(10), e0186458. https://doi.org/10.1371/journal.pone.0186458

Nakajima, R., Watanabe, F., & Kamei, M. (2021). Factors associated with medication non-adherence among patients with lifestyle-related non-communicable diseases. *Pharmacy, 9*(2), 90. https://doi.org/10.3390/pharmacy9020090

National Cancer Institute. (2024). *Financial toxicity and cancer treatment.* https://www.cancer.gov/about-cancer/managing-care/track-care-costs/financial-toxicity-hp-pdq

National Institutes of Health. (2025). *NIH clinical research trials and you.* https://www.nih.gov/health-information/nih-clinical-research-trials-you

Nipp, R.D., Lee, H., Gorton, E., Lichtenstein, M., Kuchukhidze, S., Park, E., ... Moy, B. (2019). Addressing the financial burden of cancer clinical trial participation: Longitudinal effects of an equity intervention. *Oncologist, 24*(8), 1048–1055. https://doi.org/10.1634/theoncologist.2019-0146

Office of Science Policy. (2023). *Transforming discoveries into products: Maximizing NIH's levers to catalyze technology transfer.* https://osp.od.nih.gov/wp-content/uploads/2024/03/FINAL_Innovation_Policy_Workshop_Report.pdf

Oncology Nursing Society & Oncology Nursing Certification Corporation. (2024). *Oncology clinical research nurse competencies.* https://www.ons.org/sites/default/files/2025-01/ocrn-competencies-rebrand.pdf

Panahi, S., Rathi, N., Hurley, J., Sundrud, J., Lucero, M., & Kamimura, A. (2022). Patient adherence to health care provider recommendations and medication among free clinic patients. *Journal of Patient Experience, 9,* 23743735221077523. https://doi.org/10.1177/23743735221077523

Peng, Y., Wang, H., Fang, Q., Xie, L., Shu, L., Sun, W., & Liu, Q. (2020). Effectiveness of mobile applications on medication adherence in adults with chronic diseases: A systematic review and meta-analysis. *Journal of Managed Care and Specialty Pharmacy, 26*(4), 550–561. https://doi.org/10.18553/jmcp.2020.26.4.550

Pharmaceutical Research and Manufacturers of America. (n.d.). *Research and development policy framework.* https://phrma.org/policy-issues/research-development

Poongothai, S., Anjana, R.M., Aarthy, R., Unnikrishnan, R., Venkat Narayan, K.M., Ali, M.K., ... Mohan, V. (2023). Strategies for participant retention in long term clinical trials: A participant-centric approaches. *Perspectives in Clinical Research, 14*(1), 3–9. https://doi.org/10.4103/picr.picr_161_21

Rafhi, E., Al-Juhaishi, M., Stupans, I., Stevens, J.E., Park, J.S., & Wang, K.N. (2024). The influence of patients' beliefs about medicines and the relationship with suboptimal medicine use in community-dwelling older adults: A systematic review of quantitative studies. *International Journal of Clinical Pharmacy, 46*(4), 811–830. https://doi.org/10.1007/s11096-024-01727-9

Rigatti, M., DeGurian, A.A., & Albert, S.M. (2022). "Getting There": Transportation as a barrier to research participation among older adults. *Journal of Applied Gerontology, 41*(5), 1321–1328. https://doi.org/10.1177/07334648211072537

Samper-Pardo, M., León-Herrera, S., Oliván-Blázquez, B., Méndez-López, F., Domínguez-García, M., & Sánchez-Recio, R. (2023). Effectiveness of a telerehabilitation intervention using ReCOVery APP of long COVID patients: A randomized, 3-month follow-up clinical trial. *Scientific Reports, 13*(1), 7943. https://doi.org/10.1038/s41598-023-35058-y

Shankaran, V. (2021). Mitigating the morbidity of financial toxicity in cancer care. *Journal of the Advanced Practitioner in Oncology, 12*(3), 271–274. https://doi.org/10.6004/jadpro.2021.12.3.10

Sharkiya, S. (2023). Quality communication can improve patient-centred health outcomes among older patients: A rapid review. *BMC Health Services Research, 23,* 886. https://doi.org/10.1186/s12913-023-09869-8

Shiely, F., Murphy, D., & Millar, S.R. (2023). Clinical research nurse predictions of trial failure, recruitment and retention: A case for their early inclusion in trial design. *Trials, 24*(1), 458. https://doi.org/10.1186/s13063-023-07504-9

Shih, S., & Cohen, L.L. (2020). A systematic review of medication adherence interventions in pediatric sickle cell disease. *Journal of Pediatric Psychology, 45*(6), 593–606. https://doi.org/10.1093/jpepsy/jsaa031

Torres-Robles, A., Benrimoj, S.I., Gastelurrutia, M.A., Martinez-Martinez, F., Peiro, T., Perez-Escamilla, B., ... Garcia-Cardenas, V. (2022). Effectiveness of a medication adherence management intervention in a community pharmacy setting: A cluster randomised controlled trial. *BMJ Quality and Safety, 31*(2), 105–115. https://doi.org/10.1136/bmjqs-2020-011671

Unger, J.M., Cook, E., Tai, E., & Bleyer, A. (2016). Role of clinical trial participation in cancer research: Barriers, evidence, and strategies. *American Society of Clinical Oncology Educational Book, 36,* 185–198. https://doi.org/10.1200/EDBK_156686

Verbrugghe, M., Duprez, V., Beeckman, D., Grypdonck, M., Quaghebeur, M., Verschueren, C., ... Van Hecke, A. (2016). Factors influencing adherence in cancer patients taking oral tyrosine kinase inhibitors: A qualitative study. *Cancer Nursing, 39*(2), 153–162. https://doi.org/10.1097/ncc.0000000000000250

Vrijens, B., & Urquhart, J. (2014). Methods for measuring, enhancing, and accounting for medication adherence in clinical trials. *Clinical Pharmacology and Therapeutics, 95*(6), 617–626. https://doi.org/10.1038/clpt.2014.59

Winter, N., Russell, L., Ugalde, A., White, V., & Livingston, P. (2022). Engagement strategies to improve adherence and retention in web-based mindfulness programs: Systematic review. *Journal of Medical Internet Research, 24*(1), e30026. https://doi.org/10.2196/30026

World Health Organization. (2023). *COVID-19 vaccinations shift to regular immunization as COVAX draws to a close.* https://www.who.int/news/item/19-12-2023-covid-19-vaccinations-shift-to-regular-immunization-as-covax-draws-to-a-close

Zhao, M., Ma, J., Li, M., Zhang, Y., Jiang, B., Zhao, X., ... Qin, S. (2021). Cytochrome P450 enzymes and drug metabolism in humans. *International Journal of Molecular Sciences, 22*(23), 12808. https://doi.org/10.3390/ijms222312808

Zullig, L.L., Blalock, D.V., Dougherty, S., Henderson, R., Ha, C.C., Oakes, M.M., & Bosworth, H.B. (2018). The new landscape of medication adherence improvement: Where population health science meets precision medicine. *Patient Preference and Adherence, 12,* 1225–1230. https://doi.org/10.2147/PPA.S165404

CHAPTER 18

Clinical Trial Registries

Julie McCluggage, RN, CRN-BC, OCN®

Introduction

A clinical trial registry is an online repository of information. Sponsors and investigators register new trials as evidence that a trial exists. The registration process is complete when a unique identifier number is assigned to that trial. The process sets an expectation that the sponsor or investigator will publicly disseminate results, making new research data available to improve health care. This type of registry is called a results database.

This chapter will explain the reasons why clinical trial registries are developed. An overview of the evolution of trial registries will be presented. Examples of various trial registries and samples of national, international, and commercial registries will be provided. Finally, updated trends influencing registries will be described.

The Purpose of a Clinical Trial Registry

Clinical trial registries rose out of three individual yet complementary issues: a desire to address the need for transparency or informing the public that a trial exists, an ethical concern about data censuring or influencing the development of an accurate risk–benefit profile, and concerns about scientific integrity when results were not published in the public domain (Dickersin & Rennie, 2012).

The primary purpose of creating a clinical trial registry was to announce that a clinical trial existed publicly. Through this pronouncement, the lay public, patients, and healthcare providers might consider enrollment options (Dickersin & Rennie, 2012). A secondary but equally important purpose was to minimize the negative consequences of advancing evidence-based practice when trial results are not disseminated (Dickersin & Rennie, 2012). These issues called into question the fundamental premise of why trials were conducted: to develop new knowledge, to apply that knowledge to improve the health and health outcomes of the population, and to add to the body of research literature.

As early as 1986, Simes suggested that the outcome of a trial might influence the publication of clinical trial results. This publication bias or censorship defies the basic premise of conducting human participant research in that the data collected from those who afforded the investigator to test a hypothesis were not used to generalize new knowledge. More importantly, electing not to publish trial results inhibits the advancement of evidence-based practice and care decisions based on the best available research.

Evolution of Registries

The National Cancer Institute (NCI) led the way in launching a single source of disease-specific information when it created the Physician Data Query (PDQ®) database in 1977 (Manrow et al., 2014). It developed this database to assist in the rapid dissemination of research findings, provide oncology professionals and patients with the most advanced information on cancer treatment, and facilitate recruitment into clinical trials (Manrow et al., 2014).

The PDQ portal allows access to the ClinicalTrials.gov registry. NCI-sponsored clinical trials can be located by accessing www.cancer.gov/clinicaltrials. The Health Omnibus Programs Extension of 1988, often called the HOPE Act, mandated the development of a centralized clinical trial registry specifically for AIDS and HIV interventional trials. The AIDS Clinical Trials Information Service (ACTIS) began in 1989 as a telephone call-in triage and information center located at the National Institute of Allergy and Infectious Diseases via the National Institutes of Health (NIH) (National Institute of Allergy and Infectious Diseases, 2002). In 1996, ACTIS was made available as a disease-specific database and, perhaps, the first clinical trial registry. Protocol information and lists of open and enrolling NIH- and industry-funded trials were made available to the public (National Institute of Allergy and Infectious Diseases, 2002).

As the AIDS call-in center was offering clinical trial information for patients and providers, NCI launched CancerNet, a registry focused on oncology clinical trials (Zarin et al., 2018. Oncology-specific trials were published on national clinical trial websites, making public health information available in compliance with another federal law, the National Cancer Act of 1997.

On February 29, 2000, the NIH National Library of Medicine released ClinicalTrials.gov (U.S. Food and Drug Administration [FDA], 2010). Novel in its approach, this centralized database comprises federally and privately funded interventional trials testing drugs and biologics for serious or life-threatening diseases and conditions. However, NIH primarily sponsored the bulk of the trials. Clinical trials were registered and published prospectively. This meant that registration was completed before the trial enrolled the first participant. Information posted in ClinicalTrials.gov is written in lay terminology. Required elements of trial registration are defined, called protocol data elements, as a method of standardizing the information, such as study identification, study status, description, sponsors/collaborators, and study oversight. ClinicalTrials.gov (2024a) protocol registration data elements include the following:

- Study identification
- Study status
- Sponsors/collaborators
- Oversight
- Study description
- Conditions and keywords
- Study design
- Arms, groups, and interventions
- Outcome measures
- Eligibility
- Contacts, locations, and investigator information
- Individual participant data sharing statements
- References

The FDA Modernization Act of 1997 required sponsors to register clinical trials on ClinicalTrials.gov within 21 days following protocol approval (FDA, 2010). Trials registered on ClinicalTrials.gov are given an NCT (National Clinical Trial) number. Information on how to search for trials at ClinicalTrials.gov is available at www.clinicaltrials.gov/ct2/search.

The primary purpose of the repository was to offer patients, family members, and healthcare professionals a means to locate a clinical trial of interest (ClinicalTrials.gov, 2024a). Sponsors and investigators were expected to comply with the law, register trials, and modify information in the registry as necessary. However, compliance was less than anticipated, and oversight was limited. Still, the movement toward accountability and transparency had begun.

In 2005, the International Committee of Medical Journal Editors (ICMJE) initiated a mandate requiring clinical trial registration as a condition for submission of a manuscript for publication in its journals. This was the first time an organization critical to influencing the body of scientific knowledge expanded the generally accepted and traditional author guidelines to include evidence of a professional obligation. These uniform requirements for manuscripts submitted to biomedical journals included a significant number of journals worldwide, such as *Annals of Emergency Medicine*, *Clinical Drug Investigation*, and the *American Journal of Nursing*. Any trial registry was, and still is, acceptable as long as the submission meets the data submission criteria established by that registry.

ICMJE (2014) suggested that the clinical trial registration number be identified following the manuscript abstract. Unlike ClinicalTrials.gov, ICMJE offered a broader definition of clinical trials to include "any research project that prospectively assigns people or a group of people to an intervention, with or without concurrent comparison or control groups, to study the cause-and-effect relationship between a health-related intervention and a health outcome" (ICMJE, 2014, p. 12). Just like ClinicalTrials.gov, ICMJE considered trial registration as a repository supporting open and enrolling clinical trials, not a database for trial results. However, the ICMJE mandate advanced the goal of greater transparency and reduced the chance of selective or biased publication practices. As more attention was placed on providing assurances that the existence of clinical trials was publicly announced and researchers were bearing the responsibility to conform, the lack of uniformity and standards regarding what information should be included in trial registries became evident.

To address the variability among clinical trial registry information and as the number of web-accessible registries increased, the World Health Organization (WHO) established the International Clinical Trials Registry Platform (ICTRP) in 2006 (WHO, 2006). A minimum set of data was identified as being necessary for a trial registry, offering a complete view of a clinical trial so that an informed and enlightened decision may be made. From a global perspective, the need for uniformity was as crucial as the responsibility to embrace trial registration as a universal scientific, ethical, and moral responsibility (WHO, n.d.-b). The initiative was focused on unifying each trial registry through a single global portal—the ICTRP—and defining the Trial Registration Data Set, the core set of data considered acceptable to satisfy prospective registration (WHO, n.d.-a). The 24 data items in the dataset are the minimum amount of trial information required for a fully registered trial (see www.who.int/tools/clinical-trials-registry-platform/network/who-data-set for the complete list).

The WHO registry contains interventional and phase 1–4 trials. Trials submitted to the WHO registry first receive a Universal Trial Number. Once a trial is fully registered, it is posted in the WHO portal with the registration number listed as the primary trial registry identification number and the Universal Trial Number listed as the secondary identifier.

WHO defined the criteria for the minimum dataset in a clinical trial registry internationally. This improved the quality of information available for participants, lay individuals, and health professionals when searching for an open trial. In 2007, Section 801 of the FDA Amendments Act (FDAAA) was passed, offering an essential step toward greater transparency, accountability, and publication of all trial results.

In September 2008, ClinicalTrials.gov added a results database. For all registered trials, the results database must contain aggregate or summary-level data and not patient-level data. Trial sponsors or investigators must submit summary data in tabular form no later than 12 months following trial completion (ClinicalTrials.gov, 2024b). See Figure 18-1 for a description of the results data elements.

In addition to publishing basic trial summary data, the FDAAA required the submission of Form FDA 3674, Certification of Compliance, at the time of initial registration submission (FDAAA, 2007). A copy of this form is available at www.fda.gov/about-fda/reports-manuals-forms/forms?Page=5. The FDAAA legislation furthered the goal of access to clinical trials, transparency, and facilitation of responsible scientific conduct through the public dissemination of basic trial results. Failure to comply would result in civil penalties and the inability to secure future federal funding.

Federal laws mandated that sponsors and investigators must document that a clinical trial was recruiting human participants and that all clinical trial data must be published in the public domain. However, federal law did not address the ethical imperative and responsibility that sponsors and investigators had to the participants enrolled in the clinical trials. Instead, this is addressed in the Declaration of Helsinki (World Medical Association [WMA], 2024).

In 2008, the Eighth Amendment revised the Declaration of Helsinki document, adding the expectation that clinical trial registration in a publicly accessible database occur prior to enrollment of the first participant. Moreover, the declaration supported the ICJME position paper and set the expectation that authors, regardless of the trial outcome, publish trial results in the public domain (e.g., peer-reviewed journal) (WMA, 2024). In 2013, WMA revised the document again, adding a new section titled *Research Registration and Publication and Dissemination of Results*, which stated the ethical expectation that sponsors and researchers report and disseminate trial results (WMA, 2024).

Multiple online registries housing prospective data or trial results demonstrate ethical conduct and compliance with federal laws. However, no single point of access, trial registry, or trial results database exists that is inclusive of all open clinical trials and trial results. Therefore, searching the internet is necessary to locate the most appropriate trial information.

- **Participant flow:** number of participants enrolled, withdrawing, and completed; progress of participants through each stage of a study, by study arm or comparison group
- **Baseline characteristics:** baseline data for enrolled participants by study arm; demographics, age, gender, and study-specific measures
- **Outcome measures and statistical analyses:** summary table of outcome measures by study arm, primary and secondary outcomes, post hoc outcomes, and appropriate statistical analyses
- **Adverse events:** summary table of all anticipated and unanticipated serious adverse events and anticipated and unanticipated other adverse events exceeding a specific frequency threshold

FIGURE 18-1 | Trial Results Summary Data

Note. Based on information from ClinicalTrials.gov, 2024b.

Foreign Registries

Following the development of the federally funded and operated ClinicalTrials.gov registry, many foreign countries and organizations developed similar free, open-access, web-based repositories for prospective trial registration. Although the repositories share many similarities, each database varies, reflecting the unique needs of the lay, regulatory, and scientific communities. Most of these registries are aligned with governmental agencies and support compliance with relevant local laws. Foreign-based trial registries may be found on the WHO ICTRP web portal (www.who.int/tools/clinical-trials-registry-platform/network). See Table 18-1 for a complete listing. All information posted on the WHO platform is written in the English language. Registries not included in the WHO platform may or may not be available in English.

Pharmaceutical Registries

Pharmaceutical companies have a stake in shortening the time between trial initiation and enrollment of the first participant. More importantly, as sponsors of clinical trials, they are in a position to facilitate the data analysis and dissemination activities of responsible research conduct, supporting the ethical guidelines of the Declaration of Helsinki (WMA, 2024). Some pharmaceutical companies support registration and entry of results in ClinicalTrials.gov. Others have developed company-specific portals that generally provide trial information on proprietary products or interventions. Trial types and phases may also vary.

Disease-Specific Registries

Disease-specific registries focus on certain conditions or diseases. They may serve to register prospective clinical trials or offer a repository of nonexperimental trials registered in other clinical trial registries. This allows a more focused search for open and enrolling trials. One example is the LUNGevity Foundation, which hosts a disease-specific

TABLE 18-1 | World Health Organization Foreign Registries

Name	Date	Services	Website
Australian New Zealand Clinical Trials Registry	2007	This registry offers a full spectrum of therapeutic areas of pharmaceuticals, surgical procedures, preventive measures, lifestyle devices, treatment and rehabilitation strategies, and complementary therapies.	www.anzctr.org.au
Brazilian Registry of Clinical Trials	2010/2011	Phase 1–4 studies are included in this registry.	www.ensaiosclinicos.gov.br
Chinese Clinical Trial Registry	2007	This registry is for interventional studies, prevention studies, diagnostic test studies, prognostic studies, and epidemiologic research.	www.chictr.org.cn
Clinical Research Information Service (CRiS), Republic of Korea	2010	This registry comprises any study aiming to prevent, detect, diagnose, or treat diseases (observational and interventional studies).	CRIS mobile web by entering 'cris.nih.go.kr': https://web.archive.org/web/20101121001837/http://ncrc.cdc.go.kr/cris/index.jsp
Clinical Trials Registry India	2007/2008	This registry offers information on interventions, such as investigational drugs, surgical procedures, preventive measures, lifestyle modifications, devices, educational or behavioral treatment, and rehabilitation strategies, as well as trials being conducted in the purview of the Department of AYUSH (Ayurveda, Yoga and Naturopathy, Unani, Siddha, and Homoeopathy).	www.ctri.nic.in
Cuban Public Registry of Clinical Trials	2007/2011	This registry is for interventions such as investigational drugs and medical devices.	www.rpcec.sld.cu
European Union Clinical Trials Register	2001/2011	Pediatric clinical trials, as well as phase 2–4 adult clinical trials, are covered in this registry.	www.clinicaltrialsregister.eu
German Clinical Trials Register (DRKS)	2008	This registry offers the public a complete, up-to-date overview of clinical trials in Germany; it contains more than 16,000 studies, with around 2,000 studies added each year.	www.drks.de
International Traditional Medicine Clinical Trial Registry	2023	This registry includes trials from the fields of traditional medicine from any country, including Chinese medicine, acupuncture, herbal medicine, ayurveda, homeopathy, yonani, and complementary and supplementary medicines.	https://itmctr.ccebtcm.org.cn/en-US
Japan Registry for Clinical Trials	2018	This registry was established by the Ministry of Health, Labor and Welfare based on the Clinical Trial Act (Law No.16 of Heisei 29) that took effect in April 2018. It has 3 registries that work as a network called the Japan Primary Registries Network.	https://rctportal.mhlw.go.jp/en
Lebanon Clinical Trials Registry	2019	The registry includes all human trials in various therapeutic areas in pharmaceuticals, surgical procedures, preventive measures, lifestyle, devices, treatment, and rehabilitation strategies.	https://lbctr.moph.gov.lb
Pan African Clinical Trial Registry	2007/2008	PATCR recognizes that African trialists face additional challenges in trial registration and seeks to provide feasible ways to overcome these. A common problem is limited, unreliable, and costly internet access. The registry provides alternative means of trial registration for registrants who do not have reliable internet access. Trials may be performed manually by email, post mail, or facsimile correspondence, and trial registration is free.	https://pactr.samrc.ac.za

(Continued on next page)

TABLE 18-1 | World Health Organization Foreign Registries *(Continued)*

Name	Date	Services	Website
Sri Lanka Clinical Trials Registry	2006/2008	This registry is for all trials conducted in Sri Lanka. It also comprises the first functioning clinical trials registry in South Asia. This registry only accepts clinical trials with health-related interventions and does not register observational studies. It encourages prospective registration of all clinical trials and does not accept trials for retrospective registration.	https://web.archive.org/web/20190228023836/http://slctr.lk/
Thai Clinical Trials Registry	2009/2013	The mission of this registry is to encourage all clinical trials in Thailand to be prospectively registered before participants are recruited. It aims to promote transparency, reduce redundancy, and minimize publication bias or selective reporting.	www.thaiclinicaltrials.org

Note. All trials became registered with the World Health Organization in the latter year under the Date column. More information is available at www.who.int/clinical-trials-registry-platform/network/primary-registries. Acceptable trial registries can be found at www.icmje.org.

registry and clinical trial search tool focused on lung cancer. It is reinforced by EmergingMed and provides patients with curated information about ongoing lung cancer clinical trials, including biomarker-driven and targeted therapy studies.

NCI offers free access to thousands of open and closed oncology clinical trials via its PDQ database. Visitors may sort by cancer site, trial location, treatment preferences, trial phases, and sponsor. Cooperative group trials and research funded by a specific institute, such as the National Institute of Nursing Research, are options available to refine the search. Access to the NCI oncology clinical trials repository may be found at www.cancer.gov/clinicaltrials.

Diverse Populations Recruitment

Historically, clinical trials did not recruit patients most affected by a particular disease, condition, or behavior. Most enroll White male patients, with an underrepresentation of females, older adults, and people of color (especially in regard to Black and Hispanic populations). This has led to gaps in our understanding of these diseases and conditions, preventive factors, and treatment effectiveness across diverse populations (Kelsey et al., 2022). Because of this, the quality of healthcare choices is affected, as well as the ability to educate patients on how to lower their risks, the best possible treatment responses, and the advancement of more efficient treatments or interventions.

Diversity and inclusion in clinical trials is essential, as people can experience the same disease differently based on age, biological sex, pregnancy status, life experiences, health-promoting behaviors, environmental conditions, genetic variation, geographic lineage, and underlying medical problems or comorbidities. Clinical trials must include these populations so that everyone can benefit from scientific advances. Including diverse populations in clinical trials improves care and health outcomes in racially and ethnically diverse communities (Kelsey et al., 2022).

Key stakeholders across the clinical trial ecosystem, including academia, government, patient advocacy, community leaders, healthcare providers, technology experts, and clinical research organizations, have increased their diversity, equity, and inclusion efforts around clinical trials. Examples include the following (Younossi et al., 2021):

- FDA, in the summer of 2019, drafted guidance on enhancing the diversity of clinical research participants and finalized this guidance in November 2020.
- The Multi-Regional Clinical Trials Center of Brigham and Women's Hospital and Harvard formed a workgroup in February 2018. It later published a guidance document in 2020 and a toolkit in 2021.
- The Pharmaceutical Research and Manufacturers of America published the first industrywide principles on clinical trial diversity in November 2020, *Principles on Conduct of Clinical Trials and Communication of Clinical Trial Results*. It became effective in April 2021.
- In 2021, the American Medical Association partnered with the All of Us program for "better insights into the biological, environmental, and behavioral influences on disease to enhance prevention and treatment" (Younossi et al., 2021, para. 4).
- The National Academies of Sciences, Engineering, and Medicine published a report in 2016, *Strategies for Ensuring Diversity, Inclusion, and Meaningful Participation in Clinical Trials.*

Other examples include NIH's *Minority Health and Health Disparities Strategic Plan 2021–2025*, which was developed to outline a commitment to improving minority health and reducing health disparities (Kelsey et al.,

2022). The two primary goals of this plan focus on diversity and inclusion in NIH-funded research and clinical trials.

- **Goal 7:** Ensure appropriate representation of minority and other populations experiencing health disparities in NIH-funded research.
- **Goal 8:** Promote evidence-based community engagement, dissemination, and implementation of minority health and health disparities research best practices.

The Leap Forward Research Challenges, part of the Strategic Plan, aim to redefine the science of minority health and health disparities, which include the following (Kelsey et al., 2022):

- Increase the percentage of participants from diverse populations included in NIH-funded clinical research to 40% by 2030 within specific major disease categories.
- Increase the diversity of institutions conducting genomic research and training by investing in faculty and forming curriculum-guiding partnerships. This will accelerate workforce development in underrepresented and under-resourced communities within the next 10 years.

The National Institute on Minority Health and Health Disparities sponsored a Funding Opportunity Announcement to support evidence-based efforts to increase enrollment of racial and ethnic minorities into clinical trials. Projects included the National Initiative for Minority Involvement in Neurological Clinical Trials (https://nimict.com) to evaluate strategies for enrollment, recruitment, and retention of racial and ethnic minorities in neurologic clinical trials. The Enhancing Minority Participation in Clinical Trials: Phase 2 (https://reporter.nih.gov/search/oBXtyidaq0GrrZhTE-u4IQ/projects?shared=true) project was created to test strategies to increase racial and ethnic minority enrollment in cancer clinical trials (Kelsey et al., 2022).

In 2024, the International Agency for Research on Cancer released a report on the global burden of cancer, highlighting the increasing numbers of cancers, the unequal effect on underserved populations, and the immediate need to address cancer imbalances worldwide. WHO also published a survey from 115 countries showing that the majority of countries do not, as part of their universal health coverage, prioritize or adequately finance cancer and palliative care services (WHO, 2024).

In regard to the absolute burden, the increase in the incidence of cancer is seen most significantly in low (142% increase) and medium Human Development Index countries (99%). The cancer mortality rates in these countries are estimated to double by 2050 (WHO, 2024). This increase will be felt evenly across countries of different Human Development Index levels, and those who have the fewest resources to manage cancer will bear the brunt of the global burden (WHO, 2024).

Given the increased cancer rates in these regions, the creation of registries is even more important. Despite the progress that has been made in the early detection and treatment of cancers, significant disparities in treatment outcomes exist between high- and low-income regions of the world and within countries. Tools exist to enable governments to prioritize cancer care and ensure that everyone has access to affordable, quality services. Patient registries are designed to continually observe cancer survival, treatment guidance, safety, clinical care, and patient-reported outcomes in a larger patient population and for more extended periods than clinical trials (Flick et al., 2023).

Clinical trials are often designed to have identical populations and adhere to strict eligibility criteria, which usually exclude older, frail, or sicker populations. Registries, in comparison, have fewer limitations (e.g., broad range inclusion criteria and limited exclusion criteria), which allows analysis of treatment patterns, clinical outcomes, and adverse events in more diversified patient populations, especially in specific groups of patients who are not customarily included in clinical trials or do not trust clinical trials, such as older adults, people of color, underserved populations, and patients with multiple comorbidities (Flick et al., 2023).

Connect® MM Registry analyzed 3,011 newly diagnosed patients with multiple myeloma enrolled from more than 200 community-based sites across the United States (Flick et al., 2023). It showed that 40% of these patients would not have qualified for multiple myeloma clinical trials because of the strict eligibility criteria.

With longer follow-ups and a larger patient demographic, oncology registries allow for capturing clinical outcomes of interest in smaller populations of high-risk or sick patients, such as older adults and those with high-risk disease, poor performance status, impaired hepatic or renal function, or with cytogenetics associated with poor prognosis. By including this patient population, the information learned can advise on more informed treatment guidelines (Flick et al., 2023).

Current Trends

A tremendous amount has been accomplished over the past three decades concerning the development of trial registries and databases. Several trends are noteworthy to identify, as they relate to improving the goals of clinical trial transparency, accessibility, standardization, results reporting, and informing evidence-based practice.

For example, ClinicalTrials.gov now requires registration of controlled clinical trials and trials seeking FDA approval for drugs or medical devices. Investigators can register interventional clinical trials or observational clinical studies. Once registered, they must conform to the verification and updating requirements of ClinicalTrials.gov.

A second trend involves trial matching services. Although participant recruitment may be increased from inclusion in one or more online free registries, no single web-accessible portal exists. As a result, patients, professionals, and providers may need to search several registries using a variety of search terms and individually evaluate outputs from each before making a decision. This process may result in undue frustration and perhaps too much or not enough information. More importantly, this may present a future barrier to enrollment and recruitment efforts. Gansler et al. (2012) noted that trial matching services were influential in helping to link patients with trial information, availability, and subsequent enrollment. However, other variables, such as race, insurance, stage of disease, and performance status, must be considered during the search process. Clinical trial matching services, which may be either web-accessible or available through central call centers, offer a coordinated approach to the search process. A sample list of trial matching services is found in Figure 18-3.

The question of standardization and commonalities for both registries and databases is an ongoing issue. The 12 protocol data elements used in the ClinicalTrials.gov registry are slightly different from the 24 elements required by the WHO platform. This lack of standardization in the two largest registries presents a challenge. Information deemed essential might evolve with input from users and the scientific community at large. Equally important is the monitoring of registry information to ensure accuracy and completeness and the lack of gaps, omissions, or missing data.

Ensuring that these results are submitted within the specified period of time and the issue of dissemination of the trial results must be addressed. Compliance with the results submission requirements may present a complicated enforcement issue for FDA. Title VIII of FDAAA (2007) establishes both a responsibility and a commitment to the dissemination of registered trial results. This commitment was made to the researchers, the medical community, the public at large, and, most importantly, the human participants.

In February 2012, the Agency for Healthcare Research and Quality published the *National Healthcare Quality Report*, calling for a central access site for all U.S.-based trial registries and databases and standardization of the data elements and information posted on the websites of registries (Gliklich et al., 2012). Task force members conducted multiple focused interviews among care providers, the public, and federal agencies, such as the Centers for Medicare and Medicaid Services. The recommendations addressed a single portal option, as well as enhancing access to open and closed trials, data standardization, and publications of scientific findings. The task force identified the following five objectives to improve the system (Gliklich et al., 2012, p. ES-1):

- Provide a searchable central listing of patient registries in the United States so as to enable interested parties to identify registries in a particular area of interest (to promote collaboration, reduce redundancy, and improve transparency).
- Encourage and facilitate the use of common data elements and definitions in similar conditions (to improve opportunities for sharing, comparing, and linkage) through the listing and searching of such elements.
- Provide a central repository of searchable summary results (including for registries that do not have results published in peer-reviewed literature).
- Offer researchers a search tool to locate existing data sources (from either ongoing registries or closed registries) to request for use in new studies (secondary analyses, linkage studies).
- Serve as a recruitment tool for both providers and patients.

Finally, Duke University and FDA formed a unique collaborative project called the Clinical Trials Transformation Initiative (CTTI) (Sprenger et al., 2013). More than 60 organizations have joined as paid members (CTTI, n.d.). Access to large datasets through CTTI and ClinicalTrials.gov may offer additional research avenues using secondary data.

As these issues are addressed, additional needs will be identified. A collaborative effort with input from participants, the general public, and medical communities is essential.

Implications for Oncology Clinical Research Nurses

Oncology clinical research nurses (OCRNs) play a vital role in all aspects of the research process, including protocol development, participant recruitment, trial coordination, and results dissemination and publication. Specific responsibilities and activities of OCRNs may vary among sites and settings. Performing effectively as an OCRN requires a unique skill set. The Oncology Nursing Society

- American Cancer Society: https://www.cancer.org/about-us/what-we-do/providing-support.html
- American Lung Association: www.emergingmed.com/networks/americanlungassociation
- Antidote: www.antidote.me
- Blood Cancer United: https://bloodcancerunited.org/resources/patients/clinical-trial-support-center-ctsc
- Breast Cancer Trials: www.breastcancertrials.org/bct_nation/home.seam
- Colon Cancer Alliance: https://colorectalcancer.org
- EmergingMed Clinical Trial Navigator Service: www.emergingmed.com
- Florida Cancer Trials: https://flcancer.com/participating-in-a-clinical-trial
- Mendel: https://mendel.ai
- National Library of Medicine's Clinical Trials: https://clinicaltrials.gov
- Smart Patients: www.smartpatients.com/trials

FIGURE 18-3 | Clinical Trial Matching and Support Services

(ONS) and Oncology Nursing Certification Corporation (ONCC) developed a basic set of core competencies that differentiate oncology nurses from OCRNs, titled *Oncology Clinical Research Nurse Competencies* (ONS & ONCC, 2024). The nine competencies support the intent to differentiate the contributions that OCRNs make to this practice specialty.

OCRNs integrate information concerning trial registries and databases to develop safe, compliant, and ethical care for potential and enrolled clinical research participants. OCRNs apply knowledge concerning ethical principles, guidelines, and regulations when managing trials and during the informed consent process (ONS & ONCC, 2024). Competent OCRNs employ every possible strategy to support effective participant recruitment for a diverse population while using all available resources to minimize barriers to enrollment. Finally, all nine core competencies offer novice OCRNs, advanced OCRNs, and nurses transitioning to this practice specialty the ability to develop professionally based on a minimum set of practice standards (ONS & ONCC, 2024). The OCRN core competencies recognize and differentiate the knowledge, skills, and abilities of nurses who commit to educating, caring for, and protecting clinical research participants.

Summary

A significant amount of progress has been made worldwide to address the original objectives of increasing clinical trial transparency and reducing data censuring and publication bias. The development of clinical trial registries offered researchers and sponsors the ability to document the existence of a clinical trial. Informing the public and medical community that a clinical trial was enrolling human participants led to establishing an expectation and responsibility that results generated from research should be placed in the public domain for the purposes of informing and improving healthcare decision-making.

The focus has turned to enforcement with FDAAA (2007) and with process improvements. Registering the appropriate trials into ClinicalTrials.gov no later than 21 days after enrollment of the first participant, as well as submitting summary results (e.g., adverse event information) no later than one year after a trial's (primary) completion date, will require additional resources.

Submitting results to ClinicalTrials.gov is independent of publication in a peer-reviewed journal. Incentivizing responsible parties to do both may be necessary. Finally, improving access and dissemination may be further facilitated through the concerted efforts of the Agency for Healthcare Research and Quality initiative. Together, a shared commitment to patients and ethical principles, in combination with federally regulated mandates, will improve the integrity of the research process.

Key Points

- Clinical trial registries arose out of a desire for greater transparency, a need for published trial results, and an ethical need to increase the type and amount of available information to improve informed decision-making.
- A clinical trial registry functions as a central repository for information on new or ongoing clinical trials.
- Clinical trial registries facilitate the inclusion of more diverse populations in research, which is essential for improving healthcare outcomes and informing treatment guidelines.
- Despite the advancements in early detection, treatment, and care, significant disparities in cancer outcomes persist not only between high and low-income regions worldwide but also within countries.
- Clinical trial results databases expand trial registries by linking published results summaries for public review.
- ClinicalTrials.gov was the first centralized web-accessible clinical trial registry.
- WHO advanced standardization of clinical trial registration elements through the initiation of the ICTRP and Trial Registration Data Set.
- ICMJE emphasized the publication of all trial results as a professional expectation and requirement following prospective registration of a clinical trial.
- Many clinical trial registries are available now via pharmaceutical companies, healthcare organizations, and social media sites.

The author would like to acknowledge Nina M. Trocky, DNP, RN, NE-BC, CCRA, for her contribution to this chapter that remains unchanged from the previous edition of this book.

References

Clinical Trials Transformation Initiative. (n.d.). *About CTTI.* https://ctti-clinicaltrials.org/about

ClinicalTrials.gov (2024a). *Protocol registration data element definitions for interventional and observational studies.* https://clinicaltrials.gov/policy/protocol-definitions

ClinicalTrials.gov. (2024b). *Results data element definitions for interventional and observational studies.* https://clinicaltrials.gov/policy/results-definitions

Dickersin, K., & Rennie, D. (2012). The evolution of trial registries and their use to assess the clinical trial enterprise [Editorial]. *JAMA, 307*(17), 1861–1864. https://doi.org/10.1001/jama.2012.4230

Flick, E.D., Terebelo, H.R., Fish, S., Kitali, A., Mahajan, V., Nifenecker, M., ... Grinblatt, D.L. (2023). The value of pharmaceutical industry-sponsored patient registries in oncology clinical research. *Oncologist, 28*(8), 657–663. https://doi.org/10.1093/oncolo/oyad110

Food and Drug Administration Amendments Act of 2007, Pub. L. No. 110-85, 121 Stat. 823, § 801 (2007). https://www.gpo.gov/fdsys/pkg/PLAW-110publ85/pdf/PLAW-110publ85.pdf

Gansler, T., Jin, M., Bauer, J., Dahlquist, K., Tis, L., Sharpe, K., ... Kepner, J. (2012). Outcomes of a cancer clinical trial matching service. *Journal of Cancer Education, 27*(1), 11–20. https://doi.org/10.1007/s13187-011-0296-x

Gliklich, R.E., Leavy, M.B., & Campion, D.M. (2012). *Developing a registry of patient registries: Options for the Agency for Healthcare Research and Quality* (Effective Health Care Program Research Report No.

34). https://effectivehealthcare.ahrq.gov/products/registry-of-patient-registries-development/research

International Committee of Medical Journal Editors. (2014). *Recommendations for the conduct, reporting, editing, and publication of scholarly work in medical journals.* https://www.icmje.org/icmje-recommendations.pdf

Kelsey, M.D., Patrick-Lake, B., Abdulai, R., Broedl, U.C., Brown, A., Cohn, E., ... Bloomfield, G.S. (2022). Inclusion and diversity in clinical trials: Actionable steps to drive lasting change. *Contemporary Clinical Trials, 116,* 106740. https://doi.org/10.1016/j.cct.2022.106740

Manrow, R.E., Beckwith, M., & Johnson, L.E. (2014). NCI's Physician Data Query (PDQ®) cancer information summaries: History, editorial processes, influence, and reach. *Journal of Cancer Education, 29*(1), 198–205. https://doi.org/10.1007/s13187-013-0536-3

National Institute of Allergy and Infectious Diseases. (2002). *Revamped AIDS Web site tailored to diverse users* [Press release]. https://cybercemetery.unt.edu/archive/allcollections/20090201222404/http://www3.niaid.nih.gov/news/newsreleases/2002/aidswebsite.htm

Oncology Nursing Society & Oncology Nursing Certification Corporation. (2024). *Oncology clinical research nurse competencies.* https://www.ons.org/sites/default/files/2025-01/ocrn-competencies-rebrand.pdf

Simes, R.J. (1986). Publication bias: The case for an international registry of clinical trials. *Journal of Clinical Oncology, 4*(10), 1529–1541. https://jco.ascopubs.org/content/4/10/1529.full.pdf+html

Sprenger, K., Nickerson, D., Meeker-O'Connell, A., & Morrison, B.W. (2013). Quality by design in clinical trials: A collaborative pilot with FDA. *Therapeutic Innovation and Regulatory Science, 47*(2), 161–166. https://doi.org/10.1177/0092861512458909

U.S. Food and Drug Administration. (2010, January 7). *Historical perspective on the development of* ClinicalTrials.gov, *and an overview of FDA's role in supporting the success of the database, and accessibility to clinical trials information by the public: Background.*

World Health Organization. (n.d.-a). *WHO Trial Registration Data Set (Version 1.2.1 - archived)* https://www.who.int/clinical-trials-registry-platform/network/who-data-set/archived/1-2-1

World Health Organization. (n.d.-b). *International Clinical Trials Registry Platform (ICTRP).* https://www.who.int/clinical-trials-registry-platform

World Health Organization. (2006). WHO clinical trials initiative to protect the public. *Bulletin of the World Health Organization, 84,* 10–11. https://www.ncbi.nlm.nih.gov/pmc/articles/PMC2626508

World Health Organization. (2024). *Global cancer burden growing, amidst mounting need for services.* https://www.who.int/news/item/01-02-2024-global-cancer-burden-growing--amidst-mounting-need-for-services

World Medical Association. (2024). *WMA Declaration of Helsinki—Ethical principles for medical research involving human subjects* [75th General Assembly]. https://www.wma.net/policiespost/wma-declaration-of-helsinki-ethical-principles-for-medical-research-involving-human-subjects

Younossi, A., Sanhai, W., Shah, S., Chang, C., & Overman, J. (2021, November 11). Enhancing clinical trial diversity. *Deloitte Insights.* https://www2.deloitte.com/us/en/insights/industry/life-sciences/lack-of-diversity-clinical-trials.html

Zarin, D.A., Williams, R.J., Tse, T., & Ide, N.C. (2018). The role and importance of clinical trial registries and results databases. In J.I. Callin (Ed.), *Principles and practice of clinical research* (4th ed., 111-126). Elsevier Academic Press.

CHAPTER 19

Accessibility and Underserved Populations

Alison Ivey, MS, MBA, RN, OCN®, CCRP

Introduction

Cancer clinical trials are the primary mechanism through which new drugs, devices, and other clinical approaches are tested to treat, diagnose, and prevent cancer. The ultimate goal of these investigations is to improve health outcomes through interventions aimed at various points along the cancer continuum. Although research is a major driver of progress, only a small percentage of adult patients with cancer (2%–8%) participate in clinical trials. In general, those who do participate in clinical trials tend to be less diverse than the overall population with cancer. Black, Hispanic, rural, and low-income patients are notably underrepresented in clinical trials (American Association for Cancer Research [AACR], 2024; Oyer et al., 2022). These populations are not only less likely to participate in clinical research but also face a disproportionately higher burden of cancer diagnoses and mortality compared to the general population with cancer.

In 2024, AACR released its updated report on the state of cancer health disparities in the United States. In this report, it defined *cancer disparities* as "adverse differences in the cancer burden that are experienced by, but not limited to, racially and ethnically minoritized groups, rural residents, citizens of sovereign Native Nations, those identifying as sexual and gender minorities, and those living under persistent poverty" (p. 12). Although progress has been made in the past few decades to improve health outcomes for minoritized (or underrepresented) groups, significant gaps remain, including disparities in options for clinical trial participation and subsequent rates of enrollment.

Disparities in participation have been further described by Pittell et al. (2023). Based on their analysis of oncology enrollment trends from 2017–2022, the authors synthesized data from approximately 800 sites, focusing on trials involving patients with five different cancer types: breast, colorectal, lung, myeloma, and pancreatic. Results showed persistent enrollment disparities in Black and Hispanic participants over the assessment period, which deepened during the COVID-19 pandemic.

Many factors contribute to these observed disparities among underrepresented groups, including limited access to sites offering clinical research, socioeconomic barriers, cultural and linguistic differences, historical mistrust of research, and barriers inherent within the trials themselves. A general lack of awareness about the critical role of clinical trials in cancer treatment and care among patients and healthcare providers has also contributed to lower enrollment rates (Oyer et al., 2022; Schwartz et al., 2023). Further, some underrepresented groups, including those who identify as LGBTQIA+ (lesbian, gay, bisexual, transgender, queer or questioning, intersex, and asexual) often face barriers such as discrimination, lack of inclusive trial designs, and limited research addressing specific cancer risks and outcomes. These patients may have unique needs, including culturally competent care, safe spaces for identity disclosure, and targeted support for the psychosocial challenges they encounter during cancer treatment and research participation (Ussher et al., 2022; Wheldon et al., 2024; see Chapter 20 for more information).

This chapter will help elucidate the importance of reaching historically underserved populations, barriers to clinical trial participation, and potential solutions.

Regulatory Perspectives on Diversity in Clinical Trials

The U.S. Food and Drug Administration (FDA) Safety and Innovation Act, codified in 2012, broadened the FDA's authority to advance public health. The Act included recommendations for enhancing demographic subset analyses in clinical trials across all health indications. As part of the implementation plan accompanying the Act, FDA reviewed data generated from applications for 72 medicinal products. Its subsequent report, *Collection, Analysis, and Availability of Demographic Subgroup Data for FDA-Approved Medical Products* (FDA, 2013), noted that approximately half of the applications included a subset analysis of safety by race or ethnicity. The document further noted that, even when race or ethnicity data were collected as part of the study, the quality and consistency of the demographic data included in these analyses were uneven. There was often insufficient participation by minority groups to yield meaningful data analysis.

FDA recognizes that these gaps in representation can negatively affect the ability to apply trial findings to the broader population. Although it notes a trend toward smaller, more nimble study designs, which can accelerate necessary innovations for serious and life-threatening diseases, concerns exist that a quicker pace of enrollment in these trials may further exacerbate enrollment disparities. As a result, FDA has generated several guidance documents emphasizing the need for greater attention in this space during the past decade. It should be noted that 2025 U.S. government administration changes have removed some of these documents from online search results. The references provided have been kept as is for historic context.

In 2016, FDA published guidance, *Collection of Race and Ethnicity Data in Clinical Trials*, about the importance of consistent and accurate collection of demographic data from participants. This was followed up in 2020 with a document, *Enhancing the Diversity of Clinical Trial Populations—Eligibility Criteria, Enrollment Practices, and Trial Designs*, on the need to broaden eligibility criteria, improve trial recruitment practices, and leverage community engagement to make clinical research more inclusive. More recently, FDA (2024b) released a draft guidance document, *Diversity Action Plans to Improve Enrollment of Participants from Underrepresented Populations in Clinical Studies*, outlining how the incorporation of diversity plans into clinical trials can bolster the representation of minoritized populations in clinical research.

As part of trials supporting Investigational New Drug applications, FDA encourages sponsors to declare enrollment goals for underrepresented populations and define how these goals will be assessed as part of study objectives. FDA guidance further specifies that if sponsors have evidence that a drug may work differently in a specific subgroup, focused analyses should be incorporated into statistical plans to determine if there are any impacts on safety or efficacy.

Continued dialogue from FDA about the need for enhanced attention on issues of representation in clinical trials demonstrates the importance of this topic. Enhancing the diversity of participants in oncology clinical trials is crucial for obtaining a more comprehensive clinical picture of the underlying disease process, the breadth of treatment responses, and safety data across different populations. For example, research has demonstrated that Black patients with breast cancer often have more aggressive tumors and different genomic profiles compared to White patients. These differences in tumor biology can affect response to standard therapy. When trials enroll adequate numbers of underrepresented individuals, researchers are better positioned to identify more effective therapeutic strategies for these populations (Lansey et al., 2020).

Understanding Barriers to Access

Barriers to clinical trial access can be separated into four main categories: structural, clinical, attitudinal, and demographic and socioeconomic. These categories form the basis of a framework that follows the flow of patients through the trial enrollment process. A site must have a portfolio of available trials (structural) that align with the clinical needs (clinical) of the patients it serves. The providers at that site must be willing to offer these trials to their patients, and, in turn, those patients must be willing and able to consider enrollment (attitudinal). Furthermore, demographic and socioeconomic factors may also affect decision-making during the process (Unger et al., 2016). Although there is often significant interplay between these broad categories, this framework can help simplify the identification of barriers to trial participation within a clinical practice.

Structural Barriers

The first category, structural barriers, encompasses both system- and clinic-level characteristics that can affect patient access to clinical trials. Structural barriers are quite variable and may include factors such as clinic location, insurance considerations, and research staffing. The most pervasive structural barrier, however, is a lack of available trials. A meta-analysis by Unger et al. (2019) demonstrated that the clinical trial portfolios at treatment centers served less than half of the patients with cancer. Limitations to patient enrollment included the lack of trials available for a particular disease or stage of a disease. It is worth noting that some cancers have high cure rates with available therapies, whereas others are rare. Because of resource limitations at multiple levels, from pharmaceutical companies to sites, trial development is often not pursued in these cancers.

Beyond an available portfolio of studies, additional examples of structural barriers impacting access include the following (AACR, 2024):

- **Site staffing to support clinical trials:** Sites must have adequate staffing to offer and maintain a portfolio of clinical trials that serve a patient population. Although sites may approach staffing differently, with some having

dedicated research staff and others having hybrid clinical and research staff, the effort dedicated to regulatory issues, recruitment, project management, and quality assurance activities must align with the scope of the staff and the desired depth and breadth of the clinical trial portfolio.
- **Insurance contracting and charity care availability:** Insurance can be a significant barrier to accessing trials. Oncology clinical trials often have mixed billing, meaning services provided as part of the study are considered routine care and billed to insurance. Patients who do not have insurance or are underinsured may have difficulty accessing sites that accept their care or obtaining the necessary approvals to bill insurance for certain routine services required for the study.
- **Patient distance to sites offering clinical trials:** Geographic barriers can limit access to clinical facilities and trial locations. These issues are magnified for patients who live in frontier and rural areas, as specialty care is typically centralized in more highly populated areas. For example, prior studies have shown that males with localized prostate cancer who live farther from radiation treatment facilities are less likely to receive standard radiation as part of their care plan (Arega et al., 2021).
- **Trial logistics:** Trial complexity, including the length and complexity of informed consent documents, the frequency of trial visits, the inflexibility of trial visit scheduling, and the inclusion of procedures (e.g., biopsies, other extensive specimen collections), can be a barrier to participation. Patients with transportation, childcare, work, or other personal commitments may decline participation because of the intense and rigid schedules associated with a particular clinical trial (Kumar et al., 2022).

Clinical Barriers

Cancer clinical trials often include a number of eligibility criteria that are intended to disqualify patients who might be at higher risk for experiencing severe toxicities while on the study. Although safety is paramount, some eligibility criteria can be overly restrictive and may negatively affect enrollment. Beyond contributing to slow or failed enrollment, certain underrepresented populations might be disproportionately affected by the inclusion of unnecessarily restrictive criteria (Unger et al., 2019). FDA released draft guidance in 2024 focused on laboratory value–based criteria in cancer clinical trials (e.g., strict renal and hepatic function-based criteria), which are often incorporated into trial eligibility parameters. This updated guidance, *Cancer Clinical Trial Eligibility Criteria: Laboratory Values Guidance for Industry, IRBs* [institutional review boards], *and Clinical Investigators*, reiterates prior commentary from its 2020 guidance on enhancing the diversity of clinical trial populations (FDA, 2024a). Namely, laboratory value–based criteria should be pragmatic enough so that trials do not exclude participation without solid clinical justification.

Attitudinal Barriers

The next critical step in accessing clinical trials is having providers who are willing to offer trial participation to patients as part of their clinical care. With treatment trials in particular, there is often a small window of opportunity for patients to enroll, and providers must be aware of the options at certain junctures within a patient's cancer journey. These most often occur during the initial workup or treatment phase, or when patients need to switch to a new treatment approach. At each of these points, decisions are made about whether a trial might be appropriate based on the provider's judgment of the overarching clinical picture, a patient's capacity to understand and adhere to trial requirements, and the provider's comfort level with research. Implicit biases can interfere with this decision-making process, potentially undermining efforts to diversify clinical trial enrollment.

Akimoto et al. (2023) reported that providers who are less familiar with clinical trials are less likely to offer them as a treatment option. Furthermore, providers may not opt to provide trials because of insufficient time and research staff support. Consent discussions and ongoing oversight of patients in clinical trials require more time and effort than patients receiving standard-of-care therapies. These time constraints are considered a significant challenge faced by providers across sites that participate in clinical trials (Ebrahimi et al., 2024).

Demographic and Socioeconomic Barriers

Finally, several demographic and socioeconomic factors should be considered at the patient level. Although most barriers to access are at the structural and protocol levels, the issues encountered at the patient level are disproportionately faced by underserved and underrepresented groups. Even if a patient feels a clinical trial might be the best approach for their treatment, some constraints may ultimately lead them to decline participation. The increased complexity of clinical research sometimes results in trials requiring additional or extended visits beyond what would occur with the standard of care. These factors influence the patient's decision-making process. Although not all factors can be mitigated, understanding patterns within a practice is crucial for determining potential solutions more effectively. Common reasons that patients may decline participation in clinical trials include the following (AACR, 2024; Ebrahimi et al., 2024; Unger et al., 2019):
- Lack of trust, fear of the unknown or loss of control, concerns about randomization or placebos
- Communication barriers, including a lack of access to translated materials
- Transportation issues, particularly if trial sites are geographically distant from the patient's home; some patients lack access to public transportation or do not have a means of personal transportation.
- Financial concerns, including distress about time away from work, job security, and the potential for lost wages;

these concerns are compounded for those who must travel a distance for care. Insurance coverage, including co-pays and co-insurance associated with study procedures, is also a consideration.
- Lack of access to child care or other caregiver coverage during time away from clinic visits

Assessing and Addressing Barriers to Access

In 2022, the American Society of Clinical Oncology (ASCO) and the Association of Cancer Care Centers (ACCC) published the Equity, Diversity, and Inclusion Research Site Self-Assessment to assess their practices and identify local barriers to trial participation. Prior to releasing this tool to the public, a pilot study was conducted with data generated from 75 research sites. The authors analyzed the value of the self-assessment tool as a mechanism for sites to evaluate policies, procedures, and practices in conjunction with key research metrics. Sites reported that the tool afforded new insights into their research operations. Participating sites responded favorably to the feasibility, utility, and face validity of the assessment. They agreed that it provided new insights and increased awareness about their performance, highlighting practice gaps and opportunities for improvement (Guerra et al., 2023). This tool is available at www.accc-cancer.org/home/learn/community-oncology-research/asco-accc-initiative.

The first step in assessing local barriers to trial access is to gather and evaluate site-level data. The site infrastructure, including staffing and data reporting capabilities, should be thoroughly assessed. It is essential to understand the demographics of the population within a particular service area or clinic. The breakdown of patients by cancer type and stage, along with characteristics such as age, gender, race, ethnicity, and other social determinants, should be tracked and monitored routinely. Sites should also prospectively set enrollment diversity goals that can be used to track progress over time. Once these baseline benchmarks and goals have been established, sites and study teams will have a framework for assessing whether their trials are serving their patient populations (Oyer et al., 2022).

Having thorough, accurate, and readily available data is a crucial operational necessity for sites that aim to address research barriers within their practice. These data will inform the type and number of trials that sites need to open to serve patient needs, along with the staffing necessary to oversee the research portfolio. Sites should be mindful of cancers that disproportionately affect underrepresented individuals and assess if trials for those diseases are available and appropriate for their practice. Sites also need to evaluate whether they have the necessary support and staffing to facilitate the effective conduct of clinical trials. ASCO (2019) published strategies for assessing workloads to help optimize the deployment of limited site resources. Monitoring workloads requires consistent access to data on staffing, protocols, and trial enrollments. This type of data-focused infrastructure is also necessary to evaluate research participant diversity at the site level. The ASCO/ACCC pilot study (Guerra et al., 2023) noted that access to clinical and clinical trial data was uneven across sites.

Additional strategies that sites can employ to address barriers within their practices include the following (AACR, 2024; Barrett et al., 2023; Chen et al., 2023; Ebrahimi et al., 2024; Unger et al., 2019):

- **Align clinical trial portfolios with patient populations:** Review clinical trial portfolios to ensure that opportunities are available for diverse populations to participate. Assess portfolios for the breadth of cancer types served, the restrictiveness of eligibility criteria, and the complexity of study logistics. Routinely review research metrics, including the number of patients screened, consented, and enrolled in trials, and compare these against the clinic's overall patient population metrics, including demographics. Consider activating protocols that focus on cancers more prevalent in underserved populations, have less restrictive eligibility criteria, or require fewer or less burdensome study visits.
- **Prioritize research:** Integrate clinical trials into treatment algorithms at the site level.
- **Find an appropriate workforce and navigation team**: Hire staff with diverse backgrounds who will help cultivate patient engagement efforts and enhance trust in healthcare providers and the research process. Ensure that staff are trained to assist patients through the screening process by addressing logistical challenges, connecting patients with support services, and promoting open and frequent communications.
- **Address provider biases and communication:** Implement implicit bias training for all healthcare providers and clinic staff who interact with research. Train providers on how to frame conversations around clinical research in a holistic manner.
- **Mitigate time constraints in the clinic:** Identify study opportunities in advance of clinic visits to streamline provider conversations. Foster close communication between providers and research staff, and use appropriately trained and delegated research staff to augment the consent and screening process.
- **Address geographic considerations:** Incorporate decentralized approaches to trial operationalization, including the use of local laboratories, home health care, or telehealth where appropriate.
- **Reduce financial toxicity:** Maximize sponsor support for clinical care costs during study budget negotiations. Incorporate patient travel and expense reimbursements and stipends into study budgets as allowable per institutional practice. Ensure that patients have access to clear information about study costs and financial counseling. Confirm that clinical and research staff have strong con-

nections with social workers, patient navigators, and other local patient assistance programs.

- **Foster community engagement and outreach strategies:** Engage in community education and outreach activities to improve awareness about clinical research and its role in cancer care. Provide materials tailored to the communities served and consider engaging with community advocates to ensure that messaging is developed and delivered in a culturally competent manner. Consider using social media where appropriate. Communicate trial availability through websites with clear contact information for researchers, allowing patients to seek out additional information.
- **Develop collaborative partnerships:** Establish alliances with local healthcare providers, including other oncology specialists, to enhance research awareness and facilitate seamless referrals. Consider engaging with other local healthcare organizations, such as nonprofits, health departments, and researchers, to facilitate access to oncology clinical trials.
- **Implement policy interventions:** Engage in legislative efforts to promote inclusivity in oncology clinical trial enrollment and ensure equitable access to cancer healthcare resources.

Summary

Addressing disparities in cancer clinical trial participation is essential for advancing equitable healthcare outcomes. Despite progress, significant gaps remain, particularly among racially and ethnically underserved and underrepresented groups, rural residents, and low-income patients. FDA has implemented measures to improve demographic inclusivity in trials; however, structural, clinical, attitudinal, and demographic and socioeconomic barriers persist. Practical strategies to overcome these challenges include aligning clinical trial portfolios with patient demographics, integrating trials into treatment plans, enhancing provider training, and leveraging community engagement. Additionally, addressing geographic and financial barriers, as well as fostering collaborative partnerships, are critical. By prioritizing these efforts, the healthcare community can ensure that all populations benefit from advancements in cancer research and treatment, ultimately leading to more comprehensive and effective cancer care.

Key Points

- Participation in clinical trials remains limited, with certain patient groups, including those from rural areas, lower-income backgrounds, and historically underserved populations, being less likely to enroll despite often facing a higher burden of disease.
- Barriers to enrollment are wide-ranging, including logistical challenges (e.g., distance to trial sites, insurance limitations), strict eligibility criteria, time constraints for providers, and limited awareness or trust in research among patients.
- Federal agencies have issued guidance encouraging more inclusive study designs, streamlined eligibility requirements, and clearer goals to ensure that trial findings can be applied across the broader patient population.
- Institutions are using structured tools to assess where gaps exist in trial availability and enrollment, helping them align study offerings with the needs and characteristics of the patients they serve.
- Practical solutions are available, including offering transportation and financial support, simplifying study participation requirements, enhancing communication from providers, and working with community clinics and local partners to increase awareness and referral pathways.

References

Akimoto, K., Taparra, K., Brown, T., & Patel, M.I. (2023). Diversity in cancer care: Current challenges and potential solutions to achieving equity in clinical trial participation. *Cancer Journal, 29*(6), 310–315. https://doi.org/10.1097/PPO.0000000000000675

American Association for Cancer Research. (2024). *Cancer disparities progress report 2024.* https://www.cancerdisparitiesprogressreport.org

American Society of Clinical Oncology. (2019). *Clinical trial workload assessment strategies: At a glance.* https://cdn.bfldr.com/KOIHB2Q3/as/fp8vk3qfqrct67tf533hrr4/2019-ASCORCF-Workload-Assessment

Arega, M.A., Yang, D.D., Royce, T.J., Mahal, B.A., Dee, E.C., Butler, S.S., ... Muralidhar, V. (2021). Association between travel distance and use of postoperative radiation therapy among men with organ-confined prostate cancer: Does geography influence treatment decisions? *Journal of Clinical Oncology, 39*(Suppl. 6), 24. https://doi.org/10.1200/JCO.2021.39.6_suppl.24

Barrett, N.J., Boehmer, L., Schrag, J., Benson, A.B., Green, S., Hamroun-Yazid, L., ... Guerra, C.E. (2023). An assessment of the feasibility and utility of an ACCC-ASCO implicit bias training program to enhance racial and ethnic diversity in cancer clinical trials. *JCO Oncology Practice, 19*(4), e570–e580. https://doi.org/10.1200/OP.22.00378

Chen, J., Ying, L., & Kummar, S. (2023). Increasing patient participation in oncology clinical trials. *Cancer Medicine, 12*(3), 2219–2226. https://doi.org/10.1002/cam4.5150

Ebrahimi, H., Megally, S., Plotkin, E., Shivakumar, L., Salgia, N.J., Zengin, Z.B., ... Chehrazi-Raffle, A. (2024). Barriers to clinical trial implementation among community care centers. *JAMA Network Open, 7*(4), e248739. https://doi.org/10.1001/jamanetworkopen.2024.8739

Guerra, C., Pressman, A., Hurley, P., Garrett-Mayer, E., Bruinooge, S.S., Howson, A., ... Pierce, L.J. (2023). Increasing racial and ethnic equity, diversity, and inclusion in cancer treatment trials: Evaluation of an ASCO–Association of Community Cancer Centers site self-assessment. *JCO Oncology Practice, 19*(4), e581–e588. https://doi.org/10.1200/op.22.00560

Kumar, G., Chaudhary, P., Quinn, A., & Su, D. (2022). Barriers for cancer clinical trial enrollment: A qualitative study of the perspectives of healthcare providers. *Contemporary Clinical Trials Communications, 28,* 100939. https://doi.org/10.1016/j.conctc.2022.100939

Lansey, D.G., Hefka, T.A., Carducci, M.A., & Kanarek, N.F. (2020). Problem solving to enhance clinical trial participation utilizing a framework-driven approach. *Clinical Advances in Hematology and Oncology, 18*(8), 468–476.

Oyer, R.A., Hurley, P., Boehmer, L., Bruinooge, S.S., Levit, K., Barrett, N., ... Pierce, L.J. (2022). Increasing racial and ethnic diversity in cancer clinical trials: An American Society of Clinical Oncology and Association of Community Cancer Centers joint research statement. *Journal of Clinical Oncology, 40*(19), 2163–2171. https://doi.org/10.1200/JCO.22.00754

Pittell, H., Calip, G.S., Pierre, A., Ryals, C.S., Altomare, I., Royce, T.J., & Guadamuz, J.S. (2023). Racial and ethnic inequities in US oncology clinical trial participation from 2017 to 2022. *JAMA Network Open,* 6(7), 2322515. https://doi.org/10.1001/jamanetworkopen.2023.22515

Schwartz, A.L., Alsan, M., Morris, A.A., & Halpern, S.D. (2023). Why diverse clinical trial participation matters. *New England Journal of Medicine, 388*(14), 1252–1254. https://doi.org/10.1056/nejmp2215609

U.S. Food and Drug Administration. (2012). *Food and Drug Administration Safety and Innovation Act (FDASIA).* https://www.fda.gov/regulatory-information/selected-amendments-fdc-act/food-and-drug-administration-safety-and-innovation-act-fdasia

U.S. Food and Drug Administration. (2013). *Collection, analysis, and availability of demographic subgroup data for FDA-approved medical products.* https://docslib.org/doc/4142279/fda-report-collection-analysis-and-availability-of-demographic

U.S. Food and Drug Administration. (2024a). *Cancer clinical trial eligibility criteria: Laboratory values guidance for industry, IRBs, and clinical investigators.* https://www.fda.gov/media/178013/download

U.S. Food and Drug Administration. (2024b). *Diversity action plans to improve enrollment of participants from underrepresented populations in clinical studies.* https://www.fda.gov/regulatory-information/search-fda-guidance-documents/diversity-action-plans-improve-enrollment-participants-underrepresented-populations-clinical-studies

Unger, J.M., Cook, E., Tai, E., & Bleyer, A. (2016). The role of clinical trial participation in cancer research: Barriers, evidence, and strategies. *American Society of Clinical Oncology Educational Book, 36,* 185–198. https://doi.org/10.1200/EDBK_156686

Unger, J.M., Vaidya, R., Hershman, D.L., Minasian, L.M., & Fleury, M.E. (2019). Systematic review and meta-analysis of the magnitude of structural, clinical, and physician and patient barriers to cancer clinical trial participation. *Journal of the National Cancer Institute, 111*(3), 245–255. https://doi.org/10.1093/jnci/djy221

Ussher, J.M., Power, R., Perz, J., Hawkey, A.J., & Allison, K. (2022). LGBTQI inclusive cancer care: A discourse analytic study of health care professional, patient and carer perspectives. *Frontiers in Oncology, 12,* 832657. https://doi.org/10.3389/fonc.2022.832657

Wheldon, C.W., Sklarz, T., & Frosch, Z.A.K. (2024). Advancing equity in cancer care: The critical role of sexual orientation and gender identity data collection. *JCO Oncology Practice, 20*(9), 1146–1148. https://doi.org/10.1200/op.24.00360

CHAPTER 20

Gender Identification

Gary Shelton, DNP, MSN, NP, ANP-BC, AOCNP®

Introduction

Oncology clinical research nurses (OCRNs) should have an understanding of the importance of equity and inclusion within their research studies to better affect clinical outcomes for a more generalizable public (see Chapter 19). Their recognition of implicit bias, as well as an up-to-date view of gender identity, will improve communication with and appropriate interventions for their study populations (Byrne, 2023; Dymanus et al., 2021; Korpaisarn & Safer, 2019; Lopez, 2024). Collection of sexual orientation and gender identity data within clinical trial settings will improve recognized disparities in recruitment to trials and provide targeted interventions (Wheldon et al., 2024; Zakout, 2023; Zilioto & Marcolan, 2020).

During fetal development, gender identification (or identity) and sexual orientation are programmed into the fetal brain. A testosterone surge, or lack thereof, is responsible for embedding the concept of maleness or femaleness. This occurs independently from the differentiation of the genitals; thus, there can be a disconnect, which causes confusion or dysphoria (Cooper et al., 2020; Juli et al., 2023; Korpaisarn & Safer, 2019; Rubin et al., 2020; Swaab et al., 2021). As integral members of the interprofessional clinical trial team, OCRNs must understand the need to have appropriate gender representation within studies to generalize the resultant data better, with the recognition that drug absorption and side effect profiles can be gender specific. They facilitate comprehension and adherence to therapies, document observations, and are patient advocates through expert communication skills.

This chapter will provide insight into a person's gender identity. It will help OCRNs to improve communication, better establish rapport, and decrease implicit bias. It will also highlight diversity, equity, and inclusion (DEI) programs and guidelines, which attempt to ensure access and opportunities to take part in clinical trials without concern for background, behavior, or identity (Driessnack et al., 2022; Dymanus et al., 2021; Gaedigk, 2020; Hood, 2022; Narayan, 2019; Park & Yu, 2022; Shelton, 2016; Swaab et al., 2021; Versavel et al., 2023).

Gender Identity

Gender identity relates to the perception one has of being male or female or of identifying as other less separate beings. Sexual orientation relates to one's identity as a human being. It can include heterosexuality, homosexuality, bisexuality, asexuality, and other definitions, such as non-binary, which means having an identity that lies between all male and all female or neither (Byrne, 2023; Korpaisarn & Safer, 2019; Swaab et al., 2021). Such identification is not dependent on one's genitalia, as noted at birth when one is thusly called a boy (male) or a girl (female). Sexual differentiation, as evidenced by genitalia development, occurs early in uterine development (between weeks 6 and 12). Two X chromosomes will develop as female, whereas an X and a Y chromosome become a male. A testosterone surge weeks later differentiates the brain into considerations of being male or female; thus, gender identity and sexual orientation become programmed into the brain and live there for the life of the individual. The expectation is that developing females will not have the testosterone surge, as it is the Y chromosome that produces the male hormone (Byrne, 2023; Janssen, 2023; Korpaisarn & Safer, 2019; Rubin et al., 2020; Swaab et al., 2021).

There is more at work, however, within the developing fetus than merely the development of two X chromosomes or an X and a Y chromosome. The following characteristics affect gender identification and sexual orientation beyond chromosomal imprint: hormones, genetics (genes play a role beyond regulating sex hormones), epigenetic changes affecting the nervous system that involves memory and behavior, endocrine disruptors from the environment that cross the placental barrier and interact with endogenous sex hormones and therefore the developing fetal brain, immune reactivity toward specific maternal proteins, and self-organization of the developing human brain (even identical twins differ in gender identity and sexual orientation) (Byrne, 2023; Korpaisarn & Safer, 2019; Swaab et al., 2021).

Data indicate that gender identity and sexual orientation develop during fetal development. No evidence suggests that the social environment after birth has a major effect on gender identification or sexual orientation (Byrne, 2023; Janssen, 2023; Korpaisarn & Safer, 2019; Rubin et al., 2020; Swaab et al., 2021).

Gender Dysphoria

Throughout the 1980s, scientific and behavioral thought reinforced the role of socialization after birth for sexual identity and orientation. Children born with indeterminant genitalia were immediately made female surgically, assuming such socialization would encourage female behavior and sexual orientation. Many lives were ruined, or those made female, genital-wise, reverted to living as male as they further developed their human identities.

More recent scientific inquiry has changed this understanding. Although gender identity and genital development occur at different times during fetal development and through separate mechanisms, they are present at birth. Because of endogenous and exogenous influences throughout fetal development, one can be born with an incongruent gender identity, resulting in distress secondary to gender dysphoria. This term *gender dysphoria* was classified in 2018 by the World Health Organization's *International Classification of Diseases* (ICD-10) and is now known as *gender incongruence* (Cooper et al., 2020; Juli et al., 2023; Korpaisarn & Safer, 2019; Swaab et al., 2021).

Addressing the suffering with the intent of alleviating it, or at least acknowledging and supporting these distressful emotional conflicts, requires understanding and education. Individuals with gender incongruence likely want what all humans wish for: to belong to a gender they identify with rather than their assigned gender by physical examination. The significance of this dysphoria generally leads these individuals to seek physical gender transition (Byrne, 2023; Cooper et al., 2020; Juli et al., 2023; Korpaisarn & Safer, 2019; Swaab et al., 2021).

Gender Representation in Clinical Trials

Disparities in cancer clinical trials of diverse individuals decrease the universality or usefulness of the newly learned trial evidence. Illnesses and diseases specific to certain genders or ethnicities exist; however, a review of more recent clinical trials would attest to the need for more DEI to generalize better and attribute the evidence learned. OCRNs have key roles in assessing and requesting more diverse and equitable inclusion criteria (Dymanus et al., 2021; Wheldon et al., 2024; Zakout, 2023).

Structural barriers to representation exist, such as location of facilities, available transportation, travel costs, caregiver burden, and child care. Inclusion criteria may be too restrictive, clinicians may be limited in their understanding of the needs of diverse populations, and facilities may lack interprofessional support networks. Patient-specific factors may include trust issues, fear over a lack of benefits, concern over side effects, the futility of more treatment, and lack of social support.

Disparities in cancer clinical trial participation are multifaceted and challenging. The National Institutes of Health Revitalization Act of 1993 mandated more women and underrepresented groups must be included in any National Cancer Institute–funded clinical trial. Still, challenges remain complex, and a more inclusive clinical trial mix is slow to change (Moore et al., 2023; Rubin et al., 2020; Shapiro, 2022; Wheldon et al., 2024; Zakout, 2023).

The Role of Oncology Clinical Research Nurses in Health Equity

Health equity is achieved when everyone has a fair chance at being healthy. In cancer care, this includes prevention, early detection, and the myriad of treatment modalities and therapies, including opportunities to be included in clinical trials. Health justice seeks health equity. OCRNs are key to making changes that foster inclusion for all people with a cancer diagnosis—women, diverse ethnic and racial groups, people living with disabilities, older adults, the LGBTQIA+ community (lesbian, gay, bisexual, transgender, queer or questioning, intersex, and asexual), and those with HIV and other viral etiologies. Without such representation in clinical trials, the evidence garnered is limited in generalizability, and subgroup-specific information about drug response and measures of safety and efficacy is not truly meaningful (Byrne, 2023; Dymanus et al., 2021; Lopez, 2024; Moore et al., 2023; Rubin et al., 2020; Shapiro, 2022; Wheldon et al., 2024; Zakout, 2023).

Oncology nurses excel in their abilities to connect to others in need, establish rapport, and exercise empathy and sympathy in therapeutic ways. Using Travelbee's Human-to-Human Relationship Model (Shelton, 2016) as a framework for communicating to connect, OCRNs can share their lives with other humans who happen to have a cancer diagnosis, as well as with their families and caregivers. OCRNs should practice DEI as they investigate ways to improve participation from underrepresented populations and decrease disparities in clinical trial enrollment (Byrne, 2023; Rubin et al., 2020; Shapiro, 2022; Shelton, 2016; Zakout, 2023).

OCRNs should also be aware of implicit bias, the unconscious attitudes people may have toward others that, without realizing it, can cause unintentional discriminatory behavior. Overcoming such unconscious biases facilitates our abilities to consistently adhere to the code of nursing ethics, that "nurses practice with compassion and respect for the inherent dignity, worth, and unique attributes of every person" (Narayan, 2019, p. 36).

Summary

Gender identity, sexual orientation, and physical genital development all occur in utero. No evidence exists that gender identity or sexual orientation further develops after birth. OCRNs working in cancer clinical trials are integral members of the interprofessional team. They are in a position to improve DEI for clinical trial enrollment and enhance access to underserved populations, which will, in turn, improve the safety and efficacy of data derived from trials. A person's internal and intrinsic sense of gender identity transcends any marginalized individuals but relates to how any of us interact with others.

Key Points

- OCRNs should understand the complexity of gender identity, sexual orientation, and gender incongruence, all of which occur during fetal development.
- The key to communicating is to connect by establishing immediate rapport.
- DEI improves the application of clinical trial results.
- All individuals have implicit biases. By investigating these implicit biases, one can accept other's differences.
- Being aware of the challenges and barriers to clinical trial accrual will improve participation efforts.

References

Byrne, A. (2023). The origin of "gender identity." *Archives of Sexual Behavior, 52,* 2709–2711. https://doi.org/10.1007/s10508-023-02628-0

Cooper, K., Russell, A., Mandy, W., & Butler, C. (2020). The phenomenology of gender dysphoria in adults: A systematic review and meta-synthesis. *Clinical Psychology Review, 80,* 101875. https://doi.org/10.1016/j.cpr.2020.101875

Driessnack, M., Campbell, M., & Fornero, K. (2022). Moving knowledge to action: Aware, adopt, adapt (A3). *Journal of Nurse Practitioners, 18*(5), 503–505. https://doi.org/10.1016/j.nurpra.2022.01.021

Dymanus, K.A., Butaney, M., Magee, D.E., Hird, A.E., Luckenbaugh, A.N., Ma, M.W., ... Wallis, C.J.D. (2021). Assessment of gender representation in clinical trials leading to FDA approval for oncology therapeutics between 2014 and 2019: A systematic review-based cohort study. *Cancer, 127*(17), 3156–3162. https://doi.org/10.1002/cncr.33533

Gaedigk, A. (2020). Pharmacogenetics: Chasing perfection. *Clinical Pharmacology and Therapeutics, 106*(2), 265–270. https://doi.org/10.1002/cpt.1511

Hood, B. (2022). Exploring nurses' experiences of caring for patients participating in cancer clinical trials. *British Journal of Nursing, 31*(17), S18–S24. https://doi.org/10.12968/bjon.2022.31.17.S18

Janssen, D.F. (2023). Who invented gender identity? *Archives of Sexual Behavior, 52*(7), 2713–2716. https://doi.org/10.1007/s10508-023-02650-2

Juli, G., Juli, M.R., Juli, R., & Juli, L. (2023). Gender dysphoria and DNA. *Psychiatra Danubina, 35*(Suppl. 2), 179–181.

Korpaisarn, S., & Safer, J.D. (2019). Etiology of gender identity. *Endocrinology and Metabolism Clinics of North America, 48*(2), 323–329. https://doi.org/10.1016/j.ecl.2019.01.002

Lopez, L.M. (2024). Implicit bias: More than a buzzword. *American Nurse, 19*(11), 24–28. https://doi.org/10.51256/ANJ112424

Moore, A.R., Lewis, T.H., Abah, T., Celebi, M., & Amey, F.K. (2023). Examining participation disparities in cancer clinical trials. *Oncology Nursing Forum, 50*(1), 79–89. https://doi.org/ 10.1188/23.ONF.79-89

Narayan, M.C. (2019). CE: Addressing implicit bias in nursing: A review. *American Journal of Nursing, 119*(7), 36–43. https://doi.org/10.1097/01.NAJ.0000569340.27659.5a

Park, H.-J., & Yu, S. (2022). The role of clinical trial nurses: Transitioning from clinicians to clinical research coordinators. *International Journal of Nursing Practice, 28*(1), e12943. https://doi.org/10.1111/ijn.12943

Rubin, J.D., Atwood, S., & Olson, K.R. (2020). Studying gender diversity. *Trends in Cognitive Sciences, 24*(3), 163–165. https://doi.org/10.1016/j.tics.2019.12.011

Shapiro, M. (2022). Disparity of equitable representation in cancer clinical trials: Nursing perspectives. *Clinical Journal of Oncology Nursing, 26*(4), 449–454. https://doi.org/10.1188/22.CJON.449-454

Shelton, G. (2016). Appraising Travelbee's Human-to-Human Relationship Model. *Journal of the Advanced Practitioner in Oncology, 7*(6), 657–661.

Swaab, D.F., Wolff, S.E.C., & Bao, A.M. (2021). Sexual differentiation of the human hypothalamus: Relationship to gender identity and sexual orientation. *Handbook of Clinical Neurology, 181,* 427–443. https://doi.org/10.1016/B978-0-12-820683-6.00031-2

Versavel, S., Subasinghe, A., Johnson, K., Golonski, N., Muhlhausen, J., Perry, P., & Sanchez, R. (2023). Diversity, equity, and inclusion in clinical trials: A practical guide from the perspective of a trial sponsor. *Contemporary Clinical Trials, 126,* 107092. https://doi.org/10.1016/j.cct.2023.107092

Wheldon, C.W., Sklarz, T., & Frosch, Z.A.K. (2024). Advancing equity in cancer care: The critical role of sexual orientation and gender identity data collection. *JCO Oncology Practice, 20*(9), 1146–11448. https://doi.org/10.1200/OP.24.00360

Zakout, G.A. (2023). Practicing equitable principles in cancer clinical research: Has the EU got it right? *Journal of Cancer Policy, 37,* 100435. https://doi.org/10.1016/j.jcpo.2023.100435

Zilioto, G.C., & Marcolan, J.F. (2020). Understanding prejudice of psychic suffering individuals about sexuality. *Revista Brasileira de Enfermagen, 73*(2), e20190270. https://doi.org/10.1590/0034-7167-2019-0270

SECTION IV.
Clinical Trial Participants

CHAPTER 21

Procurement, Accountability, and Administration of Investigational Agents

John Bourgeois, DNP, MMHC, RN, CCRP, OCN®, NEA-BC

Introduction

In the United States, clinical research with investigational agents is strictly regulated by the U.S. Food and Drug Administration (FDA) (2024b) under the Federal Food, Drug, and Cosmetic Act and the Public Health Services Act. Adherence with these regulations is mandatory for all parties involved in clinical trials, including the National Cancer Institute (NCI), pharmaceutical collaborators, and investigators. Additional regulations administered by the Office for Human Research Protections and the U.S. Department of Health and Human Services must also be followed to ensure the protection of the rights and welfare of research participants. These regulations include Good Clinical Practice guidelines, which provide a framework for conducting clinical trials ethically and scientifically, ensuring that the rights, safety, and well-being of research participants are protected (FDA, 2021).

Furthermore, clinical investigators and institutions are required to adhere to the Health Insurance Portability and Accountability Act (HIPAA) to maintain the privacy and confidentiality of research participants' health information. This act set standards for the protection of health information, ensuring that personal data are handled with the utmost care and confidentiality during the research process (FDA, 2024b). These stringent regulatory frameworks collectively ensure that clinical trials in the United States are conducted with the highest standards of ethical and scientific integrity, prioritizing the safety and privacy of research participants.

This chapter will address the process of investigational or research study drug procurement, accountability, and safe handling guidelines. The standards related to the administration of oncologic drugs are included to support the effective, safe, and consistent delivery of research drugs. Proper documentation is also covered to ensure adherence with policies and procedures and maintenance of records for study audits. Sites should collect source data that are Attributable, Legible, Contemporaneous, Original, Accurate, and Complete (ALCOA-C) (International Council for Harmonisation of Technical Requirements for Pharmaceuticals for Human Use [ICH], 2016).

Procurement of Research Study Drugs

Whenever possible, the pharmacy department should be responsible for drug receipt, storage, accountability, and preparation (Kay et al., 2018). The principal investigator (PI) should delegate this responsibility to the pharmacy personnel or other appropriate research study personnel. Oncology clinical research nurses (OCRNs) may be designated as the pharmacy contact if the study site does not have a pharmacist responsible for the handling of research drugs. The delegation of authority form should contain a list of the personnel who are accountable for documenting investigational product receipt, storage, accountability, preparation, destruction, and return or transfer (ICH, 2016).

Personnel Ordering of Research Drugs

For research drugs provided by the NCI Pharmaceutical Management Branch (PMB), the order must be submitted by an NCI Cancer Therapy Evaluation Program (CTEP)-approved investigator or approved designee. The order must include the investigator's NCI PI number. Any investigator who receives and administers an investigational agent supplied by NCI must be registered with the institute by submitting their curriculum vitae, the supplemental investigator data form, and a financial disclosure form (NCI CTEP, 2025).

The PI registration must be renewed annually. If the PI number is unknown, it can be obtained by submitting a question to NCI CTEP (https://ctep.cancer.gov/investigatorResources/investigator_registration_packet.htm). Investigational agents provided by NCI to a registered investigator are the direct responsibility of the PI. Secondary distribution to other registered investigators does not relieve the responsibility of the PI to whom the original shipment was made. Investigators may only order research study drugs for protocols in which their institution or group participates.

AURORA is NCI CTEP's (2024) innovative and centralized system for managing agent inventories. It will eventually and entirely replace the Online Agent Order Processing (OAOP) system for electronic submission of agent order requests in NCI-sponsored trials. AURORA facilitates the review of order request statuses and provides access to PMB documents, such as agent stock recovery notices, Investigator Brochures, and Material Safety Data Sheets. Moreover, AURORA enables clinical trial sites to create and maintain shipping addresses for Primary Shipping Designees, designate Primary Ordering Designees, and manage electronic NCI Investigational Agent Accountability Records (eDARF), along with related inventory practices. Integrated with other applications in the NCI Clinical Oncology Research Enterprise, AURORA ensures consistent recordkeeping and oversight across all trial sites, enhances adherence with regulatory requirements, and streamlines communication between sponsors and sites for NCI-sponsored trials. AURORA is also where PMB-assigned agent lot expiration dates are updated in the eDARF module when PMB issues a stock notification letter.

For non-NCI protocols (e.g., pharmaceutical sponsored), the research site must submit all required regulatory documents, sign a study contract, submit a signed Form FDA 1572, and other documents as required before research drugs can be sent to the study site. For research drugs directly provided by the pharmaceutical company sponsor, the order must be submitted by the designated investigators approved by the sponsor. The study team should always refer to the protocol or the study's pharmacy manual for specific instructions.

In protocols where commercially available agents are being used for the study, acquisition of the drugs can be handled as it is for other nonprotocol drugs. However, researchers should always refer to the protocol or check with the study coordinator to determine whether a drug accountability form should be kept for tracking the commercially available drugs used for the protocol patients.

Ordering of Research Drugs Procedures

Depending on the sponsor of the study protocol, research study drugs may be ordered from NCI PMB or directly from the pharmaceutical sponsor. For research drugs supplied by a pharmaceutical company sponsor, clinicians should refer to the instructions and guidelines provided. For sponsor trials, drugs can be ordered in some instances from a third party, such as McKesson. The information provided in this section applies to research drugs supplied by NCI.

For research drugs that are supplied by NCI's Division of Cancer Treatment and Diagnosis (DCTD) through PMB, the investigators or designees must submit agent requests through AURORA. Access to the AURORA order processing application requires establishing an NCI CTEP Identity and Access Management account (https://ctepcore.nci.nih.gov/rcr) and maintaining an active account status and current password. Submitters will receive a confirmation email for each successful order submission. The average PMB processing time for routine orders is two working days (NCI, 2021). Orders are shipped by U.S. Postal Service Priority Mail or another ground service. Agents that have special storage conditions (e.g., thermolabile agents that require refrigeration or freezing [−20°C or −70°C]) or shipping requirements (e.g., dangerous goods, infectious substances) are shipped Monday through Thursday for next-day delivery (NCI CTEP, 2014). In most instances, a starter supply of drugs is sent for NCI studies (NCI, 2021).

Best practice is to ship to the address where drugs will be stored (e.g., central or control pharmacy). This address must match the shipping address that the investigator provided on the supplemental investigator data form. For online order submissions, a confirmation email, including the order details and tracking information, is sent upon shipment. The person responsible for ordering the drug will use similar procedures for reordering, keeping in mind the processing time and appropriate amount to reorder according to the protocol's accrual rate to avoid a shortage of drug supply (NCI, 2021).

For emergency (overnight) supplies of research drugs, orders must be submitted through the online agent ordering program by 2 pm Eastern time for next-day delivery. The form should be completed with all the information as previously indicated, including the requirements for next-day delivery, the express courier name, and account number. An email will be sent to confirm the successful placement of the order. Urgent drug orders should only be made in emergencies, such as starter supplies or if the current drug supply becomes unexpectedly low. Because of the additional processing of blinded agents supplied by NCI, they cannot be shipped overnight but can be expedited for two-day delivery (NCI, 2021).

For some protocols in which the drug supply is limited or slow patient accrual is expected, a starter supply of the drug may not be available. Upon enrollment of a patient, staff should use the procedure for emergency supply of research drugs to order drugs or refer to appropriate drug transfer procedures if circumstances do not allow for the timely delivery of the drugs via the emergency ordering procedure. Initial drug orders for blinded studies are usually provided automatically following randomization of patients. Staff should always consult the protocol for details

(Southwest Oncology Group [SWOG], 2025). A survey by the National Comprehensive Cancer Network revealed that ongoing drug shortages have been affecting clinical trials at 43% of responding centers, highlighting the importance of having a process in place at these sites to address potential drug shortages (Darwin, 2024).

Accountability for Research Study Drugs

Receipt of Research Drugs

Many institutions use web-based platforms to manage investigational drug products in research studies. These systems, such as Vestigo®, offer features for electronic accountability, inventory tracking, and protocol management. Research drug shipments are accompanied by a shipment receipt. This document should be reviewed and verified with the shipment to confirm the name of the drug and dosage form, appropriate protocol number, quantity, and appropriate shipping conditions. The supplier must be contacted if the shipment is incorrect or damaged to allow for replacement of the drug in a timely manner. Drug shipment receipts should always be filed so that they are readily accessible for site audits. Study staff should refer to the protocol or shipping materials for instructions on proper handling. In many instances, clinical research drugs are sent with a temperature data logger that records the temperature of the shipment and shows an alarm if the shipment temperature is out of parameters (Ohio State University Wexner Medical Center, 2023).

Drug Accountability

For each drug supplied for a study, an NCI Investigational Agent Accountability Record (see Figure 21-1) must be maintained. This form is available on the NCI CTEP website (2025; https://dctd.cancer.gov/research/ctep-trials/for-sites/agent-management/accountability-record.pdf). The study sponsor usually provides other equivalent forms. These forms are designed to account for drug inventories and usage in clinical trials. A separate accountability form must be used for each protocol and each research drug. If more than one strength or dosage form of a drug is used for the same protocol, a separate drug accountability form is required for each drug product. Electronic drug accountability forms are allowed, provided that a print version of the log process is identical to the existing drug accountability form. Sites should develop and follow established standard operating procedures to ensure proper handling, documentation, and accountability for investigational agents across all study protocols (SWOG, 2025).

For blinded drugs supplied by NCI, the investigator or a responsible party designated by the investigator must carefully record the receipt, disposition, and return of all drugs received from PMB using the NCI Investigational Agent Accountability Record. A separate accountability record must be maintained for each patient ID number on the protocol.

When completing the drug accountability form, the following should be considered (SWOG, 2025):

- All drug supplies received must be entered into the drug log or database (i.e., drug received from NCI or other study sponsor).
- If the supply is patient-specific/blinded, an Investigational Agent Accountability Record is required for each patient on the study (see the protocol for details).
- Central or control pharmacy records must reflect returns from satellite locations.
- All shipping, return, and transfer receipts must be maintained for audit purposes.

Sponsor-specific forms are typically customized for each study. For NCI studies, a new Investigational Agent Accountability Record must be started, and the upper portion of the form should be completed with the following required information (SWOG, 2025):

- **Page No.:** Record the page number consecutively on the forms for each drug used on the protocol.
- **Control Record:** Check this box if the record is being used to account for research drugs stored at the central or control pharmacy.
- **Satellite Record:** Check this box if the record is being used to account for research drugs at a satellite pharmacy.
- **Name of Institution:** Provide the name of the location of the shipment from NCI.
- **NCI Protocol No.:** Enter the NCI protocol number; add the institutional protocol number if necessary.
- **Agent Name**
- **Dose Form and Strength**
- **Protocol Title**
- **Dispensing Area:** Provide the location where the drug is dispensed (e.g., infusion center pharmacy, satellite location, central pharmacy).
- **Investigator Name:** This is the investigator who ordered the drug from NCI.
- **CTEP Investigator ID**
- **Balance Forward:** Enter "0" if the current page is the first page, or bring the balance forward from the previous page.

Upon receiving a drug shipment, the following information should be entered in the appropriate columns to make an entry on an existing drug accountability record form (SWOG, 2025):

- **Date:** Write the date the drug is received, including the year.
- **Patient's Initials and ID No.:** Enter "Rec'd from [name of the study sponsor]."
- **Dose:** Record the dose of the medication that was dispensed.
- **Quantity Dispensed or Received:** Write "+" followed by the number of vials, ampoules, tablets, or kits received.
- **Balance:** Enter the new total obtained by adding the new quantity received.

Print Form | Save As | Reset Form

Collection of this information is authorized under 21 CFR 312.57. The information is collected to ensure compliance with Food and Drug Administration (FDA) requirements for NCI as an IND sponsor and that investigational agents are under the control and accounted for by competent authority. The information may be disclosed to researchers for investigational purposes, sponsors of clinical trials and their company collaborators, the applicable Institutional Review Board, NCI, FDA, and the Department of Health and Human Services. Submission of this information is voluntary however, in order for you to conduct a study in accordance with relevant, current protocols, you must complete all fields.

OMB No. 0925-0613
Expires: 11-30-2027

Public reporting burden for this collection of information is estimated to average 4 minutes per response, including the time for reviewing instructions, searching existing data sources, gathering and maintaining the data needed, and completing and reviewing the collection of information. **An agency may not conduct or sponsor, and a person is not required to respond to, a collection of information unless it displays a currently valid OMB control number.** Send comments regarding this burden estimate or any other aspect of this collection of information, including suggestions for reducing this burden, to: NIH, Project Clearance Branch, 6705 Rockledge Drive, MSC 7974, Bethesda, MD 20892-7974, ATTN: PRA (0925-0613). Do not return the completed form to this address.

National Institutes of Health
National Cancer Institute

Division of Cancer Treatment and Diagnosis
Cancer Therapy Evaluation Program

Investigational Agent Accountability Record

PAGE NO.
CONTROL RECORD ☐
SATELLITE RECORD ☐

Name of Institution:

NCI Protocol No.:

Agent Name:

Dose Form and Strength:

Protocol Title:

Dispensing Area:

Investigator Name:

CTEP Investigator ID:

Line No.	Date	Patient's Initials	Patient's ID No.	Dose	Quantity Dispensed or Received	Balance Forward / Balance	Manufacturer and Lot No.	Recorder's Initials
1.								
2.								
3.								
4.								
5.								
6.								
7.								
8.								
9.								
10.								
11.								
12.								
13.								
14.								
15.								
16.								
17.								
18.								
19.								
20.								
21.								
22.								

FIGURE 21-1 | Investigational Agent Accountability Record

Note. From *NCI Investigational Agent Accountability Record Form*, by National Cancer Institute Cancer Therapy Evaluation Program, 2025 (https://dctd.cancer.gov/research/ctep-trials/for-sites/agent-management/accountability-record.pdf). In the public domain.

- **Manufacturer and Lot No.:** Provide the lot number and expiration/preparation date; if the drug shipment contains more than one lot number, make separate entries for each lot number for optimal recordkeeping.
- **Recorder's Initials**

Storage of Research Drugs

Research drugs must be stored separately by protocol and have separate drug accountability forms. Because multiple protocols may use the same agent, each agent container must be labeled with the drug name, dosage form, and protocol number. Additionally, each study should maintain a unique drug accountability form. Investigational agents must be stored in a secure, locked area with limited access, following recommended storage conditions. Investigational agents should be stored separately from any commercial supplies of medications (ICH, 2016).

Quality assurance for drug storage should be maintained at all times. A daily temperature log must be kept for the refrigerator and the freezer used for storing research drugs, and it should be readily available for audit inspection. Institutional policy needs to address how to handle temperature checks if the clinic or center is not open on the weekend. Room temperature storage control should be maintained at all times to avoid excessive heating of the drugs. Whatever mechanism is used to track the temperature should also be inspected and certified at regular intervals. Light-sensitive products should be kept in their original container prior to administration, or an amber light-protection bag should be used to provide the protection required (ICH, 2016).

Recordkeeping for the Dispensing of Research Drugs

Central or Control Pharmacies

For drugs that are being prepared or dispensed at the central or control pharmacy, enter the following information in the Investigational Agent Accountability Record (SWOG, 2025) (see Figure 21-1):

- **Date:** Provide the date of dispensing and preparation, including the year.
- **Patient's Initials**: Use the same initials as for the protocol registration.
- **Patient's ID No.:** Enter the patient's study number.
- **Dose:** Record the dose.
- **Quantity Dispensed:** Enter "–" followed by the number of vials, ampoules, tablets, or kits dispensed.
- **Balance:** Enter the new total obtained when subtracting the number dispensed.
- **Manufacturer and Lot No.:** Provide the lot numbers and expiration dates of the drugs; if more than one lot number is being used, make separate entries for optimal recordkeeping.
- **Recorder's Initials**

The container of all drugs dispensed must be labeled per federal law requirements. Identification of the investigational drug or agent by the statement "Caution: New Drug—Limited by federal (or U.S.) law to investigational use" on the medication label is required (Labeling of an Investigational New Drug, 1987). Some protocols will use interactive voice response or interactive web response systems. These assist with randomizing patients and also assign vials or medications to patients for the pharmacy to dispense. Also of note, effective January 1, 2022, for studies with oral investigational agents, CTEP will allow the dispensing pharmacy to ship oral investigational agents directly to study participants (National Institutes of Health, 2022).

Satellite Pharmacies

Satellite pharmacies are limited to institutions located on the same campus as the central or control pharmacy or near where an institution employee can conduct transportation of the research drugs. Mailing of research drugs to satellite pharmacies by a commercial carrier or overnight delivery service is not permitted. A satellite pharmacy is allowed to use only the research drug supplies received by the central or control pharmacy. The central or control pharmacy and the satellite pharmacy must be tied through affiliation agreements, and the professional staff must be shared or have joint appointments. Satellite pharmacies must follow the same procedures for research drug accountability, preparation, and dispensing as the central or control pharmacy (SWOG, 2025).

Institutions separated geographically by greater distances (e.g., different cities or states) are generally referred to as affiliates and not considered satellites. Affiliates must order the research drug from the drug supplier and ship it directly to these sites. They must follow the same procedures for drug preparation and dispensing and record the documentation required for the central or control pharmacy (SWOG, 2025).

Dispensing of Research Drugs to Satellite Pharmacies

For NCI trials, if the research drug is to be prepared at a satellite location, it must first be dispensed to that location. The following information should then be entered in the central or control pharmacy's Investigational Agent Accountability Record. For other trials, the information captured may differ and will depend on the site's standard operating procedures and the specific form used (SWOG, 2025):

- **Date:** Write the date, including the year.
- **Patient's Initials and Patient's ID No.:** Enter "dispensed to [name of satellite location]."
- **Dose:** Record the dose.
- **Quantity Dispensed or Received:** Write "–" followed by the number of vials, ampoules, tablets, or kits dispensed.
- **Balance:** Enter the new total obtained when subtracting the number dispensed.
- **Manufacturer and Lot No.:** Provide the lot numbers and expiration dates of the drugs; if more than one lot

number is being used, make separate entries for optimal recordkeeping.
- **Recorder's Initials**

The package should be labeled with the drug name, protocol number, patient's name (optional), and storage condition. A similar process is followed for sponsor trials.

Upon receiving the drugs, the satellite pharmacist designated to handle the research drugs should enter the following information in the Investigational Agent Accountability Record (SWOG, 2025):
- **Date:** Write the date, including the year
- **Patient's Initials and Patient's ID No.:** Enter "Received from [name of central/control pharmacy]."
- **Dose:** Leave blank.
- **Quantity Received:** Write "+" followed by the number received.
- **Balance:** Provide the new balance obtained when adding the number received.
- **Manufacturer and Lot No.:** Enter the lot numbers and expiration dates of the drugs; if more than one lot number is being used, make separate entries for optimal recordkeeping. A similar process is followed for sponsor trials.

Documentation of Returned Drugs by Patients

For protocols that require accountability of drugs returned by patients (especially for oral medications for which adherence checks are required), a separate drug accountability log for each patient should be maintained. It is highly encouraged that clinicians should confirm the proper administration of the study medications with patients and caregivers and review the medication diaries completed by the patients, if appropriate, to ensure medication adherence and improve persistence. It is crucial to capture any discrepancies between the medication returned and what the patient has documented as taken. A clear policy should be in place to address and document these discrepancies as part of the drug accountability process. OCRNs and pharmacists can positively influence participants' adherence to a study drug schedule through frequent communication and careful listening to participants' complaints of symptoms that may be attributed to the study drug (SWOG, 2025).

Return of Research Drugs to the Supplier

For NCI-provided research drugs, investigators are required to return unused drugs under the following conditions (SWOG, 2025):
- The study is completed or terminated, and the research drugs cannot be transferred to another DCTD-sponsored trial.
- The research drug is outdated.
- The research drug is damaged (e.g., loss of refrigeration). Broken vials should not be returned. They should be destroyed on-site according to the institutional standard operating procedures, accompanied by proper documentation. The sponsor should also be contacted (SWOG, 2025).

Research drugs should be returned within 90 days of study closure or last patient activity. However, outdated or damaged drugs should be removed from inventory immediately, and the sponsor should be contacted for guidance on the next steps. For pharmaceutical-sponsored studies, protocols for specific instructions on the handling of returned or unused research drugs should be followed. Sites should develop and follow standard operating procedures to ensure consistency and adherence in managing the return, destruction, or other disposition of investigational drugs (SWOG, 2025).

The Return Investigational Agent Form (NCI CTEP, 2025) or forms provided by the study sponsor should be completed to return unused research drugs to NCI or the study sponsor. An entry should be made on the drug accountability form, subtracting the amount returned from the balance. A copy of the return drug form should be kept on file with the drug accountability form for audit purposes. For NCI-provided drugs, the original Return Investigational Agent Form should be sent to the NCI Clinical Repository at the address indicated on the form. For other sponsored studies, the drugs should be sent to the designated location as instructed by the sponsor (SWOG, 2025).

All returned research drugs must be packaged securely to prevent breakage. All drugs can be returned and shipped at room temperature using standard mail because they will be disposed of thereafter. For NCI-provided drugs, collect-on-delivery shipping should not be used (SWOG, 2025).

Research drugs that have been dispensed to patients, opened, or partially used are usually destroyed on-site according to institutional procedures after proper documentation. Study staff should always refer to the study protocol for specific instructions. The study protocol or institutional standard operating procedure should match regulatory requirements for handling and disposal of research drugs. It is essential to thoroughly document the chain of custody for study medication, particularly oral medications returned by trial participants. Research staff must return study medication to the pharmacy that dispensed it on the same day it is returned and should not store it in a different location (ICH, 2016).

Transfer of National Cancer Institute Research Drugs

For NCI-provided research drugs, the drugs can be transferred if the following criteria are met (SWOG, 2025):

- The research drugs can only be transferred within an institution.
- The drugs can only be transferred from one active protocol to another DCTD-approved protocol.
- The transferring investigator must be the investigator who originally ordered the agent or the investigator to whom the agent was previously transferred (i.e., double transfer).
- The receiving investigator must be an approved investigator on the trial to which the agent is being transferred.
- The transfer can only be made between registered active NCI investigators. For example, drug transfer may be used in the following situations:
  - The protocol is closed, and another protocol at the institution uses the same agent and formulation. However, transfer of DCTD-supplied agents to non-DCTD–approved protocols is not permitted under DCTD, NCI, and FDA policies and regulations.
  - There is excessive inventory for a protocol, and the transfer will minimize drug wastage due to outdating.
- The study drug has short dating.
- In cases of medical emergency (e.g., an urgent approval of a protocol and a very sick patient who needs to begin therapy immediately): When a drug is ordered for an individual patient under a Special Exception (compassionate use) protocol, it is no longer intended for a patient enrolled in the original study. Instead, the institution has a DCTD-approved Special Exception protocol in place that allows use of the same investigational drug for the newly identified patient under emergency or compassionate use circumstances.

Transfer of research drugs should never occur under the following circumstances (SWOG, 2025):

- Transfer of research drugs for commercial use
- Replacement of research drugs with commercial agents
- Transfer of drugs for blinded studies between protocols
- Borrowing of a study drug

Administration of Research Drugs

The administration of research drugs in clinical trials is a critical component of patient care and study integrity. Pre-entry laboratory work and baseline data collection are essential for evaluating participants' clinical responses to the study treatment (FDA, 2024a). Understanding the precise conditions under which these treatments are administered is crucial for healthcare professionals, particularly OCRNs, who play a pivotal role in managing and monitoring these protocols (Oncology Nursing Society [ONS] & Oncology Nursing Certification Corporation [ONCC], 2024).

Treatment packets should be prepared in advance that contain patient education materials regarding side effects of the protocol agent, adherence tools (e.g., calendars, diaries), and instructions regarding the reporting of side effects (Belcher et al., 2022). OCRNs should remain in close contact with the PI for each patient and notify the physician if any toxicities or adverse events occur, especially those that require dose modification, discontinuation, or interruption of the drug infusion. The study sponsor or the sponsor's representative can be a resource and ally in the clinical research process, and any problems should be discussed with them. Experiences occurring at other study sites may be significant in providing evolving information not previously known. In early development studies, such as phase 1 or 2 studies, dose-limiting toxicities may occur. These are toxic effects that are presumably related to the drugs and are considered unacceptable because of their severity or irreversibility. Dose-limiting toxicities restrict further dose escalation and should be reported expeditiously (NCI, 2024).

Patient Safety Prior to Drug Administration

Depending on the timepoint, vital signs, patient weight, and height, laboratory tests will be collected per protocol. Studies will address weight change differently, which might not be in line with the institution's standards. The research protocols may use different formulas to calculate items such as creatinine clearance and body surface area. It is important to know when there are differences. A thorough medication reconciliation should be completed to confirm that patients are not taking any contraindicated medications and are taking prescribed medications correctly (Siegel et al., 2024). A pill diary should ideally be used to ensure adherence (Belcher et al., 2022). Some studies may require electrocardiograms to detect cardiac arrhythmias and QTc prolongation. Specific assessments, such as immune effector cell–associated neurotoxicity syndrome, may need to be evaluated before dosing. Any side effects or adverse events should be assessed and graded using NCI CTEP *Common Terminology Criteria for Adverse Events* [v.5.0] (https://dctd.cancer.gov/research/ctep-trials/for-sites/adverse-events/ctcae-v5-5x7.pdf). The protocol should be reviewed to determine if any adverse events require a dose reduction or if the drug should be temporarily stopped until the adverse event improves or resolves.

From a regulatory standpoint, consent for the current protocol version should be available, along with additional items as needed, such as dose enrollment and contraception measures (ICH, 2016). In certain instances of oral medical clinical trials, drugs can be sent directly to patients, but they cannot be sent out of state.

In-service education for nursing and pharmacy staff can enhance team performance. If possible, OCRNs should be present during the initial dose calculations and administration of protocol agents (ONS & ONCC, 2024). This support allows potential problems to be identified and corrected before a protocol deviation occurs. Before each treatment, the patient's desire to continue on the protocol should be assessed and affirmed. Patients have the right to withdraw at any time when participating in clinical research. If patients decline further participation in the trial, the study coordinator should be contacted so that the study sponsor can be notified appropriately.

Research Specimen and Data Collection Tied to Dosing

Pharmacodynamics delves into the study of a drug's molecular, biochemical, and physiologic effects on the body. It examines pharmacologic impacts, such as the lowest point (nadir) of neutrophil or platelet counts, nonhematologic toxicity, and molecular correlates (Marino et al., 2023). On the other hand, pharmacokinetics investigates how the body processes and interacts with administered substances over the entire period of exposure. This includes the stages of drug absorption, distribution, metabolism, and excretion (Grogan & Preuss, 2023). Although pharmacodynamics and pharmacokinetics are closely related, they are distinct. Pharmacodynamics focuses on the drug's specific effects on the body. Furthermore, many studies gather patient experiences through quality-of-life assessments to provide a comprehensive understanding of treatment impacts (Haslam et al., 2020). Accurate timing and documentation are foundational to the scientific integrity and regulatory success of clinical trials, supporting both patient safety and high-quality data collection.

Research Drug Administration

Policies and procedures for the administration of antineoplastic clinical trial medications must be systematically developed using an evidence-based approach to ensure safe and standardized practices within institutions. Collaboration among departments, such as pharmacy, medicine, nursing, and clinical trial leadership, is essential to create comprehensive policies. These policies cover key areas, including staff qualifications, drug management, order verification, informed consent, toxicity monitoring, emergency procedures, and communication during care transitions. Given the high-alert nature of chemotherapy and antineoplastic drugs in clinical trials, which carry potential toxicities, implementing robust safety measures is essential. Errors can occur at any stage, from ordering and prescribing to drug preparation and administration. Safeguards include using standardized electronic or preprinted orders, providing independent dual verification of drug and pump settings if applicable, and performing drug and dose verifications in distraction-free settings. Additionally, institutions should ensure that emergency preparedness procedures are in place, including 24-7 triage availability and staff training in basic and advanced life support. Establishing and enforcing these comprehensive policies and procedures helps mitigate the risks associated with antineoplastic medication errors and enhances patient safety (Olsen et al., 2023; Siegel et al., 2024).

It is recommended that a policy outline the specific requirements for flushing, including variance in total volume to be infused, whether the line is primed with drug or vehicle, and the rate and volume for flushing; however, this may vary depending on protocol or sponsor requirements. Many research protocols will state "flush or administer per institution guidelines" (Kay et al., 2018). Organizations have the discretion in these instances to prime the line with a drug or another compatible solution. A case can be made either for or against priming the line with saline, depending on the clinical context and intent. Priming with the drug allows the care team to know precisely when the patient receives the drug, which some believe makes the collection times of pharmacodynamic and pharmacokinetic specimens more accurate. The other perceived benefits are that because the patient is receiving the drug from the very start of the infusion, observation of the patient for hypersensitivity or other reactions begins immediately, and one does not have to take into account how long it might take for the drug to reach the patient. Priming with a vehicle has the added safety benefit of exposure to medications where there are unknowns (ONS & Hematology/Oncology Pharmacy Association, 2019). Research has found that priming with saline can reduce the incidence of hypersensitivity reactions (Laudati et al., 2018).

Along with priming, flushing should be addressed if not in the protocol, and there should be a standard. The policy could include the total volume to be infused, whether the line was primed with a drug or vehicle, and at what rate and volume to flush with. This policy covers all drugs and may be different for hazardous and nonhazardous drugs. Administration of research drugs must be performed consistently to promote quality data.

Safe handling procedures for clinical trial drugs may or may not be included in the investigational materials. This could be provider material, the investigator brochure, or the pharmacy manual. Some organizations leverage a pharmacist to review the drug and classify it for the institution (Kay et al., 2018). In early drug clinical trials, some institutions have taken a stance to apply USP General Chapter <800> standards for safe handling, including the use of closed-system drug-transfer devices on clinical trial medications (Hodson et al., 2023).

Some early drug development clinical trials will provide supplies to administer research medication, such as tubing, IV catheters, and infusion pumps. However, it may be easier to use the materials familiar to nurses and other individuals at the trial sites. Some trials may be mandated to use certain pumps and supplies from a particular manufacturer, which may be non-negotiable.

The Role of Oncology Clinical Research Nurses in Trial Accountability

The *Oncology Clinical Research Nurse Competencies* categories for clinical research nursing encompass a diverse range of domains essential for ensuring the integrity, safety, and success of clinical research endeavors (ONS & ONCC, 2024).

These domains include adherence to ethical standards, protocol compliance, informed consent, patient recruitment and retention, management of clinical research participants, documentation and document management, data management and information technology, financial stewardship, and leadership and professional development. They collectively provide a comprehensive framework for clinical research nursing practice. Each domain represents a crucial aspect of the clinical research process, underscoring the multifaceted nature of the OCRN role.

Jones et al. (2022) estimated that 10,000 OCRNs work across a spectrum of roles and settings within the global clinical research enterprise. Ethical considerations lie at the heart of clinical research. These 10,000 OCRNs must demonstrate a steadfast commitment to upholding ethical standards throughout every phase of a study, including ensuring informed consent from participants, maintaining protocol adherence to safeguard participant rights and welfare, and overseeing patient recruitment and retention efforts with sensitivity and transparency (ONS & ONCC, 2024).

Effective management of clinical research participants is paramount for the success of any study (ONS & ONCC, 2024). OCRNs are tasked with providing specialized care tailored to the unique needs of research participants while also navigating the intricacies of protocol requirements. This requires a deep understanding of the study's objectives, procedures, and potential risks, as well as the ability to communicate and collaborate effectively with interprofessional teams.

Documentation and data management are critical components of clinical research, and OCRNs play a pivotal role in maintaining accurate and comprehensive records throughout the study life cycle. From documenting participant interactions and adverse events to managing regulatory paperwork and ensuring adherence with data protection laws, OCRNs must possess strong organizational skills and meticulous attention to detail.

In an era increasingly reliant on technology, OCRNs must also be adept at leveraging information technology tools and systems to streamline data collection, analysis, and reporting processes. This includes proficiency in electronic data capture systems, electronic health records, and other software platforms designed to enhance efficiency and accuracy in clinical research operations (ONS & ONCC, 2024).

Financial stewardship is another key responsibility of OCRNs, who must effectively manage study budgets, allocate resources judiciously, and ensure adherence with financial regulations and reporting requirements. This involves balancing the financial considerations of the research sponsor with the ethical imperative to prioritize participant safety and well-being (ONS & ONCC, 2024).

Leadership and professional development are essential for OCRNs seeking to advance their careers and make meaningful contributions to clinical research. Whether through continuing education, participation in professional organizations, or mentorship opportunities, OCRNs must actively pursue opportunities for growth and development to stay abreast of emerging trends, best practices, and regulatory updates (ONS & ONCC, 2024).

Overall, OCRNs occupy a unique and indispensable role within the clinical research landscape, serving as advocates for both participants and the scientific community. Their expertise, dedication, and commitment to excellence are fundamental to the advancement of knowledge and the improvement of patient outcomes in health care.

Summary

Stringent regulations on investigational agents ensure the ethical and scientific integrity of clinical research while safeguarding the rights, safety, and privacy of research participants. Procurement processes necessitate meticulous delegation of responsibilities, primarily handled by the pharmacy department, ensuring accurate documentation and adherence to established protocols. The use of systems such as AURORA streamlines inventory management and regulatory adherence, enhancing the efficiency and oversight of investigational drug handling.

Accountability is pivotal, with detailed procedures for ordering, receiving, storing, and documenting research drugs. Maintaining separate drug accountability forms for each protocol and ensuring secure storage conditions are critical to maintaining adherence and readiness for audits.

The administration of investigational drugs requires rigorous adherence to protocols, emphasizing patient safety and accurate data collection. Pretreatment evaluations, dose calculations, and monitoring for adverse events are essential components ensuring the efficacy and safety of the treatments.

The role of the OCRN is indispensable, providing specialized care, managing patient interactions, and ensuring protocol adherence. Through meticulous planning, stringent documentation, and a strong ethical foundation, clinical trials can achieve their goal of advancing medical knowledge while prioritizing patient safety and integrity.

Key Points

- **Investigational drug procurement is tightly controlled, with responsibilities often delegated to pharmacy teams and documentation required per protocol and sponsor-specific forms (e.g., ALCOA-C, eDARF, AURORA systems).**
- **Orders must follow sponsor-specific protocols (e.g., NCI via AURORA or pharma-sponsored pathways) and adhere to strict guidelines for storage, labeling, and chain of custody, including processes for returns, transfers, and emergency supply management.**
- **Safe administration of research drugs involves pre-dose assessments, dose verification, flushing protocols, toxicity monitoring, and adherence to institution and protocol-specific procedures to avoid deviations and ensure valid data collection.**

The author would like to acknowledge Siu-Fun Wong, PharmD, FASHP, FCSHP, Carol Anne Bales, MSN, RN, CCRP, Kathleen R. Hurtado, RPh, and Joan G. Westendorp, MSN, RN, OCN®, CCRP, CIM, for their contribution to this chapter that remains unchanged from the previous edition of this book.

References

Belcher, S.M., Mackler, E., Muluneh, B., Ginex, P.K., Anderson, M.K., Bettencourt, E., ... Morgan, R.L. (2022). ONS Guidelines™ to support patient adherence to oral anticancer medications. *Oncology Nursing Forum, 49*(4), 279–295. https://doi.org/10.1188/22.ONF.279-295

Darwin, R. (2024). New survey from NCCN finds cancer drug shortage management remains a moving target, impacting clinical trials. *National Comprehensive Cancer Network.* https://www.nccn.org/home/news/newsdetails?NewsId=4620

Grogan, S., & Preuss, C.V. (2023). *Pharmacokinetics.* In *StatPearls.* StatPearls Publishing. https://www.ncbi.nlm.nih.gov/books/NBK557744

Haslam, A., Herrera-Perez, D., Gill, J., & Prasad, V. (2020). Patient experience captured by quality-of-life measurement in oncology clinical trials. *JAMA Network Open, 3*(3), e200363. https://doi.org/10.1001/jamanetworkopen.2020.0363

Hodson, L., Ovesen, J., Couch, J., Hirst, D., Lawson, C., Lentz, T.J., MacKenzie, B., & Mead, K. (2023). *Managing hazardous drug exposures: Information for healthcare settings.* National Institute for Occupational Safety and Health (NIOSH), Centers for Disease Control and Prevention. https://doi.org/10.26616/NIOSHPUB2023130

International Council for Harmonisation of Technical Requirements for Pharmaceuticals for Human Use. (2016). *ICH harmonised guideline: Integrated addendum to ICH E6(R1): Guideline for good clinical practice: E6(R2).* https://database.ich.org/sites/default/files/E6_R2_Addendum.pdf

Jones, C.T., Griffith, C.A., Fisher, C.A., Grinke, K.A., Keller, R., Lee, H., Purdom, M., & Turba, E. (2022). Nurses in clinical trials: Perceptions of impact on the research enterprise. *Journal of Research Nursing, 27*(1–2), 50–65. https://doi.org/10.1177/17449871211073757

Kay, S.C., Luke, D.G., & Tamer, H.R. (2018). ASHP guidelines for the management of investigational drug products. *American Journal of Health-System Pharmacy, 75*(8), 561–573. https://doi.org/10.2146/ajhp170812

Labeling of an Investigational New Drug, 21 C.F.R. § 312.6 (1987). https://www.ecfr.gov/current/title-21/chapter-I/subchapter-D/part-312/subpart-A/section-312.6

Laudati, C., Clark, C., Knezevic, A., Zhang, Z., & Barton-Burke, M. (2018). Hypersensitivity reactions: Priming practice change to reduce incidence in first-dose rituximab treatment. *Clinical Journal of Oncology Nursing, 22*(4), 407-414. https://doi.org/10.1188/18.CJON.407-414

Marino, M., Jamal, Z., & Zito, P.M. (2023). Pharmacodynamics. In *StatPearls.* StatPearls Publishing. https://www.ncbi.nlm.nih.gov/books/NBK507791

National Cancer Institute. (2021). *Policy and guidelines for investigational agent ordering.* https://ctep.cancer.gov/protocoldevelopment/requisition_agents/docs/Investigational_Agent_Ordering.pdf

National Cancer Institute. (2024). *NCI guidelines for investigators: Adverse event reporting requirements for DCTD (CTEP AND CIP) INDs and IDEs.* https://ctep.cancer.gov/protocoldevelopment/electronic_applications/docs/aeguidelines.pdf

National Cancer Institute Cancer Therapy Evaluation Program. (2014). *A handbook for clinical investigators conducting therapeutic clinical trials supported by CTEP, DCTD, NCI.* https://ctep.cancer.gov/investigatorresources/docs/investigatorhandbook.pdf

National Cancer Institute Cancer Therapy Evaluation Program. (2024). *AURORA: CTEP inventory management system.* https://ctep.cancer.gov/branches/pmb/aurora.htm

National Cancer Institute Cancer Therapy Evaluation Program. (2025). *CTEP forms, templates, and documents.* https://ctep.cancer.gov/forms

National Institutes of Health. (2022). *Guidance for shipment of oral IND agents to clinical trial subjects on clinical trials sponsored by the National Cancer Institute Cancer Therapy Evaluation Program.* https://ctep.cancer.gov/content/docs/CTEP_Oral_IND_Agent_Shipment_Guideline.pdf

Ohio State University Wexner Medical Center. (2023). *Department of Pharmacy Investigational Drug Service (IDs) standard operating procedures (SOPs).* https://medicine.osu.edu/departments/pharmacy/research

Olsen, M., LeFebvre, K.B., Walker, S.L., & Dunphy, E.P. (Eds.). (2023). *Chemotherapy and immunotherapy guidelines and recommendations for practice* (2nd ed.). Oncology Nursing Society.

Oncology Nursing Society & Hematology/Oncology Pharmacy Association. (2019). *Joint position statement from the Oncology Nursing Society and the Hematology/Oncology Pharmacy Association ensuring healthcare worker safety when handling hazardous drugs.* https://www.ons.org/network-advocacy/position-statements/ensuring-healthcare-worker-safety-when-handling-hazardous-drugs

Oncology Nursing Society & Oncology Nursing Certification Corporation. (2024). *Oncology clinical research nurse competencies.* https://www.ons.org/sites/default/files/2025-01/ocrn-competencies-rebrand.pdf

Siegel, R.D., LeFebvre, K.B., Temin, S., Evers, A., Barbarotta, L., Bowman, R.M., ... Olsen, M.M. (2024). Antineoplastic therapy administration safety standards for adult and pediatric oncology: ASCO-ONS standards. *Oncology Nursing Forum, 51*(4), 297–320. https://doi.org/10.1188/24.ONF.297-320

Southwest Oncology Group. (2025). *Oncology research professional (ORP) manual.* https://txwb.crab.org/TXWB/CRA_MANUAL/Vol1/chapter%2006_Drug%20Ordering%20and%20Maintenance.pdf

U.S. Food and Drug Administration. (2021). *Good clinical practice (GCP) inspection collaboration with international regulators for drug development.* https://www.fda.gov/science-research/clinical-trials-and-human-subject-protection/good-clinical-practice-gcp-inspection-collaboration-international-regulators-drug-development

U.S. Food and Drug Administration. (2024a). *Cancer clinical trial eligibility criteria: Laboratory values (Draft guidance for industry, IRBs, and clinical investigators).* https://www.fda.gov/regulatory-information/search-fda-guidance-documents/cancer-clinical-trial-eligibility-criteria-laboratory-values

U.S. Food and Drug Administration. (2024b). *Clinical trials guidance documents.* https://www.fda.gov/science-research/clinical-trials-and-human-subject-protection/clinical-trials-guidance-documents

CHAPTER 22

Adverse Events

Elizabeth Ness, MS, RN, CRN-BC

Introduction

Identifying and monitoring adverse events (AEs) is critical to protect research participants and ensure data integrity. Assessment of AEs and timely documentation are crucial to research participant safety and Good Clinical Practice (GCP). AE surveillance during a study intervention allows for identifying events that may have an immediate effect on the safety of participants; informing regulators, investigators, and others of new and important information about events that occur during clinical trials; and providing a summary of adverse experiences to develop the drug or regimen toxicity profile (National Institutes of Health [NIH] VideoCast, 2023a).

Oncology clinical research nurses (OCRNs) are responsible for the education, protection, and safety of patients enrolled in clinical trials (American Nurses Association, 2024). As nurses, OCRNs are well-positioned to solicit, assess, collect, and provide appropriate follow-up for AEs experienced by research participants. OCRNs can also educate research participants about potential AEs and the importance of communicating to the research team any AEs they experience, serving as reinforcement of the informed consent process.

This chapter will focus on the assessment, documentation, recording, and reporting of AEs and unanticipated problems, as well as the critical role OCRNs play in identifying and monitoring AEs.

Definitions

An *adverse event* is any unwanted sign, symptom, or disease that was not seen before an individual's research participation or a worsening of a baseline symptom, regardless of the expectedness of the event or its relationship to the research. *Toxicity*, *side effects*, and related terms (e.g., *adverse drug reaction*, *adverse drug event*, *acute* or *late effect*, *complication*) imply a relationship between the event and an intervention. There are many other definitions associated with AEs (see Table 22-1). Recognizing these various definitions is the first step in understanding AEs.

Adverse Event Assessment

The principal investigator (PI) conducts the AE assessment or delegates this duty to other members of the research team (e.g., subinvestigators). This assessment includes the following (Callahan et al., 2018):

- Selecting the correct AE term
- Identifying the expectedness of the event (i.e., known to occur with the intervention)
- Assessing the severity of the event
- Determining the attribution of the event

Understanding how to collect and solicit information about AEs is crucial. OCRNs are well-positioned to assist with AE assessment, often being the patient participants' first point of contact.

Event Terminology

OCRNs must understand the importance of using appropriate terminology when assessing an AE. Using controlled vocabularies to represent clinical concepts is the best way to describe AEs. The Medical Dictionary for Regulatory Activities (MedDRA) is a clinically validated international medical terminology dictionary with each term having a unique code or concept ID. It was developed in 1994 by the International Council for Harmonisation of Technical Requirements for Pharmaceuticals for Human Use (ICH) to facilitate the sharing of regulatory information internationally. MedDRA is used by the biopharmaceutical industry and regulatory authorities for AE classification and has five hierarchical levels (MedDRA, n.d.):

- **System Organ Class (SOC):** the highest level of the terminology and distinguished by the anatomic or physiologic system, etiology, or purpose

TABLE 22-1 | Comparison of Adverse Event Terminology Among Regulatory Bodies

Terminology	Office for Human Research Protections	U.S. Food and Drug Administration	International Council for Harmonisation of Technical Requirements for Pharmaceuticals for Human Use
Adverse event (AE)	An AE is any untoward or unfavorable medical occurrence, including any abnormal sign (e.g., abnormal physical examination or laboratory finding), symptom, or disease, temporally associated with research participants. The AE may or may not be caused by the research itself. AEs encompass physical and psychological harms. They occur most commonly in biomedical research, although they can also occur in social and behavioral research.	An AE is any untoward medical occurrence associated with the use of a drug in humans, whether or not considered drug related.	An AE is any unfavorable medical occurrence in a research participant administered the investigational product. The AE does not necessarily have a causal relationship with the treatment.
Life threatening	A life-threatening AE places the participant at immediate risk of death from the event as it occurred.	An AE or suspected adverse reaction is considered life threatening if, in the view of either the investigator or sponsor, its occurrence places the patient or participant at immediate risk of death. It does not include an AE or suspected AE that, had it occurred in a more severe form, might have caused death.	–
Suspected adverse reaction	–	Any AE for which there is a reasonable possibility that the drug caused the AE. For Investigational New Drug safety reporting, reasonable possibility means there is evidence to suggest a causal relationship between the drug and the AE. Suspected adverse reaction implies a lesser degree of certainty about causality than adverse reaction, which means any AE caused by a drug.	–
Serious adverse event	A serious adverse event results in death, is life-threatening, leads to inpatient hospitalization or prolongation of existing hospitalization, causes a persistent or significant disability or incapacity, results in a congenital anomaly or birth defect, or based upon appropriate medical judgment, may jeopardize the participants health and may require medical or surgical intervention to prevent one of the other outcomes listed in this definition. This is a modified definition of serious adverse drug experience in U.S. Food and Drug Administration Code of Federal Regulations 21 CFR § 312.32(a).	An AE or suspected adverse reaction is considered serious if, in the view of either the investigator or sponsor, it results in death, a life-threatening AE, inpatient hospitalization or prolongation of existing hospitalization, a persistent or significant incapacity or substantial disruption of the ability to conduct normal life functions, or a congenital anomaly or birth defect. Important medical events that may not result in death, be life threatening, or require hospitalization may be considered serious when, based upon appropriate medical judgment, they jeopardize the patient or participant and may require medical or surgical intervention to prevent one of the outcomes listed in this definition.	A serious adverse event is an unfavorable medical occurrence that results in death, is life threatening, requires inpatient hospitalization or prolongation of existing hospitalization, causes persistent or significant disability or incapacity, or leads to a congenital anomaly or birth defect. An important medical event that may not be immediately life-threatening or result in death or hospitalization, that may jeopardize the participant, or that may require intervention to prevent serious outcomes should generally be considered as serious.

(Continued on next page)

TABLE 22-1 | Comparison of Adverse Event Terminology Among Regulatory Bodies *(Continued)*

Terminology	Office for Human Research Protections	U.S. Food and Drug Administration	International Council for Harmonisation of Technical Requirements for Pharmaceuticals for Human Use
Unanticipated adverse device effect	–	An unanticipated adverse device effect is any serious adverse effect on health or safety or any life-threatening problem or death caused by, or associated with, a device, if that effect, problem, or death was not previously identified in nature, severity, or degree of incidence in the investigational plan or application (including a supplementary plan or application), or any other unanticipated serious problem associated with a device that relates to the rights, safety, or welfare of participants.	–
Unanticipated problem	An unanticipated problem is any incident, experience, or outcome that meets all the following criteria: • Unexpected, in terms of nature, severity, or frequency given – The research procedures that are described in the protocol-related documents, such as the institutional review board (IRB)-approved research protocol and informed consent document – The characteristics of the participant population being studied • Related or possibly related to participation in the research (in this guidance document, possibly related means there is a reasonable possibility that the incident, experience, or outcome may have been caused by the procedures involved in the research) • Suggests that the research places participants or others at a greater risk of harm (including physical, psychological, economic, or social harm) than was previously known or recognized	AE observed during the conduct of a study should be considered an unanticipated problem involving risk to human subjects, and reported to the IRB, only if it was unexpected and serious and would have implications for the conduct of the study (e.g., requiring a significant, and usually safety-related change in the protocol such as revising inclusion/exclusion criteria or including a new monitoring requirement, informed consent, or investigator's brochure).	–
Unexpected adverse event or adverse drug reaction	An unexpected adverse event or adverse drug reaction is any AE occurring in one or more participants in a research protocol, the nature, severity, or frequency of which is not consistent with either of the following: • The known or foreseeable risk of AEs associated with the procedures involved in the research that are described in – The protocol-related documents, such as the IRB-approved research protocol, any applicable investigator's brochure, and the current IRB-approved informed consent document	An AE or suspected adverse reaction is considered unexpected if it is not listed in the investigator's brochure or is not listed at the specificity or severity that has been observed. If an investigator's brochure is not required or available, then *unexpected* is defined as not being consistent with the risk information described in the general investigational plan (i.e., protocol) or elsewhere in the current IND application, as amended.	An adverse reaction for which the nature or severity is not consistent with the applicable product information (e.g., investigator's brochure or other documents referencing safety information)

(Continued on next page)

TABLE 22-1 | Comparison of Adverse Event Terminology Among Regulatory Bodies *(Continued)*

Terminology	Office for Human Research Protections	U.S. Food and Drug Administration	International Council for Harmonisation of Technical Requirements for Pharmaceuticals for Human Use
Unexpected adverse event or adverse drug reaction *(cont.)*	– Other relevant sources of information, such as product labeling and package inserts • The expected natural progression of any underlying disease, disorder, or condition of the participants experiencing the AE and the participants' predisposing risk factor profile for the AE.		

Note. Based on information from IND Safety Reporting, 1987; International Council on Harmonisation for Technical Requirements for Registration of Pharmaceuticals for Human Use, 2025; Investigational Device Exemptions, 1980; Office for Human Research Protections, 2007.

- **High-Level Group Term:** subordinate to SOC
- **High-Level Term:** subordinate to High-Level Group Term
- **Preferred Term:** represents a single medical concept
- **Lowest Level Term:** lowest level of the terminology related to a single Preferred Term as a synonym, lexical variant, or quasi-synonym

See Figure 22-1 for an example of the hierarchical structure for the AE term *fatigue.*

MedDRA is owned by the International Federation of Pharmaceutical Manufacturers and Associations, which functions as a trustee for ICH and is managed by the Maintenance and Support Services Organization. It is available in more than 20 languages, including Chinese, Czech, Dutch, English, German, French, Italian, Japanese, Portuguese, and Spanish. The use of MedDRA is mandated in Europe and Japan for AE safety reporting. The U.S. Food and Drug Administration (FDA) has adopted MedDRA terminology for its web-based Adverse Event Reporting System (AERS). MedDRA is reviewed twice yearly, with a major release yearly, usually in the spring, and a minor release with additional new terms in the fall. To learn more, visit www.meddra.org (MedDRA, n.d.).

System Organ Class
- General disorders and administration site conditions

High-Level Group Term
- General system disorders not elsewhere classified

High-Level Term
- Asthenic conditions

Preferred Term
- Fatigue

Lower-Level Term
- Chronic fatigue
- Exhaustion
- Fatigue
- Tired all the time
- Washed-out
- Weariness
- Worn out

FIGURE 22-1 | Medical Dictionary for Regulatory Activities Fatigue Hierarchy

Note. Based on information from Medical Dictionary for Regulatory Activities, n.d.

Severity Rating Scales

In clinical trials, rating scales are used to measure the severity of an AE (see Table 22-2). The severity often determines if dosing interruptions, modifications, or discontinuations need to be implemented according to protocols. Rating scales can even be used for eligibility criteria (e.g., exclusion criteria to include no grade 2 or higher peripheral sensory neuropathy). The protocol should consist of how the severity of AEs is to be measured, even if only providing descriptions for mild, moderate, and severe. In oncology, the standard rating scale is a combination of an AE term and a severity rating scale, the *Common Terminology Criteria for Adverse Events* (CTCAE).

Common Terminology Criteria for Adverse Events

The National Cancer Institute Cancer Therapy Evaluation Program (NCI CTEP) developed the original *Common Toxicity Criteria* (CTC) in 1983 to aid in recognizing and assessing the severity (i.e., grading) of AEs of chemotherapy. Since CTC v1.0, the tool has been expanded, adapted internationally by the oncology community, renamed, and, with the release of v4.0 in May 2009, harmonized with MedDRA terminology (see Table 22-3). CTCAE remains a subset of MedDRA terms pertinent to the AEs seen in oncology clinical trials (Miller & Aplenc, 2021; NCI CTEP, 2024; Trotti et al., 2003, 2007).

TABLE 22-2 | Types of Severity Rating Scales

Scale	Description
Common Terminology Criteria for Adverse Events	• Developed in 1983 by the National Cancer Institute Cancer Therapy Evaluation Program to aid in the recognition and grading severity of adverse effects of chemotherapy • Originally called the *Common Toxicity Criteria* • Grading scale – Grade 1 (mild) – Grade 2 (moderate) – Grade 3 (severe) – Grade 4 (life threatening) – Grade 5 (death)
U.S. Food and Drug Administration Toxicity Grading Scale Tables	• Clinical and laboratory abnormalities – Grade 1 (mild) – Grade 2 (moderate) – Grade 3 (severe) – Grade 4 (potentially life threatening)

Note. Based on information from National Cancer Institute Cancer Therapy Evaluation Program, 2017; U.S. Food and Drug Administration, 2007.

CTCAE is an agreed-upon descriptive terminology by experts in the oncology community for the designation, reporting, and grading of AEs that occur in oncology clinical trials. The grading or severity rating scale promotes consistency among clinical researchers, facilitates a common understanding of AE data shared among academic, commercial, and regulatory entities, and provides a framework to compare AEs across different studies (Trotti et al., 2007).

Several versions of the CTCAE are found on CTEP's website (https://dctd.cancer.gov/research/ctep-trials/for-sites/adverse-events#ctep-ctcae), including other related documents (e.g., mapping CTCAE v4.0 to v5.0). OCRNs need to be aware of the CTCAE version that is being used for a protocol. Older protocols may not have transitioned to the current version of the CTCAE. At the time of this writing, CTCAE v6.0 is under development (NCI CTEP, n.d.-a).

How to Read the Common Terminology Criteria for Adverse Events

CTCAE is set up in a table format with 26 MedDRA SOCs listed alphabetically (see Figure 22-2). Within each SOC, AEs are listed alphabetically. Each AE is defined and assigned a numeric grade (grades 1–5), which describes the event that pertains to that term (see Table 22-4). Within the description of the grade, a semicolon (;) is read as an "or" statement, and an em dash (—) indicates that the grade is not available for the specific AE term. Each SOC has an "Other"| option for reporting events not listed in CTCAE

TABLE 22-3 | Historical Timeline of the *Common Terminology Criteria for Adverse Events*

Year and Version	Name	Number of Categories	Number of Terms
1983 Version 1.0	*Common Toxicity Criteria*	18	49
1998 Version 2.0	*Common Toxicity Criteria*	24	295
2003 Version 3.0	*Common Terminology Criteria for Adverse Events*	28	> 900
2010 Version 4.03	*Common Terminology Criteria for Adverse Events*	26 (Categories replaced with Medical Dictionary for Regulatory Affairs System Organ Class)	790 (Adverse event terms replaced with Medical Dictionary for Regulatory Affairs Lowest Level Term)
2017 Version 5.0	*Common Terminology Criteria for Adverse Events*	26	837

Note. Based on information from National Cancer Institute Cancer Therapy Evaluation Program, 2017; Trotti et al., 2003.

- Blood and lymphatic system disorders
- Cardiac disorders
- Congenital, familial, and genetic disorders
- Ear and labyrinth disorders
- Endocrine disorders
- Eye disorders
- Gastrointestinal disorders
- General disorders and administration site conditions
- Hepatobiliary disorders
- Immune system disorders
- Infections and infestations
- Injury, poisoning, and procedural complications
- Investigations
- Metabolism and nutrition disorders
- Musculoskeletal and connective tissue disorders
- Neoplasms benign, malignant, and unspecified (including cysts and polyps)
- Nervous system disorders
- Pregnancy, puerperium, and perinatal conditions
- Psychiatric disorders
- Renal and urinary disorders
- Reproductive system and breast disorders
- Respiratory, thoracic, and mediastinal disorders
- Skin and subcutaneous tissue disorders
- Social circumstances
- Surgical and medical procedures
- Vascular disorders

FIGURE 22-2 | System Organ Class Titles Used in the *Common Terminology Criteria for Adverse Events*

Note. Based on information from National Cancer Institute Cancer Therapy Evaluation Program, 2017.

(NCI CTEP, 2017). General guidelines should be used when assessing the severity of an AE that is not currently available (see Table 22-5).

Patient-Reported Outcomes Version of Common Terminology Criteria for Adverse Events

Many of the AE terms found in CTCAE (approximately 10%) are symptoms or subjective assessments requiring the provider and research team to translate what the patient is describing into an appropriate CTCAE term (Basch et al., 2014; Miller & Aplenc, 2021). These AEs are often referred to as patient-reported outcomes (PROs) and allow for serious events to be reported sooner than an assessment done solely by the provider. Combining patient-reported symptoms with provider assessment can lead to improved safety (Basch et al., 2014; Miller & Aplenc, 2021).

FDA is encouraging drug developers to incorporate the patient perspective in the drug development process and has developed various approaches to assist with this goal (Basch, 2013). As defined by FDA (2009b, p. 2), a PRO is

> any report of the status of a patient's health condition that comes directly from the patient, without interpretation of the patient's response by a clinician or anyone else. The outcome can be measured in absolute terms (e.g., severity of a symptom, sign, or state of a disease) or as a change from a previous measure. In clinical trials, a PRO instrument can be used to measure the effect of a medical intervention on one or more concepts (i.e., the thing being measured, such as a symptom or group of symptoms, effects on a particular function or group of functions, or a group of symptoms or functions shown to measure the severity of a health condition).

In 2008, NCI's PRO-CTCAE project, led by the Division of Cancer Control and Population Sciences, began to develop a valid, reliable, feasible, and clinically useful patient version of the CTCAE, specifically, an electronic system for patient self-reporting of symptom AEs. The PRO-CTCAE measurement system characterizes an AE based on frequency, severity, amount, interference, and presence or absence. The PRO-CTCAE Item Library includes 124 items representing 78 symptomatic events drawn from CTCAE. PRO-CTCAE is available in more than 30 languages.

A pediatric module permits self-reporting by children and adolescents aged 7–17 years. The Ped-PRO-CTCAE

TABLE 22-4 | Common Terminology Criteria for Adverse Events for Anemia

System Organ Class: Blood and lymphatic system disorders					
Adverse Event	**Grade**				
	1	**2**	**3**	**4**	**5**
Anemia	Hgb < LLN–10 g/dl; < LLN–6.2 mmol/L; < LLN–100 g/L	Hgb < 10–8 g/dl; < 6.2–4.9 mmol/L; < 100–80 g/L	Hgb < 8 g/dl; < 4.9 mmol/L; < 80 g/L; transfusion indicated	Life-threatening consequences; urgent intervention indicated	Death
Definition: A disorder characterized by a reduction in the amount of hemoglobin in 100 ml of blood. Signs and symptoms of anemia may include pallor of the skin and mucous membranes, shortness of breath, palpitations of the heart, soft systolic murmurs, lethargy, and fatigability.					

Hgb—hemoglobin; LLN—lower limit of normal

Note. From *Common Terminology Criteria for Adverse Events* [v.5.0], by National Cancer Institute Cancer Therapy Evaluation Program, 2017 (https://ctep.cancer.gov/protocolDevelopment/electronic_applications/docs/CTCA E_v5_Quick_Reference_5x7.pdf). In the public domain.

TABLE 22-5 | Common Terminology Criteria for Adverse Events: Other Adverse Event Terminology

Grade	Description
1	Mild; asymptomatic or mild symptoms; clinical or diagnostic observations only; intervention not indicated
2	Moderate; minimal, local, or noninvasive intervention indicated; limiting age-appropriate instrumental activities of daily living[a]
3	Severe or medically significant but not immediately life-threatening; hospitalization or prolongation of hospitalization indicated; disabling; limiting self-care activities of daily living[b]
4	Life-threatening consequences; urgent intervention indicated
5	Death related to adverse event

[a] Instrumental activities of daily living refers to preparing meals, shopping for groceries or clothes, using the telephone, managing money, and more.

[b] Self-care activities of daily living refers to bathing, dressing and undressing, feeding self, using the toilet, taking medications, and not being bedridden.

Note. From *Common Terminology Criteria for Adverse Events* [v.5.0], by National Cancer Institute Cancer Therapy Evaluation Program, 2017 (https://ctep.cancer.gov/protocolDevelopment/electronic_applications/docs/CTCA E_v5_Quick_Reference_5x7.pdf). In the public domain.

module is available in English, Simplified Chinese, and Italian. A version for caregiver reporting is available for use when children or adolescents aged 7–17 years are unable to self-report. The pediatric module includes 130 items representing 62 symptomatic events drawn from CTCAE. The symptoms used in PRO-CTCAE are MedDRA compliant (NCI, 2025). Updated information about PRO-CTCAE can be viewed at the Division of Cancer Control and Population Sciences website (https://healthcaredelivery.cancer.gov/pro-ctcae/overview.html).

Determining Attribution

Once the severity of the event is established, the next step is to find the cause or attribution of the event. Attribution is the relationship or association between the research and the AE, though for any AE, a cause should be determined. In clinical trials, there can be many challenges when assessing AEs. Protocols are complex and often involve multiple drugs. Patients' prior therapies, concomitant medications, or comorbid diseases may make it difficult to determine the cause of an AE (Callahan et al., 2018; George et al., 2019; NIH VideoCast, 2023b).

OCRNs are typically responsible for gathering initial information about the AE, discussing this with the investigator, and collaborating on further assessments to determine the severity of the AE and its attribution to the research (Oncology Nursing Society [ONS] & Oncology Nursing Certification Corporation [ONCC], 2024). Determining the attribution is performed by the PI with input from the research team, including OCRNs (Callahan et al., 2018; George et al., 2019; NIH VideoCast, 2023b). Figure 22-3 provides a list of questions for the PI and research team to consider when determining the attribution of the AE.

An AE may be considered unrelated or related to the study treatment according to the PI. It has been a long-standing practice in oncology clinical trials to use a five-tier approach when assigning AE attributions. However, recommendations have been made to collapse into a two-tier or three-tier system to improve attribution efficiencies (George et al., 2019). Figure 22-4 describes the three approaches for determining the causal relationship between the research and an AE.

Adverse Event Collection

The assessment of AEs comes from the review of symptoms, the physical examination, and laboratory and radiology results. Before a patient starts a clinical trial, a thorough baseline assessment needs to be conducted, including a physical examination noting any abnormal findings, signs, or symptoms the patient is experiencing at the time the trial begins, their prior medical history, and their current medications. This information is helpful in providing a baseline assessment from which an AE is identified or potentially assigning an attribution.

The collection of AE information begins at the initiation of a study intervention. AE information should be collected from the start of a placebo lead-in period or other observational period intended to establish a baseline status for the patient. The collection period and the data to be collected must be specified in the clinical protocol. AEs should be followed to resolution or stabilization. Follow-up is required for AEs that cause interruption or discontinuation of the study drug or those that are present at the end of study treatment as appropriate (NIH VideoCast, 2023b).

- What is already known about the drug, therapy, or classification of drug?
- What is the temporal relationship of the adverse event to the study therapy?
- Does the adverse event improve or disappear when the drug or therapy is stopped?
- If rechallenged with the drug or therapy, does the adverse event reappear? Does it recur at the same severity and at the same timepoint?
- Is the adverse event a result of an existing disease or condition's signs and symptoms?
- Is the adverse event a worsening of baseline symptoms?
- Is the adverse event a result of an underlying concurrent medical condition or concurrent medication?

FIGURE 22-3 | Questions to Assist in Determining Adverse Event Attribution

5-Tier Attributions
- Unrelated: The AE is clearly not related to the intervention.
- Unlikely related: The AE is doubtfully related to the intervention.
- Possibly related: The AE may be related to the intervention.
- Probably related: The AE is likely related to the intervention.
- Definitely related: The AE is clearly related to the intervention.

2-Tier Attributions
- Unrelated: The AE is clearly not or doubtfully related to the intervention; the AE is more likely related to other causes than the intervention.
- Related: The AE may be or is clearly related to the intervention; the AE is more likely related to the intervention than other causes.

3-Tier Attributions
- Unrelated: The AE is clearly not or doubtfully related to the intervention; the AE is more likely related to other causes than the intervention.
- Related: The AE may be or is clearly related to the intervention; the AE is more likely related to the intervention than other causes.
- Unknown: the AE is equally related to the intervention and other causes.

FIGURE 22-4 | Three Approaches for Adverse Event Attributions

The institutional review board and Office for Human Research Protections look for relevance to the research, and the U.S. Food and Drug Administration looks for relevance to the investigational new drug/investigational device exemption.

AE—adverse event

Note. Based on information from Callahan et al., 2018; George et al., 2019; National Cancer Institute Cancer Therapy Evaluation Program, 2024.

Patients should not be asked direct questions regarding specific events that might be anticipated during the study to prevent the biased collection of AEs. For example, if diarrhea is an anticipated event, the patient should be asked if they have had a change in their bowel habits. Based on the answer, more questions can be asked. Ideally, AEs should be spontaneously reported or elicited from a research participant during open-ended questioning, examination, or evaluation. Sometimes, AE information may need to be collected from a family member or significant other who observes a change in the participant. This may be necessary with some pediatric participants or for individuals with cognitive impairment (NIH VideoCast, 2023b).

OCRNs must assess patients prior to, during, and following treatment on a protocol (ONS & ONCC, 2024). Working in collaboration with other members of the healthcare team, OCRNs should observe, assess, evaluate, and document patients' treatment- and disease-related symptoms. Study documentation and completed case report forms (CRFs) are audited by monitors, sponsors, and FDA to ensure that toxicity assessments are accurate and that protocol treatment modifications are followed.

Patients sometimes have difficulty accurately remembering the onset, severity, and duration of symptoms experienced during therapy. One tool that is often used is a patient diary, which can be combined with a study drug self-administration diary (see Figure 22-5). The collection of AE information is just one use for a diary. Diaries can also serve as source documents and can be paper or electronic (e.g., interactive voice response systems, handheld devices). The protocol should identify the purpose of the diary, the type of diary to be used, how frequently entries are to be made, surrogate completion, and how to handle missing data. For symptom-specific diaries, a quality-of-life survey or PRO tool may be considered.

The use of diaries should also be addressed in the informed consent document and reviewed during the informed consent discussion. OCRNs play a critical role in educating patients on the use of diaries. Patients may need to be reminded to return their diaries at an appointment or to input data if using an electronic system. Diaries should be reviewed with patients and their family members or caregivers at their visit.

If patients are seen or hospitalized at an outside institution, the OCRN will need to obtain these medical records for review or to complete a serious adverse event (SAE) report. Patients may sign a release of information; however, if they are unable to or deceased when the records are sought, the Code of Federal Regulations (C.F.R.) governs the release of information. The Health Insurance Portability and Accountability Act Privacy Rule permits certain disclosures of protected health information under 45 C.F.R. § 164.512 for research purposes. Accessing information on a deceased patient falls under the same regulation; however, the request must state that the patient is deceased and that the information is to be used for research purposes only (NCI CTEP, 2024).

Adverse Event Documentation

It is important for all healthcare providers caring for patients on a clinical trial to document AEs (e.g., physical examination findings, review of systems). All AEs should be documented in the patient's medical records, including any workup or treatment needed, following good clinical research practice documentation (see Chapter 30 for more information). Therefore, a good progress note documenting an AE will contain the following (Callahan et al., 2018):
- Date the AE began, including the time of the infusion reaction
- Description of the event
- Treatment for the AE
- Attribution of the AE
- Dates the AE improved or worsened (i.e., grade changed)
- Date the AE resolved

Keeping track of AEs can be an overwhelming task at times; however, it is crucial for patient safety. Reviewing and seeing trends of AEs in a patient population may alert the PI or sponsor to serious safety concerns. Captur-

Cycle #______ Patient Name________________ Patient Study ID ____________________				
Date	Day	Drug × 10 mg (taken twice a day for 14 days)		
		Time of morning dose	Time of evening dose	Side effects
	1			
	2			
	3			
	4			
	5			
	6			
	7			
	8			
	9			
	10			
	11			
	12			
	13			
	14			

FIGURE 22-5 | Drug Administration and Side Effect Diary Sheet

ing timely and concise information is vital to the management of data. Sponsors may provide study logs to facilitate the capture and overall review of events. However, all AE-related information should be in the medical record so that all healthcare providers are aware of what is happening with their patients.

Adverse Event Recording

Recording AEs (i.e., data extraction or abstraction) onto a CRF is dependent on the protocol. For some protocols, such as phase 1 studies, all AEs will be recorded. Other protocols may only record grade 2–5 events. The protocol should clearly outline what types of AEs will be recorded. Although AE CRFs may differ from sponsor to sponsor, most forms contain the following common elements (Callahan et al., 2018; NIH VideoCast, 2023b).:

- Description of the event
- AE term (e.g., CTCAE, MedDRA)
- Date the AE began
- Treatment for the AE
- Attribution of the AE
- Outcome of the AE
- Date the AE resolved

Always refer to the protocol for events that may not need to be abstracted on the CRF, as well as the CRF completion for additional information on AE recording (Callahan et al., 2018).

Adverse Event Expedited Reporting

A subset of AEs require expedited reporting (sooner than annually) to regulatory groups (i.e., institutional review board [IRB], sponsor, FDA). This reporting includes new and unexpected AEs that impact safety (i.e., risk) and may lead to a revision in the protocol, investigator's brochure, or informed consent. It is important to understand the definitions of *suspected adverse reaction* (SAR), *SAE*, and *unexpected event* to know which types of AEs need to be reported in an expedited manner (see Table 22-1). These definitions, plus the attribution, will drive the expedited reporting requirements for regulatory groups. OCRNs should become familiar with these definitions, as they are usually delegated the responsibility for reporting AEs. Events to be reported in an expedited manner should be defined in the protocol, including the timeline and mechanism (e.g., form, database) for reporting. All expedited reports and any response information from the regulatory or oversight group are considered essential documents to be placed in the regulatory file (see Chapter 32).

Expedited Reporting to the Institutional Review Board

Office for Human Research Protections (OHRP, 2007) regulations do not specifically address AE reporting to the IRB but rather the requirement for reporting unanticipated problems involving risks to research participants (Protection of Human Subjects, 2017). FDA regulations also support the investigator reporting AEs that are unanticipated problems to the IRB, as they have implications for the study (FDA, 2009a; Institutional Review Boards, 1981; Investigational New Drug (IND) Application, 1987). Some unanticipated problems are AEs. Specific to devices, the investigator is to report unanticipated adverse device effects to the IRB within 10 working days after the investigator first learns of the effect (IND Safety Reporting, 1987). ICH (2025) GCP guidelines defer to the local regulatory requirements for reporting of unexpected AEs that are serious and related to the drug.

To meet these requirements, IRBs develop criteria for the reporting of AEs. Many IRBs will only want to have AEs that are also unanticipated problems to be reported; however, OCRNs should be aware of specific protocol requirements and which AEs need to be reported to the IRB in an expedited manner, the time frame, and the format. The time frame can range from 24 hours to 7 days. Many IRBs will use a management system for reporting, often classified as reportable new information. Paper or email documentation is a popular alternative.

Expedited Reporting to the Sponsor

FDA IND regulations and GCP guidelines require the PI to report all SAEs immediately to the sponsor, unless identified in the protocol as not needing immediate (i.e., expedited) reporting (ICH, 2025; IND Application, 1987). *Immediately* is typically within 24 hours, as defined by the sponsor's policy. For studies conducted under an Investigational Device Exemption (IDE), the investigator reporting requirements to the sponsor are the same as to the IRB: unanticipated adverse device effects must be reported to the sponsor within 10 working days after the investigator first learned of the effect (Investigational Device Exemptions, 1980). Each sponsor will have either a form or a database application for reporting expedited AEs. Often these are referred to as an SAE form. OCRNs will need to be familiar with each sponsor's requirements and report forms.

Sometimes, study staff will have limited information. Often, OCRNs or investigators will receive a phone message indicating that a research participant was hospitalized or died. To meet the investigator's reporting requirements to the sponsor, OCRNs or investigators can perform the following (NIH VideoCast, 2023c):

- Contact the treating physician or institution and document all conversations in the medical record.
- Submit what is known, including the following:
  - Most recent clinical evaluations, baseline history, and physical
  - A summary of the event and treatment to date
  - A plan for obtaining information
- Request medical records.

When additional information becomes available, the report is to be amended.

Adverse Events of Special Interest

Additional adverse events may need to be reported in an expedited manner to the sponsor that are not SAEs but could be of scientific or medical concern for the development of the IND product. These are referred to as adverse events of special interest and should be identified in the protocol (Council for International Organizations of Medical Sciences, 2005; NIH VideoCast, 2023c). For example, an IND protocol may require all bleeding AEs to be reported even if they are not an SAE. The reporting mechanism is the same as reporting an SAE to the sponsor.

Reporting to the U.S. Food and Drug Administration

OCRNs may be involved with industry-sponsored IND/IDE protocols or investigator-held IND protocols, making it important to understand the expedited reporting requirements to FDA. Per FDA IND regulations,

> The sponsor must promptly review all information relevant to the safety of the drug obtained or otherwise received by the sponsor from foreign or domestic sources, including information derived from any clinical or epidemiological investigations, animal or in vitro studies, reports in the scientific literature, and unpublished scientific papers, as well as reports from foreign regulatory authorities and reports of foreign commercial marketing experience for drugs that are not marketed in the United States. (FDA, 2009a, para. 6)

The sponsor is to notify FDA and all participating investigators, in writing, about potential serious risks from clinical trials or any other source as soon as possible, but no later than 15 calendar days. In this scenario, participating investigators include all investigators to whom the sponsor is providing drugs or biologics under its INDs or any investigator-held IND. These reports are referred to as IND safety reports (ISRs) (FDA, 2009a; IND Safety Reporting, 1987) (see Table 22-6).

In addition to the ISR, the sponsor must notify FDA of any unexpected fatal or life-threatening SARs as soon as possible, but no later than seven calendar days after the sponsor's initial receipt of the information. The initial contact is by phone or email with a written follow-up report.

TABLE 22-6 | Investigational New Drug Application Safety Reports

Type	Sponsor Responsibilities
Unexpected and suspected serious adverse reaction (SAR)	• Sponsor must report any SAR that is both serious and unexpected. • Sponsor must also report an adverse event (AE) as an SAR only if evidence suggests a causal relationship between the drug and the AE, such as the following: – Single occurrence of an event that is uncommon and known to be strongly associated with drug exposure – One or more occurrences of an event that is not commonly associated with drug exposure but is otherwise uncommon in the population exposed to the drug – Aggregate analysis of specific events observed in a clinical trial that indicates those events occur more frequently in the drug treatment group than in a concurrent or historical control group
Findings from other studies	• Sponsor must report any findings from clinical, epidemiologic, or pooled analysis of multiple studies or any findings from animal or in vitro testing that suggest a significant risk in humans exposed to the drug. • Reports are required for studies from any source, regardless of whether they are conducted under the Investigational New Drug application or by the sponsor.
Findings from animal or in vitro testing	Sponsor must report any findings from animal or in vitro testing, whether or not conducted by the sponsor, that suggest a significant risk in humans exposed to the drug, such as reports of mutagenicity, teratogenicity, carcinogenicity, or reports of significant organ toxicity at or near the expected human exposure. Ordinarily, any such findings would result in a safety-related change in the protocol, informed consent, investigator's brochure (excluding routine updates of these documents), or other aspects of the overall conduct of the clinical investigation.
Increased rate of occurrence of suspected SAR	Sponsor must report any clinically important increase in the rate of a suspected SAR over that listed in the protocol or investigator's brochure.

Note. Based on information from IND Safety Reporting, 1987.

Upon request from FDA, the sponsor must submit any additional data or information that the agency deems necessary as soon as possible, but no later than 15 calendar days after receiving the request (FDA, 2012).

FDA allows for various formats for the written report, including the following (IND Safety Reporting, 1987):

- General narrative summary for ISRs that include overall findings or pooled analyses from published and unpublished in vitro, animal, epidemiologic, or clinical studies
- MedWatch Form FDA 3500A, mandatory reporting form, which is the most common format, located on the FDA forms website (www.fda.gov/AboutFDA/ReportsManualsForms/Forms/default.htm)
- Council for International Organizations of Medical Sciences I Form, which is used with international studies
- FDA Safety Reporting Portal (www.safetyreporting.hhs.gov), which is for drugs and biologics

The sponsor's report to FDA will include all previously submitted ISRs for similar SARs and analyze the significance of the SAR, considering previous similar reports or any other relevant information (IND Safety Reporting, 1987). Sponsors will sometimes send SAE reports that do not meet the criteria to be an ISR; however, a true ISR will result in a protocol, and possibly a consent or amendment. Figure 22-6 describes what the investigator should do with an ISR.

For IDE studies, the sponsor needs to evaluate any unanticipated adverse device effects immediately, determine if there is an unreasonable risk to research participants, and terminate all investigations or parts of investigations presenting that risk as soon as possible. Termination shall occur no later than five working days after the sponsor makes this determination and no later than 15 working days after the sponsor first received notice of the effect (Investigational Device Exemptions, 1980). The report is written in a narrative format.

Report Forms

Regardless of the regulatory group to which OCRNs are reporting, each report form will have similar elements,

- Principal investigator reviews the safety report.
- Principal investigator sends to subinvestigators and clinical research nurses.
- Principal investigator assesses the need to amend the protocol and consent documents.
- Safety report is submitted to the institutional review board per local policy.
- All safety reports are placed in a regulatory file.
- Principal investigator amends protocol and consent documents as needed.
- Principal investigator or clinical research nurse informs currently enrolled patients immediately (i.e., by phone) of new potential risk and documents conversation and patients' willingness to continue on study in the medical record.
- Principal investigator or clinical research nurse reconsents patients as guided by the institutional review board or sponsor.

FIGURE 22-6 | Site Processing of an Investigational New Drug Safety Report

Note. Based on information from Callahan et al., 2018.

including reporter information, participant demographics, study agent or intervention information (e.g., dates given, dose, route of administration), events, attribution, and narrative summary (Callahan et al., 2018; NIH VideoCast, 2023c). The narrative summary is the most important part of the report and provides the background information necessary to assess the event and support the investigator's attribution. This is essential, as the individual or group receiving the report typically does not know anything about the patient. When describing the event, the reporter should provide information that puts it into perspective, including relevant patient history, such as underlying medical conditions, prior surgeries or procedures, family history, recent events that may be a contributing factor, or concomitant medications (Callahan et al., 2018; NIH VideoCast, 2023c).

Some sponsors may require other CRFs (e.g., medical history, AE) to be submitted along with the expedited report, but this is less common with an electronic reporting system. It can be beneficial to send related source documentation (e.g., discharge summary, radiology report) with the expedited report, as this can help explain the event and treatment and support the differential diagnosis or investigator's attribution. OCRNs should be aware of the sponsor and regulatory group processes for submitting additional information (NIH VideoCast, 2023c).

Voluntary Postmarketing Surveillance Programs

AEs not listed in the current labeling of a product or an SAE can be reported voluntarily by either patients or healthcare professionals via FDA's Safety Information and Adverse Event Reporting Program. OCRNs can visit the website to learn more, access a report form, and submit a report: www.fda.gov/drugs/surveillance/postmarketing-surveillance-programs.

Unanticipated Problems

Unanticipated problems are incidents, experiences, or outcomes that meet all the following criteria (OHRP, 2007):

- Unexpected, in terms of nature, severity, or frequency, given the research described in the IRB-approved protocol and informed consent documents, investigator's brochure, and the characteristics of the population being studied
- Related or possibly related to participation in the research
- Suggests the research may place participants or others at a greater risk of harm (e.g., physical, psychological, economic, social) than previously recognized

Some unanticipated problems will include AEs, but not all unanticipated problems are AEs (see Figure 22-7). The investigator can take several steps to identify if the incident, experience, or outcome is an unanticipated problem (see Figure 22-8). FDA considers AEs as unanticipated problems only if the AE was unexpected and serious and would have implications for the conduct of the study (e.g., change in protocol or investigator's brochure). In other words, it is an event that would be included in an ISR (FDA, 2009a).

Determine if the event or incident is an adverse event or non–adverse event.

- Adverse event: Any untoward medical occurrence, including any abnormal sign, symptom, or disease, associated with the patient's participation in research (e.g., an abnormal physical examination or laboratory finding).
- Non–adverse event: Nonmedical events that may involve social or economic harm rather than physical or psychological harm (e.g., breach of privacy that leads to stigma or loss of insurance coverage, false HIV-positive testing). This can include protocol deviations and noncompliance.

Determine if the event is serious or nonserious.

- Serious: Event results in death, hospitalization, significant disability, is life threatening, or requires immediate action by the principal investigator to protect the rights, safety, or well-being of the participants or others (e.g., admission to the intensive care unit, reporting a confidentiality breach).
- Nonserious: Event suggests that the participant or others may be placed at an increased risk of harm, but the event was not serious or the participant did not suffer harm. However, as a result, substantive changes to the protocol, consent, conduct of the study, or other corrective actions are required to protect participants or others. This could include a series of adverse events that occurred at a greater frequency or severity than was previously known.

Determine if the event is related to the research.

The event results from participation in research (e.g., research procedures, interventions, investigational or approved drugs/devices used for a new indication or a new method of delivery) and may also affect participant providers.

Determine if the event is expected.

The event is listed as a risk in the protocol, consent, or investigator's brochure.

FIGURE 22-7 | Steps to Determine if an Event Is an Unanticipated Problem

Note. Based on information from Office for Human Research Protections, 2007.

Once an unanticipated problem is identified, the next steps include developing a corrective action plan and reporting the problem to the IRB and other institutional officials. A corrective action plan can include any of the following activities (NIH VideoCast, 2023d; OHRP, 2007):

- Revise the protocol (e.g., modify inclusion or exclusion criteria to mitigate the newly identified risks, implement additional procedures for monitoring participants).
- Suspend enrollment of new participants.
- Revise the informed consent document (e.g., provide additional information about newly recognized risks to previously enrolled participants, inform enrolled participants).
- Increase monitoring activities.
- Provide staff training or retraining.
- Work with appropriate institutional officials to correct the problem.

Adverse Event

- A participant with chronic gastroesophageal reflux disease enrolls in a randomized, placebo-controlled, double-blind, phase 3 clinical trial evaluating a new investigational agent that blocks acid release in the stomach. Two weeks after being randomized and started on the study intervention, the participant develops acute kidney failure as evidenced by an increase in serum creatinine from 1 mg/dl prerandomization to 5 mg/dl. The known risk profile of the investigational agent does not include renal toxicity, and the institutional review board–approved protocol and informed consent document for the study do not identify kidney damage as a risk of the research. Evaluation of the participant reveals no other apparent cause for acute renal failure. The investigator concludes that the episode of acute renal failure was probably due to the investigational agent. This is an example of an unanticipated problem that must be reported because the participant's acute renal failure was unexpected, related to participation in the research, and serious.
- The fifth participant enrolled in a phase 2, open-label, uncontrolled clinical study evaluating the safety and efficacy of a new oral agent administered daily for treatment of severe psoriasis unresponsive to U.S. Food and Drug Administration–approved treatments develops severe hepatic failure complicated by encephalopathy a month after starting the oral agent. The known risk profile of the new oral agent prior to this event included mild elevation of serum liver enzymes in 10% of participants receiving the agent during previous clinical studies, but there was no other history of participants developing clinically significant liver disease. The institutional review board–approved protocol and informed consent document for the study identify mild liver injury as a risk of the research. The investigators identify no other etiology for the liver failure in this participant and attribute it to the study agent. This is an example of an unanticipated problem that must be reported because although the risk of mild liver injury was foreseen, severe liver injury resulting in hepatic failure was unexpected in severity, possibly related to participation in the research, and serious.

Non–Adverse Event

- Patients with cancer are enrolled in a phase 2 clinical trial evaluating an investigational biologic product derived from human sera. After several participants are enrolled and receive the investigational product, a study audit reveals that the investigational product administered to them was obtained from donors who were not appropriately screened and tested for several potential viral contaminants, including HIV and the hepatitis B virus. This constitutes an unanticipated problem that must be reported because the incident was unexpected, was related to participation in the research, and placed participants and others at a greater risk of physical harm than was previously known or recognized.
- An investigator conducting behavioral research collects individually identifiable sensitive information about illicit drug use and other illegal behaviors by surveying college students. The data are stored on a laptop computer without encryption, and the laptop computer is stolen from the investigator's car on the way home from work. This is an unanticipated problem that must be reported because the incident was unexpected (i.e., the investigators did not anticipate the theft), was related to participation in the research, and placed participants at a greater risk of psychological and social harm from the breach in confidentiality of the study data than was previously known or recognized.

FIGURE 22-8 | Examples of Unanticipated Problems That Must Be Reported Under the U.S. Department of Health and Human Services Regulations

Note. Based on information from Office for Human Research Protections, 2007; Protection of Human Subjects, 2017.

OHRP regulations state that the investigator should promptly report all unanticipated problems to the IRB; however, *prompt* is not defined. Instead, OHRP (2007) recommends the following based on certain criteria:

- An unanticipated problem that is also an SAE should be reported to the IRB within seven days of the investigator's notification of the event because it could have a direct impact on the protocol's risk assessment and other research participants.
- All other unanticipated problems are to be reported to the IRB within 14 days.
- All unanticipated problems need to be reported to appropriate institutional officials (as required by an institution's written procedures), the supporting agency head or designee, and OHRP within one month of the IRB's receipt of the unanticipated problem report from the investigator.

FDA defers to the IRB's process, and ICH GCP guidelines reference prompt reporting of unexpected, serious AEs related to the product (ICH, 2025; Protection of Human Subjects, 2017). The unanticipated problem report should include a detailed description of the problem, an explanation of the basis for determining that the event is an unanticipated problem, and a description of any changes to the protocol or other corrective actions that have been taken or are proposed in response. OCRNs should know how to report unanticipated problems to the various IRBs that they encounter.

National Cancer Institute–Sponsored Clinical Trials and Adverse Events

Protocols sponsored by NCI are required to follow the *NCI Guidelines for investigators: Adverse event reporting requirements for DCTD (CTEP and CIP), INDs, and IDEs* (NCI CTEP, 2024). The guidelines describe criteria for routine and expedited AE reporting, including how to report and how to handle persistent and recurrent AEs (see Figure 22-9). The PI has the primary responsibility for AE identification, documentation, grading, and assignment of attribution and will provide medical documentation needed to support the expedited AE report. The PI must report any SAE to the NCI sponsor by following expedited reporting guidelines (NCI, 2024). The protocol will include the reporting requirement outlined in the guidelines.

Expedited Reporting Requirements for Adverse Events That Occur on Studies Under an IND/IDE Within 30 Days of the Last Administration of the Investigational Agent/Intervention [1,2]

Note. Investigators MUST immediately report to the sponsor (NCI) **ANY** SAEs, whether or not they are considered related to the investigational agent(s)/intervention (21 C.F.R. § 312.64)

An AE is considered serious if it results in ANY of the following outcomes:
- Death
- A life-threatening AE
- An AE that results in inpatient hospitalization or prolongation of existing hospitalization for ≥ 24 hours
- A persistent or significant incapacity or substantial disruption of the ability to conduct normal life functions
- A congenital anomaly/birth defect
- Important Medical Events (IME) that may not result in death, be life threatening, or require hospitalization may be considered serious when, based upon medical judgment, they may jeopardize the patient or subject and may require medical or surgical intervention to prevent one of the outcomes listed in this definition (FDA, 21 C.F.R. § 312.32; ICH E2A and ICH E6).

ALL SAEs that meet the above criteria **MUST** be immediately reported to the NCI via CTEP-AERS within the timeframes detailed in the table below.

Grade 1–2 Timeframes	Grade 3–5 Timeframes
24-Hour notification, 10 Calendar Days	24-Hour notification, 5 Calendar Days

Note. Protocol-specific exceptions to expedited reporting of SAEs are found in the Specific Protocol Exceptions to Expedited Reporting (SPEER) portion of the CAEPR.

Expedited AE reporting timelines are defined as:
- "24-Hour; 5 Calendar Days"- The SAE must initially be reported via CTEP-AERS within 24 hours of learning of the SAE, followed by a complete expedited report within 5 calendar days of the initial 24-hour report.
- "24-Hour notification, 10 Calendar Days"- The SAE must initially be reported via CTEP-AERS within 24 hours of learning of the SAE, followed by a complete expedited report within 10 calendar days of the initial 24-hour report.

[1]SAEs that occur more than 30 days after the last administration of investigational agent/intervention and have an attribution of possible, probable, or definite require reporting as follows:

Expedited 24-Hour notifications are required for all SAEs followed by a complete report
- Within 5 calendar days for grade 3–5 SAEs
- Within 10 calendar days for grade 1–2 SAEs

[2]For studies using nuclear medicine or molecular imaging IND agents (NM, SPECT, or PET), the SAE reporting period is limited to 10 radioactive half-lives, rounded UP to the nearest whole day, after the agent/intervention was last administered. Footnote "1" above applies after this reporting period.

Effective Date: August 30, 2024

FIGURE 22-9 | Phase 1 and Early Phase 2 Studies

AE—adverse event; CAEPR—Comprehensive Adverse Events and Potential Risks List; C.F.R.—Code of Federal Regulations; CTEP-AERS—Cancer Therapy Evaluation Program Adverse Event Reporting System; FDA—U.S. Food and Drug Administration; ICH—International Conference on Harmonisation of Technical Requirements for Pharmaceuticals for Human Use; IDE—Investigational Device Exemption; IND—Investigational New Drug; NCI—National Cancer Institute; NM—nuclear medicine; PET—positron-emission tomography; SAE—serious adverse event; SPECT—single photon emission computed tomography

Note. From *NCI Guidelines for Investigators: Adverse Event Reporting Requirements for DCTD (CTEP and CIP) INDs and IDEs* (pp. 31–32), by National Cancer Institute Cancer Therapy Evaluation Program, 2024 (https://dctd.cancer.gov/research/ctep-trials/for-sites/adverse-events/reporting-requirements.pdf). In the public domain.

Adverse Event Reporting System

Expedited AEs are submitted through the CTEP-AERS (NCI CTEP, n.d.-b). Information about CTEP-AERS and how to subscribe to the distribution list is available at https://dctd.cancer.gov/research/ctep-trials/for-sites/adverse-events#adverse-event-reporting-aer-requirements-and-ctep-aers Note that CTEP-AERS has been integrated with CTEP's Rave database (i.e., electronic CRFs). The protocol will describe the process for initiating an SAE submission via the AE CRF in Rave. This will start the SAE report in AERS so the SAE report can be completed and submitted.

Comprehensive Adverse Events and Potential Risks List

The Comprehensive Adverse Events and Potential Risks (CAEPR) list is an NCI-generated list of reported and potential AEs associated with an agent under an NCI IND or IDE. Information contained in the CAEPR is compiled from the following (NCI CTEP, 2024):
- Investigator's brochures
- Package inserts (for investigational agents that are available commercially)
- Instructions for use (for a device)

- Company safety reports
- AEs submitted through CTEP-AERS
- Peer-reviewed publications that have safety information not included in the current investigator's brochure or package insert

Initially, the CAEPR list will not show a frequency for the events (i.e., likely [> 20%], less likely [≤ 20%], rare but serious [< 3%]), but as AE information is collected, the CAEPR list will be updated to contain AE frequency. This can be helpful to the PI and OCRNs when developing the informed consent document. The list is set up as a table and follows the CTCAE in structure (see Figure 22-10). NCI requires the inclusion of a CAEPR list in all studies conducted under an NCI IND and all studies reviewed by CTEP or the NCI Cancer Imaging Program that include investigational agents and interventions for which NCI has a CAEPR. However, other studies may use the CAEPR list.

The last column in the CAEPR list is a subset list known as the Specific Protocol Exceptions to Expedited Reporting (SPEER). The SPEER is specific to the protocol and provides guidelines on what is considered a reportable or expedited AE to report (NCI CTEP, 2024). AEs should be reported on the SPEER list only if they exceed the grade noted in parentheses next to the AE in the SPEER. If a drug specific–CAEPR is part of a combination protocol using multiple investigational agents and has an AE listed on different SPEER lists, the lower of the grades should be used to determine if expedited reporting is required. When the CAEPR list is updated, the SPEER list is also revised. The revisions are sent to all PIs registered to NCI-approved studies using the agent or agents.

Commercial agents are available to the public and are not provided under an IND. These agents may be considered investigational agents when the indication for use is not FDA approved. Protocols may contain a combination of an investigational agent and a commercial agent. When an AE occurs with a commercial agent, it may or may not be reported in CTEP-AERS and may be reported voluntarily through commercial reporting of MedWatch. When a protocol uses a commercial drug and an investigational drug

Adverse Events With Possible Relationship to Drug X (CTCAE 4.0 Term) [N = 1,141]			Specific Protocol Exceptions to Expedited Reporting (SPEER)
Likely (>20%)	**Less Likely (≤20%)**	**Rare but Serious (<3%)**	
Blood and Lymphatic System Disorders			
Anemia			Anemia (grade 4)
	Disseminated intravascular coagulation		Disseminated intravascular coagulation (grade 4)
	Febrile neutropenia		Febrile neutropenia (grade 4)
	Hemolysis		Hemolysis (grade 1)
Cardiac Disorders			
	Atrial fibrillation		Atrial fibrillation (grade 4)
	Atrial flutter		Atrial flutter (grade 1)
	Paroxysmal atrial tachycardia		Paroxysmal atrial tachycardia (grade 2)
	Sinus bradycardia		Sinus bradycardia (grade 3)
	Sinus tachycardia		Sinus tachycardia (grade 3)
	Supraventricular tachycardia		Supraventricular tachycardia (grade 4)
	Ventricular arrhythmia		Ventricular arrhythmia (grade 4)
	Ventricular fibrillation		Ventricular fibrillation (grade 4)

FIGURE 22-10 | Sample Comprehensive Adverse Event and Potential Risks List

Note. From *NCI Guidelines for Investigators: Adverse Event Reporting Requirements for DCTD (CTEP and CIP) INDs and IDEs* (p. 38), by National Cancer Institute Cancer Therapy Evaluation Program, 2024 (https://dctd.cancer.gov/research/ctep-trials/for-sites/adverse-events/reporting-requirements.pdf). In the public domain.

in a treatment arm, expedited reporting is required (NCI CTEP, 2024).

Summary

Understanding AEs and unanticipated problems takes time. There are many terms to learn and regulations to understand. Each AE may have multiple regulatory groups with their reporting requirements. OCRNs play a pivotal role in the comprehensive assessment and reporting of AEs and unanticipated problems that occur during a clinical trial. A quick way to learn about or refresh knowledge about AEs and unanticipated problems is to read the OHRP (2007) and FDA (2009a) guidance documents. OCRNs working on NCI-sponsored trials should also read the NCI CTEP (2024) guidelines. Vigilant AE assessment, monitoring, and reporting ultimately ensure the protection of research participants; OCRNs are in the best position to play a pivotal role in this process.

Key Points

- An AE is any unwanted sign, symptom, or disease that was not seen before an individual's research participation, or a worsening of a baseline symptom, regardless of expectedness of the event or relationship of the event to the research.
- AE assessment consists of selecting the correct AE term, identifying the expectedness of the event, assessing the severity of the event, and determining the attribution of the event.
- It is crucial to understand how to collect and solicit information about AEs. OCRNs are well-positioned to assist with AE assessment and are often the participants' first point of contact.
- CTCAE is an agreed-upon terminology by experts in the oncology community for the designation, reporting, and grading of AEs that occur in oncology clinical trials.
- OCRNs should refer to the protocol for the version of CTCAE that is being used.
- Events to be reported in an expedited manner should be defined in the protocol, including the timeline and mechanism for reporting.
- A unanticipated problem is an incident, experience, or outcome that is (a) unexpected (in terms of nature, severity, or frequency) given the research described in the IRB-approved protocol, informed consent documents, the investigator's brochures, and the characteristics of the population being studied; (b) related or possibly related to participation in the research; and (c) suggests the research may place the participants or others at a greater risk of harm (e.g., physical, psychological, economic, social).
- Protocols sponsored by NCI are required to follow *NCI Guidelines for Investigators: Adverse Event Reporting Requirements for DCTD (CTEP and CIP) and INDs and IDEs*.

The author would like to acknowledge Ann M. Lau Clark, MSN, RN, CCRC, CCRP, for her contribution to this chapter that remains unchanged from the previous edition of this book.

References

American Nurses Association. (2024). *Clinical research nursing: Scope and standards of practice* (2nd ed.). Author.

Basch, E. (2013). Toward patient-centered drug development in oncology. *New England Journal of Medicine, 369*(5), 397–400. https://doi.org/10.1056/NEJMp1114649

Basch, E., Reeve, B.B., Mitchell, S.A., Clauser, S.B., Minasian, L.M., Dueck, A.C., ... Schrag, D. (2014). Development of the National Cancer Institute's Patient-Reported Outcomes version of the *Common Terminology Criteria for Adverse Events* (PRO-CTCAE). *Journal of the National Cancer Institute, 106*(9), dju244. https://doi.org/10.1093/jnci/dju244

Callahan, A., Ness, E., & Chen, H. (2018). Monitoring, assessing, and reporting adverse events. In W.K. Kelly & S. Halabi (Eds.), *Oncology clinical trials: Successful design, conduct, and analysis* (2nd ed., pp. 207–220). Springer. https://doi.org/10.1891/9780826168733.0023

Council for International Organizations of Medical Sciences. (2005). *Management of safety information from clinical trials: Report of CIOMS Working Group VI.* https://cioms.ch/wp-content/uploads/2017/01/Mgment_Safety_Info.pdf

George, G.C., Barata, P.C., Campbell, A., Chen, A., Cortes, J.E., Hyman, D.M., ... Hong, D.S. (2019). Improving attribution of adverse events in oncology clinical trials. *Cancer Treatment Reviews, 76*, 33–40. https://doi.org/10.1016/j.ctrv.2019.04.004

IND Safety Reporting, 21 C.F.R. § 312.32 (1987). https://www.ecfr.gov/current/title-21/chapter-I/subchapter-D/part-312/subpart-B/section-312.32

Institutional Review Boards, 21 C.F.R. § 56 (1981). https://www.ecfr.gov/current/title-21/chapter-I/subchapter-A/part-56

International Council for Harmonisation of Technical Requirements for Pharmaceuticals for Human Use. (2025). *ICH harmonised guideline: Guideline for good clinical practice: E6(R3).* https://database.ich.org/sites/default/files/ICH_E6%28R3%29_Step4_FinalGuideline_2025_0106.pdf

Investigational Device Exemptions, 21 C.F.R. § 812 (1980). https://www.ecfr.gov/current/title-21/chapter-I/subchapter-H/part-812

Investigational New Drug Application, 21 C.F.R. § 312 (1987). https://www.ecfr.gov/current/title-21/chapter-I/subchapter-D/part-312

Medical Dictionary for Regulatory Activities. (n.d.). *Frequently asked questions.* http://www.meddra.org/faq

Miller, T.P., & Aplenc, R. (2021). Evolution of hematology clinical trial adverse event reporting to improve care delivery. *Current Hematologic Malignancy Reports, 16*(2), 126–131. https://doi.org/10.1007/s11899-021-00627-3

National Cancer Institute. (2025). *Patient-Reported Outcomes version of the Common Terminology Criteria for Adverse Events (PRO-CTCAE).* https://healthcaredelivery.cancer.gov/pro-ctcae

National Cancer Institute Cancer Therapy Evaluation Program. (n.d.-a). *Adverse events: Adverse effects.* https://ctep.cancer.gov/protocolDevelopment/adverse_effects.htm

National Cancer Institute Cancer Therapy Evaluation Program. (n.d.-b). *Adverse events: Electronic applications.* https://ctep.cancer.gov/protocolDevelopment/electronic_applications/adverse_events.htm

National Cancer Institute Cancer Therapy Evaluation Program. (2017). *Common terminology criteria for adverse events* [v.5.0]. https://dctd.cancer.gov/research/ctep-trials/for-sites/adverse-events/ctcae-v5-8x11.pdf

National Cancer Institute Cancer Therapy Evaluation Program. (2024). *NCI Guidelines for investigators: Adverse event reporting requirements for DCTD (CTEP and CIP) INDs and IDEs.* https://dctd.cancer.gov/research/ctep-trials/for-sites/adverse-events/reporting-requirements.pdf

National Institutes of Health VideoCast. (2023a, August 31). *Adverse event reporting: Part 1 of 4* [Video]. YouTube. https://youtu.be/lQr3hls5KFY?si=CkcyC32ruE0dm8Os

National Institutes of Health VideoCast. (2023b, August 31). *Adverse Event Reporting: Part 2 of 4* [Video]. YouTube. https://www.youtube.com/watch?v=EKh_V5F0ETk

National Institutes of Health VideoCast. (2023c, August 31). *Adverse Event Reporting: Part 3 of 4* [Video]. YouTube. https://www.youtube.com/watch?v=XG2JbRhjrCk

National Institutes of Health VideoCast. (2023d, August 31). *Adverse Event Reporting: Part 4 of 4* [Video]. YouTube. https://www.youtube.com/watch?v=tywN1bgjIuI

Office for Human Research Protections. (2007). *Reviewing and reporting unanticipated problems involving risks to subjects or others and adverse events: OHRP guidance.* https://www.hhs.gov/ohrp/regulations-and-policy/guidance/reviewing-unanticipated-problems/index.html

Oncology Nursing Society & Oncology Nursing Certification Corporation. (2024). *Oncology clinical research nurse competencies.* https://www.ons.org/sites/default/files/2025-01/ocrn-competencies-rebrand.pdf

Protection of Human Subjects, 45 C.F.R. § 46 (2017). https://www.ecfr.gov/current/title-45/subtitle-A/subchapter-A/part-46

Trotti, A., Colevas, A.D., Setser, A., & Basch, E. (2007). Patient-reported outcomes and the evolution of adverse event reporting in oncology. *Journal of Clinical Oncology, 25*(32), 5121–5127. https://doi.org/10.1200/JCO.2007.12.4784

Trotti, A., Colevas, A.D., Setser, A., Rusch, V., Jaques, D., Budach, V., ... Rubin, P. (2003). CTCAE v3.0: Development of a comprehensive grading system for the adverse effects of cancer treatment. *Seminars in Radiation Oncology, 13*(3), 176–181. https://doi.org/10.1016/S1053-4296(03)00031-6

U.S. Food and Drug Administration. (2007, September). *Guidance for industry: Toxicity grading scale for healthy adult and adolescent volunteers enrolled in preventive vaccine clinical trials.* http://www.fda.gov/downloads/BiologicsBloodVaccines/GuidanceComplianceRegulatoryInformation/Guidances/Vaccines/ucm091977.pdf

U.S. Food and Drug Administration. (2009a, January). *Adverse event reporting to IRBs—Improving human subject protection.* https://www.fda.gov/regulatory-information/search-fda-guidance-documents/adverse-event-reporting-irbs-improving-human-subject-protection

U.S. Food and Drug Administration. (2009b, December). *Patient-reported outcome measures: Use in medical product development to support labeling claims.* https://www.fda.gov/regulatory-information/search-fda-guidance-documents/patient-reported-outcome-measures-use-medical-product-development-support-labeling-claims

U.S. Food and Drug Administration. (2012). *Guidance for industry and investigators: Safety reporting requirements for INDs and BA/BE studies.* https://www.fda.gov/downloads/Drugs/Guidances/UCM227351.pdf

CHAPTER 23

Patient and Caregiver Education

Patricia Shannon, BS, RN, OCN®

Introduction

Patients with cancer and their caregivers require personalized education, especially when deciding to participate in a clinical trial. Oncology clinical research nurses (OCRNs) need to assess factors such as distress, learning needs, and readiness to learn to ensure that patients and caregivers understand and are fully informed. Additional elements that contribute to patients' ability to receive or absorb education that may not be readily evident are physical or learning disabilities, poor health literacy, mental health challenges, and economic and social issues (Snively, 2023). Therefore, patient and caregiver education are an ongoing process and need to be assessed and reinforced at each visit (Oncology Nursing Society, 2023).

This chapter will detail patient and caregiver education specifically related to clinical trial participation. By using health literacy tools, OCRNs can effectively assess learning needs, readiness to learn, and different learning styles. This chapter will also outline how to assess distress and psychological challenges as patients move through the healthcare continuum.

Health Literacy

Health literacy is defined as the ability to obtain, process, and understand basic health information and services, make informed healthcare decisions (act on information), and access or navigate care systems (Centers for Disease Control and Prevention [CDC], 2024b). All patients and caregivers are at risk of not understanding health information. To remedy this gap, the Agency for Healthcare Research and Quality (AHRQ) has developed a Health Literacy Universal Precautions Toolkit to help practitioners to "reduce the complexity of healthcare, increase patient understanding of health information, and enhance support for patients of all health literacy levels" (AHRQ, n.d., para. 6).

Health Literacy in Healthy People 2030 looks at health literacy from a personal and organizational standpoint. *Personal health literacy* is defined as "the degree to which individuals have the ability to find, understand, and use information and services to inform health-related decisions and actions for themselves and others" (Office of Disease Prevention and Health Promotion, n.d., para. 2). *Organizational health literacy* is defined as "the degree to which organizations enable individuals to find, understand, and use information and services to inform health-related decisions and actions for themselves and others" (Office of Disease Prevention and Health Promotion, n.d., para. 2).

The overarching goal is to "eliminate health disparities, achieve improved health for all, and attain health literacy to improve the health and well-being of all" (Office of Disease Prevention and Health Promotion, n.d., para. 1). Key benefits of health literacy have been identified as the following (CDC, 2025; World Health Organization [WHO], 2024a, 2024b):

- **Improved health outcomes:** Health-literate individuals are more likely to follow medical advice, adhere to treatment plans, and manage chronic conditions effectively, leading to better health outcomes and reduced healthcare costs.
- **Empowerment:** Health literacy empowers individuals to take control of their health. When people understand their health conditions, medications, and treatment options, they can actively participate in their care.
- **Preventive measures:** Health-literate individuals are better equipped to prevent illnesses. They understand the importance of preventive measures, such as vaccinations, screenings, and healthy lifestyle choices.
- **Reduced health disparities:** Improving health literacy can reduce disparities in health outcomes among different populations. When everyone has access to accurate health information, it promotes equity in health care.
- **Effective communication:** Health literacy enhances communication between patients and healthcare provid-

ers. Clear communication ensures that patients understand diagnoses, treatment plans, and potential risks.
- **Cost savings:** Health-literate individuals are less likely to misuse healthcare services or seek unnecessary treatments, leading to cost savings for individuals and healthcare systems.

Organizational Health Literacy

AHRQ has identified four key domains for organizations that help patients and caregivers on their journey: assessing organizational structure, policy, and leadership; enhancing patient and provider communication; improving ease of navigation; and supporting patient self-management (Brach, 2024). Organizations can help patients and caregivers by creating and providing information and services that they can understand and use most effectively with their current skillset (CDC, 2024a).

In a discussion paper published in 2012, the Institute of Medicine, now the National Academy of Medicine, detailed the 10 attributes of healthcare organizations (Brach et al., 2012, p. 3):
- Has leadership that makes health literacy integral to its mission, structure, and operations
- Integrates health literacy into planning, evaluation measures, patient safety, and quality improvement
- Prepares the workforce to be health literate and monitors progress
- Includes populations served in the design, implementation, and evaluation of health information and services
- Meets the needs of populations with a range of health literacy skills while avoiding stigmatization
- Uses health literacy strategies in interpersonal communications and confirms understanding at all points of contact
- Provides easy access to health information and services and navigation assistance
- Designs and distributes print, audiovisual, and social media content that is easy to understand and act on
- Addresses health literacy in high-risk situations, including care transitions and communications about medicines
- Communicates clearly what health plans cover and what individuals will have to pay for services

Plain Language

According to CDC, using plain language makes it easier for everyone to understand and use health information. The Plain Writing Act, signed into law on October 13, 2010, requires federal agencies to use clear communication that the public can understand (CDC, 2025). CDC also developed an interactive webpage, *Everyday Words for Public Health Communication*, which lists terms frequently used in public health materials and their common, everyday alternatives (www.cdc.gov/ccindex/everydaywords/index.html).

Examples of using plain language over complex words when speaking to patients and their caregivers include the following:
- *Stomach* instead of *abdomen*
- *Medicine* or *drug* instead of *medication*
- *Tube* instead of *catheter*
- *Treatment* instead of *therapy*

The third edition of the *AHRQ Health Literacy Universal Precautions Toolkit* provides the Communication Observation Form to give feedback to OCRNs and other healthcare providers educating patients (AHRQ, 2024a).

Effective Patient Education Messaging

One of the basic principles of the *AHRQ Health Literacy Universal Precautions Toolkit* is to treat all patients as if they may have difficulty understanding how to manage their health concerns, regardless of their educational level. OCRNs must have an understanding of the personal and learning needs of patients and caregivers. This can be accomplished by applying health literacy universal precautions and a basic assessment of the patient's desire to learn, their religious or cultural beliefs, potential emotional barriers, cognitive and physical limitations, and possible communication barriers assessing the patient's needs, concerns, preferences, and readiness to learn (Gusman, 2022; Mirabella et al., 2022).

From a patient education perspective, OCRNs need to teach all patients as if they have low health literacy (Brach, 2024; Cutilli, 2020). Research has demonstrated that a multimodal approach to educating patients is more effective than a single mode.

Learning Needs

OCRNs need to obtain a baseline assessment of patients' knowledge, skills, behaviors, and attitudes. The assessment should be taken at each patient encounter to assess the patient and caregiver understanding, learning needs, knowledge gaps, and compliance, as well as the efficacy of interventions (Anderson et al., 2020; Oncology Nursing Society & Oncology Nursing Certification Corporation, 2024). A *knowledge gap* or *learning need* refers to the difference between the current and desired levels of knowledge, skills, behaviors, or attitudes that a patient needs to effectively manage their care, maintain their health, or improve their condition. Health behavior theories suggest that people are more likely to adhere to treatment protocols when they understand the disease and treatment (Christiansen et al.,

2023). When speaking with patients and caregivers about their learning needs, OCRNs should ask open-ended questions. Asking patients and caregivers, "What are you worried about?" demonstrates that OCRNs are listening and focused on their perspective (Cutilli, 2020; Mirabella et al., 2022). Topics to consider when assessing learning needs include, but are not limited to, the following (MedlinePlus, 2023; Ohio State University, n.d.):

- Previous health instruction and experience in health care
- Learning needs and readiness to learn
- Understanding health benefits and cultural practices
- Comprehending and applying health information
- Performing a skill
- Adhering to treatment or protocol
- Learning about financial and other resources

Additionally, issues identified for families of children with cancer in accepting clinical trial participation include the following (Pritchard-Jones, 2008):

- Understanding what is meant by a clinical trial
- Understanding that a trial means that their child is not being experimented on, but is being offered the best-known treatment for their situation
- Understanding the questions that the trial is asking and what they mean for their child
- Understanding the relative risks of side effects and keeping these in proportion
- Being asked to involve a competent child in decision-making when they might not wish to worry them about the possibility of non-cure or details of treatment side effects.

The six domains of patient-centered communication are highlighted in Figure 23-1.

Learning Styles

Each patient and caregiver receives and processes information differently (see Table 23-1). Education does not automatically lead to learning. "Learning is a cognitive process by the learner that generates a change in knowledge and is influenced by experience" (Muisjsenberg et al., 2023, para. 2). OCRNs must recognize and address any implicit biases to provide inclusive cancer care, especially when it comes to patient education (Snively, 2023). One validated tool to assess a person's learning style preference is VARK (visual, aural, read/write, kinesthetic), which posits that learning styles may be influenced by a person's age, gender, and cultural background (Tomic et al., 2023).

OCRNs need to be aware of the following six basic principles when working with adult learners (CDC, n.d.):

- Adults are internally motivated and self-directed.
- Adults need to draw upon their own life experiences and knowledge.

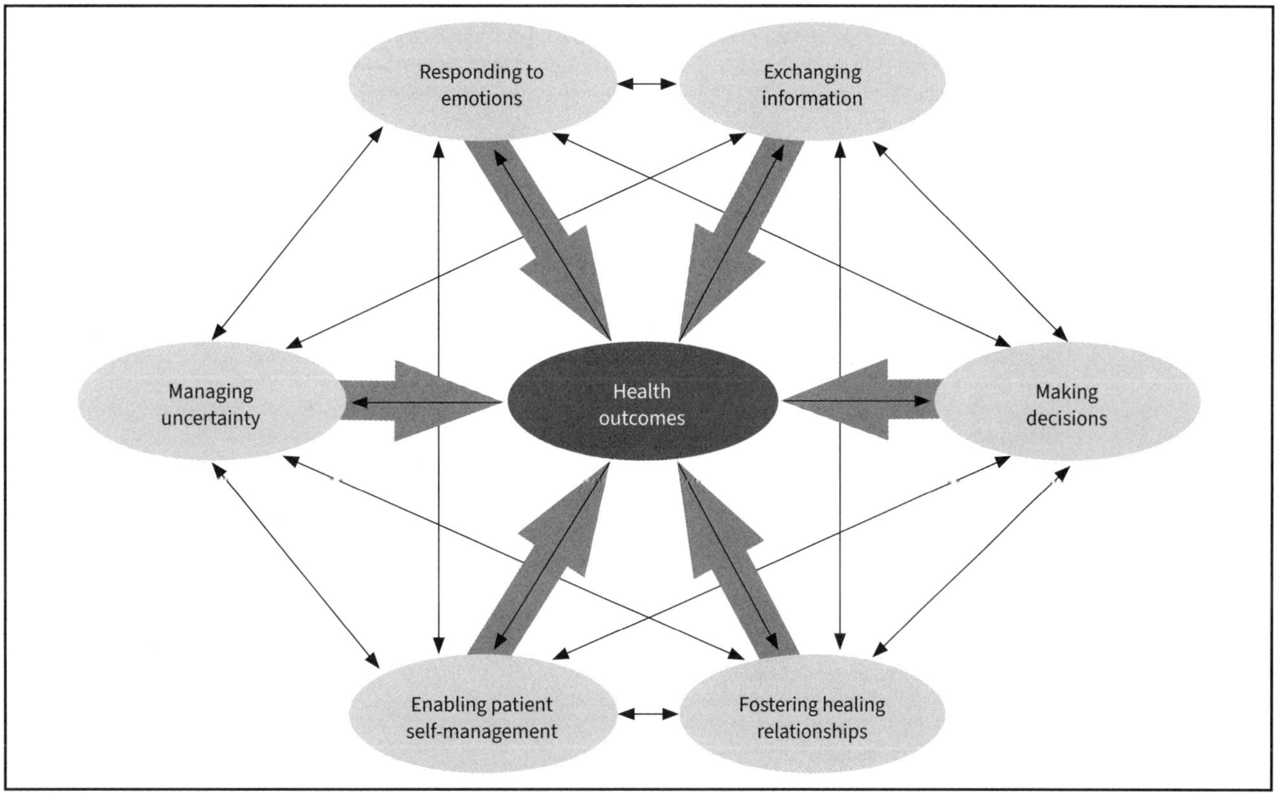

FIGURE 23-1 | The Six Domains of Patient-Centered Communication

Note. From *Health Literacy and Communication Strategies in Oncology: Proceedings of a Workshop*, by National Academies Press, 2020 (https://doi.org/10.17226/25664). In the public domain.

- Adults are goal oriented.
- Adults are relevancy oriented.
- Adults are practical.
- Adults need to be shown respect.

OCRNs should also consider these eight important characteristics of the adult learner (Pappas, 2021):

- **Self-direction:** Adults feel the need to take responsibility for their lives and decisions, and this is why they need to have control over their learning.
- **Practical and results oriented:** Adult learners are usually practical, reject theory, and need information that is immediately applicable to their situation.
- **Less open-minded:** Adult learners are more resistant to change. Maturity and profound life experiences usually lead to rigidity, the enemy of learning.
- **Slower learning, yet more integrative knowledge**: Aging does affect learning. Adults tend to learn less rapidly with age. However, the depth of learning tends to

TABLE 23-1 | Learning Styles, Characteristics of Learners, and Suggested Teaching Strategies

Learning Style	Characteristics	Suggested Teaching Strategies
Visual	Prefers written instructions rather than verbal instructions Prefers to have photographs and illustrations to view when receiving written or visual instructions Prefers a timeline, calendar, or some other similar diagram to remember the sequence of events Observes all the physical elements in the learning environment Carefully organizes their learning materials Remembers and understands through the use of diagrams, charts, and maps Studies materials by reading notes and organizing it in outline form	Provide lots of interesting visual material in a variety of formats. Make sure visual presentations are well organized. Make handouts and all other written work as visually appealing as possible, and easy to read. Make full use of a variety of technologies: computers, overhead projection, video camera, live video feeds/closed circuit TV, photography, Internet, etc.
Auditory	Remembers what they say, and what others say very well Remembers best through verbal repetition and by saying things aloud Prefers to discuss ideas they do not immediately understand Remembers verbal instructions well Finds it difficult to work quietly for long periods of time Easily distracted by noise, but also easily distracted by silence Verbally expresses interest and enthusiasm Enjoys group discussions	Rephrase points and questions in several different ways to communicate intended message. Vary speed, volume, and pitch, as appropriate, to help create interesting aural textures. Write down key points or key words before providing verbal instructions to help avoid confusion due to pronunciation. Ensure auditory learners are in a position to hear well (be sure hearing aids are inserted and functional). Incorporate multimedia applications utilizing sounds, music, or speech (use tape recorders, computer sound cards/recording applications, musical instruments, etc.).
Kinesthetic	Remembers best through getting physically involved in whatever is being learned Enjoys the opportunity to build and/or physically handle learning materials Will take notes to keep busy but will not often use them Enjoys using computers Physically expresses interest and enthusiasm by getting active and excited Has trouble staying still or in one place for a long time Enjoys hands-on activities Tends to want to fiddle with small objects while listening or working Remembers what they do, what they experience with their hands or bodies (movement and touch) Enjoys using tools or lessons which involve active/practical participation Can remember how to do things after doing them once (motor memory) Has good motor coordination	Permit frequent breaks in teaching session to allow learner to move around room. Encourage learner to write down their own notes. Encourage learner to stand or move while reciting information or learning new material. Incorporate multimedia resources (computer, video camera, overhead transparencies, photography camera, etc.) into programs (teacher presentations and student presentations). Provide lots of tactile-kinesthetic activities in the class. Have product samples available for practice. Encourage return demonstration of procedures.

Note. From "An Overview of Adult-Learning Processes," by S.S. Russell, 2006, *Urologic Nursing, 26*(5), p. 351. Copyright 2006 by Society of Urologic Nurses and Associates. Reprinted with permission.

increase over time, navigating expertise and skills to unprecedented personal levels.

- **Use personal experience as a resource:** Adults have lived longer, seen and done more, and tend to link their past experiences to anything new and validate new concepts based on prior learning.
- **Motivation:** Learning in adulthood is usually voluntary.
- **Multilevel responsibilities:** Adult learners have a lot to juggle—family, friends, work, and the need for personal quality time.
- **High expectations:** Adult learners have high expectations. They want to be taught about things that will be immediately useful to them. It is important to meet individual needs and learning challenges.

Children and Adolescent Learners

More than 15,000 children aged 19 years or younger will be diagnosed with cancer (Curesearch for Children's Cancer, 2024). According to data from 2020, 33%–86% of individuals aged 15 years who are newly diagnosed with cancer are treated on a therapeutic clinical trial (Schapira et al., 2020).

Adolescence is the phase of life between childhood and adulthood, encompassing the age range of 10 to 19 years old (WHO, 2024a). Adolescents start to become more autonomous, begin to make their own decisions about health, and become increasingly involved with their health care (Manganello et al., 2015). Clinical trial participation in adolescents is much lower, which may contribute to higher mortality and morbidity among adolescents and young adults (Schapira et al., 2020). Some of the health literacy tools developed for adolescents include the Rapid Estimate of Adolescent Literacy in Medicine, the Test of Functional Health Literacy in Adults, and the Newest Vital Sign (Tavousi et al., 2022).

Although the Test of Functional Health Literacy in Adults has not been validated for adolescents, in 2007, Chisolm and Buchanan showed that the reading comprehension portion of the tool is valid for adolescents. However, these instruments assess very specific skills that are one part of health literacy, such as reading ability, reading comprehension, and numeracy. They are also not self-administered, making them difficult to use for large survey samples (Manganello et al., 2015).

When working and educating pediatric and adolescent patients, OCRNs should ensure that the information is developmentally appropriate. All nurses should be familiar with the stages of cognitive development for these age groups when designing and implementing age-appropriate teaching.

Barriers to participation in pediatric clinical trials include a lack of understanding and mistrust of the research process and logistical challenges, such as language barriers, financial constraints, transportation barriers, and time or opportunity costs for working parents or caregivers. Study procedures that are perceived to cause discomfort or stress also negatively impact enrollment and retention (Lewandowska, 2022; Watson et al., 2022).

Parents and caregivers taking care of children with cancer face psychosocial, emotional, physical, informational, financial, educational, and spiritual needs (Lewandowska, 2022). OCRNs should assess parent or caregiver readiness to learn prior to educating them. These individuals are usually feeling overwhelmed following the initial diagnosis or with any change in a child's condition, are often suffering from sleep disturbances, and are working out logistical issues, especially if they are away from home or have other children (Rodgers et al., 2018). As with adult learners, teaching can occur with each patient encounter and is not limited to just formal education sessions. Good communication between the parent or caregiver and the healthcare team can decrease the stress of the situation and enhance achieving the goals of the teaching required.

Providing Clear and Effective Patient Education

After a patient's learning needs and readiness are determined, this information can be used as a foundation for what and how the health information is provided. To individualize health information, OCRNs should work closely with patients and families to decide what is essential, realistic, and achievable for patients. Before continuing with the teaching–learning process, OCRNs should individualize the message to present relevant material. Providing patients with opportunities to ask questions and discuss concerns, and outlining expectations and outcomes will enhance patient learning. OCRNs should communicate expected outcomes in terms of patient actions or behaviors. A well-defined outcome concentrates on a single task, and the more precise it is, the simpler it becomes to observe and evaluate progress toward achieving it.

Setting Priorities for Teaching

As clinical trials become more complex and patient conditions become complicated, there is considerably more education that is needed. OCRNs should establish teaching priorities early, be prepared, and organize their time more efficiently. The *AHRQ Health Literacy Universal Precautions Toolkit* offers tools for healthcare professionals to share information with patients and caregivers. Strategies for communicating clearly include the following (Brach, 2024):

- Engage with patients.
- Be respectful and caring.
- Ask open-ended questions.
- Listen actively and with curiosity.
- Encourage questions.
- Limit content and reinforce key points to avoid information overload.

It is well-documented that up to 80% of the medical information patients are told during office visits is forgotten immediately. Nearly half of the information patients retain is incorrect (Kessels, 2003).

Implementing Methods for Effective Teaching

Based on the patient's initial learning assessment, OCRNs should provide education materials and teaching methods. The teach-back method should be used to assess comprehension of instruction (AHRQ, 2024b; Anderson et al., 2020). It also offers the opportunity for the patient to ask additional questions and seek clarification. If a patient is an auditory learner, follow-up with written materials is necessary (Anderson et al., 2020; Campbell, 2020; Mirabella et al., 2022).

OCRNs can provide supplemental instruction materials and tools via easy-to-read materials, audio-recorded instructions, videos, closed-circuit televisions, compact discs, DVDs, interactive computer programs, models, posters, and diagrams or pictures to help facilitate patient learning (Snively, 2023). Selecting the appropriate methods will depend on the complexity of the education and the patient's or caregiver's needs.

Access to the internet and digital communication has expanded dramatically over the past 30 years. However, not all patients have access to this technology, are able to navigate the digital realm, or have the desire to use digital sources. The WHO definition of *digital health literacy* is "the ability to seek, find, understand, and appraise health information from electronic sources and apply the knowledge gained to addressing or solving a health problem" (Seidel et al., 2023, para. 1). Being health literate allows one to search for health information online easily, access telehealth services, and electronically communicate with healthcare providers (Seidel et al., 2023). OCRNs need to determine the level of digital health literacy of patients and their caregivers to address any misconceptions. To avoid misinformation, OCRNs should work with patients and caregivers to help them understand how to evaluate online resources. Patients and their caregivers can access this information online at https://medlineplus.gov/evaluatinghealthinformation.html. The National Cancer Institute website also offers access to patient education publications (www.cancer.gov/publications/patient-education).

OCRNs should be prepared to give health information by being alert to one-minute teaching opportunities. Creating a positive and supportive learning environment and organizing the material prior to giving the information are essential to enhance patient learning. OCRNs can do this by logically presenting information, limiting content to three to five of the most important points, breaking down complex instructions into smaller steps, and repeating the most essential points at the end of each instruction session. After giving the information, OCRNs can use the teach-back method to verify patient understanding (Anderson et al., 2020).

Teach-Back Method

OCRNs must ensure that patients and caregivers have a clear understanding of what they have learned. According to Tool 5 in the *AHRQ Health Literacy Universal Precautions Toolkit* (Brach, 2024) the teach-back method is a way of checking understanding by asking patients to state in their own words what they need to know or do about their health. The related show-me method allows OCRNs to confirm that patients are able to follow specific instructions, such as how to use an inhaler. The teach-back and show-me methods are valuable to use with all patients and can assist with the following (Anderson et al., 2020; AHRQ, 2024b; Gibson et al., 2022; Snively, 2023):

- Improving patient understanding and adherence
- Decreasing call backs and cancelled appointments
- Improving patient satisfaction and outcomes

The teach-back is not a test of patients' memory (Anderson et al., 2020; Mirabella et al., 2022). Patients can refer to written material when asking for teach-back, so it is imperative to ensure that they use their own words and are not just reading from the material. OCRNs should use the chunk-and-check method by not waiting until the end of the visit to initiate teach-back. Small segments of information should be taught, then patients should be requested to teach it back. Once successful, OCRNs should move to teaching the next segment of information (AHRQ, 2024b). OCRNs need to start slowly and use consistency when patients are learning the teach-back method. With practice, it becomes part of the routine, can be done without awkwardness, and does not lengthen a visit. Use of the teach-back observation tool can help individuals and organizations guide staff to become more familiar with the teach-back method and provide helpful feedback (Anderson et al., 2020; Gibson et al., 2022).

Challenges to Learning

Several patient populations are identified as requiring in-depth and highly individualized assessment, including older adult patients; those who are blind, deaf, or mentally deficient; those who are illiterate; and those do not speak the native language of the country in which they reside. Some of these patients may be ineligible for clinical trials because of comorbidities or poor performance status, and for others, informed consent may be difficult, if not impossible, to obtain (Winter et al., 2018).

When presenting clinical trial information to older adults, explanations must be simple and straightforward. Both a verbal and an easily understandable written explanation of the concept should be provided. For patients who are illiterate, education videos are helpful to facilitate learning. The informed consent document must be read aloud and explained to these individuals, as well as to the blind. Sign language interpreters and foreign language translators should be available to assist in communicating with special populations. When many individuals who speak a particular foreign language enroll in a clinical trial, a short, institutional review board–approved consent form written in the appropriate language can be used (Winter et al., 2018).

Distress in Cancer

Cancer remains one of the leading causes of death worldwide, and as such, anxiety and fear rank high among the psychological predictors of distress in this patient population. The National Cancer Institute (2025) defined *distress in cancer* as "a multifactorial unpleasant experience of a psychological (i.e., cognitive, behavioral, emotional), social, spiritual, and/or physical nature that may interfere with one's ability to cope effectively with cancer, its physical symptoms, and its treatment" (para. 11). In a 2020 study, Donovan et al. (2020) chose the word *distress* to "avoid stigmatisation and to facilitate measurement by self-report" (p. 1).

Distress is often associated with reduced survival, poor quality of life, and dissatisfaction with care. To develop more successful and effective interventions, it is imperative to identify patients at high risk for persistent distress. Physical symptoms associated with distress include fatigue, insomnia, and digestive issues (D'Andre et al., 2024).

Distress Related to Clinical Trial Discontinuation

Patients and caregivers face unique challenges at clinical trial discontinuation. Most often, patients are discontinued because of a lack of efficacy or intolerable side effects. During clinical trial participation, patients and their caregivers receive psychosocial and physical support from their care team. At treatment discontinuation, there may be feelings of isolation and abandonment. The sense of security and continuity of care that patients experience when participating in a clinical trial may produce feelings of loss when trial participation ceases.

Ulrich et al. (2021) recognized five themes in patients who were withdrawn from their study: prognostic awareness, goals of care discussions, emotional coping, burden of adverse effects, and professional trust and support. Participants expressed emotions of sadness, fear, and hope for something else, as well as mixed emotions. Patients discontinuing clinical trial participation must navigate next steps, which may include end-of-life care. This can put a tremendous amount of distress on them and their caregivers (Ulrich et al., 2021).

Carter et al. (2004) compiled a list of feelings that patients may experience when treatment has ended, such as feelings of abandonment and isolation, anxiety, depression, and coping with side effects of the treatment. In all instances, patients and caregivers experience a significant change in the frequency of clinic visits, where healthcare providers have been at the forefront and providing physical and emotional support, as well as continuous patient education.

Tools to Evaluate Distress

Distress has been characterized as the sixth vital sign (Sun et al., 2019). Since 2015, the American College of Surgeons Commission on Cancer has made distress screening an accreditation standard for cancer centers in the United States. The National Comprehensive Cancer Network has developed distress screening tools that can assist in assessing distress in patients (Deshields et al., 2018). The Edmonton Symptom Assessment Scale is another valid, reliable tool that assesses pain, activity, nausea, depression, anxiety, drowsiness, appetite, and sense of well-being (Hui & Bruera, 2017).

OCRNs should incorporate distress screening with patients and caregivers and continually reassess distress at each visit. Swift referrals can help patients and caregivers cope better and achieve better outcomes. Involvement of the interprofessional team is critical to help these individuals through their cancer journey.

Specific Informational Needs for Study Phases

Participation in a clinical trial, regardless of phase, occurs at varying points in a patient's care continuum. A patient diagnosed with early-stage or limited-stage disease may want to participate in a later phase trial (phase 2–3). Patients who have exhausted all standard of care options may look into participation in an early-stage trial. When there are no standard of care options or if patients have specific variants that have new therapies, they may be enrolled in early-stage trials (Paluri et al., 2020). Interprofessional communication between the patient and the healthcare team, including the physician and OCRN, is vital. OCRNs are tasked with understanding the patient's needs and guiding the discussion with the healthcare team. Clinical trials that focus on treatment are performed in progressive phases. Information from an earlier phase will help determine the study design and criteria for the next phase. Figure 23-2 shows the purpose, characteristics, and patient educational needs for phase 1–3 studies.

Phase 1 Studies

Phase 1 clinical trials are presented mainly to patients with advanced disease for whom standard treatment regimens have been either unsuccessful or nonexistent. These types of studies are usually the first that involve humans and are conducted to find the highest dose of the treatment that can be given safely without causing severe side effects. Patients can be either treatment naïve or have had multiple palliative treatments. Trials are performed in generally small groups of

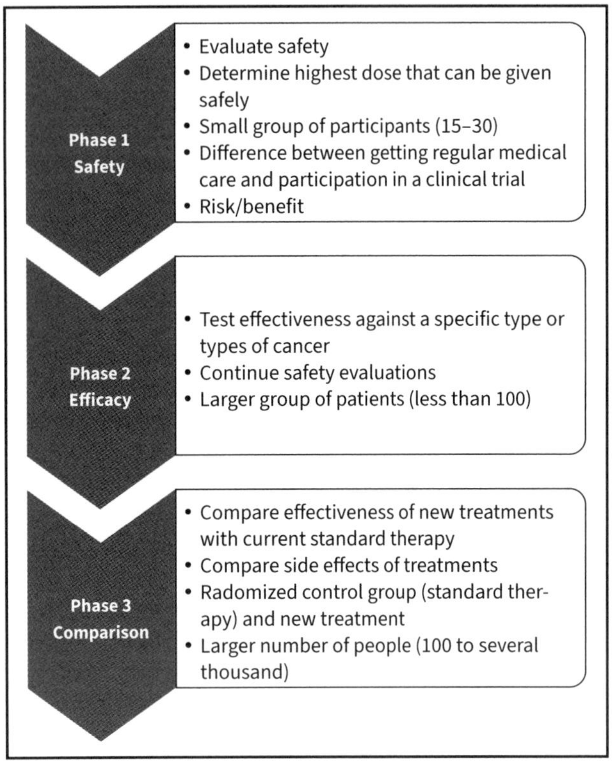

FIGURE 23-2 | Purpose, Characteristics, and Patient Educational Needs for Phase 1–3 Trials

Note. Based on information from National Cancer Institute, 2016.

people (15–30). Newer phase 1 study designs (seamless phase 1 trials), where multiple expansion arms are added, can enroll up to 1,000 patients and are sometimes used to obtain regulatory approvals (Bittlinger et al., 2022; Kandi & Vadakedath, 2023).

The majority of these investigational agents have not been tested before in humans; therefore, patient education can be difficult because the possible side effects are unknown. Research suggests there is high therapeutic misconception, misestimation, or unrealistic optimism in patients participating in phase 1 trials (Bittlinger et al., 2022).

The role of OCRNs in obtaining consent varies by institution. Once the physician has explained the protocol to the patient, it may be the responsibility of an OCRN to obtain consent. OCRNs should be available to serve as an educational resource and a patient advocate throughout a patient's participation.

Patient safety is critical, especially in a phase 1 study where side effects are unknown. Patients and caregivers must be instructed to report all side effects, whether treatment related or not, to the healthcare team. Education may include documentation of side effects in a diary, as well as methods on how to reach the healthcare team when the patient experiences an unusual symptom.

Patients and caregivers need to maintain realistic hope but must be kept informed of their current condition and response to treatment. Ferrell et al. (2019) noted the following about patients in phase 1 trials:

- Patients remain optimistic about treatment options while aware of their mortality.
- Patients need strong support systems to address quality-of-life concerns.
- Patients must understand their disease status and treatment options.

Phase 2 Studies

Phase 2 studies include a larger number of people (less than 100) to see if a new treatment seems to work against the cancer, such as by shrinking tumors or slowing their growth. Researchers want to determine how the new treatment affects the body and fights the cancer. Safety is still studied. In phase 2 studies, there is more information regarding possible side effects and risks based on the information gathered from the phase 1 studies. As in phase 1 studies, patients and caregivers need to be educated about the importance of adherence to treatment and testing schedules. They should also be advised to report side effects in a timely manner.

Phase 3 Studies

In phase 3 studies, researchers compare the treatment to the current standard therapy and evaluate side effects. Participants are randomly assigned to one of the treatments to ensure that any differences are not the result of differences in the features of the participants. Phase 3 trials include large numbers of people, any number from a hundred to several thousand individuals, to ensure that all results are valid and reliable to the study.

Patients and families are instructed about the different treatment arms of the study and the various potential side effects associated with these therapies. If a patient wishes to receive a particular treatment, they should not be entered into the study. OCRNs need to educate patients and their caregivers about what to expect when entering into a randomized clinical trial and how the randomization process works.

The treatments administered in phase 3 studies have documented toxicities, and information is collected from patients to determine any additional unexpected toxicities. Patient education focuses on the expected toxicities and interventions available to alleviate these issues. Teaching reinforces to patients that these toxicities are not to be endured but reported to the healthcare team. This will enable the appropriate medical and nursing actions to be implemented.

Other Clinical Trial Phases

Other clinical trial phases include phase 0 and phase 4 studies. Phase 0 studies are intended to expedite clinical evaluation and new molecular entities. Doses tested are usually subtherapeutic and are given to very small groups of participants, usually for no more than a week. These studies also help sponsors gather pharmacokinetic data (Newton, 2022).

Phase 4 studies, also known as postmarketing studies, are conducted after a new drug is marketed. The main objectives of this study are to check drug performance in real-world scenarios, study the long-term risks and benefits of using the drug, and discover rare side effects (Kandi & Vadakedath, 2023; Mandal, 2023).

Summary

Patients and their caregivers experience an array of personal psychological challenges as they move through the healthcare continuum. Routine assessment and intervention are imperative to provide holistic care to these individuals. It is the responsibility of OCRNs to educate patients and caregivers participating in a clinical trial.

Education should be individualized based on the patient's age, cultural background, preferred method of learning, desire for information, placement on the healthcare continuum, attitudes toward health care, and other specific considerations to determine what style of teaching will be the most effective. Knowing the patient's motivation to enter into the clinical trial can also help guide education. When developing educational materials for patients and caregivers, OCRNs must evaluate learners' communication needs; social, cultural, and religious values influence patients' and caregivers' knowledge and attitudes about the educational materials. Special populations require in-depth and individualized assessments.

Using health literacy tools to create materials should be trial and phase specific. Patients and caregivers want to understand and be involved in their treatment decisions. Education should be incorporated into each visit and should be broken up into short, easy-to-follow segments. A variety of creative materials are available to help accommodate specific learning styles, including verbal and written information, audiovisual media, and computer-assisted learning.

Key Points

- To provide effective patient education, OCRNs must assess factors such as distress, patient and caregiver learning needs, readiness to learn, and learning style.
- Identification of where a patient is along the healthcare continuum is essential for the assessment of teaching needs.
- OCRNs should work with patients and caregivers to determine how and which health information should be provided.
- Patients experience personal psychological challenges as they move through their cancer treatment continuum, especially if they are part of a clinical trial.
- OCRNs should assess distress at every visit and document their findings (e.g., vital signs).
- Teaching material should be individualized to meet patients' and caregivers' needs.
- OCRNs should set teaching priorities, determine what to teach, and select the appropriate tools to provide effective patient education, using health literacy guidelines and teach-back methods.

The author would like to acknowledge Geri L. Schmotzer, PhD, MSN, MPH, RN, for her contribution to this chapter that remains unchanged from the previous edition of this book.

References

Agency for Health Research and Quality. (n.d.). *Tools and resources.* https://www.ahrq.gov/health-literacy/improve/precautions/index.html

Agency for Healthcare Research and Quality. (2024a). *Communication observation form.* https://www.ahrq.gov/health-literacy/improve/precautions/tool4c.html

Agency for Healthcare Research and Quality. (2024b). *Use the teach-back method: Tool 5.* https://www.ahrq.gov/health-literacy/improve/precautions/tool5.html

Anderson, K.M., Leister, S., & De Rego, R. (2020). The 5Ts for teach back: An operational definition for teach-back training. *Health Literacy Research and Practice, 4*(2), e94–e103. https://doi.org/10.3928/24748307-20200318-01

Bittlinger, M., Bicer, S., Peppercorn, J., & Kimmelman, J. (2022). Ethical considerations for phase I trials in oncology. *Journal of Clinical Oncology, 40*(30), 3474–3488. https://doi.org/10.1200/JCO.21.02125

Brach, C. (Ed.). (2024). *AHRQ health literacy universal precautions toolkit* (3rd ed.). Agency for Healthcare Research and Quality. https://www.ahrq.gov/sites/default/files/wysiwyg/health-literacy/3rd-edition-toolkit/health-literacy-toolkit-third-edition.pdf

Brach, C., Keller, D., Hernandez, L.M., Baur, C., Parker, R., Dreyer, B., … Schillinger, D. (2012). *Ten attributes of health literate health care organizations.* Institute of Medicine. https://nam.edu/wp-content/uploads/2015/06/BPH_Ten_HLit_Attributes.pdf

Campbell, J. (2020). Health literacy in adult oncology: An integrative review. *Oncology Nursing Forum, 47*(1), 18–32. https://doi.org/10.1188/20.ONF.18-32

Carter, H., MacLeod, R., Brander, P., & McPherson, K. (2004). Living with a terminal illness: Patients' priorities. *Journal of Advanced Nursing, 45*(6), 611–620. https://doi.org/10.1046/j.1365-2648.2003.02953.x

Centers for Disease Control and Prevention. (n.d.). *Adult learning principles.* https://www.cdc.gov/training-development/media/pdfs/2024/04/adult-learning-principles.pdf

Centers for Disease Control and Prevention. (2024a). *Understanding health literacy.* https://www.cdc.gov/health-literacy/php/about/understanding.html

Centers for Disease Control and Prevention. (2024b). *What is health literacy?* https://www.cdc.gov/health-literacy/php/about/index.html

Centers for Disease Control and Prevention. (2025). *Plain language materials and resources.* https://www.cdc.gov/health-literacy/php/develop-materials/plain-language.html

Chisolm, D.J., & Buchanan, L. (2007). Measuring adolescent functional health literacy: A pilot validation of the Test of Functional Health Literacy in Adults. *Journal of Adolescent Health, 41*(3), 312–314. https://doi.org/10.1016/j.jadohealth.2007.04.015

Christiansen, K., Buswell, L., & Fadelu, T. (2023). A systematic review of patient education strategies for oncology patients in low- and middle-income countries. *Oncologist, 28*(1), 2–11. https://doi.org/10.1093/oncolo/oyac206

Curesearch for Children's Cancer. (2024). *Childhood cancer statistics.* https://curesearch.org/childhood-cancer-statistics

Cutilli, C.C. (2020). Excellence in patient education: Evidence-based education that "sticks" and improves patient outcomes. *Nursing Clinics, 55*(2), 267–282. https://doi.org/10.1016/j.cnur.2020.02.007

D'Andre, S., Ellsworth, L.S., Kirsch, J.L., Montane, H.N., Kruger, M.B., Donovan, K.A., ... Ehlers, S.L. (2024). Cancer and stress: Understanding the connections and interventions. *American Journal of Lifestyle Medicine.* https://doi.org/10.1177/15598276241304373

Deshields, T.L., Howrey, H.L., & Vanderlan, J.R. (2018). Distress in oncology: Not just a psychosocial phenomenon. *Journal of Oncology Practice.* https://doi.org/10.1200/JOP.18.00222

Donovan, K.A., Grassi, L., Deshields, T.L., Corbett, C., & Riba, M.B. (2020). Advancing the science of distress screening and management in cancer care. *Epidemiology and Psychiatric Sciences, 29,* e85. https://doi.org/10.1017/S2045796019000799

Ferrell, B., Williams, A.C., Borneman, T., Chung, V., & Smith, T.J. (2019). Clinical trials: Understanding patient perspectives and beliefs about treatment. *Clinical Journal of Oncology Nursing, 27*(5), 592–598. https://doi.org/10.1188/19.CJON.592-598

Gibson, C., Smith, D., & Morrison, A. (2022). Improving health literacy knowledge, behaviors, and confidence with interactive training. *Health Literacy Research and Practice, 6*(2), e113–e121. https://doi.org/10.3928/24748307-20220420-01

Gusman, N.M. (2022). Transforming patient education: effectively identifying and eliminating barriers related to culture, literacy and learning styles. *Journal of Oncology Navigation and Survivorship, 13*(1). https://www.jons-online.com/issues/2022/january-2022-vol-13-no-1/transforming-patient-education-effectively-identifying-and-eliminating-barriers-related-to-culture-literacy-and-learning-styles

Hui, D., & Bruera, E. (2017). The Edmonton Assessment System 25 years later: Past, present, and future developments. *Journal of Pain and Symptom Management, 53*(3), 630–643. https://doi.org/10.1016/j.jpainsymman.2016.10.370

Kandi, V., & Vadakedath, S. (2023). Clinical trials and clinical research: A comprehensive review. *Cureus, 15*(2), e35077. https://doi.org/10.7759/cureus.35077

Kessels, R.P.C. (2003). Patients' memory for medical information. *Journal of the Royal Society of Medicine, 96*(5), 219–222. https://doi.org/10.1258/jrsm.96.5.219

Lewandowska, A. (2022). The needs of parents of children suffering from cancer—Continuation of research. *Children, 9*(2), 144. https://doi.org/10.3390/children9020144

Mandal, D.A. (2023). What is a phase 4 clinical trial? *News Medical Life Sciences.* https://www.news-medical.net/health/What-is-a-Phase-4-Clinical-Trial.aspx

Manganello, J.A., DeVellis, R.F., Davis, T.C., & Schottler-Thal, C. (2015). Development of the Health Literacy Assessment Scale for Adolescents (HAS-A). *Journal of Communication in Healthcare, 8*(3), 172–184. https://doi.org/10.1179/1753807615Y.0000000016

MedlinePlus. (2023, October 13). *Communicating with patients.* https://medlineplus.gov/ency/patientinstructions/000456.htm

Mirabella, A., Vrana, A., Bay, R., Slater, A., & Brewer, M. (2022). SMART oncology nursing: Literacy, goals, coaching, and empowerment. *Oncology Nursing Forum, 49*(1), 37–45. https://doi.org/10.1188/22.ONF.37-45

Muisjsenberg, A.J., Bouben-Wilke, S., Yugin Zeng, M.S., & Janssen, D.J. (2023). Methods to assess adults' learning styles and factors affecting learning in health education: A scoping review. *Patient and Education and Counseling, 107*, 107588. https://doi.org/10.1016/j.pec.2022.107588

National Cancer Institute. (2016). *Taking part in cancer treatment research studies.* https://www.cancer.gov/publications/patient-education/crs.pdf

National Cancer Institute. (2025). *Adjustment to cancer: Anxiety and distress (PDQ®)–Health professional version.* https://www.cancer.gov/about-cancer/coping/feelings/anxiety-distress-hp-pdq

Newton, W. (2022). Phase 0 clinical trials: What you need to know. *Clinical Trials Arena.* https://www.clinicaltrialsarena.com/features/phase-0/?cf-view&cf-closed

Office of Disease Prevention and Health Promotion. (n.d.). *Health literacy in healthy people 2030.* https://health.gov/healthypeople/priority-areas/health-literacy-healthy-people-2030

Ohio State University. (n.d.). *Learning assessment questions and observations.* https://ogg.osu.edu/media/documents/health_lit/HOLearning_Assessment2.pdf

Oncology Nursing Society. (2023). *Health literacy huddle card.* https://www.ons.org/huddle-cards/health-literacy-huddle-card

Oncology Nursing Society & Oncology Nursing Certification Corporation. (2024). *Oncology clinical research nurse competencies.* https://www.ons.org/sites/default/files/2025-01/ocrn-competencies-rebrand.pdf

Paluri, R.K., Li, P., Anderson, A., Nandagopal, L., McArdle, T., Young, M., ... Saleh, M. (2020). First-in-human phase 1 clinical trials – A single-center experience in the era of modern oncotherapeutics. *Scientific Reports, 10,* 7935. https://www.nature.com/articles/s41598-020-64906-4

Pappas, C. (2021). 8 important characteristics of adult learners. *E Learning Industry.* https://elearningindustry.com/8-important-characteristics-of-adult-learners

Pritchard-Jones, K. (2008). Improving recruitment to clinical trials for cancer in childhood. *Lancet Oncology, 9*(4), 392–399. https://doi.org/10.1016/S1470-2045(08)70101-3.

Rodgers, C., Bertini, V., Conway, M.A., Crosty, A., Filice, A., Herring, R.A., ... Landier, W. (2018). A standardized education checklist for parents of children newly diagnosed with cancer: A report from the Children's Oncology Group. *Journal of Pediatric Oncology Nursing, 35*(4), 235–246. https://doi.org/10.1177/1043454218764889

Schapira, M.M., Stevens, E.M., Sharpe, J.E., Hochman, L., Reiter, J.G., Calhoun, S.R., ... Barakat, L.P. (2020). Outcomes among pediatric patients with cancer who are treated on trial versus off trial: A matched cohort study. *Cancer, 126*(15), 3471–3482. https://doi.org/10.1002/cncr.32947

Seidel, E., Cortes, T., & Chong, C. (2023, October 31). Digital health literacy. *Agency for Health Research and Quality.* https://psnet.ahrq.gov/primer/digital-health-literacy

Snively, A. (2023, December 5). Personalized patient education. *ONS Voice.* https://voice.ons.org/news-and-views/12-2023/personalized-patient-education

Sun, H., Yang, Y., Zhang, J., Liu, T., Wang, H., Garg, S., & Zhang, B. (2019). Fear of cancer recurrence, anxiety and depressive symptoms in adolescent and young adult cancer patients. *Neuropsychiatric Disease and Treatment, 15,* 857–865. https://doi.org/10.2147/NDT.S202432

Tavousi, M., Mohammadi, S., Sadighi, J., Zarei, F., Kermani, R.M., Rostami, R., & Montazeri, A. (2022). Measuring health literacy: A systematic review and bibliometric analysis of instruments from 1993 to 2021. *PLOS ONE, 17*(7), e0271524. https://doi.org/10.1371/journal.pone.0271524

Tomic, D., Rastovski, D., & Curic, M. (2023). *Exploring the VARK model: A review of the validity and reliability of the questionnaire and its relationship to learning outcomes.* https://www.researchgate.net/publication/371633359_Exploring_the_VARK_model_a_review_of_the_validity_and_reliablity_of_the_questionnaire

Ulrich, C.M., Knafl, K., Foxwell, A.M., Zhou, Q., Paidipati, C., Tiller, D., ... Miller, V. (2021). Experiences of patients after withdrawal from cancer clinical trials. *JAMA Network Open, 4*(8), e2120052. https://doi.org/10.1001/jamanetworkopen.2021.20052

Watson, S.E., Smith, P., Snowden, J., Vaughn, V., Cottrell, L., Madden, C.A., ... Yakes Jimenez, E. (2022). Facilitators and barriers to pediatric clinical trial recruitment and retention in rural and community settings: A scoping review of the literature. *Clinical and Translational Science, 15*(4), 838–853. https://doi.org/10.1111/cts.13220

Winter, S.S., Page-Reeves, J.M., Page, K.A., Haozous, E., Solares, A., Nicole Cordova, C., & Larson, R.S. (2018). Inclusion of special populations in clinical research: Important considerations and guidelines. *Journal of Clinical and Translational Research, 4*(1), 56–69. https://doi.org/10.18053/jctres.04.201801.003

World Health Organization. (2024a). *Adolescent health.* https://www.who.int/health-topics/adolescent-health/#tab=tab_1

World Health Organization. (2024b). *Health literacy.* https://www.who.int/teams/health-promotion/enhanced-wellbeing/ninth-global-conference/health-literacy

SECTION V.
Genetics and Genomics

CHAPTER 24

Pharmacogenetics and Pharmacogenomics

Gary Shelton, DNP, MSN, NP, ANP-BC, AOCNP®

Introduction

One of the core values of the oncology clinical research nurse (OCRN) role focuses on advancing evidence-based oncology care through the use of scientifically based research (Driessnack et al., 2022; Herzog-LeBoeuf & Willenberg, 2020; O'Brien et al., 2022). Drug development is part of oncology care, and the goal is to develop drugs that work with maximum efficacy and minimal toxicity (Portier, 2020). For a drug to become marketable, the optimum concentration needed to exert a therapeutic effect needs to be determined. This level depends on the amount of the drug administered and the amount that can be metabolized. Situations where the drug concentration is minimal or above the expected level could result in a lack of drug effect or cause an adverse drug reaction.

To avoid unwanted toxic reactions, healthcare providers must exercise their knowledge of pharmacology and pharmacogenetics. The knowledge of pharmacogenetics assists in understanding the basic drug interaction process and helps to correctly identify responders, nonresponders, and those who may be at risk of developing adverse drug reactions (Gaedigk, 2019; Luzum et al., 2021). OCRNs must be informed about current and emerging genetic discoveries to apply the genetic information in their research practice. Not only do they need to be informed, but they also need to have a working knowledge of pharmacogenomics to manage clinical trials (Hood, 2022). For treatment protocols, review the chapters on cytogenetics (Chapter 26) and tumor profiling (Chapter 27).

This chapter will provide a basic foundation for understanding genetic terms and a detailed discussion of pharmacogenetics. It will discuss how the metabolism of drugs is affected by genetic makeup and describe the OCRN's role in studies that incorporate pharmacogenetics.

Differentiation of Terminology

The terms *pharmacogenetics* and *pharmacogenomics* describe how genetic determinants affect an individual's response to a medication. The study of these variations in a single gene is called *pharmacogenetics*. However, genes interact with each other; hence, "the study of the variability of the expression of individual genes relevant to disease susceptibility as well as drug response at cellular, tissue, individual, or population level" is called *pharmacogenomics* (European Agency for the Evaluation of Medicinal Products, 2002, p. 3). These two terms are used interchangeably in the literature, and the primary difference between them is that pharmacogenomic studies look at a group of genes or the entire genome instead of a single gene (Cecchin & Stocco, 2020; Gaedigk, 2019; Luzum et al., 2021; Roden et al., 2019).

Pharmacogenomics has been studied and applied across several therapeutic delivery models for various diseases, allowing for better evaluation and prediction of responses to specific drugs based on an individual's genetic makeup. The Clinical Pharmacogenetics Implementation Consortium provides guidelines to assist those in clinical trial development in improving the evidence derived. OCRNs should be aware of these guidelines and review them with their interprofessional team members to evaluate their appropriateness (Luzum et al., 2021; Morris et al., 2022; Relling et al., 2020).

Many clinical trials are adding pharmacogenetics with pharmacokinetics (PK) (see Chapter 29) to determine how investigational drugs respond when people have already been diagnosed with a variety of diseases and conditions. The goal of pharmacogenetics is to personalize treatment based on an individual's genetic makeup. Some genetic information has been identified for use. Still, much remains unknown, even though the human genome has been sequenced (Venter et al., 2001) and new technology has generated genetic information in the laboratory that awaits application in the clinical setting (Cecchin & Stocco, 2020; Morris et al., 2022). As more is known regarding pharmacogenetics, OCRNs need additional education and training in genetics to help their patients in clinical trials to understand the basic science of treatment (Luzum et al., 2021).

The Drug Development Process

Before the introduction of a new drug into the clinical setting, extensive preclinical testing is performed in vitro using tumor cell lines and in vivo using animal models. A drug is first tested in the laboratory using human tumor cell lines to determine its spectrum of antitumor activity. It is administered to tumor-bearing animals to assess antitumor activity in vivo. If evidence of an antitumor effect exists, and the drug can be efficiently produced in large quantities, then the toxicology and PK are studied in several laboratory animal species (U.S. Food and Drug Administration [FDA], 2017). PK studies play a critical role in the drug development process. The toxicology and PK studies in animals are used to determine a starting dose and schedule for the subsequent clinical trial drugs (Nomeir, 2010) (see Chapter 2).

The objectives of a phase 1 clinical trial are to determine the appropriate route, maximum tolerated dose, and schedule of administration; to define the spectrum of drug toxicities in healthy human participants; and to study the PK of the new agent (FDA, 2017). Because phase 1 trials are single-agent studies, they provide the best opportunity to identify correlations between PK parameters and the drug's pharmacodynamics (PD) (i.e., the drug's toxicity and response). The results of PK and PD studies are important components of the Investigational New Drug application that is submitted to FDA to gain approval for commercial use of a new drug (Cecchin & Stocco, 2020; Nomeir, 2010) (see Chapter 2).

Review of Basic Genetics

For OCRNs working in drug development clinical trials, understanding genetic background can assist in the education, communication, and management of patients and their families. In addition, knowledge in this evolving area of genetics will aid communication between colleagues to ensure the accurate implementation and follow-up of potentially life-threatening therapeutic drug protocols.

In clinical settings, variations in drug dose effects and the severity of adverse effects are seen among patients. One cause for interpatient variability is differences in genetic constitution (Gaedigk, 2019; Roden et al., 2019). Proteins encoded by specific genes influence the PK and PD of a drug; variations in the constitution of these genes result in differences in drug response among individuals. Alterations in DNA sequences, through a variation in a single base pair, deletions, insertions, and gene copy number variants, contribute to genetic variability. When DNA sequences are altered, the end product (protein) of gene transcription, the protein structure, and its stability are altered. However, these changes may or may not affect the protein function depending on the location of the DNA alteration (Deenen et al., 2011).

It is well known that a gene is a molecule of DNA, which consists of four types of building blocks: adenine (A), guanine (G), cytosine (C), and thymine (T). These blocks, along with a sugar molecule and a phosphate group, are called a nucleotide (Lewis, 2012). For RNA, thymine (T) is replaced by uracil (U). RNA bases can be compared to an alphabet with three consecutive bases (letters) or nucleotides coding for (spelling) an amino acid. Multiple amino acids strung together create a protein. DNA remains in the nucleus of the cell and is passed to daughter cells when a cell undergoes division. The information in cellular DNA is transcribed to RNA and carried by RNA from the cell to the cytoplasm to bring about the instructions directed by the DNA (Lewis, 2012) (see Figure 24-1).

The human genome has approximately 20,325 protein-coding genes, with only a few thousand known to cause disorders or traits. Information about human disorders and traits is found in the Online Mendelian Inheritance in Man catalog (www.omim.org). Only 1.5% of the 3.2 billion nucleotides encode proteins. The rest of the sequences may assist in protein synthesis or the regulation of the function of a gene by turning them on or off. New components of

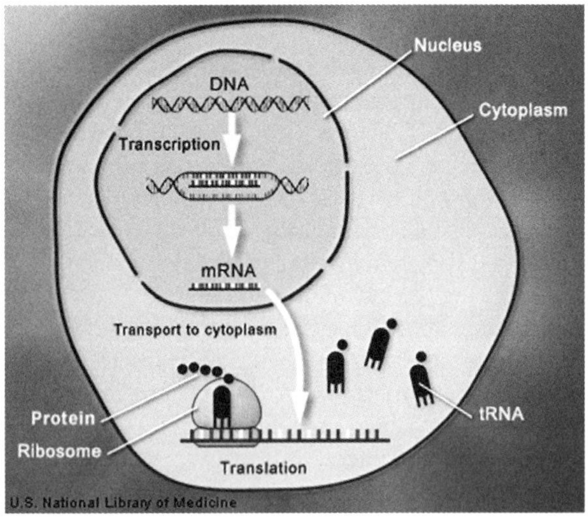

FIGURE 24-1 | Transcription and Translation

Note. From *How Do Genes Direct the Production of Proteins?*, by U.S. National Library of Medicine, n.d. In the public domain.

DNA (e.g., microRNA) and their function are still being identified, with many functions of DNA yet to be discovered (Lewis, 2012).

The collection of protein coding sequences (exons) of the genome is called an exome. Proteins are made up of long chains of amino acids known as polypeptides. To form a polypeptide, transcription occurs, enabling the RNA to enter the cytoplasm, where the information is used to manufacture proteins by arranging amino acids per the instructions in RNA (translation). Through translation, the messenger RNA (mRNA) is read as triplets called codons. Each codon corresponds to an amino acid. For example, AUG identifies methionine; UUA and UUG identify leucine.

Twenty different amino acids create proteins. The amino acids are linked to each other by a chemical bond called a peptide bond. The protein-coding genes may differ among individuals, and the alternate forms are called alleles. These DNA sequence changes are caused by polymorphisms or variants and are passed on to the daughter cells as the cell divides (Lewis, 2012). If a minor allelic variant is present in more than 1% of the population, it is called a genetic polymorphism. When there is a variation in a single base pair, it is called a single nucleotide polymorphism (SNP) (National Human Genome Research Institute, n.d.). An alteration causing a disease is called a variant.

To understand how alterations in DNA sequences affect protein function, a simple example with three-letter words may be used. The words have only three letters, similar to the codons (any three nucleotides together of adenine, guanine, cytosine, or thymine). If "THE BIG FAT BOY ATE ONE EGG" corresponds to triplet coding for a protein, then an SNP in the sequence will read as "THE BIG FIT BOY ATE ONE EGG." In this example, there is meaning to the sentence despite a change in a single letter. Similarly, proteins may not be affected even when a single nucleotide is changed in a codon. This is called a silent polymorphism, as the substitution of a nucleotide does not change the amino acid and eventually has no effect on the protein (Sauna et al., 2007). For example, AUU, AUC, AUA encodes the amino acid isoleucine. However, when there is a deletion or an insertion of a nucleotide, the reading frame shifts, and the sentence makes no sense. For example, inserting a letter "A" in the third word results in "THE BIG FAA TBO YAT EON EEG G," or deleting the letter "E" in the first word reads as "THB IGF ATB OYA TEO NEE GG." These two changes create an abnormal protein that causes altered function. In the *CYP2D6* gene, which is important in the metabolism of medications, when there is a deletion of a thymine base pair at position 1707, the frameshift variant creates a protein with no enzyme activity, causing patient problems with toxicity (Deenen et al., 2011).

A gene variant can be inherited or acquired. A germline variant is inherited from a parent. These variants are passed to new generations through the DNA in the egg or sperm, making the variants present in every cell throughout a person's lifetime. The second type of variant is a somatic variant, which is acquired during a person's lifetime when changes or damage are acquired to an individual cell. Cellular changes can be a result of environmental factors, such as smoking and ultraviolet light, or can occur during DNA transcription, where a mistake is made as DNA is being copied. Somatic (acquired) variants are not passed to future generations (Calzone & Masny, 2004; Eggert, 2017).

Chromosomal abnormalities are likely responsible for aberrations associated with how drugs are metabolized. The two types of chromosomal aberrations are structural and numerical. Structural aberrations are divided into the following four groups (Naeim et al., 2018):

- **Duplication (dup):** Part of the chromosome appears twice.
- **Deletions (del):** Part of the chromosome is missing.
- **Inversions (inv):** A segment of the chromosome is reversed.
- **Translocations (t):** Two chromosomes exchange parts.

Chromosome numerical changes include euploidy, an increased number of complete chromosomal sets, and aneuploidy, an increased or decreased number of individual chromosomes.

The International System for Human Cytogenetic Nomenclature is a naming system to identify the chromosomes and the location of abnormalities. Chromosomes are recognized by their numbers, arms (p arm [petite arm] and q arm [q follows p]), regions, bands, and sub-bands. The total number of chromosomes, including the sex chromosomes, is separated by a comma; for example, 46, XX is a female, and 46, XY a male. Sex chromosome aberrations are usually associated by autosomal (non-sex chromosomes) aberrations. When two chromosomes have abnormalities, a comma separates the designation. For instance, [46, XY, del (7q)] is a deletion in the long arm of chromosome 7, and [47, XX, +21] is a female with trisomy 21 or Down syndrome (Shaffer et al., 2012).

Basic Pharmacogenomics for Oncology Clinical Research Nurses

OCRNs should have an understanding of pharmacogenetics and the terminology related to basic physiology and pharmacology. Prodrugs (the inactive form of drugs) are primarily metabolized in the liver to their active forms. For example, tamoxifen is a prodrug that is converted to its active metabolites in the liver. Of note, the liver is where the active metabolites are converted to inactive forms for the sake of elimination (Gaedigk, 2019; Roden et al., 2019). Several enzymes and processes are involved in drug metabolism, and a superfamily among them is the cytochrome P450 enzymes, which are responsible for oxidation reactions. Well-known examples are CYP1A2, CYP2C9, CYP2C19, CYP2D6, CYP2E1, and CYP3A4 (Gaedigk,

2019; Luzum et al., 2021; Roden et al., 2019). CYP is the root symbol for the cytochrome P450 family, followed by an Arabic number for the family, a letter to denote the subfamily, and an Arabic numeral for the individual gene (Nebert et al., 1987). The most common type of gene is denoted by an asterisk followed by number 1 (*1), and the numbers thereafter identify variations in the gene caused by SNPs. The gene that encodes a particular isoenzyme follows the same nomenclature but is italicized. For example, isoenzyme CYP2C19 is a product of the gene *CYP2C19*. Populations differ in their frequency of specific alleles. In the United States, Caucasians have a high frequency of *CYP2D6*4*, and Asians have a high frequency of *CYP2D6 *10* (Luzum et al., 2021; Roden et al., 2019).

For an autosomal gene, numbered genes not associated with a sex chromosome, every individual receives two alleles from their parents for each gene. An allele has a variation, such as eye color, with an individual getting an allele from each parent. Some genes can have several copies of an allele inherited from one parent at a particular locus in a chromosome. The common form of the gene that codes for a full functioning isoenzyme is called a wild-type allele. The genotype of the individual corresponds to the allele makeup for a particular gene and is reflected in the phenotype. It is important to remember that these phenotypes can be influenced by medications, herbal remedies, and the food that an individual ingests (Louie & Russell, 2013; Scripture & Figg, 2006).

Phenotypically, individuals can be characterized as poor, intermediate, extensive, and ultra-rapid metabolizers. For poor metabolizers, the metabolism of the drug is significantly reduced, and the drug remains in the circulation for a longer duration. Therefore, the patient experiences a prolonged drug effect. If a patient is a poor metabolizer for warfarin, a prolonged drug effect can lead to severe hemorrhage (Shi et al., 2001). The intermediate metabolizers are the heterozygotes who experience decreased drug effect and suffer from toxic drug levels. However, these individuals benefit from drugs when started in low doses and gradually increased (Prows, 2011). Extensive metabolizers experience the drug effect to the expected level with or without minimal adverse drug reactions. At the other extreme to the poor metabolizers are the ultra-rapid metabolizers, who have increased efficiency in metabolizing the drug. These individuals clear the drug from their circulation at an increased level and therefore may not receive the required drug effect, causing inadequate or no cancer treatment (Prows, 2011).

Pharmacogenetics and Common Anticancer Drugs

Several well-known examples of pharmacogenetics are commonly used anticancer drugs. Although OCRNs will be managing clinical trial protocols that are different from the examples in this chapter, these have been included so that OCRNs new to research can have a better appreciation for the importance of the ability to translate molecular knowledge of pharmacogenetics into practice as it relates to potential cancer treatments.

5-Fluorouracil and Dihydropyrimidine Dehydrogenase

The dihydropyrimidine dehydrogenase (DPD) protein encoded by the *DYPD* gene is involved in the metabolism of the drug 5-fluorouracil (5-FU), well known for the treatment of solid tumors. Eighty percent of the 5-FU active drug is converted to inactive metabolites by the DPD enzyme. Hence, individuals who are deficient in DPD suffer from severe toxic effects (Houtsma et al., 2010). The most common variant found in individuals who are DPD deficient is in an intron, *DYPD*2A* (Raida et al., 2001). This is because of a G to A variant in the GT 5′ splice recognition site of intron 14. Here, the term *variant* versus *polymorphism* is used, as the change in this base pair occurs in less than 1% of the population. When compared to patients with normal DPD activity, 60% of the patients who were DPD deficient suffered from grade 3–4 toxicity, and 55% of them developed grade 4 neutropenia when administered 5-FU (Raida et al., 2001; van Kuilenburg et al., 2000). Pretreatment genetic screening may help identify patients who have deficient DPD activity. It may also aid in treatment decision-making to limit toxic effects and potentially save lives in extreme cases (Houtsma et al., 2010; Mounier-Boutoille et al., 2010). In this scenario, OCRNs would be involved in completion of the consent process, education of the patient and family about pharmacogenetics and potential side effects, collection of a DNA sample, timely collection of blood and urine samples, and careful assessment and monitoring for side effects and levels of toxicity.

6-Mercaptopurine and Thiopurine S-Methyltransferase

Thiopurine S-methyltransferase (TPMT) regulates anticancer drugs such as 6-mercaptopurine (6-MP) and 6-thioguanine that are commonly used for acute lymphoblastic leukemia (ALL) treatment. Because TPMT is an enzyme, its primary action is to inactivate the drug, thereby preventing toxicity from the drug (Coulthard & Hogarth, 2005). Studies have found that individuals who have low TPMT activity do not receive adequate treatment of ALL blast cells, causing escalating blast cells and higher concentrations of active 6-MP, leading to toxic effects. Hence, dose regulation based on the genetic test is necessary to avoid toxicities (Lennard et al., 1990; McLeod et al., 1995).

The most frequent variant alleles are *TPMT*2*, *TPMT*3A* (mostly seen in Caucasians), and *TPMT*3C* (common in Asians). These account for low or intermediate TPMT activity (Collie-Duguid et al., 1999; Hiratsuka et al., 2000). Individuals who carry the variant gene *TPMT*1* are wild-type homozygotes and have the highest TPMT activity, followed by the heterozygotes (*1/*3) with intermediate activity, and homozygotes (*3/*3) with two variant alleles that have no or trace TPMT activity (McLeod et al., 2000). The individuals with low TPMT activity have 10–15 times the accumulation of toxic metabolites compared to those with high and intermediate TPMT activity (McLeod & Siva, 2002).

Genetic tests are available to identify the individual's *TPMT* genotype to predict enzymatic activity prior to treatment; however, these are not routinely administered outside of a clinical trial because they were not found to be cost-effective (Brownstein et al., 2012; Higgs et al., 2010; Pinto et al., 2012; Stocco et al., 2008).

In this scenario, consent, education, DNA collection, and monitoring and management of the clinical trial protocol are essential. An extra addition to the monitoring would include the collection and calculation of cost measurements.

Irinotecan and UDP-Glucuronosyltransferase

Irinotecan, a prodrug commonly used in the treatment of colorectal cancers, is metabolized in the body to its active form, SN-38. UGT1A1, a major isoform, catalyzes the conversion of active SN-38 to inactive SN-38 glucuronide. This suggests that individuals who are deficient in UGT1A1 suffer from serious adverse effects when administered irinotecan (Iyer et al., 1998; Nagar & Blanchard, 2006; Palomaki et al., 2009). Studies have confirmed the presence of alleles at different frequencies among different populations. The UGT1A1*28 polymorphism in the Caucasian population (because of the addition of TA to the TATA box of the *UGT1A1* promoter) is the most common variant (Kaniwa et al., 2005). It is associated with a decrease in *UGT1A1* expression when homozygous. With decreased expression, the patient suffers from irinotecan toxicity (Bosma et al., 1995), such as grade 3–4 diarrhea and grade 3–4 neutropenia (Carlini et al., 2005; Innocenti et al., 2004; Massacesi et al., 2006). The allele *6 is specific to East Asians (Araki et al., 2006; Minami et al., 2007; Sai et al., 2004). Although information about the alleles that cause toxicity is available, not enough information exists to dictate patient management, so pharmacogenetic testing is not required.

The need for OCRNs to understand allelic nomenclature, decipher and include it in communications with staff, and discuss it with patients and their families is obvious. Patients appreciate information that can be communicated in a simple way so they can understand how their body responds to treatments and why their response may be different from others.

Drug Transporter Genes

Drug transporters are responsible for pumping out drug molecules across cell membranes. Too much or too little activity of these transporters can interfere with the efficacy of the drug. The ATP-binding Cassette (ABC) is a superfamily of transporters with one of its members encoded by the *ABCB1* gene, a P-glycoprotein (Houtsma et al., 2010; Petros & Evans, 2004). The role of P-glycoprotein is to decrease intestinal absorption and brain uptake of the drug as well as to increase the drug excretion via biliary, intestinal, or renal routes (Zhou, 2008). High P-glycoprotein levels indicate worse treatment outcomes. Low P-glycoprotein contributes to longer survival postchemotherapy (Opdam et al., 2012). Multiple polymorphisms in the *ABCB1* gene have been identified, a few with functional significance. Some are SNPs identified in exon 26 of *ABCB1*, causing altered drug disposition (Cascorbi et al., 2001), and SNPs in exon 12 of *ABCB1* associated with irinotecan PKs (Mathijssen et al., 2003). When these findings from clinical trials were submitted to FDA, it resulted in the requirement that the polymorphism information be incorporated into patient package inserts (Giacomini et al., 2007).

Pharmacogenetic Testing

When molecular diagnostics become routinely used in clinical settings by physicians and pharmacists, the concept of standardized dosing will be replaced by individualized dosing based on patient data from genetic testing (Cecchin & Stocco, 2020; Luzum et al., 2021). The present barriers are the cost of the newer genetic technologies compared to the cheaper alternatives (polymerase chain reaction [PCR]-based) and also the need for highly qualified and well-trained personnel for test result interpretation (Morris et al., 2022; Relling et al., 2020). Genotyping assays for detecting genetic polymorphisms, when compared to phenotypic assessments, have advantages, such as relatively easy sample collection (small amount of peripheral blood or buccal swab) and not being compromised by drug–drug and drug–food interactions (Shi et al., 2001).

It is possible that clinical trials could use currently available genotyping assays. These vary from testing for (a) a single genetic variation (UGT1A1 promoter polymorphism, Mayo Medical laboratory) (Ratain, 2006), (b) a series of genes (*CYP2D6* and *CYP2C19* on AmpliChipCYP450 Test) (Roche Molecular Diagnostics, n.d.), (c) hundreds to thousands of genetic variants (Agilent Human Genome CGH Microarray 244A) (Agilent Technologies, n.d.), or (d) the entire human genome (23andMe, n.d.).

Phenotyping assays that can identify genetic variability are gene expression profiling and enzyme activity tests (Huang & Ratain, 2009). Prediction markers have been generated to identify chemoresistance in children with ALL (Holleman et al., 2004). Oncotype DX is used in breast cancer diagnosis of tumors with an estrogen influence to quantify the likelihood of recurrence and assess the benefit of chemotherapy in newly diagnosed patients (Ishibe et al., 2011). TPMT enzyme activity testing was the first pharmacogenomic test that has proceeded to routine use and is completed before initiation of 6-MP (Ford & Berg, 2010). These genotyping and phenotyping assays on tumor cells may have to be repeated in an individual before repeated treatments, but not the individual's germline (sex chromosome) DNA, as it remains unchanged in one's lifetime (Riegert-Johnson et al., 2008).

Other methods include Taqman Allelic Discrimination Assay, a genotyping method that identifies SNPs related to drug resistance using the 5′-nuclease activity of Taq polymerase during or after PCRs. These assays detect SNPs related to drug resistance and mutations, such as point mutations, insertions, and large deletions (Fedick et al., 2012; Kamau et al., 2012). PCR with allele-specific oligonucleotide hybridization is a simple, cost-effective method used to detect a variant. The PCR method was used in identifying extensive and poor metabolizers of CYP2D6 in the late 1990s (De Gregori et al., 2010). Quantitative real-time PCR (QRT-PCR), although expensive, is a rapid and dependable method that simultaneously amplifies and quantifies a targeted DNA molecule. It was initially used in the identification of CYP2D6 alleles specific to poor metabolizers (De Gregori et al., 2010).

Several hundred drug-metabolizing genes can be studied using commercial or custom-made chips (a microarray technology used in genetic testing). Some available in the market are DMET chip, VeraCode ADME chip, and iPLEX ADME pharmacogenomics panel (Pinto et al., 2012). The DMET chip analyzes 230 drug-metabolizing genes for 1,936 SNPs, whereas the VeraCode ADME has 184 SNPs in 34 drug-metabolizing genes. In addition to these commercial chips, custom-made chips have been developed by research groups that contain specific SNPs for particular drug-metabolizing genes (Pinto et al., 2012).

Cisplatin-related ototoxicity in children was studied using a custom-made chip that had 1,949 variants in 220 drug-metabolizing genes. The chip identified TPMT and catechol-O-methyl transferase (known as COMT) enzymes to be significantly associated with ototoxicity, which was not known previously in relation to cisplatin metabolism (Ross et al., 2009).

Genome-wide association studies (GWASs) have identified significant findings related to predicting patients' risk of toxicity. A GWAS studies an entire genome for variations or SNPs (in 100s and 1,000s at the same time) that occur more often in people with a particular disease when compared to those without the disease. For example, a GWAS identified an SNP that was found to be overrepresented in GRIA1, associated with hypersensitivity to asparaginase, which is used in the treatment of ALL. The research looked at more than 500,000 SNPs in 485 children. This discovery would have been impossible if research were focused only on candidate genes (Chen et al., 2010).

Any of these tests, and even others in development, could potentially be used in a clinical trial. OCRNs must be cognizant of the emerging technologies available for use in clinical trials and be able to explain the rationale for their use to patients.

The Role of Oncology Clinical Research Nurses in Advancing Evidence-Based Care

OCRNs play an important role in moving the discoveries made in laboratories to the bedside. Their involvement in clinical trials spans the cancer continuum from conception through end-of-life care. It includes research to provide an evidence base for different facets, such as risk assessment, genetic testing, prevention, profiling, pharmacogenetics, and treatments, with a need for counseling and education. Although OCRNs collect a variety of data, one of the critical components of their role is to obtain careful medication and food intake histories. Other medications, herbal remedies, supplements, and a variety of foods are known to interfere with anticancer drug metabolism. They can lead to toxicity, even if the genetic test was negative for high-risk polymorphisms. Some clinical trials include pharmacogenetics testing to identify individuals with a high risk for toxicity of a new treatment agent being studied. This could include the need for the nurse to monitor for adverse effects and teach patients and family members to recognize or note any changes in how patients feel or react (Backman Lönn et al. 2022; Gaedigk, 2019; Hood, 2022; O'Brien et al., 2022; Park & Yu, 2021; Roden et al., 2019).

OCRNs can adapt their roles in compliance with the *Oncology Clinical Research Nurse Competencies* from the Oncology Nursing Society and the Oncology Nursing Certification Corporation (2024).

OCRNs will need to understand pharmacogenetics to perform the following (Backman Lönn et al. 2022; Calzone & Masny, 2004; Herzog-LeBoeuf & Willenberg, 2020; Patterson & Barber, 2020; Portier, 2020):

- Interpret individuals' results obtained from DNA chip technology.
- Perform a comprehensive health assessment in relation to personal, medical, and genetic risks, as well as modifiable risk factor behaviors.
- Counsel individuals about risk reduction related to the clinical trial (e.g., chemoprevention using tamoxifen, referral to clinical trials).
- Educate individuals about genetic events involved in tumor initiation and progress.
- Provide necessary information and assist in obtaining informed consent from individuals participating in clinical trials (see Chapter 12).
- Assess patients' knowledge about genetic terms (e.g., *variant* versus *polymorphism*) and understanding of screening results as related to the clinical trial.
- Interpret the genetic signature of the tumor to patients and families.

- Explain individualized treatment recommendations based on tumor profile with education about the dose of treatment using the individual's pharmacogenetic profile.
- Provide genetic profile results to physicians, assist patients in understanding their personalized results involved in drug metabolism, and give details about dose recommendations based on the individual's profile.

Summary

Pharmacogenetic studies of anticancer drugs have led to evidence-based drug administration schedules that have improved patient outcomes. Patients who participate in research studies make an invaluable contribution to the knowledge base of new and conventional anticancer drugs and diagnostics, such as cytogenetics or treatment discussions using tumor profiling. OCRNs play an essential role in coordinating and conducting these vital research studies that have a direct impact on the safety, effectiveness, and outcomes of anticancer drug administration. OCRNs must understand genetics, specifically pharmacogenetics (part of a drug clinical trial), so that they can partner with their colleagues and educate their patients to understand the important roles pharmacogenetic clinical trial studies have in the development of diagnostics and treatments in cancer care.

Key Points

- The goal of pharmacogenetics is to personalize treatment based on an individual's genetic makeup.
- The knowledge of pharmacogenetics not only aids in understanding the basic drug interaction process but also helps to correctly identify responders, nonresponders, and those who are at risk of developing adverse drug reactions.
- In clinical settings, patients experience variations in drug dose-effect and severity of adverse effects. Differences in genetic constitution are among the causes of interpatient variability.
- Phenotypically, individuals can be characterized as poor, intermediate, extensive, and ultra-rapid metabolizers.
- When molecular diagnostics become routinely used in clinical settings by physicians and pharmacists, the concept of standardized dosing will be replaced by individualized dosing based on patient data from genetic testing.
- OCRNs play an essential role in coordinating and conducting vital research studies that have a direct impact on the safety, effectiveness, and outcomes of anticancer drug administration.

The author would like to acknowledge Annamalar Jeyasehar, PhD(c), MSN, RN, and Julia A. Eggert, PhD, GNP-BC, AGN-BC, AOCN®, for their contribution to this chapter that remains unchanged from the previous edition of this book.

References

Agilent Technologies. (n.d.). *Human genome CGH microarrays.* http://www.genomics.agilent.com/en/product.jsp?cid=AG-PT-110&tabId=AG-PR-1079&_requestid=2731592

Araki, K., Fujita, K., Ando, Y., Nagashima, F., Yamamoto, W., Endo, H., ... Sasaki, Y. (2006). Pharmacogenetic impact of polymorphisms in the coding region of the UGT1A1 gene on SN-38 glucuronidation in Japanese patients with cancer. *Cancer Science, 97*(11), 1255–1259. https://doi.org/10.1111/j.1349-7006.2006.00321.x

Backman Lönn, B., Hajdarevic, S., Olofsson, N., Hörnsten, Å., & Stryrke, J. (2022). Clarifying the role of clinical research nurses working in Sweden, using the Clinical Trial Nursing Questionnaire – Swedish version. *Nursing Open, 9*(5), 2434–2443. https://https://doi.org/10.1002/nop2.1260

Bosma, P.J., Chowdhury, J.R., Bakker, C., Gantla, S., de Boer, A., Oostra, B.A., ... Elferink, R.P.O. (1995). The genetic basis of the reduced expression of bilirubin UDP-glucuronosyltransferase 1 in Gilbert's syndrome. *New England Journal of Medicine, 333*(18), 1171–1175. https://doi.org/10.1056/NEJM199511023331802

Brownstein, C., Fusaro, V.A., Savage, S., Clinton, C., Mandl, K., Margulies, D., ... Manzi, S. (2012). Integration of a standardized pharmacogenomic platform for clinical decision support at Boston Children's Hospital. *BMC Proceedings, 6*, P5. https://doi.org/10.1186/1753-6561-6-S6-P5

Calzone, K.A., & Masny, A. (2004). Genetics and oncology nursing. *Seminars in Oncology Nursing, 20*(3), 178–185. https://doi.org/10.1053/j.soncn.2004.04.004

Carlini, L.E., Meropol, N.J., Bever, J., Andria, M.L., Hill, T., Gold, P., ... Blanchard, R.L. (2005). UGT1A7 and UGT1A9 polymorphisms predict response and toxicity in colorectal cancer patients treated with capecitabine/irinotecan. *Clinical Cancer Research, 11*(3), 1226–1236.

Cascorbi, I., Gerloff, T., Johne, A., Meisel, C., Hoffmeyer, S., Schwab, M., ... Roots, I. (2001). Frequency of single nucleotide polymorphisms in the P-glycoprotein drug transporter MDR1 gene in White subjects. *Clinical Pharmacology and Therapeutics, 69*(3), 169–174. https://doi.org/10.1067/mcp.2001.114164

Cecchin, E., & Stocco, G. (2020). Pharmacogenomics and personalized medicine. *Genes, 11*(6), 679. https://doi.org/10.3390/genes11060679

Chen, S., Pei, D., Yang, W., Cheng, C., Jeha, S., Cox, N.J., ... Relling, M.V. (2010). Genetic variations in GRIA1 on chromosome 5q33 related to asparaginase hypersensitivity. *Clinical Pharmacology and Therapeutics, 88*(2), 191–196. https://doi.org/10.1038/clpt.2010.94

Collie-Duguid, E., Pritchard, S., Powrie, R., Sludden, J., Collier, D., Li, T., ... McLeod, H. (1999). The frequency and distribution of thiopurine methyltransferase alleles in Caucasian and Asian populations. *Pharmacogenetics, 9*(1), 37–42. https://doi.org/10.1097/00008571-199902000-00006

Coulthard, S., & Hogarth, L. (2005). The thiopurines: An update. *Investigational New Drugs, 23*(6), 523–532. https://doi.org/10.1007/s10637-005-4020-8

Deenen, M.J., Cats, A., Beijnen, J.H., & Schellens, J.H. (2011). Part 1: Background, methodology, and clinical adoption of pharmacogenetics. *Oncologist, 16*(6), 811–819. https://doi.org/10.1634/theoncologist.2010-0258

De Gregori, M., Allegri, M., De Gregori, S., Garbin, G., Tinelli, C., Regazzi, M., ... Ranzani, G.N. (2010). How and why to screen for CYP2D6 interindividual variability in patients under pharmacological treatments. *Current Drug Metabolism, 11*(3), 276–282. https://doi.org/10.2174/138920010791196274

Driessnack, M., Campbell, M., & Fornero, K. (2022). Moving knowledge to action: Aware, adopt, adapt (A_3). *Journal for Nurse Practitioners, 18*(5), 503–505. https://doi.org/10.1016/j.nurpra.2022.01.021

Eggert, J. (2017). Genetics and genomics in oncology nursing: What does every nurse need to know? *Nursing Clinics of North America, 52*(1), 1–25. https://doi.org/10.1016/j.cnur.2016.11.001

European Agency for the Evaluation of Medicinal Products. (2002, November 21). *Position paper on terminology in pharmacogenetics.* https://s3-eu-west-1.amazonaws.com/contenidos.institutoroche.es/pdf/gmbib/position_paper.pdf

Fedick, A., Su, J., & Treff, N.R. (2012). Development of TaqMan allelic discrimination based genotyping of large DNA deletions. *Genomics, 99*(3), 127–131. https://doi.org/10.1016/j.ygeno.2012.01.003

Ford, L., & Berg, J. (2010). Thiopurine S-methyltransferase (TPMT) assessment prior to starting thiopurine drug treatment: A pharmacogenomic test whose time has come. *Journal of Clinical Pathology, 63*(4), 288–295. https://doi.org/10.1136/jcp.2009.069252

Gaedigk, A. (2019). Pharmacogenetics: Chasing perfection. *Clinical Pharmacology and Therapeutics, 106*(2), 265–270. https://doi.org/10.1002/cpt.1511

Giacomini, K., Brett, C., Altman, R., Benowitz, N., Dolan, M., Flockhart, D., ... Zineh, I. (2007). The pharmacogenetics research network: From SNP discovery to clinical drug response. *Clinical Pharmacology and Therapeutics, 81*(3), 328–345. https://doi.org/10.1038/sj.clpt.6100087

Herzog-LeBoeuf, C., & Willenberg, K.M. (2020). The history of clinical trials research: Implications for oncology nurses. *Seminars in Oncology Nursing, 36*(2), 150997. https://doi.org/j.soncn.2020.150997

Higgs, J., Gambhir, N., Ramsden, S.C., Poulton, K., & Newman, W.G. (2010). Pharmacogenetic testing in the United Kingdom genetics and immunogenetics laboratories. *Genetic Testing and Molecular Biomarkers, 14*(1), 121–125. https://doi.org/10.1089/gtmb.2009.0156

Hiratsuka, M., Inoue, T., Omori, F., Agatsuma, Y., & Mizugaki, M. (2000). Genetic analysis of thiopurine methyltransferase polymorphism in a Japanese population. *Mutation Research, 448*(1), 91–95. https://doi.org/10.1016/S0027-5107(00)00004-X

Holleman, A., Cheok, M.H., den Boer, M.L., Yang, W., Veerman, A.J., Kazemier, K.M., ... Relling, M.V. (2004). Gene-expression patterns in drug-resistant acute lymphoblastic leukemia cells and response to treatment. *New England Journal of Medicine, 351*(6), 533–542. https://doi.org/10.1056/NEJMoa033513

Hood, B. (2022). Exploring nurses' experiences of caring for patients participating in cancer clinical trials. *British Journal of Nursing, 31*(17), S18–S24. https://doi.org/10.12968/bjon.2022.31.17.S18

Houtsma, D., Guchelaar, H., & Gelderblom, H. (2010). Pharmacogenetics in oncology: A promising field. *Current Pharmaceutical Design, 16*(2), 155–163. https://doi.org/10.2174/138161210790112719

Huang, R.S., & Ratain, M.J. (2009). Pharmacogenetics and pharmacogenomics of anticancer agents. *CA: A Cancer Journal for Clinicians, 59*(1), 42–55. https://doi.org/10.3322/caac.20002

Innocenti, F., Undevia, S.D., Iyer, L., Chen, P.X., Das, S., Kocherginsky, M., ... & Ratain, M.J. (2004). Genetic variants in the UDP-glucuronosyltransferase 1A1 gene predict the risk of severe neutropenia of irinotecan. *Journal of Clinical Oncology, 22*(8), 1382–1388. https://doi.org/10.1200/JCO.2004.07.173

Ishibe, N., Schully, S., Freedman, A., & Ramsey, S.D. (2011). Use of Oncotype DX in women with node-positive breast cancer. *PLOS Currents, 3,* RRN1249. https://doi.org/10.1371/currents.RRN1249

Iyer, L., King, C.D., Whitington, P.F., Green, M.D., Roy, S.K., Tephly, T.R., ... Ratain, M.J. (1998). Genetic predisposition to the metabolism of irinotecan (CPT-11). Role of uridine diphosphate glucuronosyltransferase isoform 1A1 in the glucuronidation of its active metabolite (SN-38) in human liver microsomes. *Journal of Clinical Investigation, 101*(4), 847–854. https://doi.org/10.1172/JCI915

Kamau, E., Alemayehu, S., Feghali, K.C., Tolbert, L.S., Ogutu, B., & Ockenhouse, C.F. (2012). Development of a TaqMan allelic discrimination assay for detection of single nucleotides polymorphisms associated with anti-malarial drug resistance. *Malaria Journal, 11,* 23. https://doi.org/10.1186/1475-2875-11-23

Kaniwa, N., Kurose, K., Jinno, H., Tanaka-Kagawa, T., Saito, Y., Saeki, M., ... Hasegawa, R. (2005). Racial variability in haplotype frequencies of UGT1A1 and glucuronidation activity of a novel single nucleotide polymorphism 686C> T (P229L) found in an African-American. *Drug Metabolism and Disposition, 33*(3), 458–465. https://doi.org/10.1124/dmd.104.001800

Lennard, L., Lilleyman, J., Van Loon, J., & Weinshilboum, R. (1990). Genetic variation in response to 6-mercaptopurine for childhood acute lymphoblastic leukaemia. *Lancet, 336*(8709), 225–229. https://doi.org/10.1016/0140-6736(90)91745-V

Lewis, R. (2012). *Human genetics: Concepts and applications* (10th ed.). McGraw-Hill.

Louie, S., & Russell, J. (2013). Biomarkers for safety assessment and clinical pharmacology. In H.-J. Lenz (Ed.), *Biomarkers in oncology: Prediction and prognosis* (pp. 381–400). Springer.

Luzum, J.A., Petry, N., Taylor, A.K., Van Driest, S.L., Dunnenberger, H.M., & Cavallari, L.H. (2021). Moving pharmacogenetics into practice: It's all about the evidence. *Clinical Pharmacology and Therapeutics, 110*(3), 649–661. https://doi.org/10.1002/cpt.2327

Massacesi, C., Terrazzino, S., Marcucci, F., Rocchi, M.B., Lippe, P., Bisonni, R., ... Leon, A. (2006). Uridine diphosphate glucuronosyl transferase 1A1 promoter polymorphism predicts the risk of gastrointestinal toxicity and fatigue induced by irinotecan-based chemotherapy. *Cancer, 106*(5), 1007–1016. https://doi.org/10.1002/cncr.21722

Mathijssen, R.H.J., Marsh, S., Karlsson, M.O., Xie, R., Baker, S.D., Verweij, J., ... McLeod, H.L. (2003). Irinotecan pathway genotype analysis to predict pharmacokinetics. *Clinical Cancer Research, 9*(9), 3246–3253.

McLeod, H.L., Krynetski, E.Y., Relling, M.V., & Evans, W.E. (2000). Genetic polymorphism of thiopurine methyltransferase and its clinical relevance for childhood acute lymphoblastic leukemia. *Leukemia, 14*(4), 567–572. https://doi.org/10.1038/sj.leu.2401723

McLeod, H.L., Relling, M.V., Liu, Q., Pui, C.H., & Evans, W.E. (1995). Polymorphic thiopurine methyltransferase in erythrocytes is indicative of activity in leukemic blasts from children with acute lymphoblastic leukemia. *Blood, 85*(7), 1897–1902.

McLeod, H.L., & Siva, C. (2002). The thiopurine S-methyltransferase gene locus-implications for clinical pharmacogenomics. *Pharmacogenomics, 3*(1), 89–98. https://doi.org/10.1517/14622416.3.1.89

Minami, H., Sai, K., Saeki, M., Saito, Y., Ozawa, S., Suzuki, K., ... Yamamoto, N. (2007). Irinotecan pharmacokinetics/pharmacodynamics and UGT1A genetic polymorphisms in Japanese: Roles of UGT1A1* 6 and* 28. *Pharmacogenetics and Genomics, 17*(7), 497–504. https://doi.org/10.1097/FPC.0b013e328014341f

Morris, S.A., Alsaidi, A.T., Verbyla, A., Cruz, A., Macfarlane, C., Baur, J., & Patel, J.N. (2022). Cost effectiveness of pharmacogenetic testing for drugs with clinical pharmacogenetics implementation consortium (CPIC) guidelines: A systematic review. *Clinical Pharmacology and Therapeutics, 112*(6), 1318–1328. https://doi.org/10.1002/cpt.2754

Mounier-Boutoille, H., Boisdron-Celle, M., Cauchin, E., Galmiche, J., Morel, A., Gamelin, E., & Matysiak-Budnik, T. (2010). Lethal outcome of 5-fluorouracil infusion in a patient with a total DPD deficiency and a double DPYD and UTG1A1 gene mutation. *British Journal of Clinical Pharmacology, 70*(2), 280–283. https://doi.org/10.1111/j.1365-2125.2010.03686.x

Naeim, F., Rao, P.N., Song, S.X., & Phan, R.T. (2018). *Atlas of hematopathology: Morphology, immunophenotype, cytogenetics, and molecular approaches* (2nd ed.). Elsevier Academic Press. https://doi.org/10.1016/C2015-0-05997-4

Nagar, S., & Blanchard, R.L. (2006). Pharmacogenetics of uridine diphosphoglucuronosyltransferase (UGT) 1A family members and its role in patient response to irinotecan. *Drug Metabolism Reviews, 38*(3), 393–409. https://doi.org/10.1080/03602530600739835

National Human Genome Research Institute. (n.d.). *Polymorphism.* http://ghr.nlm.nih.gov/glossary=polymorphism

Nebert, D.W., Adnesik, M., Coon, M.J., Estabrook, R.W., Gonzalez, F.J., Guengerich, F.P., ... Levin, W. (1987). The P450 gene superfamily: Recommended nomenclature. *DNA, 6*(1), 1–11. https://doi.org/10.1089/dna.1987.6.1

Nomeir, A.A. (2010). Pharmacokinetics. In M.N. Cayen (Ed.), *Early drug development: Strategies and routes to first-in-human trials* (pp. 64–65). Wiley.

O'Brien, C., Furlong, E., Coughlan, B., Fox, P., & Darley, A. (2022). Building research capacity and culture: Exploring nurses' experience of implementing a nurse-led clinical trial. *Journal of Nursing Management, 30*(4), 1002–1010. https://doi.org/10.1111/jonm.13576

Oncology Nursing Society & Oncology Nursing Certification Corporation. (2024). *Oncology clinical research nurse competencies.* https://www.ons.org/sites/default/files/2025-01/ocrn-competencies-rebrand.pdf

Opdam, F.L., Gelderblom, H., & Guchelaar, H. (2012). Phenotyping drug disposition in oncology. *Cancer Treatment Reviews, 38*(6), 715–725. https://doi.org/10.1016/j.ctrv.2011.12.003

Palomaki, G.E., Bradley, L.A., Douglas, M.P., Kolor, K., & Dotson, W.D. (2009). Can UGT1A1 genotyping reduce morbidity and mortality in patients with metastatic colorectal cancer treated with irinotecan? An evidence-based review. *Genetics in Medicine, 11*(1), 21–34. https://doi.org/10.1097/GIM.0b013e31818efd77

Park, H-J., & Yu, S. (2021). The role of clinical trial nurses: Transitioning from clinicians to clinical research coordinators. *International Journal of Nursing Practice, 28*(1), e12943. https://doi.org/10.111/ijn.12943

Patterson, C., & Barber, F.D. (2020). Clinical trial subinvestigator: An emerging role for oncology nurse practitioners. *Clinical Journal of Oncology Nursing, 24*(5), 479–481. https://doi.org/10.1188/20.CJON.479-481

Petros, W.P., & Evans, W.E. (2004). Pharmacogenomics in cancer therapy: Is host genome variability important? *Trends in Pharmacological Sciences, 25*(9), 457–464. https://doi.org/10.1016/j.tips.2004.07.007

Pinto, N., Cohn, S.L., & Dolan, M.E. (2012). Using germ line genomics to individualize pediatric cancer treatments. *Clinical Cancer Research, 18*(10), 2791–2800. https://doi.org/10.1158/1078-0432.CCR-11-1938

Portier, W.S. (2020). Caner clinical trials: Implications for oncology nurses. *Seminars in Oncology Nursing, 36*(2), 150998. https://doi.org/10.1016/j.soncn.2020.150998

Prows, C.A. (2011). Infusion of pharmacogenetics into cancer care. *Seminars in Oncology Nursing, 27*(1), 45–53. https://doi.org/10.1016/j.soncn.2010.11.006

Raida, M., Schwabe, W., Häusler, P., Van Kuilenburg, A.B., Van Gennip, A.H., Behnke, D., & Höffken, K. (2001). Prevalence of a common point mutation in the dihydropyrimidine dehydrogenase (DPD) gene within the 5′-splice donor site of intron 14 in patients with severe 5-fluorouracil (5-FU)-related toxicity compared with controls. *Clinical Cancer Research, 7*(9), 2832–2839.

Ratain, M.J. (2006). From bedside to bench to bedside to clinical practice: An odyssey with irinotecan. *Clinical Cancer Research, 12*(6), 1658–1660. https://doi.org/10.1158/1078-0432.CCR-06-0159

Relling, M.V., Klein, T.E., Gammal, R.S., Whirl-Carrillo, M., Hoffman, J.M., & Caudle, K.E. (2020). The Clinical Pharmacogenetics Implementation Consortium: 10 years later. *Clinical Pharmacology and Therapeutics, 107*(1), 171–175. https://doi.org/10.1002/cpt.1651

Riegert-Johnson, D.L., Macaya, D., Hefferon, T.W., & Boardman, L.A. (2008). The incidence of duplicate genetic testing. *Genetics in Medicine, 10*(2), 114–116. https://doi.org/10.1097/GIM.0b013e31816166a7

Roche Molecular Diagnostics. (n.d.). *AmpliChip CYP450 test.* https://molecular.roche.com/assays/Pages/AmpliChipCYP450Test.aspx

Roden, D.M., McLeod, H.L., Relling, M.V., Williams, M.S., Mensah, G.A., Peterson, J.F., & Van Driest, S.L. (2019). Pharmacogenomics. *Lancet, 394*(10197), 521–532. https://doi.org/10.1016/S0140-6736(19)31276-0

Ross, C.J., Katzov-Eckert, H., Dubé, M., Brooks, B., Rassekh, S.R., Barhdadi, A., ... Hayden, M.R. (2009). Genetic variants in TPMT and COMT are associated with hearing loss in children receiving cisplatin chemotherapy. *Nature Genetics, 41*(12), 1345–1349. https://doi.org/10.1038/ng.478

Sai, K., Saeki, M., Saito, Y., Ozawa, S., Katori, N., Jinno, H., ... Saijo, N. (2004). UGT1A1 haplotypes associated with reduced glucuronidation and increased serum bilirubin in irinotecan-administered Japanese patients with cancer. *Clinical Pharmacology and Therapeutics, 75*(6), 501–515. https://doi.org/10.1016/j.clpt.2004.01.010

Sauna, Z.E., Kimchi-Sarfaty, C., Ambudkar, S.V., & Gottesman, M.M. (2007). Silent polymorphisms speak: How they affect pharmacogenomics and the treatment of cancer. *Cancer Research, 67*(20), 9609–9612. https://doi.org/10.1158/0008-5472.CAN-07-2377

Scripture, C.D., & Figg, W.D. (2006). Drug interactions in cancer therapy. *Nature Reviews: Cancer, 6*(7), 546–558. https://doi.org/10.1038/nrc1887

Shaffer, L.G., McGowan-Jordan, J., & Schmid, M. (Eds.). (2012). *ISCN 2013: An international system for human cytogenetic nomenclature: Recommendations of the International Standing Committee on Human Cytogenetic Nomenclature.* Karger.

Shi, M.M., Bleavins, M.R., & de la Iglesia, F.A. (2001). Pharmacogenetic application in drug development and clinical trials. *Drug Metabolism and Disposition, 29*(4), 591–595.

Stocco, G., Cheok, M., Crews, K., Dervieux, T., French, D., Pei, D., ... Evans, W.E. (2008). Genetic polymorphism of inosine triphosphate pyrophosphatase is a determinant of mercaptopurine metabolism and toxicity during treatment for acute lymphoblastic leukemia. *Clinical Pharmacology and Therapeutics, 85*(2), 164–172. https://doi.org/10.1038/clpt.2008.154

23andMe. (n.d.). *Welcome.* https://www.23andme.com

U.S. Food and Drug Administration. (2017). *The FDA's drug review process: Ensuring drugs are safe and effective.* http://www.fda.gov/drugs/resourcesforyou/consumers/ucm143534.htm

van Kuilenburg, A.B., Haasjes, J., Richel, D.J., Zoetekouw, L., Van Lenthe, H., De Abreu, R.A., ... van Gennip, A.H. (2000). Clinical implications of dihydropyrimidine dehydrogenase (DPD) deficiency in patients with severe 5-fluorouracil–associated toxicity: Identification of new mutations in the DPD gene. *Clinical Cancer Research, 6*(12), 4705–4712.

Venter, J.C., Adams, M.D., Myers, E.W., Li, P.W., Mural, R.J., Sutton, G.G., ... Zhu, X. (2001). The sequence of the human genome. *Science, 291*(5507), 1304–1351. https://doi.org/10.1126/science.1058040

Zhou, S.-F. (2008). Structure, function and regulation of P-glycoprotein and its clinical relevance in drug disposition. *Xenobiotica, 38*(7–8), 802–832. https://doi.org/10.1080/00498250701867889

CHAPTER 25

Genetic Testing

Madeline Merrill, MSN, AGNP-BC

Introduction

More than 30 years ago, the Human Genome Project started with the ambitious goal of mapping the human genome. In response, the National Human Genome Research Institute (NHGRI) was created to conduct concurrent research and to foster "basic and applied research on the ethical, legal, and social implications of genetic and genomic research for individuals, families, and communities" (NHGRI, 2025, para. 1).

In 2018, the Pan-Cancer Atlas was published by the National Institutes of Health (NIH) and NHGRI, detailing the genomics of more than 10,000 tumors across 33 different cancer types and conveying information about cell origin, oncogenic processes, and oncogenic pathways (Faherty, 2018). This was a monumental accomplishment in the scientific oncology world, inconceivable on such a large scale even 10 years prior, with resulting technical, ethical, legal, and social implications for cancer care and patients worldwide.

Oncology clinical research nurses (OCRNs) whose research area includes hereditary cancer syndromes, cancer somatic and germline testing, and use of genetic information must be familiar with ethical, legal, and social implications for cancer care, identification of genetic and genomic information associated with hereditary syndromes, and sampling and storage of genetic material and information as part of primary and ancillary trials. The conduct of research studies for screening, prevention and risk reduction, diagnosis, treatment, and survivorship in the hereditary cancer population promotes oncology care in this high-risk population.

This chapter will discuss genetic testing. It will highlight hereditary cancer predisposition testing and address the integration and utility of hereditary cancer predisposition information into oncology research protocols. Further, it will explore genetic counseling, outlining the ethical considerations and costs surrounding it.

Hereditary Cancer Predisposition Testing

Genetics and Cancer Development

A gene is a tiny instruction manual located within the nucleus of a cell that tells the cell what kind of proteins to make and what function to perform. A person's genes are inherited from their parents. All the genes of a person make up their genome. Although all human genomes are similar, they have some small differences that make each person unique. NHGRI (2019, para. 9) detailed that "on average, a human gene will have 1–3 letters that differ from person to person. These differences are enough to change the shape and function of a protein, how much protein is made, when it is made, or where it's made. These variations in your genome also influence your risk of developing diseases and your responses to medications." How a person interacts with their environment also influences the expression and function of a gene; changes in DNA sequencing result in changes in the function of the cell. The overall effect of changed cell function can be harmful and cause health issues (e.g., cancer).

In hereditary cancer syndromes, a variant can pass from one or both parents to a child through the sperm or ovum, resulting in a predisposition, or increased risk, to develop cancer. Of all diagnosed cancers, 5%–10% are considered hereditary (National Cancer Institute [NCI], 2024a). Most hereditary cancer syndrome variants pass in an autosomal dominant manner, meaning that they only require one altered variant gene to pass the condition. *Penetrance* refers to "the likelihood that a clinical condition will occur when a particular genotype is present" (NCI, 2024a, para. 25). The variants associated with hereditary cancer syndromes are highly penetrant, that is, very likely to cause one or more cancers in the lifetime of the individual and often at a younger age than in the general population. Somatic variants, also known as acquired variants, are genetic variants that arise from environmental factors throughout a person's lifetime. Viruses, diet, exercise, and tobacco use can cause somatic variants in cells. This type of variant occurs after fertilization and is thus not inherited and cannot be passed down to future generations (Miles & Tadi, 2024).

Cancer risk assessment, genetic testing, and screening for cancer predisposition are valuable tools in the medical management of individuals identified with, or whose personal and family history is suggestive of, a hereditary cancer syndrome. This high-risk population has needs specific to the younger age at onset with increased screening, prevention, survivorship, treatment, and reproductive health education and support (NCI, 2025). When a cancer predisposition syndrome is suspected, further evaluation through tumor profiling, documentation of family history, and identification of any features suggestive of hereditary cancers will determine if cancer predisposition testing is appropriate. Genetic cancer predisposition testing can provide information for cancer risk management for an individual and their family. Predisposition testing provides information so that healthcare providers may tailor the treatment, screening, surveillance, prevention, and survivorship to the risks specific to the syndrome as compared to general population risks. Clinical trials, research registries for data collection, and genetic testing are sources of evidence to develop and support the unique and specific needs of this high-risk population (NCI, 2025).

Cancer Predisposition Genetic Testing

Genetic testing has rapidly evolved in the past 50 years, drastically altering the patient experience and provider services. In the 1970s, genetic information was gained entirely from a patient's family history and detailed personal medical history. Providers would create a pedigree and advise patients based on trends noted within their family histories. In the 1980s, some institutions began using fluorescence in situ hybridization, a blood test using short, single-stranded DNA identified by fluorescent dye that could show large aberrations in genetic material and isolate chromosomes affected. Although this was a significant advancement, small genetic changes were still unable to be detected.

In 1993, English-born Canadian biochemist Michael Smith and American biochemist Kary Banks Mullis won the Nobel Prize for Chemistry for the discovery of a polymerase chain reaction technique that allowed researchers to make millions of copies of a gene in a test tube. Combined with gene cloning, gene sequencing, and gene mapping, researchers were able to move rapidly from identifying a chromosomal position to recreating the gene (Mukherjee, 2017). These advancements enabled American geneticist Mary-Claire King to discover the breast cancer susceptibility gene 1 (*BRCA1*), which is responsible for 57%–66% of early-onset breast cancers and 39%–59% of ovarian cancers (NCI, 2024a).

In 1996, Myriad Genetics began marketing a test for *BRCA*. For this study, a genetic counselor evaluated a patient who then submitted a swab of mouth cells to a central laboratory where parts of the *BRCA1* gene were amplified to identify variant genes. Reports were created that labeled a woman's cells "normal," "mutant," or "indeterminate" (Mukherjee, 2017). This testing essentially launched the field of routine genetic testing, leading to the multitudes of genetic testing options available to patients for common hereditary cancer syndromes.

Completion of the Human Genome Project in 2003 and ongoing clinical trials now support the identification of less penetrant genetic alterations in cancer predisposition genes, with the U.S. Preventive Services Task Force (2024) and NCI (2024a) issuing recommendations for testing by cancer type. Genetic testing for inherited predisposition is now routine in the management and care of high-risk individuals. Germline DNA, inherited through the sperm or ovum and present in every cell, is the source for hereditary cancer predisposition testing and is typically obtained from blood or saliva. Testing for somatic or acquired variants is generally performed from a blood sample or on tumor tissue obtained via biopsy.

Hereditary Cancer Syndrome Identification

The American Society of Clinical Oncology (ASCO) has long held that the identification and management of patients with inherited susceptibility to cancer is a core tenet of oncology care, releasing its first statement recommending genetic testing as early as 1996 (Robson et al., 2015). The decision to test for hereditary cancer predisposition syndromes is determined through careful assessment and consideration of how the outcome of testing will affect the patient and family, and if the test will have clinical utility. ASCO guidelines include specific recommendations regarding the taking of a family history in an oncology practice. OCRNs are frequently the front-line clinicians meeting patients. Therefore, taking a thorough medical and familial history is an essential skill to perfect. Information collected should include the patient's personal cancer history and the history of at least three generations of immediate family members, including both first- and second-degree relatives. First-degree relatives are parents, children, and full siblings. Second-degree relatives are grandparents, aunts and uncles, nieces and nephews, grandchildren, and half-siblings. For each family member, the information collected should include the diagnosis or disease and age of onset. Ethnicity should be noted in familial history as well (Tung et al., 2024).

Ideally, a three-generation pedigree could be able to be constructed for each patient. However, ASCO guidelines acknowledge that the intensive labor required and time constraints in a busy oncology practice are limiting factors and thus encourage the use of electronic tools to construct a pedigree for review by the clinician. The addition of pathology reports, when available, can improve the accuracy of the recall of cancer history within a family and support identification of a hereditary cancer syndrome. Family history should be taken at the first visit and periodically updated. ASCO guidelines note that a necessary time to update family history is during the transition from active treatment to survivorship, as screening and prevention strategies will be discussed at that visit (Tung et al., 2024).

A targeted physical examination should be included because some hereditary cancer syndromes have associated characteristic physical features (phenotypic traits), including benign features (Lindor et al., 2008) (see Figure 25-1). OCRNs who work with hereditary syndromes in clinical trials should be familiar with other features, often referred to as *red flags*, that suggest a hereditary cancer within a family, including early onset of cancer (prior to age 50 years), multiple primary cancers in a single individual, multiple relatives or generations with the same type of cancer, occurrence of rare or uncommon tumors, and Ashkenazi Jewish heritage (Tung et al., 2024) (see Figure 25-2).

- Cutaneous findings (e.g., trichilemmomas, lipomas, keratosis, café-au-lait spots, unusual freckling, pigmentation)
- Polyposis (e.g., colon, small bowel)
- Thyroid changes
- Macrocephaly (particularly if associated with autism)
- Tumor histology suggestive of a hereditary cancer (e.g., microsatellite instability, medullary thyroid cancer)

FIGURE 25-1 | Cutaneous Features Associated With Hereditary Cancer Syndromes

Note. Based on information from Lindor et al., 2008.

- Early onset of cancers that usually occur later in life (e.g., premenopausal breast cancer, colon cancer before age 50 years, endometrial cancer before age 50 years)
- Multiple primary cancers in a single individual (e.g., colon and endometrial, breast and ovarian, thyroid and endometrial, colon cancer more than once); may be synchronous or metachronous
- Bilateral cancer in paired organs or multifocal disease (e.g., bilateral or multifocal breast or renal cancer)
- Multiple relatives or generations with the same type of cancer
- Male breast cancer
- Occurrence of rare or uncommon tumors (e.g., adrenocortical carcinoma, duodenal cancer, medullary thyroid cancer)
- Rare cancers associated with birth defects (e.g., Wilms tumor, genitourinary abnormalities)
- Ashkenazi Jewish heritage associated with a higher prevalence of *BRCA1*/*BRCA2* variants

FIGURE 25-2 | Hereditary Cancer Syndrome Red Flags

Note. Based on information from National Cancer Institute, 2025; Tung et al., 2024.

When to Test for Hereditary Cancer Syndromes: Contrasting Clinical Testing With Research Testing

Clinical utility is the primary determining factor in the decision to offer cancer predisposition testing in the clinical setting. The NCI algorithm for determining the appropriateness of testing illustrates this decision process (see Figure 25-3). This knowledge will assist OCRNs in confirming the appropriateness of genetic testing, even in a clinical trial setting.

OCRNs associated with the identification and management of hereditary cancer syndromes must understand the principles and guidelines of clinical predisposition testing to educate patients appropriately (International Society of Nurses in Genetics, 2021). A 2010 ASCO policy statement described the value of clinical research in cancer predisposition testing stating that "prospective clinical trials, large registries, and retrospective reviews are the most accurate methods for deriving relative risks of genetic variants and measuring the response to and effectiveness of clinical interventions based on genetic cancer risk assessment" (Robson et al., 2010, p. 896). In 2015, this policy was updated to account for the opportunities and challenges that arise from massive technological advancements made possible by parallel sequencing and multigene panel testing. The authors encouraged research to establish evidence bases for understanding the best use of multigene panel testing, quality assurance of the technology, and education of the providers. ASCO's position also continues to encourage research that includes the clinical implications of unexpected germline variants in high-penetrance genes and variants in moderate-penetrance genes, as well as addresses variants of unknown significance. Robson et al. (2015, p. 3664) noted that "until these questions are resolved, it remains appropriate to conduct limited testing for mutations in genes of established clinical utility suggested by the patient's history."

Benefits and Limitations

The physical risks for predisposition genetic testing are the same as for any blood draw via venipuncture (e.g., slight bruising, slight discomfort, low risk of infection at the venipuncture site) or buccal smear/swab or collection of saliva (e.g., potential for burning or stinging sensation if mouthwash is used). The laboratory performing the test will offer instructions about the preferred or alternative collection methods. When performing somatic testing, cells from the existing cancer can be taken either through biopsy of the tumor tissue or through blood draw via venipuncture, assessing circulating tumor DNA (ctDNA). Biopsy of tumor tissue will typically give more comprehensive results. However, a biopsy procedure has a higher risk of complications depending on the tumor site (e.g., bleeding, infection, pain, scarring, damage to nearby organs).

Researchers are investigating and evaluating the benefits and limitations of genetic tests associated with hereditary cancer syndromes, with most of the evidence in the high-penetrance gene variants. The existing evidence for the benefits and limitations of testing for low- or intermediate-penetrance variants is limited (National Comprehensive Cancer Network, 2025). Identification of high-penetrance variants can clarify risk, provide information for family members, and support medical management.

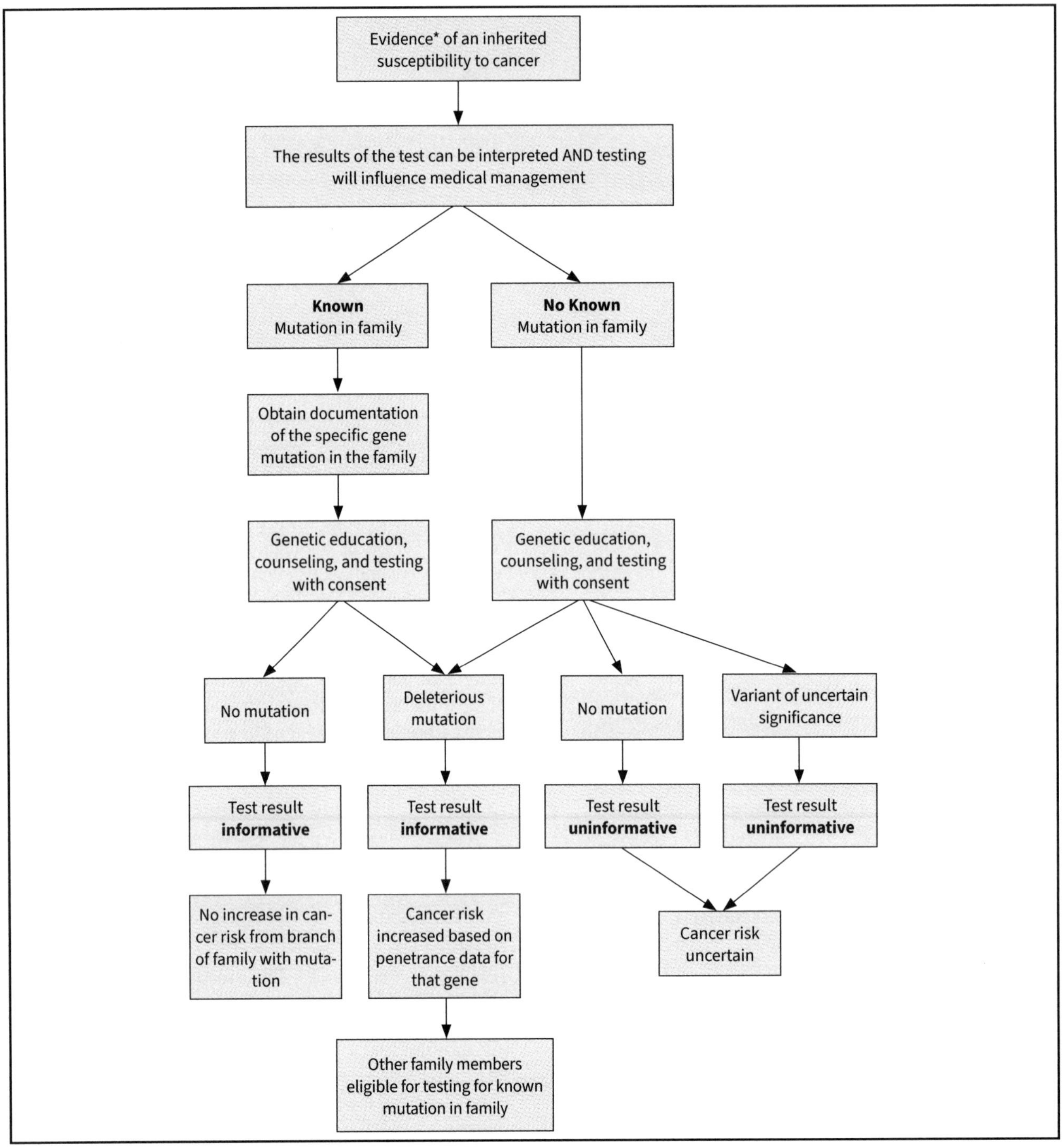

FIGURE 25-3 | Genetic Testing Algorithm for Cancer Susceptibility

Note. From *Cancer Genetics Risk Assessment and Counseling (PDQ®)–Health Professional Version*, by National Cancer Institute, 2025 (www.cancer.gov/cancertopics/pdq/genetics/risk-assessment-and-counseling/HealthProfessional). In the public domain.

Genetic Counseling

When undergoing germline and hereditary cancer testing, ASCO guidelines recommend referral of patients for genetic counseling. The term *genetic counseling* was first used in 1947 to describe advice given by American biologist and geneticist Sheldon Reed to physicians about their patients' genetic conditions. This term has evolved to include more than 5,000 professionals licensed as genetic counselors practicing in multiple specialties, with oncology being the most common (Ebott & Scalia, 2023). Typically, a genetic counseling consultation involves pretest counseling in which risks, limitations, and potential effects of results for patients and families are discussed. A results review and post-test counseling are also included, along with recommendations for the patient's health, such as increased screening, testing recommendations for family, and referrals to specialists.

Somatic genetic testing does not require the use of a genetic counselor, as these variants are not inheritable. Counseling may improve patient understanding of potential results and provide anticipatory guidance for response to results (e.g., relief, guilt, fear, anxiety). Counseling prepares patients to understand their risk for cancer when test results are uninformative or inconclusive. For example, test results are uninformative when no variant is identified in an unaffected individual (i.e., the person has not had cancer) and no affected family member (i.e., a family member with cancer) has been tested for variants. Test results are inconclusive when a variant of uncertain significance has been identified. Inconclusive results cannot be interpreted with confidence using existing information. Figure 25-4 lists the potential limitations and benefits of genetic testing.

A limited number of trained professionals are available in the United States, and more patients than ever qualify for genetic testing. Because of this, genetic counseling modalities are expanding to include telehealth, alternative counseling providers such as nurses, and artificial intelligence technology (Ebott & Scalia, 2023). These modalities continue to be closely studied, especially as they are changing clinical workflows and insurance reimbursement.

A significant development is the advent and popularity of direct-to-consumer marketing of DNA sequence–based testing. This type of testing is marketed as time-saving and frequently does not require provider visits. NHGRI (2023) notes that many of these tests are not regulated by the U.S. Food and Drug Administration, the Centers for Medicare and Medicaid Services, and the Federal Trade Commission. In 2023, the U.S. Food and Drug Administration authorized 23andMe to market a test that includes 44 pathogenetic variants in *BRCA1* and *BRCA2*. Similar authorizations are anticipated in the coming years for these at-home tests. However, direct-to-consumer testing should not be perceived as a replacement for approved germline genetic testing, as consumer testing does not fully sequence the genes being tested and can have a false positive rate of approximately 40% (Tandy-Connor et al., 2018).

Limitations

- Potential for uninformative result or result of uncertain significance
- May need to have other family members tested for clarification
- Lack of evidence-based guidance regarding prevention or surveillance associated with the result
- The financial cost of testing and the cost of increased screening or prevention measures
- Psychological distress, including anxiety, loss of self-esteem, and depression
- Alteration in family communication
- Potential guilt related to transmission to children
- Survivor guilt
- Potential or perceived insurance, employment, or social discrimination (for self or extended family)
- Misunderstanding of the meaning of a negative result, with failure to adhere to increased screening
- Adjustment to change in expected life course
- Regret over previous decisions, such as having risk-reducing surgeries
- Family coping difficulties resulting in distress
- Identification of new information, such as nonpaternity
- Feeling unprepared or not equipped to disseminate information to family
- Loss of privacy
- Failure to seek informational updates on testing advances and availability

Benefits

- May eliminate uncertainty about inherited susceptibility
- Support for additional cancer risk management strategies, such as chemoprevention, risk-reducing surgery, or increased screening
- Opportunity to provide information to the family
- Reassurance and reduction of anxiety about personal cancer risk
- Avoidance of unnecessary screening and prevention strategies
- Avoidance of aggressive interventions such as risk-reducing surgery
- Relief that children are not at increased risk
- Feeling of empowerment to obtain screening for children (in some syndromes)
- No need to rely on other family members for informative test results
- Opportunity to inform relatives about the likelihood that they have the family mutation
- Sense of overall empowerment
- Able to contribute to research
- Support for treatment decisions
- Support for family planning decisions

FIGURE 25-4 | Potential Limitations and Benefits of Genetic Testing

Note. Not all instances apply to all individual situations.

Cost of Genetic Testing

A decade ago, genetic testing cost multiple thousands of dollars, limiting participation. Since then, the cost to patients has lessened significantly. The upfront cost of next-generation sequencing may range in the thousands of dollars, versus more directed testing, which costs in the hundreds. Many insurances now cover testing if clinically indicated based on personal and family medical history. The National Comprehensive Cancer Network's annually updated guidelines for testing are used to determine the cost of coverage, though some insurances have a list of covered testing (Ebott & Scalia, 2023). The Patient Protection and Affordable Care Act of 2010 mandated that insurance cover preventive services without cost sharing, including grade A and B testing as recommended by the U.S. Preventive Services Task Force (Walcott & Dunn, 2015). Clinicians may be required to complete specific paperwork for prior authorizations before coverage is granted. Alternatively, some insurances require meetings with genetic counselors prior to covering the cost of testing (Smith, 2019). Even without insurance, many laboratories offer large, multigene panel cancer testing for an out-of-pocket cost of around $250 (Ebott & Scalia, 2023).

Additional Ethical Considerations Surrounding Genetic Testing

As genetic testing becomes more easily accessible and widely available for patients with cancer, many ethical questions, especially related to privacy, confidentiality, and disclosure, have emerged. NHGRI (n.d., para. 19) stated,

> The leaders of the Human Genome Project recognized the need to be proactive in addressing a wide range of ethical and social issues related to the acquisition and use of genomic information. They were especially aware of the potential risks and benefits of incorporating new genomic knowledge into research and medicine. Similarly, they were aware of the potential misuse of genomic information when it came to insurance and employment, among others.

OCRNs should be prepared to discuss the ethical, legal, and social implications that result from rapidly advancing genetic and genomic technologies and applications. Providers and researchers need to work with patients to explore knowledge and self-awareness about (a) personal choice, (b) limit setting in acceptable risk, (c) testing of children (especially if the disorder has or is expected to have an adult-age onset), (d) testing in vulnerable populations, and (e) equal access to those with limited economic resources.

Privacy concerns should be addressed with all patients. Genetic testing results are protected under the Health Insurance Portability and Accountability Act of 1996 (HIPAA) (U.S. Department of Health and Human Services, 2025), which protects access to a patient's personal medical history, and the Genetic Information Nondiscrimination Act of 2008 (GINA, 2011). *Genetic information* is defined in GINA (2011) as "information about an individual's genetic tests, the genetic tests of that individual's family members, the manifestation of disease or disorder in family members of the individual family (family medical history), an individual's request for, or receipt of, genetic services, or the participation in clinical research that includes genetic services by the individual or a family member of the individual" (GINA, 2011, para. 3).

GINA also defines what genetic information does not include, such as information about the sex or age of the individual, the sex or age of family members, or information about the race or ethnicity of the individual or family members that is not derived from a genetic test (Definitions Specific to GINA, 2010). This law was passed so that employers or health insurance companies would not be able to discriminate against patients based on the results of their or a family member's genetic test results. However, this law does not protect military or Native American tribe members; it also does not apply to life, disability, or long-term care insurance policies (Smith, 2019). OCRNs should be familiar with the content of this act so they can educate patients and other care providers (see Figure 25-5).

Prohibits
- Use of genetic information for decisions regarding hiring, promotion, terms of employment, compensation, or termination
- Use of genetic information to limit, segregate, or classify an employee or deprive an individual of employment opportunities
- Collection of genetic information of the individual or a family member (there are some exceptions)
- Refusal, or declining referral, of an individual for employment based on genetic information
- Use of genetic information for admission to apprenticeships or training and retraining, including on-the-job training
- Requirement of genetic information for eligibility, coverage, underwriting, or premium-setting decisions
- Use of genetic information to make either enrollment or coverage decisions
- Requirement of genetic testing for insurance purposes

Does Not
- Apply to members of the U.S. military, veterans obtaining health care through the Veterans Health Administration, the Indian Health Service, or federal employees obtaining health care through Federal Employees Health Benefits Program plans
- Apply to life, disability, or long-term care insurance
- Apply to small group insurers (less than 15 employees)
- Apply to individual manifested symptoms (regardless if genetically based)
- Override any more stringent state laws

FIGURE 25-5 | Key Points of the Genetic Information Nondiscrimination Act of 2008

Note. Based on information from Definitions Specific to GINA, 2010; Genetic Information Nondiscrimination Act of 2008.

Although this law works to protect the privacy of and prevent discrimination against patients, genetic material can never be truly anonymous, given that each person's DNA is unique. A 2013 study showed that through the use of public records and genealogic databases, patients can potentially be identified (Gymrek et al., 2013). Because of this, NIH strictly controls access to these databases and issues certificates of confidentiality to ensure that researchers protect the confidential information housed within (NHGRI, 2023). To receive information from a genetic results repository, a researcher must request access from the NIH Data Access Committee and include specifically outlined potential uses.

With direct-to-consumer testing, no federal laws exist that prohibit the companies providing testing from selling the genetic information to third parties. The Federal Trade Commission includes some protections, mostly guaranteeing against false assurances. Patients should be counseled that by downloading their genetic report, they release the company of liability regarding breach of privacy (NHGRI, 2023).

When reviewing genetic test results, OCRNs will also want to consider the psychological impact that results may have on patients. Patients may find out unwanted information about their family members or themselves, which could cause distress. A positive result could elicit a range of feelings, from empowerment regarding their personal health to fear and anxiety surrounding implications for familial health. Clinicians should consider partnering with social workers, providing access to supportive services, and preparing for lengthy discussions to adequately answer patient questions.

OCRNs whose role responsibilities include the provision of information about reproductive technology must be familiar with the associated regulatory and policy guidelines. Katz and Schweitzer (2010) identified concerns specific to healthcare provision, policy, reproductive technology, and quality assurance, including (a) diffusion of genetic testing and its impact on medical practices, (b) tension between confidentiality and transparency related to health insurance, (c) expansion of genetic testing for embryo selection, and (d) evolution of regulatory frameworks for quality assurance of genetic tests. The National Comprehensive Cancer Network (2025) recommended that patients of reproductive age should be advised about options for prenatal diagnosis and assisted reproduction, including preimplantation diagnosis, and the associated risks, benefits, and limitations of these approaches.

Informed Consent

The Commercial or Non-Research Setting

Informed consent is an element of the genetic testing process regardless of whether it occurs in a research setting, research laboratory, or a commercial laboratory. It is an opportunity for the provider and the individual presenting for the genetic testing to affirm that they have discussed essential elements of testing, including the benefits and limitations associated with the potential results of the specific test (Tung et al., 2024) (see Figure 25-6). Performing genetic testing without informed consent is illegal in the United States.

The NIH Consent and Disclosure Recommendations Workgroup created a framework for communication of key topics prior to testing, with the goal of not overwhelming patients with information while still informing them of critical concepts. Ormond et al. (2021, p. 8) suggested that all informed consents for genetic testing include eight key concepts:

- Genetic testing is voluntary.
- Why is the test recommended, and what does it test for?
- What results will be returned and to whom?
- Are there other types of potential results, and what choices exist?
- How will the prognosis and management be impacted by results?
- What is the potential family impact?
- What are the test limitations and next steps?
- What is the potential risk of genetic discrimination and legal protections?

All OCRNs should be familiar with the informed consent process, though the ability for a nurse to review this legal document with patients may vary by state and institution. Rego et al. (2020) recommend a dialogue between patients and clinicians to ensure that the patients' values and objectives are considered, as well as to provide an opportunity for patients to ask questions. Clinicians may use a teach-back method or ask questions after an informed consent discussion to ensure that patients comprehend the legal document and can autonomously give consent.

In an initial informed consent discussion, the potential range of results is limited by the number of conditions for which technology is currently able to test. Patients may find the idea that variants are not immediately actionable or that results may change over time to be confusing. Patients should be informed that future re-analysis may be required (Rego et al., 2020). Although the benefits of genetic testing (e.g., receiving a diagnosis, starting treatment) may be immediately recognizable, patients should also be counseled on the risks of testing, including learning about unexpected biological relationships and new genetic information.

A second informed consent process may be used before disclosure of genetic test results in case a patient changes

- Process of testing (e.g., amount of blood to be drawn)
- Clarification of a person's increased risk status
- Elicitation and discussion of a person's expectations, beliefs, goals, and motivations
- Potential results (e.g., positive, negative, uninformative, true negative, variant of uncertain significance)
- Benefits and limitations of testing
- Associated risks (e.g., unexpected results, genetic discrimination)
- Cancer risk assessment and management, if testing is not completed
- Options and anticipated medical management with or without testing, including prevention, risk reduction with chemoprevention and surgery, surveillance, and the risks, benefits, effectiveness, and limitations of the management strategies
- Further decision-making once genetic test results are received
- Time for results to become available, and how results will be communicated
- Communication with family members and implications for other family members, including offspring
- Potential psychological responses and availability of counseling and support services
- Costs (e.g., testing, counseling)
- Accuracy of the test, including interpretation of results
- Privacy protection and limitations to protection, release of results, confidentiality, and access to records
- Storage and potential use of DNA (e.g., for research)
- Attainment of verbal and written informed consent or clarification of the decision to decline testing

FIGURE 25-6 | Elements of Informed Consent for Genetic Testing

Note. Based on information from Giarelli et al., 2006; Jenkins & Lea, 2005; National Cancer Institute, 2025; Robson et al., 2010.

their mind about receiving the results. Once disclosure of results occurs, a third informed consent discussion can address issues regarding sharing the results with healthcare providers and interested family members, either in the present or future. Requiring written permission from the patient with the original test results to share the results with at-risk family members can avoid future problems in the event the original person is not available to release the results (NCI, 2025).

The Genetic and Genomic Research Setting

Federal regulation protects human research participants. The use of genetic data in research requires special considerations, given that a balance must be achieved between the dissemination of information for the advancement of science and the respect of patient privacy. The Federal Policy for the Protection of Human Subjects, also known as the Common Rule, requires that all participants receive informed consent prior to participating in a research study. Research that involves genetic information should explicitly state who may have access to the results and how they could be used. Institutional review boards may also raise ethical questions about specific protocols, management of genetic and genomic information, and genetic testing. Researchers and clinicians could have concerns about competent disclosure of incidental genetic findings, significant new findings, and individual research results if provisions for such disclosures were not included in the original consent document (Simon et al., 2012). Technology increases the use of genetic and genomic information and biorepository materials. Dressler et al. (2012) called for guidelines to ensure that research participants whose contributions result in actionable findings receive that information in a manner that they can use and understand.

The standard elements of informed consent (see Chapter 12) can include specific content to address concerns associated with genetic studies (NHGRI, 2024). The informed consent process also involves discussions related to the genetic aspects of the research and promotes participant understanding. The consent document clarifies the measures designed to protect the individual who is providing the genetic material and information. If samples are being collected and used for research purposes, or if samples may be associated with or linked to an individual, then informed consent must be obtained from the donor, unless waived by the institutional review board that oversees the research (NHGRI, 2024). This information should be reviewed and discussed in depth with the research participant during the consent process.

Informed consent is an important aspect of any genetic test or research study. NHGRI strongly advocates careful counseling of patients who are receiving genetic testing (NHGRI, 2022). Figure 25-7 includes recommended additions to the required components of informed consent for research using genetic material, information, and testing under the Code of Federal Regulations, effective in 2012 (NHGRI, 2022).

Language Explaining the Purpose
- Brief description of the genomic science supporting the research
- Type of any samples needed, as well as collection, storage, and length of storage
- Coding or de-identification, and the use of personal health information
- Access by other researchers
- Future contact provisions, if any
- Whether genome-wide association studies data sharing is included

Financial Information
- Compensation
- Costs
- If compensation for any research injury is available
- If the participant will receive any portion of the profit generated from a research discovery or product

Potential Benefits and Risks
- Personal versus societal benefit
- Psychological risks (may affect the participant and family)
- Disclosure of information, including unintended disclosure
- The possibility of loss of privacy

Confidentiality
- Measures taken to protect confidentiality
- Potential for and circumstances of possible disclosure

Return of Results and/or Incidental Findings
- Description of the plan to release incidental findings, new relevant discoveries, findings of no or undetermined clinical utility, and significant findings
- Plan for disclosure of individual findings
- Plan for disclosure of group findings
- Potential participants' right "not to know," if that is their election

Withdrawal, Alternatives, and Voluntary Participation
- Information specifying that the removal or elimination of data released and associated with individual DNA may not be possible if the participant withdraws
- Destruction of data and samples, if possible
- Storage and use of specific data

FIGURE 25-7 | Informed Consent Elements Tailored to Genomic Clinical Trials Research

Note. Based on information from National Human Genome Research Institute, 2022.

NHGRI (2024) summarized the essential elements and comprehensive purpose of the informed consent document, which include the following:

- Patients must be informed of the test's purpose, medical implications, alternatives, and possible risks and benefits.
- Patients must be given information about privacy rights, the location of DNA storage, and who will have access to their personal information.
- Even after signing, patients may still opt out of the test or study.
- The informed consent document is not a contract.
- A patient signature is required.

The Office for Human Research Protections (2008) *Engagement of Institutions in Human Subject Research* guidelines give directions for the conduct of human participant research and include directions for research with biologic materials. Coded information that the researcher cannot link to the participant is not considered human participant research. This definition applies to information that (a) includes no personal identifiers, (b) if coded, the researcher does not have the code, (c) if participants are alive, the code cannot be released, and (d) policies and procedures are in place that prevent release of the code (Office for Human Research Protections, 2008).

Genetic Testing of Children

Genetic testing of children in families with a history of genetically related illness remains a very complex topic that requires careful consideration of the risks and benefits. This is especially true when working with hereditary cancer syndromes that increase the risk of childhood cancers, as well as those that are not expected to increase this risk. Although parents and providers may request testing, experts recommend delaying genetic testing until a child is aged 18 years or older, unless results would have clinical care implications, such as immediate treatment, because of concerns about autonomy, discrimination, and the psychosocial impact on the child. The ASCO statement on genetic testing for cancer susceptibility states that when considering genetic testing for hereditary cancer syndromes in children, both the risk of cancer development and evidence for risk reduction associated with that disorder should be taken into account (Robson et al., 2015). Performing genetic testing on patients with a high risk of developing childhood cancer and no known risk reduction strategies remains controversial, with consequences including impaired child and parent bonding, decreased development of self-concept and self-esteem, and increased anxiety. When testing will positively impact a child's health outcomes and is therefore appropriate, careful consideration of their developmental stage for assessment of understanding and the family's psychosocial dynamics is essential prior to testing.

Hereditary Cancer Predisposition Testing in Clinical Trials

Several types of clinical trials in oncology exist and are classified based on the study's primary purpose, including treatment, prevention, screening, diagnostic, and quality-of-life or supportive care (NCI, 2024b).

Treatment Trials

Treatment trials include the use of chemotherapy, radiation therapy, surgery, vaccines, or stimulation of the immune system (NCI, 2024b). Tumor (or molecular) profiling includes the evaluation of genomic, proteomic, and epigenomic expression factors (Santos et al., 2013).

Individual characteristics, such as protein expression and DNA replication errors in healthy tissues and tumor tissues, can be indicators of an inherited increased risk for cancer and predictors of response to selected therapies. Researchers investigate single nucleotide polymorphisms, which are genetic variations on a single nucleotide base, to understand genetic variation among humans as well as epigenetics, factors that alter gene expression. This research contributed to the understanding of risk, prognosis, and responses to therapy (Santos et al., 2013).

Prevention Trials

Research to reduce the incidence of cancer in individuals with a hereditary predisposition to cancer explores many options, including risk reduction through lifestyle changes, chemoprevention, risk-reducing surgery, and increased surveillance with management (e.g., polyp removal). Many prevention studies target epigenetic factors to prevent new or recurrent cancers or precursor lesions.

Screening Trials

Red-flag features, such as earlier-age onset of cancers, bilateral occurrences in paired organs, synchronous occurrences, and the diagnosis of rare or unusual cancers, are the hallmarks of hereditary cancer syndromes. These cancers often present in organs not routinely screened for cancer in the general population. Research studies are essential to refining risks and improving cancer risk management, survivorship, and surveillance for people at high risk for cancer, including those that comprise registries that collect data and investigate the effectiveness of screening on high-risk populations (Travis et al., 2006).

Diagnostic Trials

Diagnostic trials study new tests or procedures that may help to identify or diagnose cancer more accurately. These trials usually involve people who have signs or symptoms of cancer. Some cancers with increased incidence in hereditary cancer syndromes, such as pancreatic, fallopian tube, ovarian, and small bowel cancers, are difficult to identify and diagnose in early stages. Clinical trials designed to test and establish the efficacy of diagnostic measures contribute to improved management of hereditary cancer syndromes.

Quality-of-Life or Supportive Care Trials

Quality-of-life trials focus on the comfort and quality of life of patients with cancer and cancer survivors. These trials often study new ways to decrease the number or severity of side effects of cancer or its treatment. How a specific type of cancer or its treatment affects a person's everyday life may also be studied. Ongoing studies in the development of second cancers, treatment effects, and psychosocial concerns associated with hereditary cancer syndromes can be included in quality-of-life and supportive care studies (Travis et al., 2006).

Commercial DNA Banking

Clinicians engaged in hereditary cancer syndrome assessment, testing, and research are increasingly discussing DNA banking outside of the research setting (Quillin et al., 2011). DNA banking is becoming common in both clinical trials and standard of care management. Banking allows retesting of tissue as technology evolves, which may identify new treatment options or the presence of a hereditary cancer syndrome that was initially unable to be found. OCRNs engaged in genetic testing within a clinical trial may be called on to facilitate DNA banking.

Implications for Oncology Clinical Research Nurses

The rapid evolution of genetics and genomics affects the role of OCRNs, who should be knowledgeable about the changing healthcare landscape using genetic information. In 2005, the American Nurses Association (2023) published basic competencies in genetics and genomics for all nurses in *Essentials of Genetic and Genomic Nursing: Competencies, Curricula Guidelines, and Outcome Indicators*, and recently updated this publication to a third edition in 2023. OCRNs must understand the essential competencies of genetics in conjunction with the publication *Oncology Clinical Research Nurse Competencies* by the Oncology Nursing Society and Oncology Nursing Certification Corporation (2024). Nurses participating in genetic testing for hereditary cancer predisposition should demonstrate additional expertise.

Summary

Use of genetic testing in oncology care has rapidly changed over the past decades. Testing is increasingly available for clinical trials research for germline and somatic variants, as well as directed testing versus whole-gene sequencing and multigene panel testing. Technology is rapidly advancing, with clinicians and legislature racing to catch up to the advancements. OCRNs should be aware of the different types of testing and implications for treatment. Clinicians should also ensure that patients are adequately educated regarding the testing process through use of the informed consent, are able to obtain an accurate family and medical history to identify red flags for further evaluation, relay information about cost, and help patients understand the limitations of testing, especially as direct-to-consumer testing becomes more commercially available and popular. OCRNs need a strong understanding of the basics of genetics, given that a dearth of trained professionals may result in an increased use of nurses for genetic counseling. Basic ethical and legal considerations regarding genetic testing will continue to evolve as technology does the same, making it essential that OCRNs have an understanding of the legislations that protect participants.

Key Points

- OCRNs involved in the use of genetic information must be familiar with ethical, legal, and social implications, hereditary syndromes, and sampling of genetic material and information.
- Key features of hereditary cancer syndromes are red-flag indicators to suggest patients and families for cancer predisposition genetic testing, especially when found in combination with a family history.
- Continued research is required to refine the interpretation, clinical utility, and the ethical, legal, psychosocial, global, and economic implications of genetic testing and the use of genetic information.
- Patient education and counseling (pre- and post-test) are essential elements of the management of hereditary cancer syndromes and associated genetic testing.
- Federal and state regulations are in place to protect human research participants' privacy and the use of their genetic information.
- HIPAA and GINA contain significant, although not complete, protection against discrimination and disclosure of health information without consent.
- Genetic testing in children presents unique concerns and should focus on the best interests of the child.
- Genetic testing in clinical trials supports treatment, screening, prevention, diagnosis, and quality-of-life research.
- OCRNs must have a basic understanding of genetics. Nurses working with genetic testing for hereditary cancer predisposition should demonstrate additional expertise and preparation.

The author would like to acknowledge Jacqueline M. Hale, MSN, APNC, APNG-BC, AOCN®, for her contribution to this chapter that remains unchanged from the previous edition of this book.

References

American Nurses Association. (2023). *Essentials of genetic and genomic nursing: Competencies, curricula guidelines, and outcome indicators* (3rd ed.). https://www.nursingworld.org/nurses-books/ana-books/ebook-essentials-of-genomic-nursing-competencies-

Definitions specific to GINA, 29 C.F.R. § 1635.3 (2010). https://www.ecfr.gov/cgi-bin/text-idx?SID=59748b93fd9f7038406e7a644c5c627b&node=se29.4.1635_13&rgn=div8

Dressler, L., Smolek, S., Ponsaran, R., Markey, J., Starks, H., Gerson, N., … Weisner, G. (2012). IRB perspectives on the return of individual results from genomic research. *Genetics in Medicine, 14*(2), 215–222. https://doi.org/10.1038/gim.2011.10

Ebott, J.A., & Scalia, J. (2023). A genetic revolution: Cancer genetic testing and counseling. *Rhode Island Medical Journal (2013), 106*(5), 8–11. https://www.rimed.org/rimedicaljournal/2023/06/2023-06-08-cancer-genetics-ebott.pdf

Faherty, S. (2018, April 5). *NIH completes in-depth genomic analysis of 33 cancer types.* Genome.gov. https://www.genome.gov/news/news-release/NIH-completes-in-depth-genomic-analysis-of-33-cancer-types

Genetic Information Nondiscrimination Act of 2008, 29 C.F.R. pt. 1635. (2011). https://www.gpo.gov/fdsys/pkg/CFR-2011-title29-vol4/xml/CFR-2011-title29-vol4-part1635.xml

Giarelli, E., Lea, D.H., Jones, S.L., & Lewis, J.A. (2006). Genetic technology: The frontiers of nursing ethics. In V.D. Lachman (Ed.), *Applied Ethics in Nursing* (pp. 61–80). Springer.

Gymrek, M., McGuire, A.L, Golan, D., Halperin, E., & Erlich, Y. (2013). Identifying personal genomes by surname inference. *Science, 339*(6117), 321–324. https://doi.org/10.1126/science.1229566

International Society of Nurses in Genetics. (2021). *Access to genomic healthcare: The role of the nurse* [Position statement]. https://www.isong.org/resources/Documents/PS_Access%20to%20Genomic%20Healthcare_November%202021.pdf

Jenkins, J.F., & Lea, D.H. (2005). *Nursing care in the genomic era: A case-based approach.* Jones and Bartlett Learning.

Katz, G., & Schweitzer, S.O. (2010). Implications of genetic testing for health policy. *Yale Journal of Health Policy, Law, and Ethics, 10*(1), 90–134. https://digitalcommons.law.yale.edu/yjhple/vol10/iss1/2

Lindor, N.M., McMaster, M.L., Lindor, C.J., & Greene, M.H. (2008). Concise handbook of familial cancer susceptibility syndromes—second edition. *Journal of the National Cancer Institute Monographs, 2008*(38), 3–93. https://doi.org/10.1093/jncimonographs/lgn001

Miles, B., & Tadi, P. (2024). Genetics, somatic mutation. In *StatPearls.* StatPearls Publishing. https://www.ncbi.nlm.nih.gov/books/NBK557896

Mukherjee, S. (2017). *The gene: An intimate history.* Scribner.

National Cancer Institute. (2024a). *Genetic testing for inherited cancer risk.* https://www.cancer.gov/about-cancer/causes-prevention/genetics/genetic-testing-fact-sheet

National Cancer Institute. (2024b). *What are clinical trials?* https://www.cancer.gov/research/participate/clinical-trials/what-are-clinical-trials

National Cancer Institute. (2025). *Cancer genetics risk assessment and counseling (PDQ®).* https://www.cancer.gov/publications/pdq/information-summaries/genetics/risk-assessment-hp-pdq

National Comprehensive Cancer Network. (2025). *NCCN Clinical Practice Guidelines in Oncology (NCCN Guidelines®): Genetic/familial high-risk assessment: Breast, ovarian, pancreatic, and prostate.* [v.3.2025]. https://www.nccn.org

National Human Genome Research Institute. (n.d.). *The Human Genome Project.* https://www.genome.gov/about-genomics/educational-resources/fact-sheets/human-genome-project

National Human Genome Research Institute. (2019). *Introduction to genomics.* https://www.genome.gov/About-Genomics/Introduction-to-Genomics

National Human Genome Research Institute. (2022). *Required elements of the consent form.* https://www.genome.gov/about-genomics/policy-issues/Informed-Consent/Required-Elements-of-Consent-Form

National Human Genome Research Institute. (2023). *History of genomics archive.* https://www.genome.gov/history-of-genomics-archive

National Human Genome Research Institute. (2024). *Informed consent.* https://www.genome.gov/10002332

National Human Genome Research Institute. (2025). *Ethical, Legal and Social Implications Research Program.* https://www.genome.gov/10001618

Office for Human Research Protections. (2008). *Engagement of institutions in human subjects research.* https://www.hhs.gov/ohrp/policy/engage08.html

Oncology Nursing Society & Oncology Nursing Certification Corporation. (2024). *Oncology clinical research nurse competencies.* https://www.ons.org/sites/default/files/2025-01/ocrn-competencies-rebrand.pdf

Ormond, K.E., Borensztein, M.J., Hallquist, M.L.G., Buchanan, A.H., Faucett, W.A., Peay, H.L., ... Coughlin, C.R., II. (2021). Defining the critical components of informed consent for genetic testing. *Journal of Personalized Medicine, 11*(12), 1304. https://doi.org/10.3390/jpm11121304

Quillin, J., Bodurtha, J., Siminoff, L., & Smith, T. (2011). Physicians' current practices and opportunities for DNA banking of dying patients with cancer. *Journal of Oncology Practice, 7*(3), 183–187. https://doi.org/10.1200/JOP.2010.000190

Rego, S., Grove, M.E., Cho, M.K., & Ormond, K.E. (2020). Informed consent in the genomics era. *Cold Spring Harbor Perspectives in Medicine, 10*(8), a036582. https://doi.org/10.1101/cshperspect.a036582

Robson, M.E., Bradbury, A.R., Banu, A., Domchek, S.M., Ford, J.M., Hampel, H.L., ... Lindor, N.M. (2015). American Society of Clinical Oncology Policy Statement Update: Genetic and genomic testing for cancer susceptibility. *Journal of Clinical Oncology, 33*(31), 3660–3667. https://doi.org/10.1200/JCO.2015.63.0996

Robson, M.E., Storm, C.D., Weitzel, J., Wollins, D.S., & Offit, K. (2010). American Society of Clinical Oncology Policy Statement Update: Genetic and genomic testing for cancer susceptibility. *Journal of Clinical Oncology, 28*(5), 893–901. https://doi.org/10.1200/JCO.2009.27.0660

Santos, E.M.M., Edwards, Q.T., Floria-Santos, M., Rogatto, S.R., Achatz, M.I.W., & MacDonald, D.J. (2013). Integration of genomics in cancer care. *Journal of Nursing Scholarship, 45*(1), 43–51. https://doi.org/10.1111/j.1547-5069.2012.01465.x

Simon, C., Shinkunas, L.A., Brandt, D., & Williams, J.K. (2012). Individual genetic and genomic research results and the tradition of informed consent: Exploring US review board guidance. *Journal of Medical Ethics, 38*(7), 417–422. https://doi.org/10.1136/medethics-2011-100273

Smith, L.P. (2019). The spectrum of genetic testing. *Seminars in Oncology Nursing, 35*(1), 11–21. https://doi.org/10.1016/j.soncn.2018.12.008

Tandy-Connor, S., Guiltinan, J., Krempely, K., LaDuca, H., Reineke, P., Gutierrez, S., ... Davis, B.T. (2018). False-positive results released by direct-to-consumer genetic tests highlight the importance of clinical confirmation testing for appropriate patient care. *Genetics in Medicine, 20*(12), 1515–1521. https://doi.org/10.1038/gim.2018.38

Travis, L.B., Rabkin, C.S., Brown, L.M., Allan, J.M., Alter, B.P., Ambrosone, C.B., ... Greene, M.H. (2006). Cancer survivorship—Genetic susceptibility and second primary cancers: Research strategies and recommendations. *Journal of the National Cancer Institute, 98*(1), 15–25. https://doi.org/10.1093/jnci/djj001

Tung, N., Ricker, C., Messersmith, H., Balmaña, J., Domchek, S., Stoffel, E.M., ... Vidal, G.A. (2024). Selection of germline genetic testing panels in patients with cancer: ASCO guideline. *Journal of Clinical Oncology, 42*(21), 2599–2615. https://doi.org/10.1200/jco.24.00662

U.S. Department of Health and Human Services. (2025). *Summary of the HIPAA Privacy Rule.* https://www.hhs.gov/hipaa/for-professionals/privacy/laws-regulations/index.html

Walcott, F., & Dunn, B.K. (2015). Legislation in the genomic era: The Affordable Care Act and genetic testing for cancer risk assessment. *Genetics in Medicine, 17*(22), 962–964. https://doi.org/10.1038/gim.2015.18

CHAPTER 26

Cytogenetics

Amanda Brink, DNP, APRN, FNP-BC, AOCNP®

Introduction

Cytogenetics, the study of chromosomes and their variations, is at the forefront of modern medical research, playing a pivotal role in understanding the genetic basis of diseases, particularly cancer (Mathew et al., 2024). For nurses working in clinical trials, a solid grasp of cytogenetic principles is essential for effectively managing patients and contributing to advancements in oncology care.

Understanding cytogenetics enables oncology clinical research nurses (OCRNs) to navigate the complexities of patient care with confidence and precision. Cytogenetic findings influence treatment decisions, prognosis, and the design of innovative clinical trials aimed at improving patient outcomes. Moreover, there are ethical and legal considerations inherent in cytogenetic testing and data management, and OCRNs are essential in ensuring patient privacy and adherence to regulatory standards.

This chapter will provide a historical overview of cytogenetics and its importance to the role of the OCRN. It will also cover the common molecular techniques and the typical cytogenetic alterations found in various cancer types.

Historical Overview

The field of cytogenetics traces its roots to the late 19th and early 20th centuries when pioneering researchers such as Walther Flemming, Theodor Boveri, Walter Sutton, and Thomas Hunt Morgan made significant contributions to our understanding of chromosomes and heredity. Morgan's research with fruit flies provided crucial insights into the relationship between genes and chromosomes, demonstrating that genes are located on specific chromosomes and are responsible for inherited traits. This laid the groundwork for understanding the role of chromosomes in heredity and cell division (O'Connor & Miko, 2008).

A significant milestone was reached in 1956 when Joe Hin Tijo and Albert Levan correctly identified the number of human chromosomes as 46, laying a crucial foundation for further research into human genetics and diseases (Durmaz et al., 2015). Diagnostic cytogenetics was introduced to the United States by Victor McKusick at Johns Hopkins University in 1958 (Ferguson-Smith, 2021). The 1970s saw remarkable progress with the introduction of chromosome banding techniques such as Giemsa banding (G-banding), which enabled researchers to visualize specific regions of chromosomes with greater clarity (Wan & Ma, 2024). This era also witnessed the identification of chromosomal abnormalities associated with diseases, including the discovery of the Philadelphia (Ph) chromosome in chronic myeloid leukemia (CML) (Ferguson-Smith, 2015) and the association of trisomy 21 with Down syndrome (Mégarbané et al., 2009).

Technological innovations such as fluorescence in situ hybridization (FISH), comparative genomic hybridization (CGH), next-generation sequencing (NGS), and optical genome mapping (OGM) have since revolutionized cytogenetic analysis, providing powerful tools for studying genetic abnormalities and their implications for health and disease. Advances in molecular technology have enabled the identification of several chromosome abnormalities, which have been crucial in diagnosing human diseases, particularly in hematologic oncology. Cytogenetics has had a profound impact on medicine, shaping the understanding of genetic diseases, guiding diagnostic and prognostic assessments, and informing treatment strategies. Cytogenetic analysis plays a critical role in personalized medicine and precision oncology, driving advancements in patient care and therapeutic interventions.

Importance in Clinical Trials

Cytogenetics serves a vital function in oncology clinical trials by providing valuable insights into the genetic underpinnings of diseases and guiding treatment strategies. Cytogenetic analysis serves as a vital tool for patient stratification, enabling researchers to identify subgroups with distinct genetic profiles that may respond differently to experimental therapies (Ribeiro et al., 2019). By incorporating cytogenetic data into trial design and patient selection criteria, researchers can optimize trial outcomes, enhance treatment efficacy, and minimize adverse effects. Moreover, cytogenetics facilitates the monitoring of disease progression, treatment response, and the emergence of drug resistance, allowing for real-time adjustments in therapeutic interventions. As such, OCRNs play a pivotal role in facilitating cytogenetic testing, interpreting results, and communicating findings to interprofessional teams, patients, and families. Through their expertise and collaboration, OCRNs contribute to the advancement of precision medicine and the development of innovative therapies that improve patient outcomes and quality of life (Ribeiro et al., 2019).

The Evolution From Cytogenetics to Cytogenomics and Chromosomics

The field of cytogenetics has undergone significant evolution with the advent of advanced molecular techniques. Traditionally, cytogenetics has focused on chromosome structure and abnormalities, using karyotyping and FISH. However, the integration of NGS has expanded the scope of cytogenetics into what is now termed *cytogenomics* and, more recently, *chromosomics*.

Cytogenomics is the study of chromosomes at a genomic level, incorporating molecular and sequence-based techniques to detect structural variations, copy number changes, and rearrangements with greater precision. This shift enables a more comprehensive analysis of germline and somatic variants, impacting both hereditary and acquired disorders (Ribeiro et al., 2019).

Chromosomics is an emerging concept that examines the three-dimensional organization of chromosomes within the nucleus, emphasizing how chromatin structure influences gene expression and disease processes (Liehr, 2021).

Genetics and Genomics

The distinction between genetics and genomics has become increasingly important in oncology care. Genetics is the study of individual genes and their role in inheritance (National Human Genome Research Institute, 2025a). Genetic testing typically focuses on identifying specific variants in individual genes, such as *BRCA1* and *BRCA2* in the context of breast cancer.

In contrast, genomics looks at the entire genome, including gene interactions, regulatory elements, and chromosomal rearrangements, offering a broader perspective on cancer biology (National Human Genome Institute, 2025b). Genomic testing can identify copy number variations, chromosomal translocations, and epigenetic modifications that influence tumor behavior.

Understanding the distinction between germline and somatic variants is also critical in oncology. Germline variants are inherited and present in every cell, impacting cancer risk and guiding family screening. Somatic variants, which occur exclusively in tumor cells, are pivotal in treatment decisions, particularly in precision oncology. Germline variants can be passed down to subsequent generations, whereas somatic variants cannot (Frost, 2024).

Basic Concepts in Cytogenetics

Structure and Function of Chromosomes

Chromosomes are thread-like structures located within the nucleus of cells. Each chromosome consists of a single, long DNA molecule that contains numerous genes. The DNA in chromosomes is tightly coiled around proteins, forming a complex called chromatin. Chromosomes are essential for ensuring accurate DNA replication and distribution during cell division. The proper structure and function of chromosomes are necessary for maintaining genomic stability, regulating cell cycle progression, and ensuring the accurate transmission of genetic information from one generation to the next. Any abnormalities in chromosome structure or number can lead to various genetic disorders and contribute to the development of cancers and other diseases (Hosea et al., 2024).

Chromosome Banding Techniques

Chromosome banding techniques are essential tools in cytogenetics for identifying and analyzing chromosomal abnormalities. These techniques involve staining chromosomes to produce distinct banding patterns, which allow for the visualization of specific regions and the identification of structural variations. Common banding methods include G-banding, which stains regions rich in adenine and thymine, and reverse banding (R-banding), which highlights regions rich in guanine and cytosine. Other techniques, such as quinacrine banding (Q-banding), centromeric banding (C-banding), and nucleolar organizer region staining (NOR staining), target specific chromosome features (Wan & Ma, 2024).

The G-banding method is widely used to detect chromosomal aberrations, including deletions, translocations, and insertions. This technique highlights the dark and light bands commonly seen in karyotypes. Trypsin is used to digest histones (proteins that fold DNA and aid in the formation of chromatin), allowing guanine and cytosine (GC)-rich regions in DNA to relax and absorb the Giemsa stain. The order and size of bands specific to each chromosome are then visualized and can be compared to other homologous chromosomes. The G-banding method is straightforward, and the stained DNA can be stored for an extended period (Wan & Ma, 2024).

Q-banding was the first banding method and requires a fluorescence microscope. Quinacrine mustard, an alkylating agent, is used for this technique. The Q-banding method stains guanine- and cytosine-rich regions of DNA, similar to G-banding. One disadvantage of this technique is that the stain fades quickly and is not permanent (Nabil, 2013).

The C-banding method is specialized for heterochromatin staining and uses the Giemsa stain. The cell is treated with acid and then with alkali. The C-banding method is used to identify centromeres. Centromeres play a crucial role in chromosome segregation during cell division, and their identification is essential in karyotype analysis (Zhu et al., 2019).

R-banding stains chromosomes in the opposite way to Q-banding and G-banding. It is specifically helpful for staining rearrangements at the ends of chromosomes. The cells are treated with a hot salt solution to denature the adenine- and thymine-rich regions of DNA, which are then stained with Giemsa (Wan & Ma, 2024).

NOR staining is a specialized technique used to visualize regions associated with ribosomal RNA synthesis, particularly on acrocentric chromosomes (13, 14, 15, 21, and 22). This method relies on silver staining (AgNOR), which binds to argyrophilic proteins associated with NORs, allowing researchers to assess chromosomal activity in both healthy and malignant cells. Although NOR staining was historically used in cytogenetics, its clinical application has diminished with the advent of more advanced molecular techniques such as FISH and NGS (Zhu et al., 2019).

These banding patterns are critical for diagnosing genetic disorders, identifying chromosomal rearrangements, and conducting detailed karyotype analyses.

Application of Cytogenetics in Cancer Research

Role of Cytogenetics in Cancer Diagnosis and Prognosis

Cancer is a group of disorders resulting from gene alterations. These gene variants are categorized into the following three types (Brown et al., 2023):

- Inherited cancer genes caused by germline variants present in every cell
- Somatic variants acquired over time, found in some cells, and that lead to sporadic cancers
- Variants associated with viral infections

The hallmark of all cancers is the abnormal growth of cells. This uncontrolled growth, driven by variations, can result in the formation of malignant tumors (Brown et al., 2023).

The nomenclature of tumors is based on their tissue of origin: carcinomas arise from epithelial tissue, lymphomas from lymphatic tissue, sarcomas from connective tissue, leukemias from hematopoietic cells, and gliomas from neuroglial cells, primarily in the central nervous system (Cancer Research UK, 2023; National Cancer Institute, n.d.).

Knowledge growth in genetics and molecular signaling, especially since the completion of the human genome sequencing in 2003, has significantly improved oncology care through clinical trials focusing on the prevention, early detection, diagnosis, and treatment of cancer. Cytogenetics plays a pivotal role in the diagnosis and prognosis of cancer by enabling the identification of chromosomal abnormalities that drive oncogenesis. Variants in oncogenes and tumor suppressor genes are precursors to changes in signaling pathways that result in cancer development. Cytogenetics enables the detailed analysis of cancer cell karyotypes, revealing specific translocations, deletions, amplifications, and other chromosomal alterations that contribute to excessive growth and tumor formation.

These abnormalities not only aid in the precise classification of cancer subtypes, such as identifying the Ph chromosome in CML, but also provide critical prognostic information. For example, the presence of certain chromosomal changes can indicate a more aggressive disease course or predict response to specific therapies. Thus, cytogenetic analysis is integral to developing personalized treatment plans, guiding clinical decision-making, and ultimately improving patient outcomes in oncology (Krzyszczyk et al., 2019).

Cytogenetic Abnormalities in Various Types of Cancer

Leukemia

Leukemias are a group of cancers that develop in blood cells and manifest in both children and adults. Essentially, there are four different categories of leukemias found in the lymphocytic and myeloid cell lineages. The myeloid lineages generally include acute myeloid leukemia (AML) and CML, whereas the lymphoid lineages encompass chronic lymphocytic leukemia (CLL) and acute lymphoblastic leukemia (ALL). AML, CML, and CLL are most common in adults. ALL is predominantly observed in children (Chennamadhavuni et al., 2023).

Acute Myeloid Leukemia

Changes in hematopoietic progenitor cells and the accumulation of acquired genetic alterations lead to AML. The karyotype is crucial for establishing the genetic background for staging AML and identifying personalized treatment strategies as quickly as possible. These abnormalities help classify AML subtypes and guide treatment decisions. For instance, the t(15;17) translocation is associated with acute promyelocytic leukemia, which responds well to all-trans retinoic acid therapy. The following chromosomal aberrations are linked to AML (Jimenez et al., 2020):

- t(8;21)(q22;q22)
- Abnormal bone marrow eosinophils and inv(16)(p13;q22) or t(16;16)(p13;q22)
- t(15;17)(q22;q12)
- 11q23 (MLL) abnormalities.

Several clinical trials study AML, and different cytogenetic factors are critical for their inclusion and exclusion criteria, requiring OCRNs to understand how to interpret bone marrow results. For example, high-risk AML in a patient with one or more risk factors, including Fms-like tyrosine kinase 3 (FLT-3) variant, complex cytogenetics, abn(3q), -5/5q, -7/7q, abn(12p), abn(17p), and secondary AML (Quessada et al., 2021).

Chronic Myeloid Leukemia

The hallmark cytogenetic abnormality in CML is the Ph chromosome, which results from a reciprocal translocation between chromosomes 9 and 22, specifically t(9;22)(q34;q11). This translocation creates the *BCR-ABL* fusion gene, a potent oncogene that drives the disease. Detection of the Ph chromosome is crucial for diagnosis and treatment with tyrosine kinase inhibitors (Soverini et al., 2019).

Acute Lymphoblastic Leukemia

The Ph chromosome can also be found in ALL. It is associated with a more aggressive form of the disease and typically indicates a poorer prognosis compared to Ph-negative ALL. The presence of the Ph chromosome in ALL is designated as Ph-positive ALL and involves the same translocation as in CML, namely t(9;22)(q34;q11), which results in the *BCR-ABL* fusion gene (Soverini et al., 2019).

Burkitt Lymphoma

This type of lymphoma is associated with a translocation involving the *MYC* gene on chromosome 8, typically t(8;14)(q24;q32), which leads to its overexpression. Identifying this translocation is important for diagnosing Burkitt lymphoma and differentiating it from other types of non-Hodgkin lymphoma (Fang et al., 2025).

Follicular Lymphoma

The characteristic cytogenetic abnormality in follicular lymphoma is t(14;18)(q32;q21), which results in the overexpression of the *BCL2* gene, promoting cell survival. The detection of this translocation aids in diagnosing follicular lymphoma and determining prognosis (Kurz et al., 2023).

Multiple Myeloma

Multiple myeloma, characterized by the proliferation of plasma cells, presents with varying severity, which the genetic factors of the plasma cells can influence. Cytogenetic analysis of multiple myeloma reveals several translocations, deletions, trisomies, and other abnormalities (Clarke et al., 2024). These genetic changes are used to stratify patients into different risk categories, guiding treatment decisions and prognosis.

One example of a cytogenetic abnormality in multiple myeloma is t(4;14). This translocation involves a rearrangement between chromosome 4 and chromosome 14, resulting in the fusion of the fibroblast growth factor receptor 3 (*FGFR3*) gene on chromosome 4 with the immunoglobulin heavy chain (*IGH*) gene on chromosome 14. The translocation leads to the overexpression of the *FGFR3* gene, which can promote cell proliferation and survival pathways, contributing to the pathogenesis of multiple myeloma. Patients with this translocation may exhibit aggressive disease behavior and poorer outcomes compared to those without it. Consideration of targeted therapies aimed at inhibiting *FGFR3* signaling pathways may improve treatment response and outcomes for patients with t(4;14) (Tsukamoto et al., 2023).

Breast Cancer

In breast cancer, common cytogenetic abnormalities include amplifications of the *HER2* gene on chromosome 17q12 and deletions on chromosome 13q. *HER2* amplification is particularly significant, as it indicates a more aggressive tumor and guides the use of targeted therapies, such as trastuzumab (Qiu et al., 2025).

Ewing Sarcoma

This cancer is often characterized by the presence of the *EWS-FLI1* fusion gene, resulting from a translocation between chromosomes 11 and 22, or t(11;22)(q24;q12). The detection of this translocation confirms the diagnosis of Ewing sarcoma and aids in tailoring the treatment approach (Bayanjargal et al., 2024).

Oral Cancers

Chromosomal aberrations, such as 8q24 amplification (associated with the *MYC* oncogene) and deletions in 9p21 (affecting the *CDKN2A* gene), have been implicated in the progression of oral squamous cell carcinoma (Sowmya et al., 2022). These findings have led to research into the development of targeted therapies aimed at disrupting oncogenic signaling pathways.

Melanoma

Cytogenetic analysis has identified variants in the *BRAF* gene (mostly *BRAF V600E*) as among the most common in melanoma. This discovery has led to the development of personalized treatment approaches using BRAF and MEK inhibitors. Additionally, cytogenetic analysis plays a key role in distinguishing cutaneous melanoma from uveal melanoma by examining karyotypic abnormalities and common chromosomal alterations unique to each type of melanoma (Ottaviano et al., 2021).

Molecular Techniques in Cytogenetics

Fluorescence In Situ Hybridization

FISH is a powerful cytogenetic technique used to detect and localize specific DNA sequences on chromosomes. By using fluorescently labeled probes that bind to particular chromosome regions, FISH enables the visualization of genetic abnormalities, such as deletions, duplications, and translocations, under a fluorescence microscope (Ramos, 2022). This technique is highly valuable in both research and clinical settings because of its ability to provide rapid and precise identification of chromosomal changes. In oncology, FISH is widely used for diagnosing and prognosticating various cancers, including the identification of the Ph chromosome in CML and HER2 amplification in breast cancer. Its application extends to prenatal diagnosis, genetic counseling, and the study of genetic disorders, making FISH an indispensable tool in modern cytogenetics (Ramos, 2022).

Comparative Genomic Hybridization

CGH is a molecular cytogenetic technique used to detect and map changes in DNA copy numbers across the entire genome. Unlike traditional karyotyping, which requires dividing cells, CGH can be performed on DNA extracted from any tissue, making it a versatile tool for analyzing genetic material. In CGH, test DNA and reference DNA are marked with different fluorescent colors and then combined and applied to normal chromosomes or a microarray, a small, chip-like device containing many DNA segments. Differences in fluorescence intensity between the test and reference DNA indicate regions of genomic gain or loss. CGH is particularly useful in cancer research and diagnosis, where it helps identify chromosomal imbalances associated with tumor development and progression. By revealing amplifications, deletions, and other structural variations, CGH provides critical insights into the genetic underpinnings of various cancers, aiding in diagnosis, prognostication, and the development of targeted therapies (Baumgartner et al., 2019).

Next-Generation Sequencing

NGS in cytogenetics has revolutionized the field by providing a comprehensive and high-resolution method for analyzing genetic material. It enables the simultaneous sequencing of millions of DNA fragments, providing detailed insights into chromosomal abnormalities, mutations, and structural variations that are not detectable by traditional cytogenetic techniques. This technology is particularly valuable in oncology, where it helps identify specific genetic changes driving cancer, enabling personalized treatment strategies. NGS has enhanced our ability to detect rare genetic events, understand tumor heterogeneity, and monitor disease progression, thereby significantly improving diagnostic precision and therapeutic outcomes (Satam et al., 2023).

Optical Genome Mapping

OGM is an emerging cytogenetic technology that has gained traction. Unlike traditional karyotyping and FISH, OGM provides a high-resolution, label-free method for detecting structural variations in the genome. OGM uses ultra-high molecular weight DNA molecules to identify deletions, duplications, inversions, and translocations with greater precision than conventional techniques. Studies have demonstrated its utility in hematologic malignancies, particularly in identifying cryptic rearrangements that may influence prognosis and treatment selection (Smith et al., 2022). Given its growing role in clinical and research settings, OGM may complement or even replace some traditional cytogenetic techniques in the future.

Summary

Cytogenetics plays an indispensable role in modern medicine, particularly in the fields of oncology and hematology. The advancements in cytogenetic techniques, such as G-banding, Q-banding, C-banding, FISH, CGH, NGS, and OGM, have significantly enhanced our ability to detect and understand chromosomal abnormalities. These techniques provide critical insights into the genetic basis of diseases, enabling precise diagnosis, risk stratification, and the development of personalized treatment plans.

In the context of cancer, cytogenetic analysis has a central role in identifying specific chromosomal translocations, deletions, amplifications, and other alterations that drive oncogenesis. This information is essential for diagnosing various cancer subtypes, predicting disease prognosis, and informing therapeutic interventions.

OCRNs are instrumental in managing cytogenetic data, from ensuring accurate sample collection and documentation to facilitating the communication of test results and integrating genetic findings into patient care. Their expertise in interpreting cytogenetic reports and understanding chromosome abnormalities is vital for the effective management of clinical trials and the delivery of high-quality patient care.

Overall, the integration of cytogenetics into clinical practice and research underscores its significance in advancing personalized medicine and improving patient outcomes. As our understanding of genetic components and their implications continues to grow, the role of cytogenetics will undoubtedly expand, offering new avenues for diagnosis, treatment, and prevention of genetic diseases.

Key Points

- Cytogenetics involves the study of chromosomes and their variations.
- Chromosome banding techniques aid in the identification of chromosome abnormalities.
- Cancer genetics focuses on gene variants and their association with cancer.
- Chromosome alterations in cancer elucidate the molecular mechanisms of mutations and their correlation with diseases, including cancer.
- OCRNs need to understand and be proficient in using chromosomal nomenclature to effectively manage their patients in clinical trials involving hematologic malignancy protocols.

The author would like to acknowledge Sourat Darabi, PhD(c), and Julia A. Eggert, PhD, GNP-BC, AGN-BC, AOCN®, for their contribution to this chapter that remains unchanged from the previous edition of this book.

References

Baumgartner, A., Hartleb, V., & Taylor, J.D. (2019). Comparative genomic hybridization (CGH) in genotoxicology. *Methods in Molecular Biology, 2031,* 209–234. https://doi.org/10.1007/978-1-4939-9646-9_11

Bayanjargal, A., Taslim, C., Showpnil, I.A., Selich-Anderson, J., Crow, J.C., Lessnick, S.L., & Theisen, E.R. (2024). DBD-α4 helix of EWSR1::FLI1 is required for GGAA microsatellite binding that underlies genome regulation in Ewing sarcoma. *bioRxiv* [Preprint], 2024.01.31.578127. https://doi.org/10.1101/2024.01.31.578127

Brown, J.S., Amend, S.R., Austin, R.H., Gatenby, R.A., Hammarlund, E.U., & Pienta, K.J. (2023). Updating the definition of cancer. *Molecular Cancer Research, 21*(11), 1142–1147. https://doi.org/10.1158/1541-7786.MCR-23-0411

Cancer Research UK. (2023). *Glioma.* https://www.cancerresearchuk.org/about-cancer/brain-tumours/types/glioma-adults

Chennamadhavuni, A., Lyengar, V., Mukkamalla, S.K.R., & Shimanovsky, A. (2023). Leukemia. In *StatPearls.* StatPearls Publishing.

Clarke, S.E., Fuller, K.A., & Erber, W.N. (2024). Chromosomal defects in multiple myeloma. *Blood Reviews, 64,* 101168. https://doi.org/10.1016/j.blre.2024.101168

Durmaz, A.A., Karaca, E., Demkow, U., Toruner, G., Schoumans, J., & Cogulu, O. (2015). Evolution of genetic techniques: Past, present, and beyond. *BioMed Research International, 2015,* 461524. https://doi.org/10.1155/2015/461524

Fang, H., Wang, W., & Medeiros, L.J. (2025). Burkitt lymphoma. *Human Pathology, 156,* 105703. https://doi.org/10.1016/j.humpath.2024.105703

Ferguson-Smith, M.A. (2015). History and evolution of cytogenetics. *Molecular Cytogenetics, 8,* 19. https://doi.org/10.1186/s13039-015-0125-8

Ferguson-Smith, M.A. (2021). Human cytogenetics at Johns Hopkins Hospital, 1959–1962. *American Journal of Medical Genetics. Part A, 185*(11), 3236–3241. https://doi.org/10.1002/ajmg.a.62366

Frost, A. (2024). *Constitutional (germline) vs somatic (tumour) variants.* https://www.genomicseducation.hee.nhs.uk/genotes/knowledge-hub/constitutional-germline-vs-somatic-tumour-variants/

Hosea, R., Hillary, S., Naqvi, S., Wu, S., & Kasim, V. (2024). The two sides of chromosomal instability: Drivers and brakes in cancer. *Signal Transduction and Targeted Therapy, 9*(1), 75. https://doi.org/10.1038/s41392-024-01767-7

Jimenez, J.J., Chale, R.S., Abad, A.C., & Schally, A.V. (2020). Acute promyelocytic leukemia (APL): A review of the literature. *Oncotarget, 11*(11), 992–1003. https://doi.org/10.18632/oncotarget.27513

Krzyszczyk, P., Acevedo, A., Davidoff, E.J., Timmins, L.M., Marrero-Berrios, I., Patel, M., ... Yarmush, M.L. (2019). The growing role of precision and personalized medicine for cancer treatment. *Technology, 6*(3–4), 79–100. https://doi.org/10.1142/S2339547818300020

Kurz, K.S., Kalmbach, S., Ott, M., Staiger, A.M., Ott, G., & Horn, H. (2023). Follicular lymphoma in the 5th edition of the WHO-classification of haematolymphoid neoplasms–Updated classification and new biological data. *Cancers, 15*(3), 785. https://doi.org/10.3390/cancers15030785

Liehr, T. (2021). Molecular cytogenetics in the era of chromosomics and cytogenomic approaches. *Frontiers in Genetics, 12,* 720507. https://doi.org/10.3389/fgene.2021.720507

Mathew, M.T., Babcock, M., Hou, Y.C., Hunter, J.M., Leung, M.L., Mei, H., ... Akkari, Y. (2024). Clinical cytogenetics: Current practices and beyond. *Journal of Applied Laboratory Medicine, 9*(1), 61–75. https://doi.org/10.1093/jalm/jfad086

Mégarbané, A., Ravel, A., Mircher, C., Sturtz, F., Grattau, Y., Rethoré, M.O., & Mobley, W.C. (2009). The 50th anniversary of the discovery of trisomy 21: The past, present, and future of research and treatment of Down syndrome. *Genetics in Medicine, 11*(9), 611–616. https://doi.org/10.1097/GIM.0b013e3181b2e34c

Nabil, A. (2013). Q-banding. In S. Maloy & K. Hughes (Eds.), *Brenner's encyclopedia of genetics* (2nd ed., pp. 1–3). Elsevier Academic Press. https://doi.org/10.1016/B978-0-12-374984-0.01246-8

National Cancer Institute. (n.d.). *Disease classification.* SEER Training Modules. https://training.seer.czncer.gov/disease/categories/classification.html

National Human Genome Research Institute. (2025a). *Genetics.* https://www.genome.gov/genetics-glossary/Genetics

National Human Genome Research Institute. (2025b). *Genomics.* https://www.genome.gov/genetics-glossary/Genomics

O'Connor, C., & Miko, I. (2008) Developing the chromosome theory. *Nature Education, 1*(1), 44. https://www.nature.com/scitable/topicpage/developing-the-chromosome-theory-164/

Ottaviano, M., Giunta, E.F., Tortora, M., Curvietto, M., Attademo, L., Bosso, D., ... Simeone, E. (2021). BRAF gene and melanoma: Back to the future. *International Journal of Molecular Sciences, 22*(7), 3474. https://doi.org/10.3390/ijms22073474

Qiu, X., Tarantino, P., Li, R., Grinshpun, A., Gupta, H., Hughes, M.E., ... Jeselsohn, R. (2025). Molecular characterization of HER2-negative breast cancers reveals a distinct patient subgroup with 17q12 deletion and heterozygous loss of ERBB2. *ESMO Open, 10*(2), 104111. https://doi.org/10.1016/j.esmoop.2024.104111

Quessada, J., Cuccuini, W., Saultier, P., Loosveld, M., Harrison, C.J., & Lafage-Pochitaloff, M. (2021). Cytogenetics of pediatric acute myeloid leukemia: A review of the current knowledge. *Genes, 12*(6), 924. https://doi.org/10.3390/genes12060924

Ramos, J.M. (2022). Fluorescent in situ hybridization (FISH). *Methods in Molecular Biology, 2422,* 179–189. https://doi.org/10.1007/978-1-0716-1948-3_12

Ribeiro, I.P., Melo, J.B., & Carreira, I.M. (2019). Cytogenetics and cytogenomics evaluation in cancer. *International Journal of Molecular Sciences, 20*(19), 4711. https://doi.org/10.3390/ijms20194711

Satam, H., Joshi, K., Mangrolia, U., Waghoo, S., Zaidi, G., Rawool, S., ... Malonia, S.K. (2023). Next-generation sequencing technology: Current trends and advancements. *Biology, 12*(7), 997. https://doi.org/10.3390/biology12070997

Smith, A.C., Neveling, K., & Kanagal-Shamanna, R. (2022). Optical genome mapping for structural variation analysis in hematologic malignancies. *American Journal of Hematology, 97*(7), 975–982. https://doi.org/10.1002/ajh.26587

Soverini, S., Bassan, R., & Lion, T. (2019). Treatment and monitoring of Philadelphia chromosome–positive leukemia patients: Recent advances and remaining challenges. *Journal of Hematology and Oncology, 12*(1), 39. https://doi.org/10.1186/s13045-019-0729-2

Sowmya, S.V., Augustine, D., Haragannavar, V.C., Khudhayr, E.A., Matari, M.H., Elagi, W.A., ... Patil, S. (2022). Cytogenetics in oral cancer: A comprehensive update. *Journal of Contemporary Dental Practice, 23*(1), 123–131. https://www.thejcdp.com/abstractArticleContentBrowse/JCDP/28055/JPJ/fullText

Tsukamoto, T., Kinoshita, M., Yamada, K., Ito, H., Yamaguchi, T., Chinen, Y., ... Kuroda, J. (2023). Imaging flow cytometry-based multiplex FISH for three *IGH* translocations in multiple myeloma. *Journal of Human Genetics, 68*(7), 507–514. https://doi.org/10.1038/s10038-023-01136-2

Wan, T.S.K., & Ma, E.S.K. (2024). Chromosome bandings and recognition. *Methods in Molecular Biology, 2825,* 137–150. https://doi.org/10.1007/978-1-0716-3946-7_7

Zhu, J.J., Qi, H., Cai, L.R., Wen, X.H., Zeng, W., Tang, G.D., ... Zhang, S.Q. (2019). C-banding and AgNOR-staining were still effective complementary methods to identify chromosomal heteromorphisms and some structural abnormalities in prenatal diagnosis. *Molecular Cytogenetics, 12,* 41. https://doi.org/10.1186/s13039-019-0453-1

CHAPTER 27

Tumor Profiling

Monique Tarrant, MSN, MPH, RN, AGCNS-BC

Introduction

Tumor profiling uses various methods to check for the presence of specific genes, proteins, or other molecules in a sample of blood, body fluid, or a specimen of tumor tissue obtained from a biopsy (National Cancer Institute [NCI], n.d.-c). It can also be a tool used to determine the risk of cancer recurrence or development based on genes or chromosomes (NCI, 2021).

As tumor profiling methods become more advanced, the impact and volume of biomarker-driven clinical trials continue to expand (Fountzilas et al., 2022; Portier, 2020). Over the past decade, oncology treatment trials have evolved from focusing on treatment based on tumor type to treatment based on a tumor's molecular characteristics (Veninga & Voest, 2021). Portier (2020) described the progression of umbrella trials, basket (bucket) trials, and super umbrella trials. Umbrella trials target one cancer type with multiple genetic variants. These studies test different variants with multiple drugs simultaneously (e.g., Lung-MAP trial) (Fountzilas et al., 2022). Basket (bucket) trials test the same drug or treatment across multiple types of cancer for a common genetic variant or biomarker (Fountzilas et al., 2022). Super umbrella trials combine umbrella trials with basket trial designs (e.g., NCI-MATCH trial) (Flaherty et al., 2020; Portier, 2020).

Biomarkers have emerged as fundamental tools in modern medicine, providing critical insights that substantially enhance diagnostic accuracy, forecast disease progression, and predict therapeutic responses. By leveraging molecular, histologic, and radiographic features, biomarkers help to inform personalized clinical decision-making. This multifaceted use underpins the clinical integration of biomarkers in various settings, from initial disease screening to the longitudinal monitoring of treatment efficacy.

This chapter will provide an overview of biomarker types (e.g., prognostic, predictive, diagnostic) used in precision oncology, outline somatic testing methodologies, and detail key techniques in genetic versus genomic testing.

Prognostic Biomarkers

Prognostic biomarkers are instrumental in estimating the likelihood of disease recurrence and overall progression. Their application is particularly prominent in oncologic care, where understanding the risk of tumor recurrence is paramount in determining long-term management strategies. These biomarkers assist clinicians in stratifying patients according to risk profiles. For example, individuals with biomarkers indicative of high recurrence probability may receive more vigorous surveillance and preemptive therapeutic interventions. In contrast, those with a favorable prognostic profile might warrant a more limited monitoring regimen. The risk stratification enabled by biomarkers is essential for optimizing follow-up care and guiding clinical trial design and therapeutic research (Gadade et al., 2024; NCI, n.d.-b). In this context, prognostic markers provide clinicians with a framework that enhances the precision of patient management and supports the implementation of individualized treatment regimens.

Predictive Biomarkers

In contrast to prognostic biomarkers, predictive biomarkers are used to forecast a patient's responsiveness to specific treatments. These indicators have garnered considerable attention for their role in guiding therapeutic choices, particularly in the context of targeted therapies. By delineating the molecular and genetic profile of a patient's disease, predictive biomarkers can help identify those individuals most likely to benefit from a particular therapeutic agent while simultaneously reducing the risk of unnecessary exposure to ineffective treatments (NCI, n.d.-a). This approach maximizes therapeutic efficacy and aligns with the principles of personalized medicine, where treatment specificity based on individual molecular characteristics is central. For example, in targeted cancer therapies, the presence or absence of specific genetic variants can directly influence the decision to administer specific kinase inhibitors or monoclonal antibodies, thereby improving clinical outcomes and reducing adverse effects.

Somatic Driver Variants and Considerations in Somatic Testing

Somatic driver variants are caused by tumor cells that contribute to oncogenesis and cancer progression. The detection and analysis of these variants are critical for understanding tumor heterogeneity—the complex mosaic of genetically diverse cell populations within a tumor (Gadade et al., 2024; Kiran et al., 2024; Passaro et al., 2024). As tumors evolve, their genomic landscape may shift, necessitating repeated somatic testing to capture these dynamic changes. Such repeated assays are particularly relevant when new tumor samples can be obtained, allowing for an updated evaluation of the tumor's molecular profile.

Several approaches and methodologies for somatic testing exist, each with its inherent advantages and limitations:

- **Tumor-only testing:** This method involves analyzing a tumor sample without concurrent germline testing. The assay identifies both somatic and germline variants present in the tumor. Without additional comparative analysis, distinguishing between the two sources of variants can be challenging (Li et al., 2020).
- **Paired somatic/germline testing (germline subtraction):** In this approach, both tumor and germline samples are analyzed, and variants present in the germline are subtracted from the tumor profile. The final report focuses on tumor-specific (somatic) alterations. This method enhances diagnostic precision by filtering out inherited variants, thereby refining the list of actionable somatic variants (Liu & Stadler, 2021).
- **Paired somatic/germline testing (comprehensive reporting):** In some cases, both somatic and germline variants are reported concurrently. Although this comprehensive approach can provide broader insights into both inherited and acquired variants, it raises ethical issues regarding patient consent and the potential disclosure of incidental germline findings. Consequently, clear ethical guidelines and robust informed consent processes are required to address the implications of such testing (Gadade et al., 2024; Liu & Stadler, 2021; Passaro et al., 2024).

The methodologic choices in somatic testing, including whole-exome sequencing, whole-genome sequencing, or targeted gene panels, are dictated by the clinical context, desired resolution, cost considerations, and the specific advantages and disadvantages of each test or technique. Notably, results from somatic testing may eventually indicate the need for confirmatory or supplementary testing, particularly when unexpected or clinically significant inherited variants are detected.

Diagnostic Biomarkers

Diagnostic biomarkers play a crucial role in establishing the most appropriate treatment modalities for individual patients. These tests enable the alignment of patient-specific disease characteristics with corresponding therapeutic agents, thus facilitating a personalized approach to treatment (Sankar et al., 2022; Twomey & Zhang, 2021). By accurately predicting which patients are likely to respond to a targeted therapy, biomarker diagnostics help in optimizing treatment selection and further enable real-time monitoring of therapeutic responses. Ongoing assessments provide clinicians with timely feedback on treatment efficacy, allowing for prompt modifications to therapeutic strategies if needed (Sankar et al., 2022; Twomey & Zhang, 2021). The real-time nature of these assays is particularly beneficial in complex clinical scenarios, promoting a dynamic treatment approach that evolves in response to the patient's clinical progress.

Implications for Oncology Clinical Research Nurses

Advancements in tumor profiling and biomarker detection have had a profound impact on clinical trials, especially in the field of oncology (Sankar et al., 2022). Oncology clinical research nurses require an in-depth understanding of the principles underlying biomarker applications and various tumor profiling techniques. These healthcare professionals play a central role in administering biomarker-driven treatments, providing ongoing assessment of individuals receiving investigational agents, and determining the effectiveness of planned interventions to address side effects related to responses to treatment during the clinical trial (Sankar et al., 2022; Twomey & Zhang, 2021). Their expertise is pivotal in optimizing trial protocols and ensuring that the insights gained from advanced tumor profiling are translated into improved patient outcomes. Consequently, there is an increasing demand for continuing education and training opportunities for nurses, particularly oncology clinical research nurses, regarding the evolving landscape of tumor profiling and precision medicine.

Genetic Testing Versus Genomic Testing

Although the terms *genetic testing* and *genomic testing* appear similar, they have different definitions. Genetic testing is the study of one's genes and how certain genetic conditions may be hereditary (National Human Genome Research Institute, 2018). With genetic testing, the laboratory can identify genetic variants, gene amplifications, and gene fusions (National Human Genome Research Institute, 2018).

Genomics is an interprofessional field that refers to the study of the expression of the entire set of genes within the human genome (National Human Genome Research Institute, 2018). Genome-wide profiling is the process of examining the allelic structure (the genotype) of hundreds of thousands or millions of single nucleotide polymorphisms (SNPs), which occur as an individual's genes interact with other genes and the environment. Molecular profiling is a type of genomic testing that identifies abnormal gene changes within cancer cells.

Within the field of genomics, genome-wide association studies represent a significant methodologic paradigm (Harris et al., 2025). These observational genetic mapping studies are designed to investigate the potential associations between genetic variants, notably SNPs, and heritable traits or diseases throughout the genome. This typically requires individually testing for differences in genotype, allowing genome-wide comparison with a specific identified phenotype or risk of disease. Genome-wide association studies attempt to determine the frequency of association between individuals with a heritable trait (cases) by comparing them to individuals who do not express the trait (controls) across hundreds of thousands of common SNPs. This comparative analysis enhances the understanding of genetic predisposition and provides valuable insights into the underlying biologic pathways involved in various health conditions.

Molecular profiling tests continue to evolve as methodology, technological advancements, and new cancer assays are developed (Magaki et al., 2019). Most kits will require a specific amount of tissue to perform the molecular testing/tumor profiling. Liquid biopsies usually require cell-free DNA, or circulating tumor, which are DNA fragments shed by the tumor. This is typically obtained from cerebrospinal fluid or a blood sample (Ray & Mukherjee, 2022); however, many kits include saliva or cheek swab samples, as genes can be found in all body fluids. The input amount or requirement is specific to the test performed, so it is vital to understand the specific volume of blood or cerebrospinal fluid required for the tumor profiling or biomarker testing.

Advancements in Testing

Several technological advancements in cancer assays have occurred since 1970. Over time, tumor profiling tests have increased in variety and accuracy.

Karyotyping

Karyotype testing is the diagnostic methodology used in examining the number and appearance of chromosomes in a single sample of cells (Drost & Clevers, 2018). It is used to detect abnormalities in chromosome number, large chromosomal duplications and deletions, and other large DNA structural rearrangements, such as translocation, inversion, or insertion of chromosomes (Ozkan & Lacerda, 2023). In comparison to karyotype testing, fluorescence in situ hybridization (FISH) is used for more targeted studies to confirm or rule out specific genetic aberrations, including gene variants, amplifications, and fusions.

Fluorescence in Situ Hybridization

FISH is a commonly used technique in detecting or diagnosing genetic aberrations. Gene amplification or duplication occurs when the copies of a gene increase or duplicate abnormally. Gene fusion occurs when a portion of two distinct genes is joined or fused. A genetic variant is a change to a specific portion of routine DNA sequencing. FISH uses DNA or RNA probes attached to fluorescence to detect nucleic acids in a sample. It is a powerful tool that can be used to target a specific DNA sequence or messenger RNA transcription (Chrzanowska et al., 2020).

The Cancer Genome Atlas was established by the National Institutes of Health in 2006 (Ganini et al., 2021). It began as a pilot study and expanded into a large-scale, pan-cancer trial with a sample size of more than 10,000 individuals (Chen et al., 2021; Ganini et al., 2021). The Cancer Genome Atlas investigated 33 cancer types and genomically characterized more than 24, concluding that 80% of cancer samples can be characterized by examining somatic variants and copy number changes.

Single Nucleotide Polymorphism Profiling

SNP profiling is a molecular genetic technique that examines variations at single nucleotide positions within the genome. These are the most common types of genetic variations among individuals and can have significant implications for disease susceptibility, drug response, and cancer development. By analyzing SNP patterns, researchers and clinicians can gain valuable insights into genetic predisposition and tumor characteristics, thereby informing personalized medicine approaches. Two commonly employed methodologies for SNP profiling in clinical and research settings are immunohistochemistry and quantitative polymerase chain reaction.

Immunohistochemistry

Immunohistochemistry is a laboratory technique that uses antibodies to detect specific markers in a tissue sample acquired from a biopsy. It assists in the clinical diagnosis of cancer and can be used to distinguish between different types of cancer. Immunohistochemistry is particularly useful for poorly differentiated cancers or those with an unknown primary site, as it can help determine a definitive diagnosis (Magaki et al., 2019).

Quantitative Polymerase Chain Reaction

Quantitative polymerase chain reaction takes trace amounts of DNA from blood or bone marrow and allows synthetic DNA fragments to signal gene amplification. This technique is useful because it requires a small sample volume to detect the presence of cancer cells. It can detect cancer in low concentrations of blood cells, often in an amount that is too small even to be seen using a microscope (Columbo et al., 2024).

Molecular Profile Testing in Specific Cancers

Gene expression analysis, or germline testing, plays a vital role in the diagnosis and treatment of patients with cancer. It can be used to provide important information about the clinical features of the cancer. This information often assists in the discussion of risks and benefits of treatment between clinicians and patients with cancer. It is important to note that not all identifiable biomarkers have an approved targeted therapy. Tumor profiling results are considered actionable variants when there is enough evidence from clinical trials to support the implementation of a targeted monotherapy or combination therapy. This section focuses on both actionable variants and prognostic markers.

Breast Cancer

Individualized treatment for breast cancer has become more common. Treatment for breast cancer depends on many factors, such as staging, extent of disease, tumor status, lymph node involvement, and presence of metastases. It may include any single treatment or a combination of surgery, radiation therapy, chemotherapy, immunotherapy, or hormone therapy. Biomarker or germline testing has become a routine practice for individuals diagnosed with breast cancer.

Phosphoinositide 3-kinase (PI3K), estrogen receptor I (ESRI), and AKT are emerging as critical components in the molecular landscape of breast cancer. Studies have found that the PI3K pathway is frequently activated in breast cancer, as the variant in the *PIK3CA* gene is among the most common alterations observed in this malignancy (Khatpe et al., 2021; Madsen et al., 2021). This activation leads to sustained AKT signaling, which, in turn, promotes tumorigenesis (Bertucci et al., 2023; Mosele et al., 2020).

Elevated levels of ESRI are associated with increased metastatic potential in several studies, suggesting a link between the marker, epithelial-mesenchymal transition, and tumor aggressiveness or metastasis. Moreover, these biomarkers can provide insights into the risk stratification for targeted therapies. For example, patients exhibiting high levels of AKT activation may be more likely to benefit from treatments aimed at inhibiting the PI3K/AKT pathway, such as PI3K inhibitors or AKT antagonists (Bertucci et al., 2023; Madsen et al., 2021; Mosele et al., 2020). Additionally, patients with high ESRI expression could require alternative therapeutic strategies, particularly aimed at addressing the likelihood of metastatic disease. Further investigation into the molecular dynamics of PI3K, ESRI, and AKT expression is imperative for advancing precision medicine options in breast cancer treatment.

Breast cancer researchers use biomarkers to stratify patients (i.e., by receptor-positive or receptor-negative status for both prognostic and predictive purposes). The presence or absence of estrogen receptors (ERs), progesterone receptors, and HER2 receptors is routinely used as a predictive marker to determine patient-specific treatment of breast cancer (Rakha & Pareja, 2021). Furthermore, multigene biomarkers from the breast tumor are used as prognostic markers, predicting the risk of recurrence. These prognostic markers, including Oncotype DX® Oncotype Breast Cancer Assay, MammaPrint®, Mammostrat®, Breast Cancer Index®, and Prosigna® PAM50 (Rakha & Pareja, 2021), can help practitioners determine treatment types to use based on patients' personal recurrence risk. This approach offers each patient personalized medicine.

The Oncotype DX Breast Cancer Assay is a 21-gene assay that uses reverse transcription polymerase chain reaction technology on paraffin-embedded tumor tissue to calculate a recurrence score that correlates with the likelihood of breast cancer recurrence within 10 years of initial diagnosis (Rakha & Pareja, 2021). The National Surgical Adjuvant Breast and Bowel Project B-14 trial validated the correlation of the recurrence score as "quantifying the likelihood of distant recurrence in tamoxifen-treated patients with node-negative, estrogen-receptor-positive breast cancer" (Paik et al., 2004, p. 2817). The population used to validate the Oncotype DX assay was patients with early-stage breast cancer, defined as stage I or II, lymph-node negative, ER-positive disease (Paik et al., 2004).

An Oncotype DX Breast Cancer Assay recurrence score is a number between 0 and 100 (Rakha & Pareja, 2021). It is calculated from 16 cancer-related genes and five reference genes, which normalize the expression of cancer-related genes (Paik et al., 2004). The score places patients into one of three categories: low risk, defined as a score of less than 18; intermediate risk, defined as a score of 18–30; and high risk, defined as a score of 31 or higher (Paik et al., 2004). Using this score, a practitioner can determine if a type of treatment will provide a longer disease-free survival time. The Oncotype DX assay was validated independently in two studies, the B-14 study, which validated its use as a predictor of recurrence, and B-20, which validated its use for females with ER-positive, node-negative disease and tumors larger than 0.5 cm (McVeigh & Kerin, 2017).

MammaPrint is another prognostic multigene assay. It targets 70 genes associated with breast cancer and uses microarray technology to determine a recurrence score for early-stage breast cancer (Rakha & Pareja, 2021). Its related study focused on females with early-stage breast cancer, defined as invasive stage I or II (T1 or T2), smaller than 5 cm, and including both node-positive and node-negative disease (Rakha & Pareja, 2021). MammaPrint stratified the results into two prognostic groups, good or poor, based on a correlation coefficient predicting recurrence during the first five years after therapy (Rakha & Pareja, 2021). Other studies evaluating the predictive value of MammaPrint concluded that chemotherapy plus endocrine therapy had a significant clinical benefit in the high-risk, poor-prognosis groups. The addition of chemotherapy was not shown to be beneficial to the good-prognosis group (Rakha & Pareja, 2021).

Mammostrat is a third prognostic test for stage I and II, node-negative, ER-positive breast cancer. It is a five-antibody immunohistochemistry panel targeting expression levels of the tumor proteins SLC7A5, HTF9C, p53, NDRG1, and CEACAM5 (Rakha & Pareja, 2021). An algorithm calculates a risk index score to classify patients into one of three categories based on the percentage of cancer recurrence in 10 years. The categories include low-, moderate-, and high-risk for relapse. Females at low risk would probably not receive additional benefit from chemotherapy, but those at high risk would have long-term benefit from chemotherapy plus hormone therapy. Validation studies have not incorporated the status of other hormone receptors, but more evidence supports the ER-positive ranking (Rakha & Pareja, 2021).

Since 2007, the mortality associated with breast cancer has plateaued in females aged 50 years or younger. There has also been a decrease in mortality in females aged older than 50 years. These favorable changes may be the result of early detection, increased awareness, and better treatments, in part, because of germline testing. Precision oncology has led to a better understanding of targeted treatment options and improved clinical outcomes for patients with breast cancer (McVeigh & Kerin, 2017; Rakha & Pareja, 2021).

Non-Small Cell Lung Cancer

Biomarker testing has become a routine practice at initial diagnosis for patients with non-small cell lung cancer. The findings from this testing aid in treatment planning discussions. Clinicians may also use repeat testing on tumor tissue or circulating tumor cells obtained via liquid biopsy. The most frequently identified biomarkers in non-small cell lung cancer are epidermal growth factor receptor (EGFR), Kirsten rat sarcoma virus (KRAS), and anaplastic lymphoma kinase (ALK) (Ettinger et al., 2022).

EGFR is a transmembrane receptor that is known to have a predictive treatment benefit from EGFR tyrosine kinase inhibitor therapy with the presence of an exon 19 deletion or exon 21 p.L858R variant (Ettinger et al., 2022). EGFR variants and copy number changes were positively correlated with a higher response rate and progression-free survival. These patients are typically treated with EGFR inhibitor tyrosine kinase inhibitor–sensitizing monotherapies, such as osimertinib, erlotinib, gefitinib, afatinib, or dacomitinib, or in combination with a monoclonal antibody, such as bevacizumab (nonsquamous) or ramucirumab.

The *KRAS* oncogene has been shown to be prognostic of survival and is associated with cigarette smoking (Ettinger et al., 2022). Studies have demonstrated that a *KRAS* variant has an unfavorable prognostic value with shorter survival. Patients with a *KRAS* G12C variant may be offered adagrasib or sotorasib after disease progression or unacceptable toxicity resulting from upfront systemic therapy.

The *ALK* oncogene has been shown in studies to have a predictive value of response to alectinib, brigatinib, ceritinib, crizotinib, and lorlatinib (Ettinger et al., 2022).

Programmed cell death-ligand 1 (PD-L1) testing via immunohistochemistry is recommended by the National Comprehensive Cancer Network (NCCN) for all patients with metastatic non-small cell lung cancer, given that U.S. Food and Drug Administration–approved immunotherapies are available for individuals with this targeted immune biomarker (Riely et al., 2024). PD-L1 is a co-regulatory molecule that can be expressed on tumor cells. Testing for the expression of PD-L1 can provide prognostic and predictive information. For patients who are PD-L1 negative or have low PD-L1 expression ($\leq 1\%$), first-line therapy includes pembrolizumab monotherapy or in combination with nivolumab/ipilimumab. Patients with high PD-L1 ($\geq 50\%$) expression may be offered atezolizumab or cemiplimab in addition to the first-line options for patients who are PD-L1 negative. Atezolizumab is known to have more immune-related adverse events; therefore, clinicians may rely on PD-L1 expression to help identify patients who have a higher likelihood of responding to immunotherapy (Riely et al., 2024).

Thyroid Cancer

Molecular diagnostic testing can be helpful in disease management and treatment planning for thyroid cancer. Diagnostic testing can be performed via multigene assay analysis or focused on detecting an individual variant (i.e., *BRAF* V600E, *RET/PTC*, *RAS*, *PAX8/ PPARγ*). *BRAF* V600E is the most common biomarker (about 45%) for papillary thyroid cancer (Haddad et al., 2018). In medullary thyroid cancer, the most common associated biomarker is the *RET* oncogene, which has a known inheritable familial pathway in multiple endocrine neoplasia type 2. In conjunction with additional testing and genetic counseling, this information may be helpful to patients and their families if an inherited risk of thyroid cancer is identified (Haddad et al., 2022).

Colorectal Cancer

Prior to 2020, there were fewer than 15 U.S. Food and Drug Administration–approved drugs for treating colorectal cancer. Only four of those drugs were biomarker driven: cetuximab and panitumumab with an antibody against EGFR, and pembrolizumab and nivolumab with an antibody against programmed cell death protein 1 (PD-1) (Louie et al., 2022; Messersmith, 2019). In 2019, NCCN guidelines were updated to include treatment options based on BRAF/MEK and NTRK fusion targets (Messersmith, 2019).

Similar to breast cancer, colon cancer has genomic profiling options to predict recurrence risk, including Oncotype DX, ColoPrint®, and ColDx® (Columbo et al., 2024; Krishnamurthi, 2022). The Oncotype DX Colon Cancer Assay is a 12-gene panel consisting of seven cancer genes and five reference genes (Colombo et al., 2024; Krishnamurthi, 2022).

Another profiling approach, ImmunoScore™, relied on the relationship between tumor gene expression and risk of cancer recurrence in four individualized cohorts to evaluate surgery alone versus surgery plus adjuvant 5-fluorouracil plus leucovorin in both stage II and III disease (Columbo et al., 2024; Krishnamurthi, 2022). These researchers used the quantitative reverse transcription polymerase chain reaction technique to identify 48 genes associated with recurrence risk and 66 genes related to the benefit of 5-fluorouracil/leucovorin (Columbo et al., 2024; Krishnamurthi, 2022). From this, seven of the recurrence genes and six of the treatment-benefit genes were identified and are the foundation of the algorithm used to categorize patients with stage II–III colon cancer into three categories: low, intermediate, and high risk of recurrence (Colombo et al., 2024; Krishnamurthi, 2022). The development of this assay was validated and confirmed for stage II colon cancer in the QUASAR and Cancer and Leukemia Group B 9581 studies (Colombo et al., 2024; Formica et al., 2022). The use of the gene expression levels of the cancer genes allows for the calculation of a recurrence score. A report is generated with a colon cancer recurrence score that ranges from 0 to 100: a score less than 30 has a recurrence risk of 15% or less; a score of 30 or greater indicates a recurrence risk greater than 15%; and a recurrence score of 41 or greater indicates a recurrence risk greater than 18% that overlaps with T4 patients (Colombo et al., 2024; Formica et al., 2022). The report also includes information on mismatch repair status.

Mismatch repair is a conserved process during DNA replication that corrects mismatches of bases (Krishnamurthi, 2022). Patients with colorectal cancer can be categorized based on tumors with mismatch repair deficiency (dMMR) and mismatch repair proficient (pMMR) colorectal cancer. Immunotherapy is becoming standard of care in dMMR colorectal cancer (Riedesser et al., 2022), whereas the majority of metastatic colorectal cancers (95%) are categorized as pMMR. Additionally, anti–programmed cell death protein 1 immunotherapies (e.g., pembrolizumab, nivolumab) are approved for metastatic colorectal cancer with dMMR or microsatellite instability–high (Louie et al., 2022).

ColoPrint is an assay that quantifies the expression of 18 genes and is a prognostic marker that classifies patients into low or high risk of recurrence (Columbo et al., 2024; Krishnamurthi, 2022). In the development of this assay, 188 tumor samples consisting of stage I–III colon cancers were categorized into A, B, and C groups based on the variant status of BRAF (Columbo et al., 2024; Krishnamurthi, 2022). Then, using the B group, an 18-gene optimal assay was developed and validated using a sample of 206 participants. In this study, researchers assessed the variants for *BRAF*, *KRAS*, and *PI3KCA* in addition to running the 18-gene assay. Based on the analysis, patients were categorized as having either low or high risk of recurrence using five-year survival. The study concluded that ColoPrint improves prognostic accuracy and was able to identify patients with stage II disease that could be managed without chemotherapy (Columbo et al., 2024; Krishnamurthi, 2022).

ColDx is a DNA microarray multigene assay that uses 634 probes to stratify patients as having either high or low risk of recurrence. Studies showed that patients with stage II colon adenocarcinoma can be predictively categorized into either group based on recurrence risk at five years (Krishnamurthi, 2022).

Precision oncology has affected the field of colorectal medicine. Based on the results of the HERACLES and the MyPathway trials, Riedesser et al. (2022) suggested fresh tumor biopsy and introduction of HER2-targeted therapy in patients with colorectal cancer refractory to standard therapy. *BRAF* somatic variants are found in 5%–10% of colorectal cancers; mostly the V600E type is a positive predictive marker for the introduction of the combination therapy of encorafenib and cetuximab (Kopetz et al., 2019; Riedesser et al., 2022). However, *BRAF* V600E variant colorectal cancer is associated with poor prognosis and poor response to therapy. Given advancements in genomic sequencing, more knowledge is available about the molecular predictive markers related to colorectal cancer (Kiran et al., 2024). However, because colorectal cancer is characterized by complex molecular profiles and resistance to many systemic agents and targeted monotherapies, several challenges remain in determining actionable variants with targeted therapies.

Prostate Cancer

Prostate cancer is the most frequently diagnosed cancer type among males older than age 60 years (Adamaki & Zoumpourlis, 2021). Genomic variants associated with increased risk and severity of prostate cancer have been identified, including *BRCA1*, *BRCA2*, *HOB13*, and Lynch syndrome–associated DNA mismatch repair genes (Giunta et al., 2021; Patel et al., 2020). Prostate cancer gene 3 (PCA3) is a non-coding RNA that is exclusively overexpressed in prostate cancer with commercially available testing (Adamaki & Zoumpourlis, 2021). Additionally, there are some specific genotype–phenotype correlations based on familial history, ancestry, and other factors that are being explored via clinical trials (Patel et al., 2020).

NCCN recommends germline testing at initial diagnosis for patients with a family history, high risk for metastatic cancer at time of diagnosis, Ashkenazi Jewish ancestry, and any individual with rare intraductal or cribriform prostate cancer (Mohler & Antonarakis, 2019). In addition to immunotherapy to treat prostate cancer, clinical trials have also begun to include germline testing to identity targeted biomarkers.

Precision Medicine

Precision oncology is the discipline in which information generated from molecular profiling is used in clinical diagnosis to determine targeted cancer treatments. Although precision oncology has progressed from isolated genomic analysis to pan-cancer genomic testing approaches, several barriers interfere with the application of the various clinical testing methodologies and widespread implementation of precision medicine, including the following (Malone et al., 2020):

- **Cost:** Gene sequencing is expensive; however, evidence suggests that as cost declines, clinical use is expected to increase.
- **Sample requirement (quantity and quality):** To perform testing, a sufficient quantity of tissue or high-quality DNA/RNA is required.
- **Laboratory expertise:** Technical expertise is required to perform testing and develop clinical trial study designs that are meaningful and lead to tangible results.
- **Clinician knowledge:** Several studies have suggested that knowledge amongst clinicians (e.g., nurses, physicians) must be improved to optimize the implementation of precision oncology. Additionally, several studies have explored the use of technology, tools, and databases to aid in matching patients with particular treatment options and planning care that is individualized and specific based on biomarker results (Dickman et al., 2024).
- **Patient attitudes and expectations:** Shirdarreh et al. (2021) found that patients possess relatively little knowledge or awareness about genomics. They have unrealistic expectations regarding tumor profiling and the associated clinical implications of testing results. However, this can be appropriately addressed by engaging patients in shared decision-making and providing patient education and counseling about testing and actionable results (Pichler et al., 2024; Shirdarreh et al., 2021).

The integration of diagnostic, prognostic, and predictive biomarkers into clinical practice underscores a significant paradigm shift toward precision medicine. By tailoring therapeutic strategies to the individual molecular and genetic makeup of each disease, biomarkers facilitate a more personalized approach to patient care. As tumor profiling techniques continue to advance, diagnostic, monitoring, and therapeutic processes are optimized, thereby enhancing overall patient care. The role of the oncology clinical research nurse becomes ever more critical in bridging the gap between complex molecular testing and practical clinical applications. The continued evolution of biomarker research promises to refine the delivery of precision medicine further, ultimately contributing to superior patient outcomes and the advancement of oncologic care.

Organoids

Tumor organoids are three-dimensional, multicellular in vitro tumors derived from individual patient DNA that can be used as a tool in the application of translational research into novel oncologic precision medicine regimens (Veninga & Voest, 2021). The first organoids were derived from stem cells. In 1907, Henry Van Peters Wilson published the earliest attempts at in vitro organism regeneration (Corrò et al., 2020). Since this discovery, three-dimensional culture models have evolved from complex cell aggregates to organoids. Organoids, also known as mini organs, are dynamic in comparison to other preclinical cancer models, such as patient-derived tumor xenografts or cancer cell lines, in that they are able to self-organize and engage in self-renewal (Corrò et al., 2020; Veninga & Voest, 2021). Studies suggest that organoids contain the characteristics of the original tumor specimen, therefore providing a sample for laboratory testing that is a phenotypical and a genetic match with the same genetic variants (Veninga & Voest, 2021). In the laboratory setting, organoids can be generated from various types of specimens, such as embryonic stem cells, neonatal stem cells, adult stem cells, or induced pluripotent stem cells from a somatic cell (Corrò et al., 2020).

The success rates of growing organoid cultures vary, and there is a lack of consensus regarding methodology (e.g., specimen required for culture, resection versus biopsy, best culture medium). Table 27-1 outlines the strengths and weaknesses of tumor organoids for preclinical research and precision medicine applications. The state of molecular profiling suggests that patient-derived tumor organoids are not entirely reliable for timely decision-making or as a tool in everyday precision medicine.

NCI has spearheaded an innovative initiative to establish a national repository of patient-derived models, the Patient-Derived Models Repository. This repository encompasses a diverse array of biologic resources, including organoids, xenografts, in vitro tumor cell cultures, and cancer-associated fibroblasts, all derived from patient samples. The establishment of this repository represents a significant step forward in fostering collaboration across the scientific community. It is intended to serve as a critical resource for both public–private partnerships and academic drug discovery efforts.

Additionally, via the Human Cancer Models Initiative (HCMI), NCI, in collaboration with Cancer Research UK,

Wellcome Sanger Institute, and the Hubrecht Organoid Technology foundation, is developing 1,000 patient-derived cancer models, including organoids for international community use. This resource is being developed to increase accessibility and advance scientific discovery via biobanks and translational cancer research worldwide. The field of tumor organoids is continually evolving, and any application of testing results on treatment-based decisions requires regulatory approval.

TABLE 27-1 | Relevance and Suitability of Organoids

Pros	Cons
Timing and Rate of Success	
Organoids have a higher success rate of initiation compared to cell lines. Organoids can grow faster compared to patient-derived tumor xenografts.	The success rate of initiation depends on several factors, such as the cancer type and assay used for culture growth.
Maintenance	
Organoids can be easier and more affordable to maintain compared to patient-derived tumor xenografts.	–
Resource Consumption	
–	Culturing organoids requires training and staffing of professional laboratory personnel with technical expertise. The culture medium and growth factors used can be expensive. Culture media formulated with growth factors may interfere with genomic sequencing results.
Three-Dimensional Growth	
–	The growth rate of a culture varies. Slow-growing three-dimensional samples could lead to a delay in timely decision-making.
Representation of Individual Cancer Treatment Prediction and Response	
Organoids allow for comparison between pretreatment and post-treatment reactions.	Although organoids retain the characteristics of the original tumor, the tumors lack vascularity and immune cells.

Note. Based on information from Corrò et al., 2020; Drost & Clevers, 2018; Veninga & Voest, 2021.

Summary

Molecular profiling has the potential to improve diagnosis and identify targets for treatment. Gene expression analysis is valuable because it can detail the prognosis and recurrent and metastatic risk of certain cancers. The identification of clinically significant actionable germline and somatic variants has progressively facilitated the integration of genomic knowledge into treatment planning and therapeutic decision-making by healthcare professionals. The evolution of genomic testing and precision medicine indicates that further studies are on the horizon to examine oncogenic pathways and the application of targeted drug therapies.

Key Points

- Tumor profiling is an advanced diagnostic approach that examines specific molecular characteristics of cancer through various methods, including analysis of genes, proteins, and other molecular markers.
- Tumor profiling represents a transformative approach in oncology care, shifting from generalized treatments to personalized, molecular-based strategies to inform treatment decisions.
- By leveraging advanced biomarker analysis, healthcare professionals can develop targeted, effective cancer treatments tailored to individual patient profiles.

The author would like to acknowledge Elizabeth Hassen, MSN, OCN®, and Julia A. Eggert, PhD, GNP-BC, AGN-BC, AOCN®, for their contribution to this chapter that remains unchanged from the previous edition of this book.

References

Adamaki, M., & Zoumpourlis, V. (2021). Prostate cancer biomarkers: From diagnosis to prognosis and precision-guided therapeutics. *Pharmacology and Therapeutics, 228*, 107932. https://doi.org/10.1016/j.pharmthera.2021.107932

Bertucci, A., Bertucci, F., & Gonçalves, A. (2023). Phosphoinositide 3-kinase (PI3K) inhibitors and breast cancer: An overview of current achievements. *Cancers, 15*(5), 1416. https://doi.org/10.3390/cancers15051416

Chen, F., Wendl, M.C., Wyczalkowski, M.A., Bailey, M.H., Li, Y., & Ding, L. (2021). Moving pan-cancer studies from basic research toward the clinic. *Nature Cancer, 2*(9), 879–890. https://doi.org/10.1038/s43018-021-00250-4

Chrzanowska, N.M., Kowalewski, J., & Lewandowska, M.A. (2020). Use of fluorescence in situ hybridization (FISH) in diagnosis and tailored therapies in solid tumors. *Molecules, 25*(8), 1864. https://doi.org/10.3390/molecules25081864

Colombo, A., Gebbia, V., Borsellino, N., & Porretto, C.M. (2024). Molecular biomarkers in colorectal cancer in the era of precision medicine: A review. *International Journal of Advanced Multidisciplinary Research and Studies, 4*(3), 38–51. https://doi.org/10.62225/2583049X.2024.4.3.2738

Corrò, C., Novellasdemunt, L., & Li, V.S.W. (2020). A brief history of organoids. *American Journal of Physiology-Cell Physiology, 319*(1), C151–C165. https://doi.org/10.1152/ajpcell.00120.20206-8

Dickman, E., Schmitt, M.L., Marty, K., & Mahon, S.M. (2024). Oncology Nursing Society's genomics and precision oncology learning library resources for nursing practice. *Clinical Journal of Oncology Nursing, 28*(2), 133–141. https://doi.org/10.1188/24.CJON.133-141

Drost, J., & Clevers, H. (2018). Organoids in cancer research. *Nature Reviews Cancer, 18*(7), 407–418. https://doi.org/10.1038/s41568-018-0007-6

Ettinger, D.S., Wood, D.E., Aisner, D.L., Akerley, W., Bauman, J.R., Bharat, A., ... Hughes, M. (2022). Non–small cell lung cancer, version 3.2022, NCCN clinical practice guidelines in oncology. *Journal of the National Comprehensive Cancer Network, 20*(5), 497–530. https://doi.org/10.6004/jnccn.2022.0025

Flaherty, K.T., Gray, R.J., Chen, A.P., Li, S., McShane, L.M., Patton, D., ... Conley, B.A. (2020). Molecular landscape and actionable alterations in a genomically guided cancer clinical trial: National Cancer Institute Molecular Analysis for Therapy Choice (NCI-MATCH). *Journal of Clinical Oncology, 38*(33), 3883–3894. https://doi.org/10.1200/JCO.19.03010

Formica, V., Sera, F., Cremolini, C., Riondino, S., Morelli, C., Arkenau, H.T., & Roselli, M. (2022). KRAS and BRAF mutations in stage II and III colon cancer: A systematic review and meta-analysis. *Journal of the National Cancer Institute, 114*(4), 517–527. https://doi.org/10.1093/jnci/djab190

Fountzilas, E., Tsimberidou, A.M., Vo, H.H., & Kurzrock, R. (2022). Clinical trial design in the era of precision medicine. *Genome Medicine, 14*(1), 101. https://doi.org/10.1186/s13073-022-01102-1

Gadade, D.D., Jha, H., Kumar, C., & Khan, F. (2024). Unlocking the power of precision medicine: Exploring the role of biomarkers in cancer management. *Future Journal of Pharmaceutical Sciences, 10*(1), 5. https://doi.org/10.1186/s43094-023-00573-2

Ganini, C., Amelio, I., Bertolo, R., Bove, P., Buonomo, O.C., Candi, E., ... Melino, G. (2021). Global mapping of cancers: The Cancer Genome Atlas and beyond. *Molecular Oncology, 15*(11), 2823–2840. https://doi.org/10.1002/1878-0261.13056

Giunta, E.F., Annaratone, L., Bollito, E., Porpiglia, F., Cereda, M., Banna, G.L., ... Rescigno, P. (2021). Molecular characterization of prostate cancers in the precision medicine era. *Cancers, 13*(19), 4771. https://doi.org/10.3390/cancers13194771

Haddad, R.I., Bischoff, L., Ball, D., Bernet, V., Blomain, E., Busaidy, N.L., ... Darlow, S. (2022). Thyroid carcinoma, version 2.2022, NCCN clinical practice guidelines in oncology. *Journal of the National Comprehensive Cancer Network, 20*(8), 925–951. https://doi.org/10.6004/jnccn.2022.0040

Haddad, R.I., Nasr, C., Bischoff, L., Busaidy, N.L., Byrd, D., Callender, G., ... Gurski, L.A. (2018). NCCN guidelines insights: Thyroid carcinoma, version 2.2018. *Journal of the National Comprehensive Cancer Network, 16*(12), 1429–1440. https://doi.org/10.6004/jnccn.2018.0089

Harris, L., McDonagh, E.M., Zhang, X., Fawcett, K., Foreman, A., Daneck, P., & Fitzgerald, T. (2025). Genome-wide association testing beyond SNPs. *Nature Reviews. Genetics, 26*(3), 156–170. https://doi.org/10.1038/s41576-024-00778-y

Khatpe, A.S., Adebayo, A.K., Herodotou, C.A., Kumar, B., & Nakshatri, H. (2021). Nexus between PI3K/AKT and estrogen receptor signaling in breast cancer. *Cancers, 13*(3), 369. https://doi.org/10.3390/cancers13030369

Kiran, N.S., Yashaswini, C., Maheshwari, R., Bhattacharya, S., & Prajapati, B.G. (2024). Advances in precision medicine approaches for colorectal cancer: From molecular profiling to targeted therapies. *ACS Pharmacology and Translational Science, 7*(4), 967–990. https://doi.org/10.1021/acsptsci.4c00008

Kopetz, S., Grothey, A., Yaeger, R., Van Cutsem, E., Desai, J., Yoshino, T., ... Tabernero, J. (2019). Encorafenib, binimetinib, and cetuximab in BRAF V600E-mutated colorectal cancer. *New England Journal of Medicine, 381*(17), 1632–1643. https://doi.org/10.1056/NEJMoa1908075

Krishnamurthi, S.S. (2022). Updates in the treatment of patients with colorectal cancer. *Journal of the National Comprehensive Cancer Network, 20*(5.5), 1–4.

Li, M.M., Chao, E., Esplin, E.D., Miller, D.T., Nathanson, K.L., Plon, S.E., ... Stewart, D.R. (2020). Points to consider for reporting of germline variation in patients undergoing tumor testing: A statement of the American College of Medical Genetics and Genomics (ACMG). *Genetics in Medicine, 22*(7), 1142–1148. https://doi.org/10.1038/s41436-020-0783-8

Liu, Y.L., & Stadler, Z.K. (2021). The future of parallel tumor and germline genetic testing: Is there a role for all patients with cancer? *Journal of the National Comprehensive Cancer Network, 19*(7), 871–878. https://doi.org/10.6004/jnccn.2021.7044

Louie, B.H., Kato, S., Kim, K.H., Lim, H.J., Lee, S., Okamura, R., ... Kurzrock, R. (2022). Precision medicine–based therapies in advanced colorectal cancer: The University of California San Diego Molecular Tumor Board experience. *Molecular Oncology, 16*(13), 2575–2584. https://doi.org/10.1002/1878-0261.13202

Madsen, R.R., Erickson, E.C., Rueda, O.M., Robin, X., Caldas, C., Toker, A., ... Vanhaesebroeck, B. (2021). Positive correlation between transcriptomic stemness and PI3K/AKT/mTOR signaling scores in breast cancer, and a counterintuitive relationship with *PIK3CA* genotype. *PLOS Genetics, 17*(11), e1009876. https://doi.org/10.1371/journal.pgen.1009876

Magaki, S., Hojat, S.A., Wei, B., So, A., & Yong, W.H. (2019). An introduction to the performance of immunohistochemistry. *Methods in Molecular Biology, 1897*, 289–298. https://doi.org/10.1007/978-1-4939-8935-5_25

Malone, E.R., Oliva, M., Sabatini, P.J.B., Stockley, T.L., & Siu, L.L. (2020). Molecular profiling for precision cancer therapies. *Genome Medicine, 12*(1), 1–19. https://doi.org/10.1186/s13073-019-0703-1

McVeigh, T.P., & Kerin, M.J. (2017). Clinical use of the Oncotype DX genomic test to guide treatment decisions for patients with invasive breast cancer. *Breast Cancer, 9*, 393–400. https://doi.org/10.2147/BCTT.S109847

Messersmith, W.A. (2019). NCCN guidelines updates: Management of metastatic colorectal cancer. *Journal of the National Comprehensive Cancer Network, 17*(5.5), 599–601. https://doi.org/10.6004/jnccn.2019.5014

Mohler, J.L., & Antonarakis, E.S. (2019). NCCN guidelines updates: Management of prostate cancer. *Journal of the National Comprehensive Cancer Network, 17*(5.5), 583–586. https://doi.org/10.6004/jnccn.2019.5011

Mosele, F., Remon, J., Mateo, J., Westphalen, C.B., Barlesi, F., Lolkema, M.P., ... André, F. (2020). Recommendations for the use of next-generation sequencing (NGS) for patients with metastatic cancers: A report from the ESMO Precision Medicine Working Group. *Annals of Oncology, 31*(11), 1491–1505. https://doi.org/10.1016/j.annonc.2020.07.014

National Cancer Institute. (n.d.-a). Predictive factor. *In NCI dictionary of cancer terms.* Retrieved August 28, 2025, from https://www.cancer.gov/publications/dictionaries/cancer-terms/def/predictive-factor

National Cancer Institute. (n.d.-b). Prognostic factor. *In NCI dictionary of cancer terms.* Retrieved August 28, 2025, from https://www.cancer.gov/publications/dictionaries/cancer-terms/def/prognostic-factor

National Cancer Institute. (n.d.-c). Tumor profiling. *In NCI dictionary of cancer terms.* Retrieved August 28, 2025, from https://www.cancer.gov/publications/dictionaries/cancer-terms/def/tumor-profiling

National Cancer Institute. (2021). *Biomarker testing for cancer treatment.* https://www.cancer.gov/about-cancer/treatment/types/biomarker-testing-cancer-treatment

National Human Genome Research Institute. (2018). *Genetics vs. genomics fact sheet.* https://www.genome.gov/about-genomics/fact-sheets/Genetics-vs-Genomics

Ozkan, E., & Lacerda, M.P. (2023). Genetics, cytogenetic testing and conventional karyotype. In *StatPearls*. StatPearls Publishing. https://www.ncbi.nlm.nih.gov/books/NBK563293

Paik, S., Shak, S., Tang, G., Kim, C., Baker, J., Cronin, M., ... Wolmark, N. (2004). A multigene assay to predict recurrence of tamoxifen-treated, node-negative breast cancer. *New England Journal of Medicine, 351*(27), 2817–2826. https://doi.org/10.1056/NEJMoa041588

Passaro, A., Al Bakir, M., Hamilton, E.G., Diehn, M., André, F., Roy-Chowdhuri, S., ... Peters, S. (2024). Cancer biomarkers: Emerging trends and clinical implications for personalized treatment. *Cell, 187(*7), 1617–1635. https://doi.org/10.1016/j.cell.2024.02.041

Patel, V.L., Busch, E.L., Friebel, T.M., Cronin, A., Leslie, G., McGuffog, L., ... Matricardi, L. (2020). Association of genomic domains in BRCA1 and BRCA2 with prostate cancer risk and aggressiveness. *Cancer Research, 80*(3), 624–638. https://doi.org/10.1158/0008-5472.CAN-19-1840

Pichler, T., Mumm, F., Dehar, N., Dickman, E., Díez de Los Ríos de la Serna, C., Dinkel, A., ... Moore, A.C. (2024). Understanding communication between patients and healthcare professionals regarding comprehensive biomarker testing in precision oncology: A scoping review. *Cancer Medicine, 13*(3), e6913. https://doi.org/10.1002/cam4.6913

Portier, W.S. (2020). Cancer clinical trials: Implications for oncology nurses. *Seminars in Oncology Nursing, 36*(2),150998. https://doi.org/10.1016/j.soncn.2020.150998

Rakha, E.A., & Pareja, F.G. (2021). New advances in molecular breast cancer pathology. *Seminars in Cancer Biology, 72*, 102–113. https://doi.org/10.1016/j.semcancer.2020.03.014

Ray, S.K., & Mukherjee, S. (2022). Cell free DNA as an evolving liquid biopsy biomarker for initial diagnosis and therapeutic nursing in cancer—An evolving aspect in medical biotechnology. *Current Pharmaceutical Biotechnology, 23*(1), 112–122. https://doi.org/10.2174/1389201021666201211102710

Riedesser, J.E., Ebert, M.P., & Betge, J. (2022). Precision medicine for metastatic colorectal cancer in clinical practice. *Therapeutic Advances in Medical Oncology, 14*, 17588359211072703. https://doi.org/10.1177/17588359211072703

Riely, G.J., Wood, D.E., Ettinger, D.S., Aisner, D.L., Akerley, W., Bauman, J.R., ... Hang, L. (2024). Non–small cell lung cancer, version 4.2024, NCCN clinical practice guidelines in oncology. *Journal of the National Comprehensive Cancer Network, 22*(4), 249–274. https://doi.org/10.6004/jnccn.2204.0023

Sankar, K., Ye, J.C., Li, Z., Song, W., & Hu-Lieskovan, S. (2022). The role of biomarkers in personalized immunotherapy. *Biomarker Research, 10*(1), 32. https://doi.org/10.1186/s40364-022-00378-0

Shirdarreh, M., Aziza, O., Pezo, R.C., Jerzak, K.J., & Warner, E. (2021). Patients' and oncologists' knowledge and expectations regarding tumor multigene next-generation sequencing: A narrative review. *Oncologist, 26*(8), e1359–e1371. https://doi.org/10.1002/onco.13783

Twomey, J.D., & Zhang, B. (2021). Cancer immunotherapy update: FDA-approved checkpoint inhibitors and companion diagnostics. *AAPS Journal, 23*(2), 39. https://doi.org/10.1208/s12248-021-00574-0

Veninga, V., & Voest, E.E. (2021). Tumor organoids: Opportunities and challenges to guide precision medicine. *Cancer Cell, 39*(9), 1190–1201. https://doi.org/10.1016/j.ccell.2021.07.020

CHAPTER 28

Storage of Genetic Material

Gabriele Urschel, DNP, FNP-C, AOCNP®

Introduction

The pathway of identifying, diagnosing, and treating cancer has significantly changed over the past few decades due in large part to the initiation of the Human Genome Project in 1990. Not only did this research expand the collection of genetic material, but it also established the criteria for a healthy human genome, allowing for the detection of early genetic changes that can lead to cancer. Organizations, such as the U.S.-based Cancer Genome Atlas and the U.K.-based Catalogue of Somatic Mutations in Cancer, have expanded upon the initial Human Genome Project to determine the genomic sequencing of many cancer types, leading to further enhancements in diagnosis and treatment (National Human Genome Research Institute, 2018). In this rapidly changing field of personalized medicine, oncology clinical research nurses (OCRNs) must advocate for participants' rights regarding the donation of genetic material (i.e., blood and tissue).

This chapter will focus on the regulations involved in protecting the rights of clinical research participants when storing their genetic material.

Regulatory Agencies

Multiple agencies within the United States focus on protecting the rights of research participants as part of the U.S. Department of Health and Human Services (HHS). The Office for Human Research Protections (OHRP) and the U.S. Food and Drug Administration (FDA) are each in charge of specific aspects of the research process on participant samples. The Office for Human Research Protections provides overall leadership to the 17 federal agencies that conduct research involving humans under the Federal Policy for the Protection of Human Subjects (the Common Rule) regulations (National Institutes of Health, n.d.; OHRP, 2024). The Common Rule outlines the basic provisions for the institutional review board (IRB), assurance of compliance, and informed consent. These regulations are outlined in Title 45 of the Code of Federal Regulations (C.F.R.) and protect participants from risks in studies conducted by federal departments or agencies (Protection of Human Subjects, 2019).

The IRB, which is under FDA regulations, is an additional layer of protection for participants in human research. It has the authority to approve, require modifications, or reject human research. The IRB's goal is to ensure that human rights and welfare are protected throughout the research process by reviewing research protocols and other materials (e.g., informed consent, investigator brochures) (FDA, 2025).

The Health Insurance Portability and Accountability Act (HIPAA) of 1996 is a federal law that created national standards to protect patient health information from being disclosed without patient consent or knowledge, including genetic material. Additionally, the HIPAA Privacy Rule created national standards to protect patients' identifiable health information and medical records and is applicable to healthcare plans, clearinghouses, and providers that conduct certain healthcare transactions. This rule created certain safeguards that set limits on the use and disclosure of patient information without authorization (Centers for Disease Control and Prevention, 2024; OHRP, 2024). Each state may have additional regulations that restrict the use of genetic materials or claims related to tissue sampling (Reymond et al., 2002). For example, California requires a fee for researchers to use stored umbilical cord, newborn blood, or pregnancy blood to cover the costs of the program (National Human Genome Research Institute [NHGRI], 2024a). OCRNs should be aware of the statutes that are in place within their state by accessing the NHGRI website to review (www.genome.gov/about-genomics/policy-issues/Genome-Statute-Legislation-Database).

Informed Consent

Obtaining informed consent is critical when participating in research. The three key features that must be met when obtaining consent from a participant are providing them with important information, confirming the participant understands the information, and ensuring that their decision to participate is entirely voluntary (NHGRI, 2024b). Compliance with 45 C.F.R. 46(a) (Protection of Human Subjects, 2019), along with the eight required elements when obtaining informed consent, is enforced by the IRB within a research facility (OHRP, 2024). When obtaining consent for genomic research, careful consideration must be taken to explain how the participants' genomic information will be used during and after the study has ended, as well as possible implications from the donation of the material.

As of 2018, participants will need to be informed if their biospecimens will undergo whole-genome sequencing during the informed consent process (NHGRI, 2024b).

For the benefit of human research participants, an informed consent document outlining important issues and risks in straightforward language should be developed and implemented. The informed consent document should specify the following:

- That patients have the right to refuse biospecimen donation, and that this will in no way influence their treatment or eligibility to participate in research studies or clinical trials.
- Why particular biospecimens and data are being sought and why human research participants are being asked to participate.
- The source of the biospecimens that will be collected for research; for example, whether the biospecimen will come from leftover tissue from a surgical procedure or from an additional procedure (e.g., an extra blood draw).
- Who will be the custodian of the biospecimens and what will be the custodian's role.
- How the obtained biospecimens will be used and whether they may be used in secondary research.
- How data collected or generated in the research will be shared.
- Whether biospecimens will continue to be stored in an identifiable or non-identifiable manner and shared as long as they are potentially useful for research, respectfully destroyed when no longer useful for research, or transferred to another established resource in accordance with the terms of the informed consent.
- Who may access biospecimens and associated data, including whether for-profit researchers may seek access and, if so, any policies regarding disposition of potential commercial profits.
- Whether there is a policy or plan for producing a lay summary of the aggregate study findings.
- Whether there is a policy or plan for offering the return of any individual research results, and whether these results will be placed in the medical record.
- The nature of any special risks associated with proposed genomic research technologies such as whole genome or exome sequencing.

FIGURE 28-1 | Informed Consent Inclusions for Biospecimens

Note. From *NCI Best Practices for Biospecimen Resources* (p. 37), by National Cancer Institute Office of Biorepositories and Biospecimen Research, 2016 (https://biospecimens.cancer.gov/bestpractices/2011-NCIBestPractices.pdf). In the public domain.

Sample language to address special considerations when discussing genomic-relevant information can be accessed at www.genome.gov/about-genomics/policy-issues/Informed-Consent/Special-Considerations-for-Genome-Research. The National Cancer Institute (NCI) Biorepositories and Biospecimen Research Branch offers 11 issues that should be specified during the informed consent process (see Figure 28-1).

Obtaining informed consent for the storage, collection, and future research of biospecimens can be challenging because the specifics of potential future research are not known when the sample is collected. Under certain situations, research using previously collected biospecimens may not be considered human participant research that requires obtaining informed consent (NCI, 2016). Additionally, under 45 C.F.R. 46(a), informed consent might not be required, even if the research is deemed human participant (subject) research if it qualifies as exempt human subject research under the regulations of 45 C.F.R. 46.101(b) or the research is deemed nonexempt human subject research that was granted a waiver of the requirements for the informed consent by the IRB under 45 C.F.R. 46.116(c) or (d) (General Requirements for Informed Consent, 2017; NCI, 2016; OHRP, 2024). Informed consent is not required under the Common Rule if the samples collected do not identify the participant or donor (e.g., samples stored in biobanks) or when using samples from deceased participants (NHGRI, 2024b). For studies that started after January 25, 2015, the informed consent for prospective data collection has to state what data types will be shared and for what purpose (e.g., genome sequence data) (National Human Genome Research Institute, 2025).

The informed consent should also highlight the participants' right to discontinue participation in the research study and outline what will happen if they decide to withdraw. When a participant discontinues enrollment, policies and procedures should be in place at the research institute that outline how the request will occur and the necessary follow-up to verify that the request was respected in accordance with governmental bodies (NCI, 2016).

Human Specimen Collection

Specimens used in research can be from any donation the participant provided, such as blood, urine, cells, tissue, organs, hair, or nail clippings. Each of these is considered personal healthcare information if it is not de-identified (National Institute of Allergy and Infectious Diseases, 2025; OHRP, 2024). When handling this material, NCI (2016) guidelines outline the technical and operational best practices for biospecimen resource management and operations; biospecimen collection, processing, storage, retrieval, and dissemination; quality management; biosafety; collecting and managing clinical data; and biospecimen resource informatics, including data management and inventory control and tracking.

When reviewing this information, OCRNs must be aware of and able to implement these best practices so as not to compromise the biospecimen collected. It should be the aim of every research institute to collect, maintain, and disseminate the highest quality biospecimen. This means the biospecimens collected should closely resemble the biology of the biospecimen prior to its removal from the human participant. If the biospecimen is exposed to the surrounding environment, its characteristics can begin to change, compromising the data collected (NCI, 2016). OCRNs can help maintain the integrity of the specimens collected by intervening with the correct collection and storage information for the specific tissue taken from the participant. Resources on how to maintain the highest quality biospecimens can be found in Table 28-1.

Collection of Biospecimens

Multiple factors can affect biospecimen quality and, subsequently, research results. Maintaining the quality of the specimen can be divided into two categories: preanalytic factors and analytic factors. Preanalytic factors refer to the collection, processing, and storage variations that can affect biospecimen integrity prior to its removal from the participant. This continues until the specimen is ready for testing. Analytic factors reference variations that affect the performance of a testing procedure (NCI, 2016). OCRNs should evaluate both preanalytic and analytic factors to determine variations while also following protocol requirements. Standardized practice at a research institution should be established for the processing and handling of biospecimens to foster data integrity (FDA, 2018; NCI, 2016).

Uniformity in collection is also imperative to maintaining the integrity of the biospecimen. Varying methods used to remove and collect the biospecimen may influence the quality of the tissue collected and subsequent results. For example, data have shown that biospecimens surgically removed may have different levels and molecular profiles depending on how long the cessation of blood flow to an organ occurred prior to its removal. Any biospecimen collected should be appropriately preserved as quickly as possible after its removal from the participant to ensure the most accurate results (FDA, 2018; NCI, 2016). A plan should be in place to handle the specimen and have the supplies needed to store the tissue adequately. Biospecimens, such as frozen tissue, wet tissue, paraffin-embedded tissue, blood, glass slides, serum, and urine, each have different best practice standards to obtain the highest-quality biospecimen results. Standards of practice should always be followed for the specific research institution (NCI, 2016). Further information on how to maintain the integrity of these specimens can be accessed at https://biospecimens.cancer.gov/bestpractices/2016-NCIBestPractices.pdf.

OCRNs should confirm the research team is maintaining adherence in appropriately retrieving and storing the biospecimen material. They can also assist in documenting the timing, method, location, and condition under which samples are collected for future review when testing the tissue (FDA, 2018; NCI, 2016).

Biospecimens should always be stored in a stabilized state. Unnecessary thawing and refreezing should be avoided. Additionally, in selecting biospecimen storage temperature, consideration of the biospecimen type can

TABLE 28-1 | Resources for Best Practices of Tissue Repositories

Resource	Website
American College of Medical Genetics and Genomics	www.acmg.net
European Medicines Agency *Guideline on Good Pharmacogenomic Practice*	www.ema.europa.eu/en/documents/scientific-guideline/guideline-good-pharmacogenomic-practice-first-version_en.pdf
International Society for Biological and Environmental Repositories: *ISBER Best Practices, Fifth Edition: A New Process for Relevance in an Evolving Landscape*	www.isber.org/page/BPR
National Cancer Institute (2016) *NCI Best Practices for Biospecimen Resources*	https://biospecimens.cancer.gov/bestpractices/2016-NCIBestPractices.pdf
Updating International Society for Biological and Environmental Repositories Best Practices, Fifth Edition: A New Process for Relevance in an Evolving Landscape (Snapes et al., 2023)	https://doi.org/10.1089/bio.2023.0140
U.S. Food and Drug Administration (2018) *E18 Genomic Sampling and Management of Genomic Data Guidance for Industry*	www.fda.gov/files/drugs/published/E18-Genomic-Sampling-and-Management-of-Genomic-Data-Guidance-for-Industry.pdf

affect the length of storage, the biomolecules of interest, and whether the research goal includes preserving cells. For example, paraffin blocks should be stored at temperatures below 80°F (27°C) in an area with humidity and pest control. If the samples are exposed to high temperatures, it can compromise the integrity of the results and provide inaccurate diagnostic information (NCI, 2016).

Each biospecimen collected should have a unique identifier firmly affixed to the holding container. The writing should be clear, legible, and able to endure storage conditions. Containers and facilities that store these biospecimens should have automated security alarm systems in place to monitor the function of the storage equipment and appropriately alert them to any malfunction. If the specimens need to be shipped, the research team needs to consider the shipping time, distance, climate, season, method of transport, and regulations prior to the shipment (NCI, 2016). A sample material transfer agreement can be accessed at https://dctd.cancer.gov/drug-discovery-development/services/next/resources/next-screening-material-transfer-agreement.pdf within Appendix 4.

Data Sharing

When human research is being conducted, it is imperative that responsible data sharing is a priority to maximize the contributions of the participants and promote trust in the research process. If data shared are derived from human research participants, the information should be adequately de-identified prior to releasing it to ensure the protection of the participant, maintain privacy, and mitigate risk. In instances where it is challenging to de-identify data and the participant is at risk of being identified, a controlled-access mechanism needs to be in place to maintain participant protection. Research investigators are not required to share scientific data if the privacy or safety of the participant would be compromised and if protective measures, such as de-identification, are insufficient. The National Institute's of Health (n.d.) policy on data sharing includes the following:

- Develop and provide a plan for sharing genomic data as a part of the Data Management and Sharing Plan.
- Provide an Institutional Certification form at Just-in-Time, if working with human data.
- Submit genomic data in a timely manner to an appropriate repository.
- Responsibly use controlled-access data.
- Appropriately cite controlled-access data in publications and presentations.

Along with the increase in genetic testing, healthcare providers are also faced with the challenge of disclosing secondary findings that do not address patients' immediate clinical questions. Initially, the American College of Medical Genetics and Genomics recommended disclosing any secondary findings that could have health implications for participants or their loved ones. The organization later adjusted this stance to provide the participant with an option to decline to receive the secondary results, even if they have implications for their future (Clayton et al., 2019).

Genetic Information Nondiscrimination Act of 2008

With advances in technology, more genome-based testing has occurred nationwide because of its increasing accuracy and affordable cost. This has led many to undergo genome-based sequencing, but it also can compromise the individual's privacy and create future implications with the data collected (Clayton et al., 2019). An individual's genomic data create information that can uniquely identify them and remain static throughout their life (Bonomi et al., 2020). With the growing world of genome testing, it is challenging to create broad, applicable legal principles that protect individuals (Clayton et al., 2019).

The Privacy Rule created under HIPAA protects health information, but not if it is re-identified. The Genetic Information Nondiscrimination Act of 2008 created protections against discrimination by employers and health insurers based on health information discovered during genetic testing by making genetic information "health information" protected under the Privacy Rule (Bonomi et al., 2020; Clayton et al., 2019). It prohibits health insurers from requesting or requiring genetic information or using this information for decisions regarding coverage (OHRP, 2024). The Genetic Information Nondiscrimination Act defines *genetic material* as an individual's genetic test results, genetic results of a family member, genetic tests of any fetus, family history of a disease or disorder, and any request for genetic services as participation in a clinical trial. Many states have regulations regarding discrimination based on genetic testing. OCRNs should review state guidelines when advising patients on this matter.

Implications for Oncology Clinical Research Nurses

OCRNs play a vital role in the collection and storage of genetic materials. This process begins with the informed consent process and ensures that the initial consent process is in accordance with regulatory bodies (Lubejko et al., 2011). OCRNs are also essential in educating trial research participants on the consent and donation of biospecimen material and identifying barriers that could impede understanding during the trial process. (Godskesen et al., 2023).

OCRNs also have the unique opportunity to verify adherence with the appropriate collection and storage of the genetic material so as not to compromise the tissue. Additionally, OCRNs can help with correct documentation when collecting the biospecimen and with any storage or shipping of the genetic material (Lubejko et al., 2011; Xing et al., 2024). OCRNs are responsible for training new members of the clinical team on adherence to the appropriate collection and storage of genetic material (Xing et al., 2024).

In the rapidly expanding world of genetic material collection, OCRNs can help guide patients through the process of consenting, collecting material, and understanding results. They are also an advocate for patients, especially if they need further information regarding their rights to their genetic results. OCRNs can change the landscape of the future of genomic testing.

Summary

The storage of genetic material is constantly changing and expanding in private, academic, and industry settings. Many private and governmental bodies are in place to protect participants. OCRNs must be aware of these regulatory bodies and participant rights so they can educate and disseminate information appropriately. As personalized medicine continues to focus on genetic findings for the diagnosis and management of diseases, OCRNs also need to stay updated on the best practices in biobanking and the use of biospecimens in research.

Key Points

- The Human Genome Project revolutionized cancer diagnosis and treatment, making treatments more personalized.
- Because genome testing has undergone rapid changes, regulatory bodies such as HHS and OHRP are actively working to protect the rights of participants.
- OCRNs can facilitate the process of obtaining informed consent, which requires participants to understand what they are consenting to, the implications of proceeding with the study, and the potential donation of their genetic material.
- The integrity of research relies on the appropriate collection, handling, and storage of genetic samples.

The author would like to acknowledge Kathy Wilkinson, BSN, RN, OCN®, and Julia A. Eggert, PhD, GNP-BC, AGN-BC, AOCN®, for their contribution to this chapter that remains unchanged from the previous edition of this book.

References

Bonomi, L., Huang, Y., & Ohno-Machado, L. (2020). Privacy challenges and research opportunities for genomic data sharing. *Nature Genetics, 52*(7), 646–654. https://doi.org/10.1038/s41588-020-0651-0

Clayton, E.W., Evans, B.J., Hazel, J.W., & Rothstein, M.A. (2019). The law of genetic privacy: Applications, implications, and limitations. *Journal of Law and the Biosciences, 6*(1), 1–36. https://doi.org/10.1093/jlb/lsz007

General Requirements for Informed Consent, 45 C.F.R. § 46.116 (2017). https://www.ecfr.gov/current/title-45/subtitle-A/subchapter-A/part-46/subpart-A/section-46.116

Godskesen, T., Björk, J., & Juth, N. (2023). Challenges regarding informed consent in recruitment to clinical research: A qualitative study of clinical research nurses' experiences. *Trials, 24*(1), Article 801. https://doi.org/10.1186/s13063-023-07844-6

Lubejko, B., Good, M., Weiss, P., Schmieder, L., Leos, D., & Daugherty, P. (2011). Oncology clinical trials nursing: Developing competencies for the novice. *Clinical Journal of Oncology Nursing, 15*(6), 637–643. https://doi.org/10.1188/11.CJON.637-643

National Cancer Institute. (2016). *NCI best practices for biospecimen resources.* https://biospecimens.cancer.gov/bestpractices/2016-NCIBestPractices.pdf

National Human Genome Research Institute. (2018). *Cancer genomics.* https://www.genome.gov/dna-day/15-ways/cancer-genomics

National Human Genome Research Institute. (2024a). *Genome statute and legislation database.* https://www.genome.gov/about-genomics/policy-issues/Genome-Statute-Legislation-Database

National Human Genome Research Institute. (2024b). *Why is informed consent required?* https://www.genome.gov/about-genomics/educational-resources/fact-sheets/why-is-informed-consent-required#:~:text=Informed%20consent%20is%20crucial%20in,by%20several%20regulations%20and%20policies

National Human Genome Research Institute. (2025). *Data sharing policies and expectations.* https://www.genome.gov/about-nhgri/Policies-Guidance/Data-Sharing-Policies-and-Expectations

National Institute of Allergy and Infectious Diseases. (2025). *Research using human subjects.* https://www.niaid.nih.gov/grants-contracts/human-subjects

National Institutes of Health. (n.d.). *Genomic data sharing policy overview.* https://sharing.nih.gov/genomic-data-sharing-policy/about-genomic-data-sharing/gds-policy-overview

Office for Human Research Protections. (2024). *Regulations.* https://www.hhs.gov/ohrp/regulations-and-policy/regulations/index.html

Protection of Human Subjects, 45 C.F.R. § 46 (2019). https://www.ecfr.gov/current/title-45/subtitle-A/subchapter-A/part-46

Reymond, M., Steinert, R., Escourrou, J., & Fourtanier, G. (2002). Ethical, legal, and economic issues raised by the use of human tissue in postgenomic research. *Digestive Diseases, 20*(3–4), 257–265. https://doi.org/10.1159/000067677

Snapes, E., Astrin, J.J., Krüger, N.B., Grossman, G.H., Hendrickson, E., Miller, N., & Seiler, C. (2023). Updating International Society for Biological and Environmental Repositories Best Practices, Fifth Edition: A new process for relevance in an evolving landscape. *Biopreservation and Biobanking, 21*(6), 537–546. https://doi.org/10.1089/bio.2023.0140

U.S. Centers for Disease Control and Prevention. (2024). *Health Insurance Portability and Accountability Act of 1996.* https://www.cdc.gov/phlp/php/resources/health-insurance-portability-and-accountability-act-of-1996-hipaa.html

U.S. Food and Drug Administration. (2018). *E18 genomic sampling and management of genomic data: Guidance for industry.* https://www.fda.gov/files/drugs/published/E18-Genomic-Sampling-and-Management-of-Genomic-Data-Guidance-for-Industry.pdf

U.S. Food and Drug Administration. (2025). *Institutional review boards frequently asked questions: Guidance for institutional review boards and clinical investigators.* https://www.fda.gov/regulatory-information/search-fda-guidance-documents/institutional-review-boards-frequently-asked-questions#Informed%20Consent%20Process

Xing, Y., Wang, X., Zhang, C., Yuan, W., Chen, X., & Luan, W. (2024). Characteristics and duties of clinical research nurses: A scoping review. *Frontiers in Medicine, 11,* 1333230. https://doi.org/10.3389/fmed.2024.1333230

CHAPTER 29

Pharmacokinetic and Pharmacodynamic Testing

Laura S. Wood, MSN, RN, OCN®

Introduction

Correlative testing, including pharmacokinetics (PK), pharmacodynamics (PD), and biomarkers, is incorporated into all phases of clinical research. PK/PD testing is critical to clinical trials, as results inform decisions regarding drug dose and administration schedules to ensure therapeutically effective concentrations at the site of action, particularly when administering drugs with a narrow therapeutic index (Khan et al., 2023).

Pharmacokinetics is the study of the absorption, distribution, metabolism, and excretion of a drug, evaluating how the drug concentration changes over time; it is described as "what the body does to the drug" (Southwood et al., 2018) (see Table 29-1). *Pharmacodynamics* is the relationship between the drug concentration at the site of action and the resulting effect, including both therapeutic and adverse effects; it is described as "what the drug does to the body" (Southwood et al., 2018). Direct measurement of drug concentration at the site of action is not feasible, so the concept of kinetic homogeneity is used to describe the relationship between plasma drug concentration and concentration at the site of drug action (Southwood et al., 2018) (see Figure 29-1).

TABLE 29-1 | Absorption, Distribution, Metabolism, and Excretion of Drugs

Process	Definition
Absorption	Refers to the method by which a drug is administered, such as IV injection or infusion, ingestion, inhalation, or dermal application
Distribution	Where the drug goes in the body and how long it takes to reach the target organ or tissue
Metabolism	How the drug is broken down by the body (e.g., liver, kidney, skin, digestive tract) so it can be excreted
Excretion	The process by which the metabolized drug is eliminated from the body

Note. Based on information from Gleichmann et al., 2024.

Monitoring drug levels using PK testing is employed in various clinical settings, including the use of busulfan in transplantation settings. Busulfan PK data are used to determine subsequent dosing and can impact clinical outcomes (Seydoux et al., 2022).

The clinical research team is responsible for obtaining blood samples in accordance with protocols and laboratory manual specifications, enabling the use of PK/PD data to analyze drug dose and correlate results with efficacy, safety, and toxicity data. PK testing can also help providers understand the potential for drug–drug interactions and identify the need to adjust the dose or select an alternative drug in specific situations, such as when using anticoagulants with cancer therapies (Van der Linden et al., 2023).

This chapter will provide the necessary information to collect, process, and document the important data required to meet the research objectives involved in cancer therapeutic drug development.

Pharmacokinetic Models

PK models employ quantitative analysis to determine the time courses of drug concentration following the administration of various drug formulations, thereby quantifying the dose–concentration relationship over a specific period (Zou et al., 2020). Models used in pharmacologic clinical trials include compartmental, noncompartmental, popula-

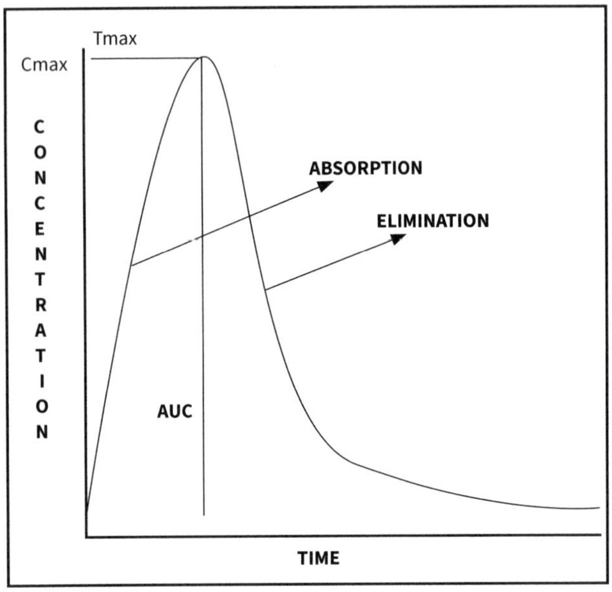

FIGURE 29-1 | Pharmacokinetic Parameters

AUC—area under the curve; Cmax—maximum drug concentration; Tmax—maximum time

tion, and physiologically based PK models. The compartmental model divides the body into a single compartment where the drug is rapidly distributed throughout or into multiple compartments with different rates of absorption, metabolism, and excretion. The advancement of technology and the diversity of drug delivery systems and molecules have led to more complex drug absorption and disposition processes, resulting in changes in the types of modeling used in drug development (Zou et al., 2020). The sponsor and the testing laboratory determine the specific collection and processing requirements for each clinical trial. Details are included in the protocol and the trial lab manual.

Pharmacokinetic and Pharmacodynamic Parameters

During dose escalation studies (most often in phase 1), PK/PD parameters are measured at different dose levels, in addition to assessing toxicities and concomitant medications. The parameters include the elimination half-life of the drug, maximum drug concentration, bioavailability, clearance, area under the curve, and volume of distribution (see Table 29-2). Phase 2 and 3 studies may include PK/PD testing based on data from earlier studies and the need to expand the data to evaluate interpatient PK variability further.

PK/PD testing is used to demonstrate the safety and toxicity profiles of new drug formulations and improve clinical outcomes, such as with liposomal drug formulations as monotherapy or in combination with chemotherapy. Liposomal doxorubicin was the first oncologic therapeutic agent approved with this unique formulation, demonstrating a longer half-life and slower clearance of free doxorubicin, which resulted in a lower peak concentration of free drug and a lower incidence of doxorubicin-induced cardiac toxicity (Gabizon et al., 2003).

In 2024, liposomal irinotecan, in combination with oxaliplatin, 5-fluorouracil, and leucovorin, received U.S. Food and Drug Administration approval as first-line treatment for adult patients with metastatic pancreatic adenocarcinoma. It also received approval in combination with 5-fluorouracil and leucovorin after disease progression following gemcitabine-based therapy (Ipsen, 2024). Data from PK testing of this agent demonstrated an increased incidence of grade 3 diarrhea but no increased risk of grade 3 or higher neutropenia for liposomal irinotecan. This guidance provides patient education and adverse event monitoring in patients receiving liposomal irinotecan (Brendel et al., 2021). PK/PD testing also guides the appropriate sequence for multiagent oncolytic regimens to maximize efficacy and minimize toxicity (Morales et al., 2020).

TABLE 29-2 | Definitions of Pharmacokinetic Parameters

Parameter	Definition
Area under the curve	Area under the plasma level-time curve
Bioavailability	The amount of drug absorbed and available to the target tissue or site of drug action
Clearance	The volume of drug cleared from the plasma per unit of time
Elimination half-life (t1/2)	The time needed to reduce the drug concentration or amount of drug in the body by one-half
Maximum drug concentration (Cmax)	Maximum drug concentration after a dose at steady state, reaching its maximum level in plasma
Maximum time (Tmax)	Time to maximum or peak drug concentration
Minimum effective concentration (MEC)	The lowest plasma drug concentration needed to achieve the desired therapeutic effect
Prodrug	An inactive drug dosage form converted to an active metabolite by biochemical reactions in the body
Steady state	The point in time when the rate of drug administration equals the rate of elimination
Volume of distribution	The ratio of the total drug administered to the total amount of plasma concentration

Note. Based on information from Murphy, 2022.

The oncology clinical research nurse, clinical research coordinator, and research laboratory technician are responsible for developing a worksheet or other site-specific trackers for blood sample collection time-points based on the clinical trial protocol and laboratory manual. Any deviations from the protocol or processing are recorded and documented in the clinical trial case report forms. Orders for sample collection are entered into the electronic health record and include specific details regarding the type of venipuncture tube, blood collection (i.e., a speckled-top tube is to be collected last), and transport instructions (i.e., place the venipuncture tube upright or in ice following collection). Clinical trials managed by a clinical research organization may provide correlative testing documentation forms to be used by all sites participating in the study. The research team creates these forms for other clinical trials, including investigator-initiated studies (see Figure 29-2).

Patient Name:	**Today's Date:**
Study ID:	**Drug Name:**
Date of Birth:	**Dose (mg or mg/m^2)**
Weight (kg):	**Actual Dose (mg)**
Height (cm):	**Dose Start Time (IV) or Dose Time (Oral):**
BSA (m^2):	**End of Infusion Time (IV Drug only):**
Time of most recent food intake:	
Comments (infusion interruption, IV infiltration, etc):	

Sample #	Post-Dose Time	Target Time	Actual Time	Comments
1	Pre-dose			
2	5 min			
3	15 min			
4	30 min			
5	1 hr			
6	2 hr			
7	4 hr			
8	6 hr			
9	8 hr			
10	24 hr	Date: Time:		
11	48 hr	Date: Time:		

FIGURE 29-2 | Monotherapy Sample Pharmacokinetic Worksheet

BSA—body surface area; hr—hour

The Target Time in the third column of the table is calculated from the End of IV infusion time and the Post Dose Time for each sample. For example, if an infusion ends at 9 am, then the Target Time for Sample #2 is 9:05 am.

Note. Figure courtesy of Frank M. Balis. Adapted with permission.

The Research Team

The research team comprises a diverse group of individuals, and each clinical trial site has its unique organizational structure. Work involved in the organization, collection, documentation, processing, and shipment of PK/PD samples can be performed by oncology research nurses, clinical research assistants, or other individuals who have received training to meet Good Clinical Practice requirements (U.S. Food and Drug Administration, 2021). The roles and responsibilities of the research team member may begin prior to receiving the formal clinical trial protocol, ensuring that the site and research personnel are qualified and have the necessary facility and equipment resources to meet the requirements defined in the protocol and laboratory procedures manual. Once the protocol and laboratory manual have been received, the research team must conduct a detailed review to clarify any questions prior to agreeing to serve as an investigational site. Site initiation visits occur prior to a clinical trial site opening a study, and a significant amount of time will be spent reviewing the specimen collection and documentation to ensure that the research team has been educated on the expectations regarding accurate procedures and documentation processes.

Protocol and Laboratory Manual Review

The protocol and laboratory manual review includes a comparison of the schedule of events to ensure that the collection timepoint requirements are consistent in both documents, including a review of the window of time allowed for PK/PD sampling (i.e., 3 minutes before or after or less than 10 minutes prior to the dose). Dietary and medication restrictions should be noted, as they impact patient education, documentation, and compliance with blood sampling requirements. Communication with the principal investigator, clinical research associate, clinical research organization, and study sponsor should occur if discrepancies are found, as resolving these is critical prior to the start of study enrollment. In some cases, email communication or administrative letters from the sponsor may be sufficient for clarification; however, significant discrepancies will require amendments to the protocol or laboratory manual to be written and approved prior to participant enrollment. Changes in collection timepoints or other processes during the clinical trial will require amendments, which must be approved by an institutional review board prior to implementation.

Equipment necessary for the collection and storage of PK/PD samples must be reviewed by the research team. It may need to be incorporated into the clinical trial budget if additional supplies or equipment are required. Some studies use a central laboratory for clinical and correlative testing when multiple clinical sites are involved, ensuring consistent analysis of samples. Kits, requisitions, labels, and supplies provided by the central laboratory must be compared to the protocol and laboratory manual to ensure consistency with timepoints and sample requirements. Some studies require the immediate shipment of samples, whereas others require samples to be shipped in batches, necessitating additional storage space at the site. Backup specimens may be stored at the investigational site until the sponsor requests shipment. Storage equipment logs must be completed to document temperature settings on refrigeration and freezer equipment used to store study samples. These logs will be reviewed during study monitoring visits.

Specimen Collection Procedures

Assessment of IV access should be included when screening patients for clinical trials that require PK/PD or other timed blood samples. Placement of a central access device prior to initiation of treatment is also appropriate for patients with poor venous access. Several principles must be followed when collecting PK/PD timed samples, including collecting from a site other than the vein used for IV drug infusion and collecting approximately 5 ml of blood from an existing IV line as a waste sample to avoid dilution of the blood sample caused by admixture with the IV solution.

If a patient has central line access (catheter or IV access device), it is helpful to administer the study drug via peripheral access and use the central line access for collecting PK/PD samples. If two peripheral IV lines are necessary, it is recommended to infuse the drug via IV access in the patient's dominant arm to minimize the risk of dislodging the catheter during the extended time frame required for blood sampling. The IV in the patient's dominant arm can be discontinued after the drug infusion, providing comfort by allowing the patient to use their dominant arm freely when PK sampling is performed via IV access in their nondominant arm. Single-timepoint PK/PD collections can be drawn from a peripheral venipuncture and do not require an additional waste tube, as no IV fluids have been infused, eliminating the concern for dilutional effects.

On the day of PK/PD testing, the research team should review the patient's use of concomitant medications, over-the-counter products, and complementary and alternative supplements to ensure that the medication record is accurate and that no prohibited products are being ingested, as these may impact the testing results. The protocol or laboratory manual provides instructions on necessary actions if prohibited medications or supplements have been taken or are not held in accordance with the sample collection guidelines. Patients must be informed prior to consenting to participate in a clinical trial about any prohibited medications, over-the-counter products, and complementary and alternative supplements. They should also be instructed to notify the research team if any prescription medications are prescribed or over-the-counter medications are initiated at any time during their participation in the clinical trial. Concomitant medication and supplement use should be reviewed at each visit, including those that should be held prior to the PK/PD testing visit.

Documentation and Specimen Labeling

Documentation must be accurate and legible, as the information noted on the source document will be transcribed onto laboratory specimen processing forms, shipping forms, and electronic case report forms—often by another member of the research team. This includes demographic information, vital signs, and any medication or dietary requirements that must be noted for protocol compliance, as well as any comments regarding delayed or missed sampling timepoints. IV access or drug infusion issues must also be documented, as they affect the PK/PD sampling results.

Proper labeling of blood samples collected is critical to ensuring that information is legible and will not smear if the label becomes wet. A thin, black permanent marker should be used; white-out should never be used for corrections. Errors should be crossed out, dated, and initialed, and the correct information should then be written on the label. Specimen labeling must be accurate and consistent with the study laboratory manual. Samples should be drawn in the order specified in the manual, and the collection time should be documented on each specimen label. Completing initial information (subject ID, visit timepoint, and collection timepoint) should always be performed prior to the initiation of study drug administration to minimize the potential for documentation errors.

Specimen Handling and Processing

Following PK/PD sample collection, careful attention must be given to ensure that processing is completed according to the study laboratory manual. The research team should always communicate upcoming PK/PD sampling schedules with the processing staff to ensure that necessary personnel and equipment are available. Staffing needs may be adjusted if early or late-day specimen collection is required. Labels for cryovial storage should be made available to the processing laboratory in advance. It is helpful to share a copy of the sample collection schedule and treatment appointment schedule with the research laboratory team.

Potential Problems and Errors

Accuracy regarding timing, documentation, processing, and shipping of PK/PD samples is critical, ensuring that cumulative data from all study participants accurately represent the results. Inaccurate collection results in drug monitoring can impact clinical outcomes, especially when monitoring drugs such as busulfan in the hematologic transplant setting. Unanticipated events, misinterpretation of the protocol or laboratory manual, errors in collection or documentation, or incorrect specimen processing and storing procedures can affect results. Although not an inclusive list, Table 29-3 identifies many of the more common errors that may occur. Protocol deviations must be submitted if errors occur during PK/PD testing. These may lead to corrective actions for the site or amendments to the protocol or laboratory testing processes. Instructions regarding the completion and submission of deviation reports are discussed during site initiation visits and throughout the study period.

Communication

Effective communication with all members of the research team is crucial to ensure that the study conduct meets the requirements of the clinical trial sponsor, the International Council for Harmonisation of Technical Requirements for Pharmaceuticals for Human Use's Good Clinical Practice guideline (2025), and the U.S. Food and Drug Administration (2021). Open communication with the clinical research organization for the study will facilitate clarification of discrepancies, concerns, or issues regarding compliance with the protocol and laboratory manual.

- The patient does not adhere to the dosing regimen of oral anticancer therapy, including missing doses, taking doses outside the recommended dosing window, and failing to take doses as required, either with or without food.
- The nurse does not administer the oral or IV dose at the time prescribed.
- Drug administration documentation is not consistent with the actual dosing time.
- The incorrect dose is administered.
- The complete dose is not administered prior to sample collection due to patient problems (e.g., infiltration of the IV line).
- The blood sample is not collected at the correct time.
- Inaccurate documentation of the sample collection time occurs.
- Inaccurate documentation of the end of infusion time occurs.
- Inaccurate documentation of oral dosing time occurs.
- An inadequate or insufficient blood sample is collected.
- The blood sample is hemolyzed due to difficulties with venous access or vein patency.
- A waste tube is not drawn, so the IV fluid dilutes the blood sample.
- The blood sample is collected from the same IV line that was used to infuse the drug.
- Blood sample is not stored correctly immediately following collection (e.g., placed on ice, not on ice, kept upright).
- The processing equipment is not correctly calibrated, or there is an error with another piece of equipment.
- A venipuncture tube is broken in the centrifuge.
- The sample is not placed in cryo vials correctly (i.e., the sample is not split and placed in submission backup cryo vials).

FIGURE 29-3 | Potential Errors That Can Occur During Pharmacokinetic and Pharmacodynamic Testing

Summary

PK/PD testing is a significant component of early clinical trials but may also be included in phase 2 or 3 trials when additional information is needed. This testing provides information on the absorption, distribution, metabolism, and excretion of drugs and may provide insight into drug–drug interactions and the use of drugs in specific populations. Testing results may also provide sponsors with information regarding the appropriate sequencing of multidrug administration, as the order of IV anticancer drugs may impact efficacy or toxicity. Preparation, starting with a detailed review of the protocol and laboratory manual, along with ongoing communication with the site's research team, study clinical research assistant, clinical research organization, and sponsor, will help ensure that testing results facilitate meeting clinical trial objectives and study end points.

Key Points

- Having a clear understanding of the PK/PD testing requirements in the protocol and laboratory manual prior to opening a study to enrollment will minimize the risk of errors in sample collection, processing, and shipment.
- Assessing potential IV access at the time of study screening is important to ensure adequate access for the completion of protocol-required blood collection. This allows time for intravascular access device placement when extensive blood collection is required or when peripheral IV access is limited.
- Effective communication among the research team and with the clinical research organization is essential for accurate sample collection, processing, and shipment.

The author would like to acknowledge Ashish Thakkar, MS, for his contribution to this chapter that remains unchanged from the previous edition of this book.

References

Brendel, K., Bekaii-Saab, T., Boland, P.M., Dayyani, F., Dean, A., Macarulla, T., ... Zhang, B. (2021). Population pharmacokinetics of liposomal irinotecan in patients with cancer and exposure—Safety analyses in patients with metastatic pancreatic cancer. *CPT: Pharmacometrics and Systems Pharmacology, 10*(12), 1550–1563. https://doi.org/10.1002/psp4.12725

Gabizon, A., Shmeeda, H., & Barenholz, Y. (2003). Pharmacokinetics of pegylated liposomal doxorubicin: Review of animal and human studies. *Clinical Pharmacokinetics, 42*(5), 419–436. https://doi.org/10.2165/00003088-200342050-00002

Gleichmann, N. (2024, May 8). *What is ADME?* Technology Networks. https://www.technologynetworks.com/drug-discovery/articles/what-is-adme-336683

International Council for Harmonisation of Technical Requirements for Pharmaceuticals for Human Use. (2025). *ICH harmonised guideline: Guideline for good clinical practice: E6(R3).* https://database.ich.org/sites/default/files/ICH_E6%28R3%29_Step4_FinalGuideline_2025_0106.pdf

Ipsen. (2024). *Onivyde® (liposomal irinotecan)* [Package insert].

Khan, A., Ahmad, L., Raza, F., Khan, S.A., & Ali, T. (2023). Editorial: The practical implication of clinical pharmacokinetics in drug development, pharmaceutical analysis, and clinical research. *Frontiers in Pharmacology, 14,* 1252030. https://doi.org/10.3389/fphar.2023.1252030

Morales, A.S.R., Joy, J.K., & Zbona, D.M. (2020). Administration sequence for multi-agent oncolytic regimens. *Journal of Oncology Pharmacy Practice, 26*(4), 933–942. https://doi.org/10.1177/1078155219895070

Murphy, J.E. (2022). *Clinical pharmacokinetics* (7th ed.). American Society of Health-System Pharmacists. https://doi.org/10.37573/9781585286607

Seydoux, C., Battegay, R., Halter, J., Heim, D., Rentsch, K.M., Passweg, J.R., & Medinger, M. (2022). Impact of busulfan pharmacokinetics on outcome in adult patients receiving an allogeneic hematopoietic cell transplantation. *Bone Marrow Transplantation, 57*(6), 903–910. https://doi.org/10.1038/s41409-022-01641-6

Southwood, R.L., Fleming, V.H., & Huckaby, G. (Eds.). (2018). Lesson 1: Introduction to pharmacokinetics and pharmacodynamics (pp.1–20). *Concepts in Clinical Pharmacokinetics* (7th ed.). American Society of Health-System Pharmacists.

U.S. Food and Drug Administration. (2021). *Regulations: Good Clinical Practice and clinical trials.* https://www.fda.gov/science-research/clinical-trials-and-human-subject-protection/regulations-good-clinical-practice-and-clinical-trials

Van der Linden, L., Vanassche, T., Van Cutsem, E., Van Aelst, L., & Verhamme, P. (2023). Pharmacokinetic drug–drug interactions with direct anticoagulants in the management of cancer-associated thrombosis. *British Journal of Clinical Pharmacology, 89*(8), 2369–2376. https://doi.org/10.1111/bcp.15785

Zou, H., Banerjee, P., Leung, S.S.Y., & Yan, X. (2020). Application of pharmacokinetic-pharmacodynamic modeling in drug delivery: Development and challenges. *Frontiers in Pharmacology, 11,* 997. https://doi.org/10.3389/fphar.2020.00997

SECTION VI. Documentation and Data Management

CHAPTER 30

Documentation

Tasha Hall, PhD, RN

Introduction

Data generated from a clinical trial are analyzed to determine the results of the trial. U.S. Food and Drug Administration (FDA) regulations state that it is the responsibility of the investigator to "prepare and maintain adequate and accurate case histories that record all observations and other data pertinent to the investigation on each individual administered the investigational drug or employed as a control in the investigation" (Case Histories, 2014, § 312.62(b)). Documentation is key in clinical research because it verifies both the accuracy and the authenticity of the data collected. Essential documents are those that individually and collectively permit evaluation of the conduct of a trial and the quality of the data produced. These documents demonstrate the compliance of the investigator with Good Clinical Practice guidelines (International Conference on Harmonisation of Technical Requirements for Pharmaceuticals for Human Use [ICH], 2025). Information from a participant's (patient's) clinical record is extracted to specific case report forms (CRFs) for the clinical trial. This extraction process may be performed by oncology clinical research nurses (OCRNs), clinical research coordinators, or clinical data managers. Chapter 31 provides more information about managing data, but documentation is the first step. The basic rules of documentation apply to all work performed by members of the research team.

This chapter will provide an overview of the basic rules for documentation in clinical trials and define source records.

The Basic Rules of Documentation in the Health Record

The basic principle underlying clinical care documentation is that "if it was not documented, it was not done." This includes procedures performed and discussions between the healthcare team and patients and families (National Cancer Institute [NCI], 2021). Examples of discussions that need to be documented include the informed consent process and patient education. In clinical research, it is critical to document everything that does and does not occur. Each interaction that OCRNs have with the study participants should be documented in the patient records.

OCRNs must legibly and legally document patient records. When using physical medical records with paper and pen, erasing or covering mistakes is prohibited. To correct an error, one single horizontal line should be drawn through it. Then, the writer must initial and date the crossed-out information. The writer may need to document why there is a change. Most often, writing "error" is sufficient. All documentation in patient records should be completed in ink, not pencil. Correction fluid and correction tape should not be used. No abbreviations may be used on the forms for a clinical trial unless the specific protocol indicates that they are appropriate (Bargaje, 2011).

Although these practices do not apply to electronic health records, some universal guidelines should be followed when entering interactions in both media. The date and time should be recorded with each entry. Items that are observed and assessed during the interaction should be documented in the health record. OCRNs should use a patient's own words in the documentation note when describing patient-reported symptoms.

Electronic records and electronic signatures used in FDA-regulated research are covered in the Code of Federal Regulations (21 C.F.R. § 11) (Electronic Records; Electronic Signatures, 1997). Part 11 applies to records in electronic form that are created, modified, maintained, archived, or transmitted under any requirements set forth in FDA regulations. It addresses electronic CRFs, electronic patient diaries, electronic health records, software validation, and source records.

Parameters exist for both open and closed systems to ensure that the authenticity, integrity, and confidentiality of the electronic records are included in the regulation. A closed system is an environment in which content owners control access to the content of the electronic records on the system. An open system is not controlled by the individuals responsible for the content of the electronic records. Certification of all electronic signatures is required (FDA, 2003). For corrections in an electronic health record, the system will retain who made the correction, when it was made, the original record, and the updated record. For more on electronic records, see Chapter 31.

The European equivalent of 21 C.F.R. 11 is Annex 11, which covers computerized electronic records and signatures for FDA-regulated activities. Annex 11 also covers all computerized systems used in good manufacturing practice–regulated activities and notes that the computer infrastructure should be qualified and the software applications validated to comply with this guidance (European Commission, 2011).

Although OCRNs are practicing under nursing licenses in a research setting, they need to continue to follow the state's nurse practice act, which typically includes documentation of participant encounters. The same standards maintained for medical documentation should be followed for research documentation.

ALCOA

The acronym ALCOA (Attributable, Legible, Contemporaneously recorded, Original or a true copy, and Accurate) is synonymous with key attributes for good documentation and quality data applied throughout the drug development process (e.g., manufacturing practices and clinical trials). It is referenced in the FDA guidance *Data Integrity and Compliance with CGMP* [current good manufacturing practice]*: Guidance for Industry*. Over time, other regulatory agencies (e.g., World Health Organization, European Medicines Agency) have adapted ALCOA. The European Medicines Agency has added the attributes *enduring*, *available* and *accessible*, *complete*, *consistent*, *credible*, and *corroborated* (Bargaje, 2011). The terms *ALCOA+* and *ALCOA-C* are used to describe these key attributes for documentation.

When considering if documentation is attributable, a question to ask is, "Is the information recorded traceable to a person, date, and participant visit?" Everything that is handwritten needs to be in ink and legible. Electronic source records solve for illegible handwriting. Data in a research record should be recorded when it occurs. There should be no predating or postdating of notes within the research record (contemporaneously recorded). The source record should be the first place where data are recorded, making it the source. For source data to be accurate, all details need to be correct and a true representation of facts. To be complete, a source record needs to be up-to-date and provide a full picture of every aspect of the study treatment. The ALCOA principles need to be applied to both paper and electronic source data and followed by all members of the research team.

Source Records

Per ICH (2025, p. 77), *source records* are "original documents or data (which includes relevant metadata) or certified copies of the original documents or data, irrespective of the media used."

Data reported on the CRF that are derived from source records should be consistent. Any discrepancies and missing or incomplete data should be explained with a signed note to file, which provides additional information or clarification when other documentation in the research records is not adequate. A note to file can be written by any member of the study team. It should contain the study name and IRB (institutional review board) number, the participant's ID (if applicable), the purpose of the note to file, a description of the issue, and the author's signature. A note to file should not be used in place of source records (Hazra, 2011).

Source records serve to substantiate the integrity of the clinical trial data, confirm observations that are recorded, and verify the existence of study participants (Sather, 2019). A source record is needed to support any information documented on a CRF for a clinical trial. An example is a rating scale or questionnaire completed by the patient. The purpose of source records is to serve as a tool to reconstruct the clinical trial as it happened for an independent observer. It also affirms adherence to the protocol and the integrity of the data. Accurate documentation in the source record supports the protection and safety of participants (Bargaje, 2011). The source record also serves as an audit trail to recreate a patient's progress on a clinical trial. CRFs may be used as a source record only when this practice is clearly outlined in the protocol.

Each participant has a medical record, either electronic or paper, and a research record. Some documents serve as source records that are often not allowed to be placed in a medical record (e.g., blinding information); however, these still need to be maintained. Creating a research record allows the research team to save these types of source records (NCI Center for Cancer Research, n.d). See Figure 30-1 for examples of documents maintained in either the medical or research record.

Many source records for clinical trials are maintained electronically. Electronic recordkeeping ensures transferability of participant data from one clinic location to another and can be used for real-time data transfer to an electronic CRF.

Research-Specific Records

Documentation that is acceptable in clinical practice may need additional details when a patient, now a

Medical Record
Includes all hospital records, medical charts, and clinical or office charts
- Physical examination findings
- Consent process
- Diagnostic reports
- Operative reports
- Laboratory reports
- Data recorded from automated instruments

Research Record
- Copy of signed informed consent document
- Participant diaries
- Quality-of-life or other surveys or tools
- Pharmacokinetic worksheets
- Eligibility checklists

FIGURE 30-1 | Medical Record Versus Research Record

Note. From *Documentation in Clinical Research* [PowerPoint slides], by National Cancer Institute Center for Cancer Research, n.d. (https://ccrod.cancer.gov/confluence/download/attachments/71041052/Documentation6.pdf). In the public domain.

research participant, enters a clinical trial. Some clinical trial–specific events must be documented for these participants. OCRNs do not have to provide all the records, but they should ensure that they all exist (NCI Center for Cancer Research, n.d.).

Informed Consent Process and Eligibility Confirmation

The informed consent process should be documented with a note that the patient received a signed copy of the informed consent. The discussion of the protocol treatments, adverse events (AEs), follow-up required, and any patient or family concerns should be included in the pretreatment notes. A note verifying eligibility needs to be made that consists of the statement that the patient meets all of the inclusion criteria and has no exclusionary criteria. All laboratory results, pathology, and any other procedures required to confirm eligibility should be in the appropriate section of the medical record (paper or electronic) (NCI Center for Cancer Research, n.d.). The patient's past medical history and previous therapies need to be noted in a summary of the initial history and physical. Outside reports and records that confirm the prior therapies and pathology need to be placed in the medical record per organizational policy (NCI Center for Cancer Research, n.d.).

Baseline Symptoms and Concomitant Treatments

Information about baseline symptoms and concomitant treatments (e.g., medications, oxygen use) needs to be documented in the medical record. All baseline symptoms caused by either the patient's disease or prior therapies should be noted, including the start date and severity of each symptom. In addition to a list of the concomitant medications with dose and frequency given, the start date of each medication needs to be documented. Any changes to concomitant medications, including dose adjustments and discontinuation, need to be noted. The date for concomitant medications taken prior to enrollment can be indicated as "month/year." Once the patient has begun study treatment, the date should also include the day in addition to the month and year. The reason the patient is on the medication should also be noted. Some medications are given for indications not approved by FDA, so OCRNs should not assume that the patient is taking them for the condition indicated in the package insert. This is referred to as off-label use. Patients may be taking over-the-counter and complementary medicines that a physician has not prescribed. These need to be included in the concomitant medication list because of the potential impact on the study treatment. Any new concomitant medications that the patient begins to take during the study treatment need to be documented (NCI Center for Cancer Research, n.d.).

Protocol-Specific Activities

All protocol-specific activities (e.g., clinic visits, physical examinations, blood draws) need to be documented in the medical record, including when they occurred, any results, and any follow-up that may be required. Some of the information may be on the final report (e.g., laboratory result, radiology report). If a scheduled visit is missed, it needs to be noted, including the reason and any follow-up that needs to occur (NCI Center for Cancer Research, n.d.).

Any unscheduled visits (i.e., visits not per protocol) need to be documented. The location of the visit, reason for the visit, and any follow-up should be included. Examples may include a patient visit for AE management at the oncology office or a visit to the emergency department. Telephone calls with the patient should be documented, including the reason for the call and outcome (NCI Center for Cancer Research, n.d.). The use of telehealth visits has increased in clinical settings after the COVID-19 pandemic. These visits should be documented with the same level of detail used for in-person visits in the medical record.

If a patient is asked to complete any forms as a part of the clinical trial (e.g., quality-of-life questionnaire, AE diary), OCRNs must ensure that the documentation includes who completed the form and the date and time it was completed. If the form or questionnaire is completed by someone other than the patient, the document should include who completed the form and how the information was obtained.

Adverse Events

For each AE, the following information should be documented (NCI Center for Cancer Research, n.d.):
- When the AE started
- Description of the event, including its severity: This information is used to select the correct AE term and

grade using the NCI *Common Terminology Criteria for Adverse Events* [v.5.0].

- How the AE was treated, if applicable
- Attribution of the AE
- Date the severity of the AE improved or worsened, if applicable
- When the AE was resolved

Study Drug Administration

All study drugs, including any pre- or post-study medications and hydration administered, must be recorded in the medical record by the licensed practitioner who gave the drugs. This documentation should include the date, time, amount, and route of administration. The time should note the start and stop times for IV medications. Any missed doses and the reason the dose was missed should be noted. This documentation is typically performed by the nurse who administers the medication. If an OCRN is not administering the drugs, they should ensure that documentation is completed in a timely manner (NCI Center for Cancer Research, n.d.).

Documentation of self-administered study drugs (i.e., when patients take the drug on their own) should include instructions for proper use, administration, and storage, as well as adherence to regimen and whether the correct amount of drug was returned (NCI Center for Cancer Research, n.d.). For example, if a participant is to take 10 mg of study drug ABC123, then an entry in the medical record needs to state, "The patient states she took 10 mg of ABC123 every day for the past 28 days; denies missing any doses; correct amount of drug returned." Some studies will have patient diaries that are completed and included in the research record. However, a note in the medical record is still needed to communicate this information to other members of the healthcare team.

Off Treatment

When a study medication or other intervention (e.g., radiation therapy) is discontinued, the patient comes off treatment. The reason that the intervention is discontinued and the date should be noted. It is also important to document the last dose of study treatment. This date is often used as a reference for safety follow-up and long-term/survival follow-up. The date is the day that the investigator or treating physician decided that no further treatment was warranted. This might be a result of the patient completing the planned treatment, or it might be because of disease progression, patient choice, or physician decision. Protocols routinely require ongoing follow-up after treatment is discontinued to monitor the duration of current AEs and the onset of new AEs (NCI Center for Cancer Research, n.d.).

Off Study

A patient is considered off study when they have completed all study-related procedures, tests, or follow-up visits. Off-study documentation needs to include the date and reason (e.g., completed six cycles of therapy, completed follow-up, died from disease progression). For protocols that have long-term follow-up, all attempts to locate the patient should be documented before deeming the patient off study (NCI Center for Cancer Research, n.d.). The protocol will often dictate how many attempts and the manner of the attempts (e.g., telephone calls, certified mail) prior to deeming a patient lost to follow-up.

Discrepancy Documentation

If at any time there is conflicting documentation or discrepancies in source records, a clarification note is required. OCRNs are usually responsible for looking for these discrepancies and facilitating a resolution, which may include talking with the authors or writing a note to clarify the correct documentation. For example, conflicting documentation can occur when two healthcare providers provide different dates or descriptions of events. OCRNs can contact the patient and ask for clarification and then document that interaction (NCI Center for Cancer Research, n.d.).

Summary

Clinical trials occur over a long period, with many members of the healthcare team documenting data in the source records. Maintaining continuity of documentation practice over time can be difficult. Documentation for clinical research can be more extensive than what is performed as part of routine clinical practice. Patients are treated in multiple locations, and all of these documents are considered source records (Bargaje, 2011).

The quality of the study data is directly affected by the quality of the study documentation (NCI, 2021). OCRNs are frequently responsible for ensuring that documentation is available and accurate so that CRFs are accurately completed. Although this can be viewed as a mundane task, it is vital to the success of clinical trials. Data recorded on CRFs are used, for example, to evaluate the efficacy of an investigational agent. All source records need to be completed accurately and in a timely manner to ensure the successful completion of the study.

Key Points

- OCRNs should document all participant (patient) encounters per their region's nurse practice act.
- Documentation for clinical research can be more extensive than what is performed as part of routine clinical practice.
- Source records serve as an audit trail to recreate the research participant's progress on a clinical trial.
- The quality of the study data is directly affected by the quality of the study documentation.

References

Bargaje, C. (2011). Good documentation practice in clinical research. *Perspectives in Clinical Research, 2*(2), 59–63. https://doi.org/10.4103/2229-3485.80368

Case Histories, 21 C.F.R. § 312.62(b) (2014). https://www.accessdata.fda.gov/scripts/cdrh/cfdocs/cfcfr/CFRSearch.cfm?fr=312.62

Electronic Records; Electronic Signatures, 21 C.F.R. § 11 (1997). https://www.ecfr.gov/current/title-21/chapter-I/subchapter-A/part-11

European Commission. (2011). *EudraLex: The rules governing medicinal products in the European Union. Volume 4: Good manufacturing practice medicinal products for human and veterinary use, Annex 11 Computerized Systems.* https://health.ec.europa.eu/document/download/8d305550-dd22-4dad-8463-2ddb4a1345f1_en?filename=annex11_01-2011_en.pdf

Hazra, A. (2011). Use, abuse and misuse of notes to file. *Perspectives in Clinical Research, 2*(1), 38–40. https://doi.org/10.4103/2229-3485.76289

International Council for Harmonisation of Technical Requirements for Pharmaceuticals for Human Use. (2025). *ICH harmonised guideline: Guideline for good clinical practice: E6(R3).* https://database.ich.org/sites/default/files/ICH_E6%28R3%29_Step4_FinalGuideline_2025_0106.pdf

National Cancer Institute. (2021). *Monday morning practice pearls #2: What is good documentation practice (GDP)?* https://ccrod.cancer.gov/confluence/display/CCRCRO/M2P2s

Sather, S. (2019). *The CRC's guide to coordinating clinical research.* CenterWatch. https://cms.centerwatch.com/wp-content/uploads/sites/2/2024/10/TheCRCsGuide-4htEd.pdf

U.S. Food and Drug Administration. (2003, August 28). *Guidance for industry: Part 11, electronic records; electronic signatures—Scope and application.* https://www.fda.gov/downloads/RegulatoryInformation/Guidances/ucm125125.pdf

CHAPTER 31

Data Management

Ashley Webb, MS, MN, RN, CRN-BC, OCN®

Introduction

Oncology clinical trials generate a vast amount of data. Laboratory values, vital signs, genetic markers, administration details, and other information collected as part of a clinical trial can connect a single patient with thousands of data points. Careful management of these data is essential to the conduct of clinical trials. The use of quality data management and sharing plans (DMSPs), systems, and processes ensures that data from trials can be accurately interpreted and generalized, contributing to advancements in the care of patients with cancer.

In addition to ensuring the efficient conduct of a clinical trial, data management is also essential in protecting the privacy of human participants. Oncology clinical research nurses (OCRNs) should be aware of the data management policies and procedures of their institutions. They must have a thorough understanding of the numerous regulations and laws that address the management of clinical trial data, such as the International Conference for Harmonisation of Technical Requirements for Pharmaceuticals for Human Use (ICH) publication *ICH Harmonised Guideline: Guideline for Good Clinical Practice E6(R3)*, the Health Insurance Portability and Accountability Act (HIPAA) (1996), and Title 21 Code of Federal Regulations § 11.200 (Electronic Records; Electronic Signatures, 2014).

This chapter will provide an overview of data management, DMSPs, and the role of OCRNs in ensuring high-quality data while protecting human participants.

Data Management Processes

Data management in clinical trials can be summarized in six steps: case report form (CRF) design and database definition, data collection and transfer, coding, data query and editing, data lock and analysis, and data reporting and sharing (see Figure 31-1). The involvement of OCRNs in each of these steps will vary depending on their roles and the institutions they represent. This entire process is informed and guided by a DMSP.

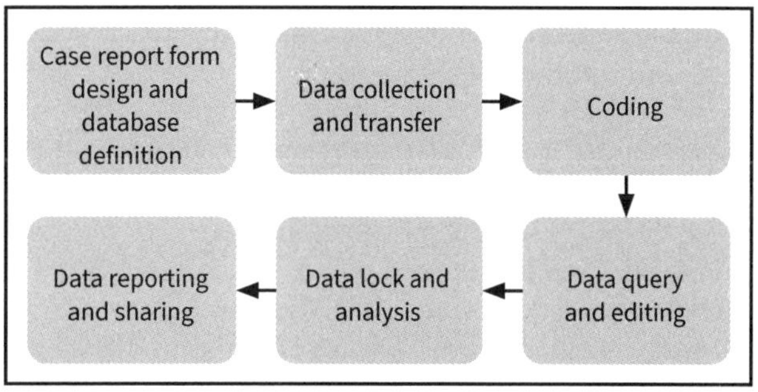

FIGURE 31-1 | Data Management Steps

Note. Based on information from Nourani et al., 2019.

Case Report Form Design and Database Definition

Once a clinical trial protocol has defined the study objectives, the corresponding CRFs are designed to collect the relevant data. Quality CRFs are crucial in ensuring that study end points are met (Hills et al., 2021). OCRNs may be involved in the creation of these forms and can verify that the data collected are complete. For example, if a trial involves assessing disease response at day 28 post-intervention, there must be CRFs at that timepoint that collect the relevant data (e.g., imaging, bone marrow biopsy). Ideally, CRFs are designed to be used in an electronic data capture (EDC) system.

In addition to the data collected in CRFs, how the data are collected is also important. CRFs should be designed so that the field format matches the data type. Automatic systems should be in place to notify when entered data does not conform to the expected format (ICH, 2025). For example, if a field is expected to capture the date of birth, then a date picker tool or a specific date format (e.g.,

DD-MMM-YYYY) should be required. If July 26, 1986, is entered, the EDC system should automatically request conformant data (i.e., 26-JUL-1986). Similarly, if a date of birth for an enrolled patient is entered as 26-JUL-1886, the system should issue an automatic query or mark the data as nonconforming, as the age would be higher than the expected possible range.

In addition to designing CRFs, a plan should be in place to capture other relevant data. For example, patient-reported outcome data may be transferred directly to the data management system when patients complete electronic surveys, eliminating the need for research personnel to enter these data into CRFs. Data from electronic health records (EHRs), such as laboratory values and vital signs, may also be transmitted directly. This prevents transcription errors and reduces the time required for research staff (Cheng et al., 2022). Transmitting data directly from EHRs presents a promising approach to increasing efficiency in data collection. However, researchers should recognize that data entered in the EHR for patient care may not meet the quality standards required for clinical trials without adjustments to EHR documentation practices (McCord & Hemkens, 2019).

Just as it is essential to collect the necessary information to achieve the study end points, it is also crucial not to include extraneous data in CRFs. The sharing of unnecessary information presents a risk to patient confidentiality.

Database definition is another key component of data collection, establishing the framework through which data will be housed, managed, and accessed. This includes the description of metadata, which are the data that describe the data. For example, in a spreadsheet with rows representing each study participant and columns with vital signs, the metadata would include the column headers describing the type of vital sign, the timepoint where it was taken, and the format or units of the data (e.g., is temperature reported in Celsius or Fahrenheit?). This provides context for the information provided and allows databases to be combined or compared. A variety of infrastructures exist to support the creation, use, and management of metadata, including the Cancer Data Standards Registry and Repository II (National Cancer Institute Center for Biomedical Informatics and Information Technology, 2022).

Data Collection, Entry, and Transfer

Once CRFs are created and a database is defined, study teams are ready to collect data. OCRNs are often heavily involved in data collection, entry, and transfer. The original data generated for a clinical trial are referred to as source data. The original documentation of these data is described as the source records (ICH, 2025). For example, the recording of vital signs in the EHR is considered a source record. A paper drug diary filled out by a patient would also be considered a source record. The source data are then entered into the CRF (usually via an EDC system but occasionally via a paper form) and transferred to a database.

Data should be entered directly into the CRF from the source record without any intervening steps. For example, when a participant's chemistry panel results are entered into the EHR, the person performing data entry should review the EHR directly to ensure accurate entry into the CRF. Staff should avoid transcribing results onto an alternate document for later entry into the CRF (ICH, 2025).

According to the U.S. Food and Drug Administration (FDA, 2013), the CRF can also function as the source record if source data are entered directly by the data originator. For example, an OCRN could assess a participant's performance status and record it directly in the CRF, which would then be considered the source.

Guidance on supporting quality data entry can be found in the CRF completion guidelines. These are referenced in the EDC system and provided to study teams at the start of the study. They provide specific directions for completing each field within the CRFs, along with other considerations for data entry, and should be referenced frequently by study teams (Hills et al., 2021).

Data Coding

Data coding transforms data into a consistent format, allowing for comparisons and summaries. This is especially important for free-text data. Adverse events, medical histories, concomitant medications, and other data elements are often collected using a free-text field, allowing the same event to be reported in many different ways. For example, patients with respiratory syncytial virus could have the adverse event described as "respiratory syncytial virus," "RSV," or "upper respiratory infection (RSV)." Coding standardizes this language, making it possible to categorize and quantify the frequency of these events. In this case, these events could all be coded as "upper respiratory infection." This may be performed automatically via the data management system or manually by data management staff. For a list of standard terminologies used to code data, see Figure 31-2. Data coding is generally the responsibility of specific data management staff, although it may sometimes be performed by OCRNs.

Common Terminology Criteria for Adverse Events (CTCAE): https://ctep.cancer.gov/protocolDevelopment/electronic_applications/ctc.htm

International Classification of Diseases (ICD-10): www.cms.gov/Medicare/Coding/ICD10/index.html?redirect=/icd10

Logical Observation Identifiers Names and Codes (LOINC®): www.loinc.org

Medical Dictionary for Regulatory Activities (MedDRA®): www.meddra.org

National Drug Code (NDC): https://dps.fda.gov/ndc

RxNorm: www.nlm.nih.gov/research/umls/rxnorm

Systematized Nomenclature of Medicine—Clinical Terms (SNOMED CT®): www.nlm.nih.gov/research/umls/Snomed/snomed_main.html

World Health Organization Drug (WHODrug) Portfolio—UMC Drug Dictionary: www.who-umc.org/whodrug/

FIGURE 31-2 | Examples of Standard Terminologies

Data Query and Editing

Although standard processes for data collection and entry contribute to a high-quality dataset, discrepancies or errors will always arise that need to be addressed. This process is referred to as data query and editing. Data queries may be automated (issued automatically by the data management system) or manual (issued by data management staff). For example, if study staff enter a 34-year-old patient's weight as 10.3 kilograms (22.7 lbs), the system may issue an automatic query of "Weight is outside of the expected range, please confirm." Manual queries may be issued based on inconsistencies within the CRFs or as part of source data verification, which is often performed by clinical research associates (CRAs) from the sponsor or a third party. For example, data management staff reviewing the laboratory CRF and noting a hemoglobin value of 6.2 g/dl may issue a query as to whether the event of anemia should be added to the adverse event CRF. Similarly, when performing source data verification, a CRA may note that the EHR reflects the patient had a temperature of 101.3°F (38.5°C), but the CRF reflects a temperature of 103.1°F (39.5°C). The CRA may issue a query requesting the site confirm the temperature. Queries should be objective and not lead sites to a particular response.

After a query is issued, the study team may respond by confirming the entry is correct or updating the data if necessary. Most electronic systems include methods for tracking open queries and resolution timelines, allowing study teams to prioritize their responses. OCRNs play an important role in query resolution. They may respond directly to queries in the EDC or provide nursing expertise to assist other study staff in resolving queries. Timely responses to queries and adequate query resolution help ensure data quality.

Data Lock and Analysis

Once the data have been reviewed and their accuracy confirmed, they are finalized through a process called data lock. After this time, the locked data cannot be revised. A study may have multiple data locks at different timepoints when interim data analysis is conducted. Study teams will be required to resolve all queries and complete all applicable CRFs prior to the data lock. At this point, the data can be converted into a format that supports analysis using statistical software tools. This enables assessments of effect, safety analysis, and required regulatory reporting to be conducted. OCRNs should be aware of the outcomes of these interim analyses as they may impact continued enrollment or study conduct. Sponsors should keep study teams updated on the timing of data locks and provide progress reports to ensure that data are properly cleaned prior to being finalized.

Data Reporting and Sharing

Once data are collected, cleaned, and analyzed, it is time to report and share findings. Information from clinical trials may be shared in summary form as journal articles or conference presentations. However, there is also an increasing movement to encourage the sharing of raw data (or minimally transformed data) via data repositories. The use of data repositories enables the generation of additional knowledge. For example, the Database of Genotypes and Phenotypes (dbGaP) archives and shares data from studies addressing the interaction between genotype and phenotype in humans. Once data from a study are shared with the database, other investigators can request access to their research projects (National Library of Medicine, n.d.). The inclusion of study data in repositories must be noted in the informed consent form, and patients must agree to this method of data sharing.

In addition to sharing data with other researchers, it is crucial to share it with participants and the broader public. This level of transparency can foster trust within communities and encourage participation in clinical trials. For example, the All of Us Research Program, sponsored by the National Institutes of Health (NIH), studies patterns in health across a diverse population. As part of this project, participants have access to their data and can also access the public database for the study (The All of Us Research Program Investigators, 2019).

Data Management and Sharing Plans

Data management should be considered throughout the life cycle of a clinical trial. From the development of CRFs to data lock and reporting, careful attention should be paid to data quality. Clinical research teams must keep in mind the data they hope to generate to achieve their objectives. This begins with the development of a thoughtfully constructed DMSP.

NIH (2020) defines a DMSP as "a plan describing the data management, preservation, and sharing of scientific data and accompanying metadata." The use of DMSPs is not only a best practice but also a requirement for certain funding bodies, including NIH and the U.S. National Science Foundation. Funders want to ensure that project data are managed appropriately and shared when possible, allowing for future research or knowledge generation from the dataset.

In addition to research sponsors and funders, regulatory bodies are also interested in reviewing DMSPs. Details included in these plans describe not only how data are acquired, manipulated, and shared to support quality results from the research study but also how data from human participants are protected to ensure ethical research conduct. Although institutions may have standard operating procedures surrounding data management and sharing, DMSPs should be study specific, as they should document the unique requirements for each trial. For example, plans should specify which specific repositories can be used to store data for future use.

The DMSP for the study should be the first resource that study teams use when questions arise about data management and sharing for a particular trial. Lebedys et al. (2021, p. 6) explained that the DMSP should be used as a "job aid for study personnel" and should be "concise and written in plain language." They also noted that, as part of the essential records, the DMSP should be managed as a controlled document with proper versioning and annual review. OCRNs should understand how to access DMSPs for studies at their institutions.

Components of a Data Management and Sharing Plan

The format and specific components of a DMSP will vary based on the use case. For an example format, see Figure 31-3. Experts note that these plans should support compliance with relevant regulations and oversight agencies; describe all operations performed on data; include involvement from a variety of groups, such as statistical operations, project management, and clinical and scientific leadership; and be approved prior to the start of the work described (Lebedys et al., 2021). Ultimately, the contents of the DMSP will depend on the policies of the stakeholders involved (e.g., sponsors, sites, funders, contract research organizations) and the particulars of the research being conducted.

Roles and Responsibilities

The DMSP should clearly indicate who is responsible for data management activities to ensure that accountability and attribution can be maintained (Lebedys et al., 2021). This includes verifying that access is limited to authorized individuals, as per FDA regulations for electronic records (Electronic Records; Electronic Signatures, 2014). The roles and responsibilities section should describe the qualifications of personnel delegated data management activities as required by *E6(R3)* (ICH, 2025).

- Data type
  - Types and amount of scientific data expected to be generated in the project
  - Scientific data that will be preserved and shared
  - Metadata, other relevant data, and associated documentation
- Related tools, software, and/or code
  - What tools will be used to access or manipulate shared data and how
- Standards
  - What common data standards will be used to enable interoperability
- Data preservation, access, and associated timelines
  - Repository where data will be archived
  - Describe how data will be findable and identifiable
  - When and how long will data be available
- Access, distribution, or reuse considerations
  - Factors affecting subsequent use of data
  - Whether/how data access will be controlled
  - Human research participant protections for privacy, rights, and confidentiality
- Oversight of data management and sharing

FIGURE 31-3 | National Institutes of Health Data Management and Sharing Plan Elements

Note. From *Data Management and Sharing Plan Format Page*, by National Institutes of Health, 2022 (https://grants.nih.gov/grants-process/write-application/forms-directory/data-management-and-sharing-plan-format-page). In the public domain.

Description of Data Collected

A description of the data to be collected should be included in the DMSP, specifying the source of the data, as well as the type and amount of data to be collected (NIH, 2020). The plan should account for all data to be collected as part of the study.

List of Standards and Terminology Dictionaries

The standard terminologies used for coding data, such as adverse events, should be included in the DMSP. This consists of the versions to be used and how updates to these standard terminologies will be managed.

Data Handling Rules

This section should describe how data are entered and cleaned to enable data provenance (i.e., the ability to reconstruct the data trail back to the source) (Richesson et al., 2023). This should include how changes to the data will be managed, consistent with Good Clinical Practice. Considerations should be made for how data points may be extrapolated (e.g., calculating age from birth year).

Data Sharing or Access

Data sharing has become an increasing priority in oncology clinical research. The NIH Data Management and Sharing Policy requires that scientific data from most funded projects be shared by the time of peer-reviewed publication (NIH, 2020). Specific publications, including the *Journal of Clinical Oncology*, also require transparency regarding how data will be shared for the research they publish (Cannistra, 2019). The data sharing section of the DMSP should describe how and when data will be shared. This should include the name of the data repository that will be used, if applicable.

Maintenance and Approval of a Data Management and Sharing Plan

The DMSP is considered a living document and should be updated as needed throughout the life of the trial. Institutional policies should dictate how often the plan is updated (e.g., annually), the process for updating the plan, the approval process for changes, and the method for communicating changes.

Clinical Data Management Systems and Clinical Trial Management Systems

A variety of tools exist to support the conduct of quality clinical trials, including clinical data management systems

(CDMSs) and clinical trial management systems (CTMSs). The key difference between these systems lies in their focus. Whereas a CDMS focuses on the collection, validation, maintenance, and retrieval of clinical trial data, a CTMS focuses on clinical trial operations, including managing documents and sites, patient enrollment, financial tracking, and regulatory activities. Often, these systems may be integrated, with one vendor offering a comprehensive solution for data management and operations. For this section, CDMS will be used to describe a standalone system for data management or the data management component of a comprehensive CTMS.

When selecting a software tool, the first step is understanding the needs of the end users. In the case of a CDMS, the end users include OCRNs and other members of research teams. In addition to understanding the needs of end users, staff involved in selecting a tool must also comprehend the functionality of the available tools (Vitharana & Basu, 2020). OCRNs may be involved in critically appraising tools when choosing a software solution. Depending on their level of involvement in this process, OCRNs may require an in-depth understanding of CDMS product functionality and how it aligns with their organization's specific needs.

Access and Tracking

Access to the CDMS will vary depending on the team member's role. For example, a CRA may have the authority to issue queries, but an OCRN would not. Alternatively, the OCRN would have the ability to enter data, but the CRA would not. The CDMS should feature an audit trail that identifies the user responsible for all entries, queries, and changes. The audit trail will also include the date and time of entry or change. Personnel should be trained on how to use the audit trail to investigate changes and maintain accountability. The audit trail is also a valuable tool for quality assurance; trends in the audit trail can identify opportunities for improving the CDMS itself or training needs for clinical trial sites and data entry staff.

Data Transmission and Exchange

Throughout a clinical trial, data may be transmitted and exchanged in various ways. When data are transferred between systems, it is essential to understand the origins of each data point and how it may have been transformed during its journey from data generation to transfer to the current system. Quality documentation of all these steps ensures data provenance.

Data Storage

Data for clinical trials can be both sensitive and irreplaceable; thus, care should be taken to ensure adequate plans for data storage. Servers hosting data should have the capability for backup and recovery in the event of an emergency. According to *E6(R3)*, Section 3.16.3, records should be retained securely in accordance with applicable regulatory requirements (ICH, 2025).

Funders and sponsors may have additional requirements for data and document retention. For example, studies funded by NIH must comply with federal retention requirements as mandated by the Freedom of Information Act. Clinical research sites should maintain relevant data and documentation until notified by the sponsor that these records are no longer needed.

Data Privacy and Security

Data privacy and security are always a priority in clinical trials. Confidentiality is an important component of "respect for persons" as outlined in *The Belmont Report*. It is thus imperative for OCRNs to maintain data privacy (National Commission for the Protection of Human Subjects of Biomedical and Behavioral Research, 1979). With the increase of digital data, privacy and security have become a complex technological problem—it is not as simple as installing a lock on a file cabinet. Study teams need information technology experts to support systems that ensure data privacy and security.

The Federal Information Security Modernization Act (FISMA) of 2014 outlines specific privacy and security requirements for clinical trials that receive federal funding. The act requires each federal agency to implement programs to support data security and manage risk (FISMA, 2014). This means federal funders may require documentation to ensure that data management systems for funded projects meet FISMA requirements. Requirements of FISMA include a process for detecting and managing security incidents, risk assessment and monitoring, and security awareness training.

Study teams and OCRNs can support data confidentiality and privacy by de-identifying personal information before transmitting data whenever possible. This includes using a study ID number to identify patients and redacting identifying information when appropriate. However, sometimes this is not possible. For example, complex genomic information collected for oncology clinical trials is a crucial component of the dataset, yet it is so inherent to the individual that it could be considered identifiable. This is why systems must have strong infrastructure and controls for managing access.

Protected Health Information

The HIPAA Privacy Rule governs how protected health information (PHI) can be transmitted and maintained (U.S. Department of Health and Human Services, 2025). The rule applies to "covered entities," which include health plans, healthcare clearinghouses, and healthcare providers who transmit PHI electronically. Most oncology clinical research involves covered entities (i.e., healthcare providers) and thus HIPAA often applies to data collected for research purposes. Though some access to PHI is essential to the conduct of research, it is important to limit unnecessary sharing of PHI. Patients must consent to the sharing of PHI for research via a HIPAA authorization form.

FAIR Data Principles and Reusability

Data reusability, the use of previously generated data for future purposes, has been of increasing interest. In 2016, an article published in *Scientific Data* by diverse stakeholders identified four core characteristics of data that ensure reusability, dubbed the FAIR data principles. FAIR stands for Findable, Accessible, Interoperable, and Reusable (Wilkinson et al., 2016). These principles support the use of technology in accessing and reusing data (see Table 31-1).

TABLE 31-1 | FAIR Data Principles

Principle	Description
Findable	• F1. (Meta)data are assigned a globally unique and persistent identifier. • F2. Data are described with rich metadata (defined by R1 below). • F3. (Meta)data clearly and explicitly include the identifier of the data it describes. • F4. (Meta)data are registered or indexed in a searchable resource.
Accessible	• A1. (Meta)data are retrievable by their identifier using a standardized communications protocol. – A1.1. The protocol is open, free, and universally implementable. – A1.2. The protocol allows for an authentication and authorization procedure where necessary. • A2. (Meta)data are accessible, even when the data are no longer available.
Interoperable	• I1. (Meta)data use a formal, accessible, shared, and broadly applicable language for knowledge representation. • I2. (Meta)data use vocabularies that follow FAIR principles. • I3. (Meta)data include qualified references to other (meta)data.
Reusable	• R1. (Meta)data are richly described with a plurality of accurate and relevant attributes. – R1.1. (Meta)data are released with a clear and accessible data usage license. – R1.2. (Meta)data are associated with detailed provenance. – R1.3. (Meta)data meet domain-relevant community standards.

Note. Based on information from Wilkinson et al., 2016.

Findable

For data to be used for future research, they must first be findable. To be findable, data should be assigned unique and persistent identifiers (GO FAIR Initiative, n.d.). For example, a website URL points to a single, unique location, and, as long as it remains hosted, it remains persistent. If the URL went to multiple web pages or if the hosting expired and the website could no longer be located using the URL, the data would not be findable.

Data should also be described with rich metadata. This allows humans and machines to understand whether the data are relevant to the question being asked. Finally, data should be registered in a searchable resource (e.g., a data repository).

Accessible

To reuse data, researchers must also be able to access the data they find. It is not possible to have all data freely available, especially in clinical research, where some data need to remain protected and private. In these cases, it should be clear which process can be used to access the data (e.g., authentication, authorization). FAIR principles dictate that, even if the original data become unavailable, the metadata should remain accessible. This would enable future researchers to understand how the original data were collected and processed, allowing them to replicate the study or contact relevant personnel if needed.

Interoperable

Interoperability is defined as the "ability of two or more systems or components to exchange information and to use the information that has been exchanged" (IEEE, 1991, p. 114). This is a crucial attribute of any CDMS, data repository, or other system that aims to share or aggregate data. *Semantic interoperability* refers to the exchange of meaning, not just information. Systems with semantic interoperability enable the recipient to accurately understand and interpret transmitted information (Kush, 2023). Interoperability relies on having adequate metadata describing the data being transmitted.

Interoperability with regard to cancer data is particularly important, given the increased complexity and volume of data involved. There has been a movement to develop a cancer data ecosystem that would create a national infrastructure for sharing cancer data as part of the Cancer Moonshot initiative (NCI, 2016). One step toward developing this ecosystem is identifying and defining common data elements (CDEs). A CDE is a description of a particular data point to be collected, how it will be measured, and how it will be represented in a dataset. For example, an important CDE could be performance status, measured by a physician's assessment of the Eastern Cooperative Oncology Group Performance Status Score, entered as an integer from 0 to 5.

One CDE set, Minimal Common Oncology Data Elements (mCODE), was created in 2018 to develop CDEs specifically for cancer. In all, 90 data elements have been identified (Osterman et al., 2020). The use of CDEs can improve interoperability within clinical trials and is also beneficial for the clinical care of patients. For example, CDEs within EHRs across different systems could support continuity of care. For examples of mCODE CDEs, see Table 31-2.

Reusable

The final FAIR principle is reusability. This is highly reliant on the quality and volume of metadata included to describe the data. The metadata should adhere to any domain-relevant standards (e.g., mCODE), have detailed provenance, and clearly describe the licensing and legal implications. Researchers need to understand the relevant usage rights associated with the data to facilitate their reusability.

Implications for Oncology Clinical Research Nurses

The complexity of oncology clinical research is increasing, and with it, so is the need for additional tools and processes to support the management of the important data generated by this research. Possible future directions include increased data sharing, new methods for directly transferring data from EHRs and other tools to research databases, and the application of artificial intelligence and machine learning in data management. The movement toward forming a cancer data ecosystem will create more opportunities and efficiency within clinical research, but it will also require a level of collaboration not seen before.

OCRNs must stay current with these developments to support the implementation of oncology clinical trials. They are well-suited to bridge the gap between clinical knowledge and the technology expertise required to achieve quality data management. OCRNs specializing in data and informatics are needed to contribute to the future of oncology clinical research by understanding how technology can improve research conduct and monitoring of patient participants (Barlow, 2020).

TABLE 31-2 | Example of Minimal Common Oncology Data Elements Consensus Data Element Standards

Profile Title	Data Element Name	Clinical Data Definition	Permissible Values Set
Myeloma Revised International Staging System (RISS) Stage Profile	Value	The stage, stage group, category, or classification resulting from the staging evaluation	Codeable: stage 1; stage 2; stage 3
Radiotherapy Course Summary	Actual Number of Sessions	The number of sessions in a course of radiation therapy	Positive integer
Primary Cancer Condition Profile	Onset	Estimated or actual date the condition began, in the opinion of the clinician	Date
Human Specimen Profile	Type	The kind of material that forms the specimen	Codeable: whole blood; sputum; marrow; skin

Note. Based on information from mCODE FHIR Implementation Guide, n.d.

Summary

Data management is woven through all stages of a clinical trial. Robust data management processes, along with an effective DSMP and CDMS, are essential for ensuring high-quality data. The FAIR data principles, emphasizing that data are findable, accessible, interoperable, and reusable, illustrate how the field will move toward managing data in ways that maximize the impact of clinical trials. This is not only an emerging best practice, but also an imperative of certain funders of research, including NIH.

Although technology is constantly improving our ability to gain insights from collected data, it is not a replacement for the knowledge and skills of experienced research professionals. It will become increasingly necessary for OCRNs to master new technology in order to harness the power of these tools fully.

Key Points

- Understanding the steps in the data management process, from CRF design to data reporting, can help study teams ensure that their final dataset is complete, accurate, and usable.
- DMSPs are living documents that describe the personnel, processes, and procedures needed to promote quality data management practices for a clinical trial.
- CTMSs and CDMSs are tools to support the conduct of clinical trials. It is important to consider both the functionality of the tool and the needs of end users when selecting a tool to use.
- Increasingly complex and inherently identifying (i.e., genomic) data require new technology and processes to support data collection and use.
- Data sharing and reuse can enable others to build upon prior discoveries, leading to increased knowledge generation.
- The FAIR principles can maximize the impact of data, and adherence to these principles should be a priority for study teams.
- Technology will lead to increased efficiency in clinical trials; OCRNs and other study team members need to develop expertise to support the use of these tools.

The author would like to acknowledge Dianne M. Reeves, MSN, RN, and Anita Walden, BS, CHI, for their contribution to this chapter that remains unchanged from the previous edition of this book.

References

Barlow, C. (2020). Oncology research: Clinical trial management systems, electronic medical record, and artificial intelligence. *Seminars in Oncology Nursing, 36*(2), 151005. https://doi.org/10.1016/j.soncn.2020.151005

Cannistra, S.A. (2019). *Journal of Clinical Oncology's* Data Sharing Policy for Clinical Trials. *Journal of Clinical Oncology, 37*(35), 3333–3334. https://doi.org/10.1200/JCO.19.02889

Cheng, A.C., Banasiewicz, M.K., Johnson, J.D., Sulieman, L., Kennedy, N., Delacqua, F., ... Harris, P.A. (2022). Evaluating automated electronic case report form data entry from electronic health records. *Journal of Clinical and Translational Science, 7*(1), e29. https://doi.org/10.1017/cts.2022.514

Electronic Records; Electronic Signatures, 21 C.F.R. § 11.200 (2014). https://www.accessdata.fda.gov/scripts/cdrh/cfdocs/cfcfr/CFRSearch.cfm?fr=11.200

Federal Information Security Modernization Act of 2014, Pub. L. No. 113–283, 128 Stat. 3073 (2014). https://www.congress.gov/113/plaws/publ283/PLAW-113publ283.pdf

GO FAIR Initiative. (n.d.). *FAIR principles.* https://www.go-fair.org/fair-principles/

Health Insurance Portability and Accountability Act of 1996, Pub. L. No. 104-191, § 264, 110 Stat.1936 (1996).

Hills, K., Bartlett, T., Leconte, I., & Zozus, M.N. (2021). CRF completion guidelines. *Journal of the Society for Clinical Data Management, 1*(1). https://doi.org/10.47912/jscdm.117

IEEE. (1991). IEEE standard computer dictionary: A compilation of IEEE standard computer glossaries (IEEE Std 610, pp. 1–217). https://doi.org/10.1109/IEEESTD.1991.106963

International Council for Harmonisation of Technical Requirements for Pharmaceuticals for Human Use. (2025). *ICH harmonised guideline: Guideline for good clinical practice: E6(R3).* https://database.ich.org/sites/default/files/ICH_E6%28R3%29_Step4_FinalGuideline_2025_0106.pdf

Kush, R.D. (2023). Data sharing and reuse of health data for research. In R.L. Richesson, J.E. Andrews, & K. Fultz Hollis (Eds.), *Clinical research informatics* (3rd ed., pp. 147–167). Springer.

Lebedys, E., Famatiga-Fay, C., Bhatkar, P., Johnson, Dr., Viswanathan, G., & Zozus, M.H. (2021). Data management plan. *Journal of the Society for Clinical Data Management, 1*(4). https://doi.org/10.47912/jscdm.116

McCord, K.A., & Hemkens, L.G. (2019). Using electronic health records for clinical trials: Where do we stand and where can we go? *Canadian Medical Association Journal, 191*(5), E128–E133. https://doi.org/10.1503/cmaj.180841

mCODE FHIR Implementation Guide. (n.d.). *HL7 International.* https://build.fhir.org/ig/HL7/fhir-mCODE-ig

National Cancer Institute. (2016). *The Cancer Moonshot.* https://www.cancer.gov/research/key-initiatives/moonshot-cancer-initiative/history/blue-ribbon-panel-report-2016.pdf

National Cancer Institute Center for Biomedical Informatics and Information Technology. (2022). *caDSR II.* https://cadsr.cancer.gov/onedata/Home.jsp

National Commission for the Protection of Human Subjects of Biomedical and Behavioral Research. (1979). *The Belmont Report: Ethical principles and guidelines for the protection of human subjects of research.* https://www.hhs.gov/ohrp/regulations-and-policy/belmont-report/read-the-belmont-report/index.html

National Institutes of Health. (2020). *Final NIH policy for data management and sharing.* https://grants.nih.gov/grants/guide/notice-files/NOT-OD-21-013.html

National Library of Medicine (n.d.). *dbGaP Cumulative Requests Counts.* https://www.ncbi.nlm.nih.gov/gap/summary/DAR_Stats/cumulative_counts

Nourani, A., Ayatollahi, H., & Dodaran, M.S. (2019). A review of clinical data management systems used in clinical trials. *Reviews on Recent Clinical Trials, 14*(1), 10–23. https://doi.org/10.2174/1574887113666180924165230

Osterman, T.J., Terry, M., & Miller, R.S. (2020). Improving cancer data interoperability: The promise of the minimal common oncology data elements (mCODE) initiative. *JCO Clinical Cancer Informatics, 4*, 993–1001. https://doi.org/10.1200/CCI.20.00059

Richesson, R.L., Lynch, C.O., & Hammond, W.E. (2023). Developing and promoting data standards for clinical research. In R.L. Richesson, J.E. Andrews, & K. Fultz Hollis (Eds.), *Clinical research informatics* (3rd ed., pp. 389–412). Springer.

The All of Us Research Program Investigators. (2019). The "All of Us" research program. *New England Journal of Medicine, 381*(7), 668–676. https://doi.org/10.1056/NEJMsr1809937

U.S. Food and Drug Administration. (2013). *Guidance for industry: Electronic source data in clinical investigations.* https://www.fda.gov/downloads/Drugs/GuidanceComplianceRegulatoryInformation/Guidances/UCM328691.pdf

Vitharana, P., & Basu, A. (2020). Examining end users' ability to select business services: A conceptual framework and an empirical study. *Information and Management, 57*(6). https://doi.org/10.1016/j.im.2019.103241

Wilkinson, M., Dumontier, M., Aalbersberg, I., Appleton, G., Axton, M., Baak, A., ... Mons, B. (2016). The FAIR Guiding Principles for scientific data management and stewardship. *Scientific Data, 3*, 160018. https://doi.org/10.1038/sdata.2016.18

SECTION VII.
Quality Assurance

CHAPTER 32

Creating and Maintaining a Regulatory File

Brittany Stith, BSN, RN, OCN®, CCRP

Introduction

Coordinating clinical trials requires immense organizational skills, a keen eye for the smallest details, and a solid understanding of the various aspects of the trial. Even the most organized coordinators struggle with keeping track of the voluminous pages of communications, queries, approvals, and other documents associated with each trial. A key strategy for successful document management is creating and maintaining a regulatory file in which all essential protocol documents are kept. A critical step in creating the file is identifying which documents need to be saved. Every investigator who conducts a clinical trial must keep a record of all the essential documents related to the conduct of the study.

Many terms are used to describe the regulatory file, including but not limited to *study binder*, *investigator binder*, *administrative binder*, *institution regulatory file*, *regulatory files*, *investigator site file*, and *investigator study files*. Although the maintenance of regulatory files is a part of Good Clinical Practice (GCP) guidelines and is not legally binding, it has become best practice for all interventional trials to have a regulatory file regardless of sponsorship. The U.S. Food and Drug Administration (FDA) has adopted the International Conference on Harmonisation of Technical Requirements for Pharmaceuticals for Human Use's (ICH) *Guideline for Good Clinical Practice E6(R2)* as guidance (FDA, 2018). The creation and maintenance of a regulatory file may also be governed by an institution's standard operating procedures (SOPs). ICH officially released its *E6(R3)* update on January 6, 2025. FDA announced guidance for this revision on September 9, 2025.

This chapter will offer a systematic approach to creating and maintaining an investigator's or institution's regulatory file in a manageable way. It will not address the role of sponsors or the documents that they should maintain.

Contents of the Regulatory File

An investigator site file is a repository for important documents. Appendix C of *E6(R3)* states the following:

> The essential records permit and contribute to the evaluation of the conduct of a trial in relation to the compliance of the investigator and sponsor with Good Clinical Practice (GCP) and applicable regulatory requirements and the reliability of the results produced. The essential records are used as part of the investigator oversight and sponsor oversight (including monitoring) of the trial. (ICH, 2025 p. 63)

These documents are reviewed by the sponsor, contract research organization, and other regulatory authorities as part of the monitoring, auditing, or inspection process.

Appendix C of *E6(R3)* includes a nonexhaustive listing of essential records that may be produced during a trial. Table 32-1 describes the different documents that should be maintained in the regulatory file and may be helpful for oncology clinical research nurses (OCRNs) who have to develop their files. Depending on the study, not all items may apply. Table 32-1 also introduces training records, another element not listed in the guidance document.

Institutions holding an Office for Human Research Protections–approved Federalwide Assurance are responsible for verifying that investigators conducting U.S. Department of Health and Human Services (HHS)–supported human participant research understand and act in accordance with HHS regulations on the protection of human participants (Office for Human Research Protections, 2024).

TABLE 32-1 | Components of a Regulatory File

Title of Essential Document	Purpose of Document or Relevant Information	Helpful Tips
Investigator and Institution Information		
Form FDA 1572 or Individual Investigator Agreement	Document the Individual Investigator Agreement to conduct the study according to FDA regulations. Update as investigators change or other pertinent information changes (e.g., address of laboratories or IRBs). Form FDA 1572 can be found at www.fda.gov/downloads/AboutFDA/ReportsManualsForms/Forms/UCM074728.pdf. For National Cancer Institute Cancer Therapy Evaluation Program–sponsored studies, use Form FDA 1572 found on the Registration and Central Repository website: https://ctepcore.nci.nih.gov/rcr.	All versions of Form FDA 1572 should be maintained. Some sponsors may require that the original document be sent to them and a copy maintained by the study team. For National Cancer Institute Cancer Therapy Evaluation Program–sponsored studies, maintain all investigators' individual Form FDA 1572 documentation provided by the Cancer Therapy Evaluation Program as part of investigator registration.
Updated curriculum vitae for the principal investigator and each subinvestigator	Document the investigators' qualifications to conduct the study.	Keep current and historical copies. The current version should be initialed or signed and dated within 2 years. This document is amenable to centralization.
Copy of medical license for the principal investigator and each subinvestigator (if applicable)	Document the investigators' qualifications to conduct the study.	This document is amenable to centralization.
Training certificates	Document that there is adequate training for all staff participating in the conduct of the study. Keep evidence of training, such as human participant protection, Good Clinical Practice, and International Air Transport Association dangerous goods regulations training certificates.	Documentation should be kept for each investigator, the oncology research nurse, study coordinator, and other key research staff associated with the study. These documents are amenable to centralization. Study-specific training should be maintained within the study-specific regulatory binder or electronic regulatory file.
Study staff responsibilities and signature form	Document that the principal investigator has delegated specific study-related tasks to others. This log should list all individuals (including signature, initials, and time span) to whom the principal investigator has delegated study-related activities. The principal investigator should sign the log. Revise as needed when study staff join or leave and when study roles change.	This document may also be referred to as a Delegation of Duties/Authority log (see Chapter 10).
Financial disclosure and certification statements	Document that the investigators are compliant with FDA regulations in 21 C.F.R. § 312.64(d).	The sponsor will often provide forms for the principal investigator to complete.
Clinical trial agreement or other contract or legal agreements (if applicable)	A clinical trial agreement is a contractual agreement entered into between the sponsor and the institution for all industry-sponsored trials. This category could include other types of agreements, such as a confidential disclosure agreement, a material transfer agreement, and cooperative research and development agreements.	If this does not include an insurance or indemnification statement and data use agreement, these documents should also be kept.
Site selection assessment (e.g., feasibility questionnaire)	Document the site's selection by the sponsor and oversight of the service providers conducting important trial-related activities.	–
Maintenance and calibration records	Document for demonstrating fitness for purpose for the equipment for important trial activities.	–

(Continued on next page)

TABLE 32-1 | Components of a Regulatory File *(Continued)*

Title of Essential Document	Purpose of Document or Relevant Information	Helpful Tips
Investigator's Brochure and Device Manual		
Investigator's brochure and updates	Document that the investigator is informed in a timely manner of relevant information. Documentation includes scientific information for the investigational product. For FDA-approved agents, file a copy of the package insert.	Keep all versions in the investigator file.
Protocol Versions and Other Protocol Information		
Protocol and amendments	Documentation includes the initial version, every protocol amendment, and a signed protocol signature page for each version (if applicable).	Save the IRB-approved protocol versions.
Study manual of procedures and updates (if applicable)	Documentation includes the laboratory procedures manual, laboratory specimen handling instructions, test article handling and preparation, and protocol-specific instructions.	If this is not kept in the regulatory file, create a note to file and indicate its location. If there is no manual of procedures, indicate this in a note to file.
Approved Informed Consent Documents and Information Given to Participants		
Informed consent documents • Initial version • Every revised version	Documentation includes a copy of all versions of the IRB-approved informed consent document and IRB-approved authorization for use and disclosure of protected health information (if separate from informed consent documents).	All versions should contain a version date and number and must be approved by the IRB of record.
Advertisements, recruitment materials, and participant educational materials	Documentation includes any written information provided to participants.	Documentation must be approved by the IRB of record.
IRB or Independent Ethics Committee Documentation		
Federalwide Assurance number and expiration date	Document that the institution is registered with the Office for Human Research Protections. The information may be found by searching the following website: https://ohrp.cit.nih.gov/search.	This documentation should be kept on file for both local IRBs and central IRBs, as applicable. This document is amenable to centralization.
IRB/institutional ethics committee membership roster	Document that the IRB is compliant with 45 C.F.R. § 46.107.	Membership lists should be updated as changes are made during the study. Historical lists should also be maintained. This document should be kept on file for both local IRBs and central IRBs, as applicable. This document is amenable to centralization.
IRB approvals of • Initial protocol, ICF • Amendments to protocol and ICF • Continuing review • Written information given to participants (if applicable) • Advertisements for participant recruitment (if applicable) • Authorization for use and disclosure of protected health information (if separate from ICF) • Authorization to use the short-form consent procedure (if applicable)	Document appropriate approval by the IRB of record prior to use and identify the version number and date of the documents.	All correspondence regarding the approval process of the protocol, including submissions to the IRB, IRB stipulations, and the response to stipulations, should be kept. It is not necessary to keep the entire package; enough documentation should be kept to provide evidence of the approval process. Documentation should be kept on file for both local IRBs and central IRBs, as applicable.

(Continued on next page)

TABLE 32-1 | Components of a Regulatory File *(Continued)*

Title of Essential Document	Purpose of Document or Relevant Information	Helpful Tips
IRB or Independent Ethics Committee Documentation *(Cont.)*		
Continuing review of the IRB and IRB approval for study continuation	–	Documentation must be compiled following IRB regulations. It may not be required for all trials, and the needed frequency may differ between trials. Documentation should be kept on file for both local IRBs and central IRBs, as applicable.
Notification to IRB of adverse events	–	Follow institutional and central IRB SOPs, as applicable.
Notification to IRB of unanticipated problems involving risks to participants and others	For U.S. Department of Health and Human Services guidance on reporting unanticipated problems, see www.hhs.gov/ohrp/policy/advevntguid.html.	Follow institutional and central IRB SOPs, as applicable.
Notification to IRB of protocol deviations	–	Follow institutional and central IRB SOPs, as applicable.
Notification to IRB of study completion and final study report	–	Follow institutional and central IRB SOPs, as applicable.
Safety Information		
Copy of serious adverse event reports sent to sponsor (if applicable)	The originating investigator gives notification to regulatory authorities of unexpected serious adverse drug reactions.	All correspondence between the sponsor or contract research organization and the site that concerns serious adverse event reports and any safety information should be kept.
Investigational New Drug safety reports received from the sponsor	The sponsor notifies the investigator of safety information.	If IRB policy is only to receive the Investigational New Drug safety report when an amendment is needed, the sponsor report should still be filed in the regulatory file.
Safety and data monitoring committee reports and correspondence	–	–
Other Regulatory Agency and Committee Documentation		
Approvals and authorizations of protocol, ICF, and amendments from additional regulatory agencies (if applicable)	Examples include the Radiation Safety Committee, Office of Biotechnology Activities, and Institutional Biosafety Committee.	–
Correspondence with regulatory agencies regarding safety information (if applicable)	–	–
Clinical Trial Material Documentation		
Records of receipt of clinical trial material and trial-related materials (if applicable)	This may include laboratory kits, electronic tablets, an electrocardiogram machine, and other matrials.	–
Samples of labels attached to investigational product containers and relabeling (if applicable)	–	–

(Continued on next page)

TABLE 32-1 | Components of a Regulatory File *(Continued)*		
Title of Essential Document	**Purpose of Document or Relevant Information**	**Helpful Tips**
Clinical Trial Material Documentation *(Cont.)*		
Temperature log (if applicable)	Log to record the temperature of the freezer or refrigerator used to store the test article.	This document is amenable to centralization. Temperature monitoring reports may be provided by your institution daily, weekly, or monthly and should be filed as they are received.
Clinical trial material dispensing and accountability records	Document that the investigational products and devices have been used according to the protocol.	If dispensing and accountability records are filed in the pharmacy, photocopies of these records should be made at study completion and inserted into the regulatory file. Create a note to file and indicate the location of the original records.
Documentation of clinical trial material destruction if performed at site	–	–
Biologic Samples Documentation		
Copies of the biologic sample transmittal forms that accompanied the shipment to the external laboratory	This may include research laboratory requisition forms and other documentation.	If these are not kept in the regulatory file, create a note to file and indicate the location of the records.
Correspondence regarding biologic samples	–	–
Record of retained body fluids and tissue samples (if applicable)	Document the location and identification of retained samples.	–
Laboratory Documentation		
Laboratory certification and accreditation	Document the competence of the facility to perform required tests and support the reliability of results.	Include updates throughout the study duration and keep historical records. These must be kept for all laboratories used in the study and listed on Form FDA 1572. These documents are amenable to centralization.
Laboratory normal reference ranges	Document normal values for laboratory tests to be performed for the clinical trial.	Keep a copy of normal ranges for all laboratory tests included in the protocol. Include updates throughout the study duration. Laboratory results with reference ranges from a participant may be used if all personally identifiable information is redacted. These documents are amenable to centralization.
Laboratory director's curriculum vitae	–	If multiple laboratories are used in a study, obtain the curriculum vitae for each laboratory director. These documents are amenable to centralization.

(Continued on next page)

TABLE 32-1 | Components of a Regulatory File *(Continued)*

Title of Essential Document	Purpose of Document or Relevant Information	Helpful Tips
Study or Participant Accountability Records		
Participant screening and enrollment logs	List participants screened for entry, as well as those enrolled in the study.	This may be one document or 2 separate lists. The screening log should document why potential participants were not included in the study. These documents may be kept electronically or on paper.
Subject identification code list	List participants enrolled in the study and identified by a unique number.	This allows the investigator or institution to identify study participants in the case of an emergency quickly. This is a confidential list and should be maintained only at the site.
Treatment allocation and decoding documentation	Decoding procedures may be detailed in the protocol itself.	–
Blank set of C.R.F.s	–	–
Signed IRB-approved ICF and authorization for use and disclosure of protected health information for each participant screened for entry into the study	–	If this is not kept in the regulatory file, create a note to file and indicate its location.
Copy of completed C.R.F.s for each participant with any related data clarification requests (if applicable)	Document that the investigator or authorized member of the investigator's staff confirms the observations recorded.	If this is not kept in the regulatory file, create a note to file and indicate its location.
Copy of completed C.R.F. transmittal forms (if applicable)	–	If this is not kept in the regulatory file, create a note to file and indicate its location.
Copy of completed C.R.F. edit logs (if applicable)	–	If this is not kept in the regulatory file, create a note to file and indicate its location.
Source records	Documentation contains original documents or data or certified copies of the original documents or data (e.g., medical records, notes, electronic patient-reported outcomes).	–
Documents related to data finalization	These documents may include query resolutions, serious adverse event reconciliations, quality control reports, coding completion, output datasets, and more.	–
Computer system validation (trial specific and non-trial specific)	Documentation includes system specifications, testing, validation reports, change control, and more.	–
Monitoring and Auditing Activities		
Site initiation visit report	–	–
Final trial closeout monitoring report	Document that all activities required for trial closeout are completed, and copies of essential documents are held in the appropriate files.	–

(Continued on next page)

TABLE 32-1 | Components of a Regulatory File *(Continued)*

Title of Essential Document	Purpose of Document or Relevant Information	Helpful Tips
Monitoring and Auditing Activities *(Cont.)*		
Monitoring logs and reports	This document contains the monitor's information for each visit, including name, date of the visit, and more. Site staff should document confirmation that the visit occurred by signing the log.	–
Monitor correspondence	This documentation contains site visit confirmation and follow-up correspondence.	–
Protocol deviations, noncompliance, and corrective and preventive actions	Documents capture information related to all protocol deviations, including the implementation of appropriate measures to prevent recurrence (if applicable).	–
Audit documentation	Document includes the observations and findings of the audit.	–
General and Sponsor Correspondence		
All correspondence between the sponsor, contract research organization, and the site concerning the study	Document any agreements or significant discussions regarding trial administration, protocol violations, trial conduct, and adverse event reporting.	–
Site-generated telephone contact reports or logs	–	–
Clinical Study Report		
Clinical study reports (if applicable)	Document the results and interpretation of the trial.	–
Notes to File		
Notes to file (if applicable)	Provide documentation of unusual events that occur during a clinical trial. Reasons to write a note to file include the following: • When a correction was made to a document that could raise questions • When there is a change or correction to a process or policy Improper uses of notes to file include the following: • Noting something previously documented elsewhere • Identifying a problem with no resolution • Using in place of recordkeeping In general, notes to file are used in the following instances: • To document the reason for missing, delayed, or erroneous documents in the clinical trial master file or the principal investigator file • To explain protocol deviations or investigator site practices that are different from the norm or from what is prescribed in the protocol	The question to ask when writing a note is, "What are the chances that a data query, site monitor, auditor, or inspector will ask a question and find this note useful in understanding what happened in the study?" A good note to file includes the following: • Date, author, and participant of note • What happened (who, what, where, why) • Why the incident is important • What has been or will be done to address this incident • What will be done to prevent or mitigate similar incidents in the future
Other information felt necessary to retain but not filed elsewhere in the regulatory file	–	–

C.F.R.—Code of Federal Regulations; FDA—U.S. Food and Drug Administration; ICF—informed consent form; IRB—institutional review board; SOP—standard operating procedure

Note. Based on information from International Council for Harmonisation of Technical Requirements for Pharmaceuticals for Human Use, 2025; Investigator Reports, 1987; IRB Membership, 2017; Protection of Human Subjects, 2017.

Additionally, FDA (2009) requires that investigators ensure adequate training for all staff involved in the conduct of a clinical trial. Study staff members should be familiar with the purpose of the study, have an understanding of the protocol requirements, acknowledge regulatory requirements and standards for conducting clinical trials and protecting human participants, have the training to perform the tasks they are delegated, and be informed of pertinent changes to the study. Training records may include a human participant protection course, a GCP course, sponsor meetings, protocol-specific staff meetings, sponsor-required training, or staff in-service exercises.

Feehan & Garcia-Diaz (2020) described how the oversight of staff training is crucially important. They detailed that FDA assesses for adequate principal investigation supervision, if the study staff are qualified to perform delegated tasks and have received adequate training and explanation of protocols, the principal investigator's involvement is adequate and ongoing, and involved third parties and contract research organizations are appropriately supervised.

Formatting Regulatory Files

Regulatory files can be found in various formats and organizational styles, ranging from paper binders to electronic files. HHS states that records may be preserved in hard copy, electronic, or other media forms and must be accessible for inspection and copying by authorized HHS representatives (Office for Human Research Protections, 2024). Often, sponsors or institutions have a required format and organization that must be followed. Regardless of the format, the file must be organized in a manner that allows for specific documents to be found easily.

An important rule of thumb with filing is consistency. The organization method of files should be easily understood by a person not familiar with the study. Developing a standard naming convention is critical for consistency and ease in finding documents for studies that are using an electronic regulatory file (e.g., protocols, amendments, financial disclosures, safety reports). Table 32-2 provides an example of standard nomenclature. Institutions are also likely to have SOPs on file management.

In all regulatory files, patient confidentiality should be maintained. It is crucial to clearly identify all documents that include protected health information (PHI) and withhold the information from those who do not have permission to view it. This may include removing or redacting the PHI from reports (e.g., expedited adverse event reports, laboratory reference ranges). Paper files are often kept in binders that must be stored in a secure location, such as a locked file or secured office. Electronic files should be kept on a secure server that is backed up daily or on a secure web-based system with limited access. At the time of monitoring visits (remote or on-site), electronic files can be shared by providing direct access to the monitors via shared cloud-based platforms and secure file-sharing systems (e.g., e-regulatory binder systems) or downloaded to a secure memory device (e.g., thumb drive, read-only compact disc) and given to monitoring personnel.

TABLE 32-2 | Suggestions for Standard Naming Conventions for Protocol Documents When Using an Electronic Regulatory File

Document Name	File Name
Initial protocol document	Protocol number_initial protocol_version_date [DD-MMM-YYYY]
Initial consent document	Protocol number_initial consent_version_clean or tracked_date [DD-MMM-YYYY]
Continuing institutional review board (IRB) review	Protocol number_CR_date [DD-MMM-YYYY]
Investigator's brochure	Drug Name_IBversion_date [DD-MMM-YYYY] (date = date of version) (i.e., MDX010_IBv6.2_10-DEC-2009)
IRB approval document	Protocol number_IRB approval letter_date [DD-MMM-YYYY]
Financial disclosure document	Form FDA 3455_Investigator name_date [DD-MMM-YYYY] or FDF_Investigator name_date (if using a sponsor-provided financial disclosure form)
Curriculum vitae	CV_Investigator name_date [DD-MMM-YYYY]
IRB membership roster	IRB Name_roster_date [DD-MMM-YYYY]
Unanticipated problem	Protocol number_event_date of event [DD-MMM-YYYY]

Centralizing Essential Documents

Some essential documents may be applied to multiple studies and, therefore, may be centralized at the study site level. For example, laboratory reference ranges, laboratory certifications (e.g., Clinical Laboratory Improvement Amendments, College of American Pathologists), curriculum vitae, and medical licenses may be kept in a central file to ease the burden of duplication. If a central file is used, a note to file should be placed in each study's regulatory file indicating that centralized files exist and where they are located.

Maintaining Regulatory Files

Essential records will be produced prior to the start of, during, and after the completion or termination of the trial. In *E6(R3)*, Section 3.3 provides a listing of documents that, if produced, are considered essential and should be retained (ICH, 2025). Source data should follow the ALCOA+ principles (Attributable, Legible, Contemporaneous, Original, and Accurate + Complete, Consistent, Enduring, and Available). ALCOA+ contains the guiding principles for ensuring data integrity that act as the cornerstone of good documentation practice. Every clinical research site should follow these principles to verify that source documentation is maintained at the highest standard (Adkins, 2024). Study team personnel should ensure audit trails are maintained if data corrections are made; this applies to both written and electronic records. The investigator and institution should take measures to prevent accidental or premature destruction of these documents. Regulations for award recipients (45 C.F.R. § 75.361) require that research records be maintained for at least three years after completion of the research and submission of the last expenditure report (Retention Requirements for Records, 2014).

Per GCP guidance, essential records should be retained for the required retention period following applicable regulatory requirements or until the sponsor communicates that the records are no longer needed, whichever is longer. Sponsors are responsible for notifying the investigator and institution when documents no longer need to be retained (ICH, 2025).

The Health Insurance Portability and Accountability Act regulations require that related records (e.g., authorizations, documentation of waiver approvals) be maintained for six years (Security and Privacy, 2000). It is important to plan for long-term storage of these documents, including their location, either in electronic or paper forms or a combination of both, to ensure the confidentiality and availability of the records should these documents be requested by regulatory agencies, outside parties with authority, and publishers. For example, a phase 1 clinical trial may take 10 years until FDA approves the drug; therefore, records need to be maintained and easily accessible if requested. The principal investigator of a study is ultimately responsible for the maintenance of the regulatory file. However, this task is often delegated to other members of the research team. OCRNs are most often assigned to perform this function.

Summary

Although creating regulatory files may seem daunting, once a process is established and clear expectations are set for document naming, it becomes a manageable part of the job. It is important to remember that these files become an invaluable and required resource and serve a number of critical functions. Most importantly, they individually and collectively permit evaluation of the conduct of a trial and the quality of the data produced.

Key Points

- OCRNs should know what documents are considered essential and file them as soon as possible.
- OCRNs should ensure that files are available during an audit or inspection and have a plan for long-term storage.
- Management of essential records and the regulatory file is not governed by regulatory agencies but is recommended per GCP guidelines and may be dictated by an institution's SOPs.
- Essential records will be produced prior to the start, throughout the duration, and after the completion of a clinical trial.
- It is acceptable to centralize some documents in a regulatory file. However, the file must include a note that states where the individual elements are available.
- All regulatory files, including source documentation with participants' personal health information, should be kept in a secure location.
- Electronic regulatory files are becoming more common as the industry moves away from reliance on paper forms. Files should be kept on a secure server with restricted access.
- Developing a standard naming convention is critical for consistency and ease in finding documents. Naming files is generally considered a challenge that is almost as difficult to determine as remembering the name of a file that was saved.
- At the time of monitoring visits, an electronic file can be shared by providing direct access to the monitors (e.g., e-regulatory binder systems), granting permission to use a secure cloud-based platform, or downloading it to a secure memory device and giving it to monitoring personnel.

The author would like to acknowledge Nicole Grant, MPH, BSN, RN, and Therese White, MSN, RN, for their contribution to this chapter that remains unchanged from the previous edition of this book.

References

Adkins, L. (2024). Best research documentation practices (GCP, GDocP, ALCOA+): Tips, tricks, and tools from a monitoring perspective. *SOCRA Source*, 2024, 15–26.

Feehan, A.K., & Garcia-Diaz, J. (2020). Investigator responsibilities in clinical research. *Ochsner Journal, 20*(1), 44–49. https://doi.org/10.31486/toj.19.0085

International Council for Harmonisation of Technical Requirements for Pharmaceuticals for Human Use. (2025). *ICH harmonised guideline: Guideline for good clinical practice: E6(R3).* https://database.ich.org/sites/default/files/ICH_E6%28R3%29_Step4_FinalGuideline_2025_0106.pdf

Investigator Reports, 21 C.F.R. § 312.64 (1987). https://www.ecfr.gov/current/title-21/chapter-I/subchapter-D/part-312/subpart-D/section-312.64

IRB Membership, 45 C.F.R. § 46.107 (2017). https://www.ecfr.gov/current/title-45/subtitle-A/subchapter-A/part-46/subpart-A/section-46.107

Office for Human Research Protections. (2024). *Investigator responsibilities FAQs.* https://www.hhs.gov/ohrp/regulations-and-policy/guidance/faq/Investigator-responsibilities/index.html

Protection of Human Subjects, 45 C.F.R. § 46 (2017). https://www.ecfr.gov/current/title-45/subtitle-A/subchapter-A/part-46

Retention Requirements for Records, 45 C.F.R. § 75.361 (2014). https://www.ecfr.gov/current/title-45/subtitle-A/subchapter-A/part-75/subpart-D/subject-group-ECFR7492b9ccc78b4d5/section-75.361

Security and Privacy, 45 C.F.R. § 164 (2000). https://www.ecfr.gov/current/title-45/subtitle-A/subchapter-C/part-164

U.S. Food and Drug Administration. (2009). *Investigator responsibilities—Protecting the rights, safety, and welfare of study subjects: Guidance for industry.* https://www.fda.gov/regulatory-information/search-fda-guidance-documents/investigator-responsibilities-protecting-rights-safety-and-welfare-study-subjects

U.S. Food and Drug Administration. (2018). *E6(R2) Good Clinical Practice: Integrated addendum to ICH E6(R1): Guidance for industry.* https://www.fda.gov/media/93884/download

CHAPTER 33

Data and Safety Monitoring Plans

Jazel Dolores Sugay, MSN, RN, OCN®

Introduction

Data and safety monitoring plans (DSMPs) are a key component of clinical research design, protecting the safety of research participants and data integrity (Wakim & Shaw, 2018). Safety monitoring plans ensure that the conduct of the trial follows the protocol, Good Clinical Practice (GCP), and applicable regulatory requirements. Research institutions are affiliated with institutional review boards (IRBs) that have specifications on monitoring the data for patient safety as described in the following Code of Federal Regulations (C.F.R.) documentation: 45 C.F.R. § 46.111(a)(6) and 21 C.F.R. § 56.111(a)(6) (Criteria for IRB Approval of Research, 2018, 2023). DSMPs may be developed by the investigator and research team, the research organization, or the clinical trial sponsor.

According to the International Conference for Harmonisation of Technical Requirements Pharmaceuticals for Human Use (ICH) publication Guideline for Good Clinical Practice E6(R3), "The sponsor should determine the appropriate extent and nature of monitoring based on identified risks. Factors such as the objective, purpose, design, complexity, blinding, number of trial participants, investigational product, current knowledge of the safety profile and end points of the trial should be considered" (ICH, 2025, p. 31).

This chapter will summarize the DSMP policy and guidance documents, the purpose of the DSMP, monitoring types, and the benefits of having a DSMP. It will also review DMC (data safety monitoring boards or committees) history, composition, responsibilities, meetings, and best practices. Finally, this chapter will discuss the role of oncology clinical research nurse (OCRNs) in safety monitoring.

Stakeholders in Data and Safety Monitoring

Communication of updated safety information among stakeholders ensures trial participant safety and minimizes and manages risks (Yao, 2013). DMCs are key stakeholders in trial oversight (see Figure 33-1 for other key stakeholders). Although every clinical trial requires oversight and monitoring, not all necessitate independent DMCs. DSMPs detail whether a protocol will use an external, independent DMC and include details on the DMC plan.

DMCs are required in trials (a) with an intervention with relatively high or unknown risk, (b) with a concern about a disease or condition with potentially serious implications, (c) conducted on a vulnerable population, (d) with

- **Clinical research sponsors**, typically pharmaceutical companies, develop the protocol, which details the safety reporting procedures and monitoring plans, as well as the informed consent form to disclose the risks associated with the investigational drug and procedures.
- **Clinical research participants** are informed of the potential risks associated with the trial, as outlined in the informed consent form. They are responsible for reporting any new adverse events they experience while participating in the trial.
- **Investigators** provide oversight and notify the institutional review board and sponsor about issues that can compromise the safety and well-being of the trial participants.
- **The institutional review board or ethics committee** has the authority to approve, disapprove, or require modifications to protocols in order to protect the rights and welfare of research participants.
- **Data safety monitoring boards or committees** are independent expert committees chartered to review data collected from the trial, confirming the continued safety of research participants and advising the sponsor on the validity and scientific merit of the trial. These boards have exclusive access to interim unblinded safety and efficacy data.
- **Regulatory authorities,** such as the U.S. Food and Drug Administration, issue guidance on the safety reporting requirements of drugs held by an Investigational New Drug application.

FIGURE 33-1 | Key Stakeholders in Clinical Trial Safety Oversight

Note. Based on information from Yao et al., 2013.

a large enough sample size that the trial may be stopped early, or (e) that are controversial. Most late-phase (3–4) and multicenter trials typically need DMCs. Early-phase (1–2), single-site, and low-risk trials may not need DMCs. Trials not using DMCs depend on the investigator, research team, or sponsor to perform monitoring functions. An institution may have standard operating procedures (SOPs) defining the requirements for the DSMP to ensure participant safety and data integrity (Wakim & Shaw, 2018).

Policy and Guidance Documents

Regulatory organizations offer guidance documents, policies, and laws to perform effective and efficient data and safety monitoring. Keeping up to date with the regulations and guidance surrounding safety monitoring is beneficial in developing monitoring plans that ensure patient safety and data integrity at all stages of the clinical trial.

U.S. Food and Drug Administration

In 2006, the U.S. Food and Drug Administration (FDA) published *Guidance for Clinical Trial Sponsors—Establishment and Operation of Clinical Trial Data Monitoring Committees* to provide recommendations to clinical trial sponsors on when to use a DMC for trial monitoring and procedures and practices to guide their operation. The guidance was revised in 2024 to *Use of Data Monitoring Committees in Clinical Trials: Guidance for Industry* and includes significant changes in DMC structure and practice because of the increased use of DMCs (whole clinical trials instead of one), longer charters, and the expansion of DMC functions into data safety review on Investigational New Drugs.

In addition to DMCs, other clinical trial oversight groups, such as IRBs, clinical trial steering committees, end point assessment and adjudication committees, and site and clinical monitoring groups, are described within the guidance. The collaboration between DMCs and these oversight groups can promote trials that produce valid, reliable, and credible results (FDA, 2024).

Systematic management of data quality can help ensure data integrity while keeping trial participants safe. In August 2013, FDA issued *Guidance for Industry: Oversight of Clinical Investigations—A Risk-Based Approach to Monitoring.* In April 2023, it released a revision, *A Risk-Based Approach to Monitoring of Clinical Investigations: Questions and Answers Guidance for Industry,* to provide more information on the implementation of risk-based monitoring.

Risk assessment should begin in the protocol design phase, with identified risks considered when developing the protocol, specifically the monitoring plan, to mitigate risks to trial participant safety and data integrity. It should then continue throughout the life cycle of the clinical trial, with monitoring plans revised as these risks are identified (FDA, 2023). This document can serve as a resource for implementing a risk-based monitoring approach in clinical trial design and conduct throughout the trial.

Clinical Trials Transformation Initiative

The Clinical Trials Transformation Initiative (CTTI) is a public–private partnership that values the improvement of the quality and efficiency of clinical trials. In 2016, the CTTI Data Monitoring Project Team, comprising representatives from across the clinical trial enterprise, released *Recommendations for Data Monitoring Committees From the Clinical Trials Transformation Initiative.* This document defines the purpose of DMCs, identifies best practices for DMC conduct, outlines effective communication practices, and provides recommendations for developing training strategies for DMC members (Calis, 2017; CTTI, 2016).

International Council for Harmonisation of Technical Requirements for Pharmaceuticals for Human Use

Released in 1996, *ICH E6(R1)* outlined the responsibilities and expectations associated with conducting clinical trial research on human participants. The Monitoring section of this document reviewed key aspects of a DSMP, including its purpose, frequency, responsibilities, procedures, methods, and reporting requirements. *ICH E6(R2)* was published in 2016 to keep pace with the increasing scale, complexity, and cost of clinical trials, as well as the evolution of technology and risk-based processes (ICH, 2016). *ICH E6(R3)* was published in 2025 and introduced a new structure for the document—a "fit for purpose" approach to the quality and design of a trial. It established new principles surrounding risk proportionality and roles and responsibilities for clinical trials and addressed technological advances in clinical trials (ICH, 2025).

ICH identifies DSMPs as a risk control strategy wherein the study sponsor identifies the plan, and the site conducting the study collects the source documentation and reports to be monitored. The 2016 revision recommended the development of a DSMP using a systematic, prioritized, risk-based approach to improve the effectiveness and efficiency of monitoring. Guidance included a selection of on-site monitoring, central (remote) monitoring, and a combination of both methods. With the increased use of central monitoring as a by-product of the COVID-19 pandemic, the 2016 revision offered additional standards for electronic data system validation through the implementation of SOPs covering data system setup, installation, use, training, and data migration (Daher, 2023; ICH, 2016). Increased standards surrounding electronic data capture help to maintain the data integrity of these studies. The 2025 revision added the consideration of decentralized clinical trials into monitoring plans. Monitoring of data or processes occurring outside the investigator site that contribute to study end points or patient safety should be addressed in the DSMP (ICH, 2025).

National Institutes of Health

The National Institutes of Health (NIH) first issued its recommendations for data safety and monitoring provisions in clinical trials in 1979. In June 1998, the NIH Policy for Data and Safety Monitoring was released, requiring all NIH-supported or conducted human research clinical trials to have oversight and monitoring to ensure patient safety and confirm the validity and integrity of data. In 2000, NIH released Further Guidance on a Data and Safety Monitoring for Phase I and Phase II Trials, adding the requirement for DMCs in NIH-supported and conducted trials based on the following (NIH, 2000):

- Assessed as more than minimal risk to the trial participants
- Likely to have early termination for safety or efficacy reasons
- Involved in phase 3 clinical trials
- For earlier phase 1–2 clinical trials
  - With multiple clinical sites
  - When blinded
  - First in human
  - When using high-risk interventions or vulnerable populations

NIH Policy 3014-203—Data and Safety Monitoring, revised in 2019, established requirements for the inclusion of DSMPs in NIH-supported protocols for nonexempt human participant research. Within the protocols, the DSMP must be described and submitted for IRB review, and the system for oversight and monitoring the conduct of clinical trials must also be included (NIH, 2019).

National Cancer Institute

The National Cancer Institute (NCI) requires a DSMP for all NCI-designated cancer centers conducting NIH-supported clinical trials (NCI, 2014). The monitoring method depends on the degree of risk for the research participants and the size and complexity of the trial. Monitoring can be performed at the research site level, the clinical trial sponsor level, or through the use of an independent DMC (NCI, 2014). NCI-designated cancer centers should check with this policy when developing DSMPs for clinical trials.

Data and Safety Monitoring Plans

Human participant research involving investigational agents or devices requires proper oversight and monitoring. Clinical trial sponsors develop monitoring plans to describe the details surrounding the scope and methods used for monitoring (FDA, 2023).

Love et al. (2022) compiled guidance documents from organizations commonly referred to when running clinical trials. The documents available from these organizations were searched for materials related to the purpose of trial monitoring. The data synthesized the purpose of clinical trial monitoring into five key principles, which can assist in creating clear monitoring guidelines and tools (Love et al., 2022):

- Keeping participants safe and respecting their rights
- Having data that can be trusted
- Making sure the trial is being run as it was meant to be
- Improving the way the trial is run
- Preventing problems before they happen

Monitoring Types

The clinical trial sponsor, research institution, or DMC can perform monitoring procedures. It is recommended that monitoring procedures have SOPs detailing staff responsibilities. A risk assessment must be performed to determine the extent and nature of monitoring required. Factors affecting risk include disease area, trial design, number of sites, study population, the type of investigational product, data management systems, and oversight mechanisms (FDA, 2023). A trial can be monitored through both on-site and off-site procedures (e.g., DMC, central monitoring). In on-site monitoring, a designated monitor (e.g., trial manager, contracted independent monitors) travels to the site where the trial is being conducted and performs data monitoring procedures. Central (e.g., remote) monitoring is a form of off-site monitoring that can be performed independently or in combination with on-site monitoring to supplement data at prespecified timepoints.

Data Monitoring Committees

Historical Perspective

The use of DMCs dates back to the 1960s, when federally run agencies (e.g., NIH, Department of Veterans Affairs) sponsored large multicenter randomized trials with the primary objectives of assessing reduced risk and improved survival of a major disease. In 1967, recommendations from an NIH external advisory group led to the establishment of a formal committee to review ongoing data, with the goal of monitoring safety, effectiveness, and trial conduct. It was not until the 1990s that DMCs in industry-sponsored clinical trials started to become more common. In combination with interim monitoring, statistical methods were being used to analyze trial data and assess safety and efficacy for trial futility (FDA, 2024).

Structure and Composition

The DSMP includes details of the DMC plan. The sponsor selects a DMC chairperson, and the sponsor or chairperson can choose the other members of the DMC. Members are individuals coming from an interprofessional background who have expertise in clinical specialties, clinical trial conduct, and statistics. Prior experience on DMCs or regulatory boards is beneficial. The number of members in a DMC is dependent on the complexity of the clinical trial but usually comprises 3–15 individuals (Wittes &

Schactman, 2014). Conflicts of interest must be disclosed when serving on a DMC, as financial or intellectual relationships with a clinical trial sponsor can alter the outcome of the trial. A DMC must exist independently of the sponsor to ensure that sponsor interests do not influence decisions, that the validity of trial conclusions is increased, and that modifications based on the DMC recommendations are made without bias (FDA, 2024).

A DMC charter is a written document that includes member selections and responsibilities, meeting information, schedules and formats, questions that the DMC will address, the processes for reporting recommendations to the sponsor, and operating procedures surrounding data review, especially unblinded data. Charters can be written by the trial sponsor or DMC members (FDA, 2024).

Responsibilities

The responsibilities of a DMC may include monitoring the following (FDA, 2024):

- Trial conduct, including enrollment, eligibility, data integrity, collaboration between site and sponsor, balance of trial arms, and site compliance with the protocol
- Safety via primary end point review, rates of adverse events, and review of serious adverse events
- Efficacy using prespecified monitoring statistical plans to guide the recommendations for early trial termination if needed
- Futility through interim data analysis
- The need for adaptations to the design of the trial

Meetings and Recommendations

An initial organizational DMC meeting can be held to review member roles and responsibilities, the charter, the protocol, and statistical analysis plans. The chairperson should be the primary point of contact with the trial sponsor; the sponsor should have minimal contact with other team members outside of meetings (Calis et al., 2017).

The timing of subsequent meetings depends on the trial's progression, level of risk, and requirements for interim analysis. Longer trials can meet every 6–12 months, whereas shorter trials can meet more often. Ad hoc meetings can also be held if a need arises due to unexpected adverse events or threats to data integrity.

DMC members convene in an open session, a closed session, or an executive session. Open sessions include the trial sponsor, leadership, and DMC members. Masked data are presented in these sessions, including recruitment status, ineligibility rate, protocol adherence, administrative data, and any other data relevant to trial monitoring (FDA, 2024; Wakim & Shaw, 2018).

Closed sessions include only the DMC members and the study statistician preparing the data for review. Statisticians are not considered members of the DMC, but statisticians who are not involved in data analysis can be members. Data relating to primary end points, safety, or futility of the trial are discussed in closed sessions (FDA, 2024; Wakim & Shaw, 2018).

Voting members of the DMC determine whether an executive session is required. Executive sessions convene after the presentation of study data and include only the chairperson and voting members. During the executive session, a discussion of the study data and any recommendations being made to the trial sponsor are presented (Wakim & Shaw, 2018).

Minutes for open and closed sessions are taken separately, and written reports to the sponsor, including any recommendations, are sent following the meeting. Recommendations from the DMC encompass their responsibilities to maintain trial conduct and ensure patient safety. An interim data review should also be considered in the recommendation for the trial to continue. Written and oral communication of the DMC recommendations, along with supporting data, should be clearly expressed to the sponsor. The sponsor decides whether to accept or reject the recommendation. Sponsors may discuss with the IRB, FDA, and other stakeholders before deciding on recommendations, as this influences patient safety. Commonly, a DMC's recommendation is to continue the trial as written; however, other possible recommendations include the following (FDA, 2024):

- Termination of the trial
- Continuation of the trial with minor or major modifications
- Suspension of trial enrollment or trial intervention
- Modification of trial population or eligibility criteria
- Modification of trial end points

External information may also be presented to the DMC when appropriate. The sponsor or steering committee must review the external data prior to the DMC review to minimize any influence it may have on study data recommendations. An example of external data is the release of unexpected safety issues in investigational drug or medical device studies.

DMC recommendations from external data consideration may include the following (FDA, 2024):

- Termination of the trial
- Termination of the trial arm or arms
- Modification of trial population, dose, and administration of study intervention
- Modification of monitoring procedures
- Concomitant medication use
- Modification of the consent form or investigator's brochure
- Issuance of a protocol letter from the sponsor to the research participants

A sponsor's decision to agree with the DMC recommendation should be communicated to the IRB, institutions conducting the study, and any regulatory authorities as needed. Any disagreements with the DMC recommendations are managed as described in the DMC charter. DMC meeting minutes (including those from closed sessions) and reports are available to the sponsor at the conclusion of the trial (Calis, 2017).

Best Practices

Because DMCs play an important role in preserving trial patient safety and data integrity of the clinical trial, recommendations on best practices for effective DMC functioning include the following (Fleming, 2017):

- Training of prospective DMC members
- Indemnification for DMC members when faced with litigation and when writing DMC charters with guiding principles instead of rigid requirements
- Independence of the DMC meetings and order of sessions from sponsor and investigator influence
- Opportunities for regulatory authorities to observe or serve on the DMC to help guide recommendations and give insight into future policy revision.

Benefits of Data and Safety Monitoring Plans

Monitoring takes on a proactive approach to patient safety evaluation. Vigilant and well-planned monitoring can also strengthen the validity and credibility of trial-produced results (Wakim & Shaw, 2018). Having a DMC independent of the sponsor removes the risk of bias and increases the validity of the trial conclusions (FDA, 2024). Using a risk-based approach in the development of monitoring plans and throughout the trial is beneficial in identifying unanticipated risks as they arise and subsequently modifying the monitoring plans to ensure that the investigation continues to protect the rights, safety, and welfare of research participants and maintain data integrity (FDA, 2023).

The Role of Oncology Clinical Research Nurses in Safety Monitoring

OCRNs can play a role in safety monitoring, from the research site level to the top of a broader oversight committee (Oncology Nursing Society & Oncology Nursing Certification Corporation, 2024).

- At the research site level, OCRNs can help develop the SOPs surrounding monitoring plans. OCRNs must also be aware of the policies surrounding the requirements for monitoring NIH and NCI trials.
- When assigned to the research team for a specific protocol, OCRNs conduct adverse event assessments on trial participants, document data collection of these events as a potential source of data verification during monitoring visits, and are responsible for protocol-specific reporting criteria for serious adverse events.
- On a broader oversight level, OCRNs can also show value as interprofessional members of the DMC. They can also review safety data for a protocol as members of the IRB.

Summary

The main goal of DSMPs is to protect patient safety and data integrity. Effective communication between key stakeholders responsible for overseeing safety monitoring will help achieve this goal. Regulatory bodies and organizations have guidance and policies available to assist in the development of DSMPs. Sponsors and research institutions may have SOPs surrounding the development and execution of monitoring plans. External DMCs are beneficial in trials with more than minimal risk because they eliminate the risk of bias and increase the validity of trial data. OCRNs can play key roles in monitoring plans that can span from data collection to membership in safety oversight committees.

Key Points

- Key stakeholders in clinical trial safety oversight must have effective communication to ensure patient safety and data integrity.
- The development of DSMPs is guided by the policies of regulatory bodies and organizations, such as FDA, CTTI, ICH, NIH and NCI.
- Safety monitoring plans are in place to ensure that trial conduct adheres to the protocol, Good Clinical Practice, and applicable regulatory requirements.
- The use of a DMC independent of the trial sponsor may reduce the risk of bias and increase the validity of trial conclusions.
- OCRNs can play key roles in safety monitoring, including the development of DSMPs, collecting trial patient data, and participating in safety committees.

The author would like to acknowledge Carol Anne Bales, MSN, RN, CCRP, and Gloria Adams, RN, CCRP, OCN®, for their contribution to this chapter that remains unchanged from the previous edition of this book.

References

Calis, K.A., Archdeacon, P., Bain, R., DeMets, D., Donohue, M., Elzarrad, M.K., ... Lewis, R.J. (2017). Recommendations for data monitoring committees from the Clinical Trials Transformation Initiative. *Clinical Trials, 14*(4), 342–348. https://doi.org/10.1177/1740774517707743

Clinical Trials Transformation Initiative. (2016, May). *CTTI recommendations: Data monitoring committees.* https://ctti-clinicaltrials.org/wp-content/uploads/2021/06/CTTI_DMC_Recs.pdf

Criteria for IRB Approval of Research, 21 C.F.R. § 56.111 (2023). https://www.accessdata.fda.gov/scripts/cdrh/cfdocs/cfcfr/CFRSearch.cfm?fr=56.111

Criteria for IRB Approval of Research, 45 C.F.R. § 46.111 (2018). https://www.hhs.gov/ohrp/humansubjects/guidance/45cfr46.html#46.111

Daher, A., Castro-Alves, J., Amparo, L., Pacheco de Moraes, N., Araújo Dos Santos, T.R., Gram Dos Santos, K.R., ... Correa Oliveira, R. (2023). A code for clinical trials centralized monitoring, sharing open-science solutions to high-quality data. *PLOS ONE, 18*(11), e0294412. https://doi.org/10.1371/journal.pone.0294412

Fleming, T.R., DeMets, D.L., Roe, M.T., Wittes, J., Calis, K.A., Vora, A.N., ... Ellenberg, S.S. (2017). Data monitoring committees: Promoting best practices to address emerging challenges. *Clinical Trials, 14*(2), 115–123. https://doi.org/10.1177/1740774516688915

International Conference for Harmonisation of Technical Requirements for Pharmaceuticals for Human Use. (2016). *ICH harmonised guideline: Integrated addendum to ICH E6(R1): Guideline for good clinical practice E6(R2).* https://database.ich.org/sites/default/files/E6_R2_Addendum.pdf

International Conference for Harmonisation of Technical Requirements for Pharmaceuticals for Human Use. (2025). *ICH harmonised guideline: Guideline for good clinical practice E6(R3).* https://database.ich.org/sites/default/files/ICH_E6%28R3%29_Step4_FinalGuideline_2025_0106.pdf

Love, S.B., Yorke-Edwards, V., Ward, E., Haydock, R., Keen, K., Biggs, K., ... Meakin, G. (2022). What is the purpose of clinical trial monitoring? *Trials, 23*(1), 836. https://doi.org/10.1186/s13063-022-06763-2

National Cancer Institute. (2014). *Policy of the National Cancer Institute for data and safety monitoring of clinical trials.* https://www.cancer.gov/research/participate/clinical-trials/safety/data-safety-monitoring.pdf

National Institutes of Health. (2019, August 30). *NIH manual chapter 3014-503 – Data and safety monitoring.* https://policymanual.nih.gov/3014-503

National Institutes of Health. (2000). *Further guidance on a data and safety monitoring for phase I and phase II trials.* https://grants.nih.gov/grants/guide/notice-files/not-od-00-038.html

Oncology Nursing Society & Oncology Nursing Certification Corporation. (2024). *Oncology clinical research nurse competencies.* https://www.ons.org/sites/default/files/2025-01/ocrn-competencies-rebrand.pdf

U.S. Food and Drug Administration. (2023, April). *A risk-based approach to monitoring of clinical investigations—Questions and answers: Guidance for industry.* https://www.fda.gov/media/121479/download

U.S. Food and Drug Administration. (2024, February). *Use of data monitoring committees in clinical trials: Guidance for industry.* https://www.fda.gov/media/176107/download

Wakim, P.G., & Shaw, P.A. (2018). Chapter 10 - Data and Safety Monitoring. In J.I. Gallin, F.P. Ognibene, & L.L. Johnson (Eds.), *Principles and practice of clinical research* (4th ed., pp. 127–140). Elsevier Academic Press. https://doi.org/10.1016/B978-0-12-849905-4.00010-1

Wittes, J., & Schactman, M. (2014). On independent data monitoring committees in oncology clinical trials. *Chinese Clinical Oncology, 3*(3), 40. https://cco.amegroups.org/article/view/3973

Yao, B., Zhu, L., Jiang, Q., & Xia, H.A. (2013). Safety monitoring in clinical trials. *Pharmaceutics, 5*(1), 94–106. https://doi.org/10.3390/pharmaceutics5010094

CHAPTER 34

Preparing for Audits, Inspections, and Monitoring Visits

Ginnette Watkins-Keller, DNP, RN, NEA-BC, OCN®

Introduction

Cancer researchers are dedicated to safeguarding the rights, safety, and welfare of the participants enrolled in their studies and ensuring that the study data collected are credible and verifiable. To do this, they must adhere to Good Clinical Practice (GCP) and document data results accurately and adequately. These data are subject to review via audits, inspections, and monitoring visits. Such reviews are conducted by federal agencies (National Cancer Institute [NCI], U.S. Food and Drug Administration [FDA], Office for Human Research Protections), sponsors (i.e., Investigational New Drug [IND] application and investigational device exemption [IDE] studies), accreditation bodies (e.g., Association for the Accreditation of Human Research Protection Programs), and internal sources (i.e., those conducted by research sites or institutions as part of a quality management program). Preparation for these reviews is fundamentally the same regardless of the format (see Figure 34-1).

This chapter will provide guidance and information for oncology clinical research nurses (OCRNs) on how to prepare for the varying types of study reviews. Additionally, it will discuss the terms and concepts associated with audits, inspections, and monitoring visits. The term *audit* will be used generically throughout this chapter for ease of reference.

Purpose of an Audit

An audit aims to ensure the trustworthiness of clinical trial data and the protection of research participants' rights, welfare, and safety (International Council for Harmonisation of Technical Requirements for Pharmaceuticals for Human Use [ICH], 2018, 2025). It differs from a routine monitoring visit, assessing the compliance and effectiveness of the study in relation to the protocol (ICH, 2018, 2025). OCRNs are crucial in ensuring the conduct of the trial, compliance with applicable regulations and guidelines (i.e., federal, state, and local), and the scientific integrity and credibility of the collected data (ICH, 2018, 2025).

Various entities may audit a clinical study site, including the study sponsor (e.g., a pharmaceutical company), a federal sponsor (e.g., NCI, U.S. Department of War), or an internal auditing group (e.g., a compliance office, a quality assurance office). Regardless of the auditing body, the purpose is the same—to ensure that the study aligns with the protocol; that research participants' rights, safety, and wel-

Audit: An independent and systematic review of trial-related activities to determine compliance with standard operating procedures, Good Clinical Practice, and applicable regulatory requirements

Routine (not-for-cause) audit/review: The review, inspection, and verification of ethical conduct in human participant research with the possibility or intention of implementing change if necessary

Directed (for-cause) audit/review: An inspection triggered when complaints are received regarding quality issues or to assess the implementation of previous corrections for violations

Monitoring: Ensures that a clinical trial complies with the protocol, standard operating procedures, Good Clinical Practice, and other applicable requirements. The sponsor's representative often conducts it.

Inspection: A formal evaluation conducted by a regulatory authority to review the documents, facilities, and records related to the clinical trial to ensure compliance with Good Clinical Practice and other applicable standards

FIGURE 34-1 | Audit and Monitoring Definitions

Note. Based on information from Coquia, 2023; International Council for Harmonisation of Technical Requirements for Pharmaceuticals for Human Use, 2018, 2025; Ness, n.d.; Ohio State University, n.d.; U.S. Food and Drug Administration, 2024c.

fare are protected; and that standard operating procedures, GCP, and applicable regulatory requirements are followed (ICH, 2018, 2025). The goals listed in Figure 34-2 apply to all audits of clinical research.

U.S. Food and Drug Administration Inspections: Routine and For Cause

FDA oversees clinical trials through the Bioresearch Monitoring Program to ensure that they are designed, conducted, analyzed, and reported in accordance with regulations and GCP guidelines (FDA, 2020b; Meeker-O'Connell, 2023). This program is a component of the FDA's preapproval process for new medicines and medical devices, performed by inspecting clinical investigators, sponsors, and institutional review boards (IRBs) to determine if they comply with FDA regulations (Coquia, 2023). These on-site inspections, remote inspections, and sometimes remote assessments—depending on the circumstances—help protect research participants from undue hazards and verify that research data supporting new human product approvals are reliable (FDA, 2010, 2023b, 2024a). A remote FDA inspection requires the facility to agree to being evaluated remotely, allowing for the transfer of records and interaction with FDA staff (FDA, 2023b).

Two types of inspections can occur: routine/surveillance (generally preannounced) and for-cause/directed (generally unannounced). Most inspections are routine, and foreign inspections are generally announced (Coquia, 2023). Routine inspections are performed (data inspections) because FDA bases important decisions on clinical data submitted as an IND or IDE. Events that could trigger a for-cause inspection include a complaint to FDA, sponsor concerns, a request from a review division within FDA, potential regulatory violations, or ongoing public health issues (Coquia, 2023).

- To ensure that research participants' rights, safety, and welfare are properly protected
- To verify the accuracy, completeness, and integrity of clinical trial data and documentation and ensure it follows the protocol, Good Clinical Practice, the site's standard operating procedures, and applicable regulatory requirements
- To ensure that local, state, and federal regulatory requirements and procedures are followed
- To provide recommendations for improvement that assist site personnel in developing useful procedures to guide research endeavors
- To identify knowledge gaps that aid in educating research staff and initiate follow-up mechanisms for problem resolution to ensure compliance, improve data quality, enhance documentation practices, promote Good Clinical Practice, and facilitate continuous improvement

FIGURE 34-2 | Audit Purposes

Note. Based on information from International Council for Harmonisation of Technical Requirements for Pharmaceuticals for Human Use, 2018, 2025.

The appropriate FDA center (e.g., Center for Drug Evaluation and Research, Center for Biologics Evaluation and Research, Center for Devices and Radiological Health) determines which clinical studies and study centers will be inspected. Although the center does not release explicit details of how it selects studies and sites for inspection, it will likely be inspected if a clinical trial is a pivotal trial used for the IND application portfolio. FDA reviewers consider the number of trial participants enrolled at a particular site, the number of participants who withdrew early, and the response rates at those sites, which can be very high or very low. The reviewers will use this information to select one or several clinical sites for inspection (FDA, 2010).

FDA staff conduct on-site inspections in accordance with the agency's compliance manuals and the *Investigations Operations Manual* (FDA, 2024c). These manuals are made available to the public to ensure transparency regarding the expectations of FDA for investigators, IRBs, and sponsors. The *Compliance Program* manual used by FDA staff when monitoring clinical investigators can be found at www.fda.gov/downloads/ICECI/EnforcementActions/BioresearchMonitoring/ucm133773.pdf, with attention paid to Part III—Inspectional (FDA, 2025a). This section instructs FDA staff to assess whether the investigator followed the protocol regarding participant selection, the number of participants enrolled, required procedures and evaluations, the administration of the investigational product, and the frequency of observations and testing to be performed during participant follow-up. Staff verifies that the investigator followed the IRB-approved protocol, submitted necessary amendments, reported adverse events promptly, obtained informed consent from every participant, administered the study drug only to those enrolled in the study, properly recorded and documented data, and reported deviations appropriately. The Clinical Investigator Inspection List, a publicly available list of the FDA deficiency codes, has been replaced with a compliance dashboard for inspections (FDA, n.d.), which shows the results of inspections with classifications of no action indicated (NAI), voluntary action indicated (VAI), and official action indicated (OAI).

Routine inspections are scheduled as follows (FDA, 2025b):

- The FDA center chooses a clinical site for inspection.
- The local FDA office nearest the site is notified that a site inspection must be scheduled.
- The local investigator contacts the site principal investigator (PI) and requests an inspection date, which can be scheduled one to two weeks prior to the contact date. However, it may be as soon as three to five days after the contact date. It is essential to ensure that a system exists for communicating information quickly so that all staff have access to the necessary information regarding the FDA inspection and can start preparing for it.

- The local inspector arrives on the agreed-upon date, presents their FDA credentials, and issues Form FDA 482: Notice of Inspection.

At the conclusion of the inspection, when an FDA investigator has observed conditions that may constitute a violation of FDA regulations, Form FDA 483: Inspectional Observations will be issued (FDA, 2024c). The *483* is the FDA inspector's report to the site of those things that, in the inspector's opinion, may include violations. Receiving a *483* does not represent the FDA's final position on the inspection; it may be overturned upon review. The *483* is used to develop an inspection report, which will include a more detailed description of the violations uncovered during the site inspection (if any) (FDA, 2020a). This report is then reviewed at the FDA center, and the inspection results will be classified in one of three ways (FDA, 2024b):

- NAI: No conditions or practices were found during the inspection.
- VAI: Conditions or practices were identified during the inspection; however, the agency does not require regulatory or administrative action.
- OAI: Conditions or practices were found during the inspection that the agency recommends regulatory or administrative actions.

Both NAI and VAI classifications result in "untitled letters," not meeting the regulatory significance of a warning letter (FDA, 2020b). The district office has 15 working days after the inspection to submit the report to the center. The center then has 15 working days from when it is issued to agree or disagree. An OAI classification typically results in the issuance of a warning letter for violations of regulatory significance; these are available under the Freedom of Information Act at www.fda.gov/ICECI/EnforcementActions/WarningLetters/default.htm (FDA, 2025c). FDA will ask the investigator to respond to the warning letter with a remedial action plan to address the compliance issues.

It is essential to consider the deadline and submit timely responses, as delays can impact the FDA's decision. Additionally, the response to the warning letter should address each observation separately, whether there is agreement or disagreement with the findings, corrective action plans and timelines for those plans, verification or monitoring of the plans, and any associated documentation of the plan (Anantha, 2019). The PI, often in conjunction with OCRNs, will develop and initiate a corrective and preventive action plan. It is essential that this plan is straightforward, demonstrates leadership commitment, and includes corrective actions to address the identified issues. The PI then submits the plan to the center within 15 working days of receiving the letter.

It will usually take the site longer to implement the plan, but FDA wants to see what is proposed and will then reinspect to assess the outcome. When violations are observed on-site during an FDA inspection, it can result in warning letters and clinical holds. In extreme cases of severe noncompliance, FDA can disqualify investigators from ever conducting FDA-regulated research again, impose fines, and possibly impose prison time on investigators and study staff (FDA, 2023a).

Investigational New Drug Application and Investigational Device Exemption Sponsors

Sponsor Audits

Sponsors sometimes conduct audits as part of their quality assurance checks (e.g., ensuring the quality performance of their study monitors), but most often, sponsor audits are performed in preparation for an FDA inspection by a drug manufacturer or pharmaceutical sponsor audit team (ICH, 2018, 2025). The auditors assist the investigational site in preparing for the inspection. The auditing team will ensure that source records are complete and well-organized and may conduct further verification of source records to identify potential problems. No data changes should be made after the study is closed. The audit team will also address site concerns and questions about the pending audit and may offer tips and suggestions on how staff should conduct themselves during the audit. An audit report is typically generated; however, the report itself is exempt from FDA review. The investigational site should not make this report available to the FDA inspector.

Sponsor Visits

The study sponsor (i.e., the IND or IDE holder) may conduct various visits as follows (ICH, 2018, 2025; Ness, n.d., 2016):

- Prestudy qualification visit
- Initiation visit
- Routine monitoring visit
- Close-out visit

Prestudy Qualification Visit

The prestudy qualification visit, which can last up to three hours and may include tours of the pharmacy, clinical, and clinical trial laboratory areas, is conducted to assess the site's suitability for conducting a clinical trial before the investigation begins (Ness, n.d.). The visit includes the PI, clinical trial staff, and OCRNs. The goal of the prestudy visit is to inspect the site, meet the staff, and assess whether the site meets the requirements for conducting the study. The sponsor must evaluate whether the PI is qualified, based on their education, experience, and training, to undertake the responsibility of conducting the study (ICH, 2018, 2025). A sponsor may choose to perform this type of visit if using a new site or a site with a good reputation that has not previously participated in a particular type of study (e.g., a phase 1 study).

Initiation Visit

The initiation visit is the sponsor's first visit to discuss aspects of the study (Peepliwal, 2023). It is conducted after all necessary legal agreements have been finalized and allows the sponsor's representatives and site staff to meet and review the following (Ness, n.d., 2016):

- Roles, responsibilities, and regulatory obligations
- Protocol procedures
- Case report form (CRF) completion instructions
- Requirements for records management and retention
- Drug handling requirements
- Review of laboratory manual
- Enrollment and consent procedures
- Adverse event reporting procedures
- Patient recruitment plan

This visit also presents an opportunity to identify and address potential problems and concerns. The PI, along with study staff, including OCRNs, will attend the initiation meeting. Preparation for the visit, as outlined in Figure 34-3, should be completed in advance to ensure a smooth visit. Initiation visits can run as long as six hours (Ness, n.d.). After the visit, the site may need to follow up with the sponsor on any outstanding issues (e.g., missing curricula vitae, missing supplies) and will also be sent a visit report, which should be placed in the protocol's regulatory file (Ness, n.d.; Peepliwal, 2023) (see Chapter 32).

- Review the protocol and any other documents received from the sponsor (e.g., case report forms and investigator's brochure).
- Become familiar with the study's procedures.
- Confirm supplies received (i.e., drugs, binders, test tubes, regulatory binder).
- Write down questions for the sponsor or contract research organization when reviewing documents.
- Secure a room or set up a remote meeting (e.g., Webex, Zoom, Microsoft Teams).
- Ensure staff availability for the visit.
- The oncology clinical research nurse can remind staff involved a few days in advance.

FIGURE 34-3 | Preparing for a Sponsor Site Initiation Visit

Note. Based on information from Ness, n.d.

Routine Monitoring Visit

The purpose of a routine monitoring visit is to ensure that the rights, safety, and welfare of clinical research participants are protected; that the data provided to the sponsors is verified, accurate, complete, and can be validated against source records; and that the conduct of the trial is in compliance with the IRB-approved protocol and relevant regulatory requirements (NCI, 2024). In addition, the sponsor must ensure that trials are adequately monitored throughout the trial and may include remote or on-site monitoring visits before, during, and after enrollment is complete (ICH, 2018, 2025).

The monitor will work with the investigator and staff to arrange a mutually agreed-upon date and time for the monitoring visit. If the visit is to be conducted on-site, a room will need to be made available to the monitor to review records and meet with research team members. If the visit is conducted remotely, study staff must ensure that the electronic health record (EHR) and any other required document access (e.g., electronic regulatory files) are available for the monitor. Additionally, some facilities may require the monitor to sign a use agreement or carry a certificate of insurance to be given access to systems, such as the EHR or electronic regulatory binder, regardless of whether the monitor is using the system on-site or remotely. The staff must ensure that all requested source records and trial-related documents are available to the monitor during the visit. Staff should remind the monitor to sign and date the site visit monitoring log at each visit (Ness, n.d.).

The monitor will review and verify that each research participant's informed consent document is executed correctly, the investigator has adequate qualifications and resources to conduct the trial, investigational products are stored and maintained appropriately, investigational products are only dispensed to eligible research participants, the investigator and staff follow the IRB-approved protocol, records are accurate and complete, events are promptly reported to the IRB and sponsor, and CRFs are accurate and complete (ICH, 2018, 2025).

The regulations do not address the timing or frequency of routine monitoring visits. The sponsor will consider the following when determining the timing and frequency (ICH, 2018, 2025):

- Protocol complexity
- Disease being studied
- Rate of recruitment
- PI and staff experience
- Site performance

FDA's guidance document, *Oversight of Clinical Investigations—A Risk-Based Approach to Monitoring,* describes various risk-based monitoring strategies focusing on critical study parameters. The guidance suggests the use of a combination of differing monitoring activities, including centralized monitoring methods, depending on the study design and monitoring strategy (FDA, 2013).

After the visit, the monitor should provide the site with a report that includes a summary of the items reviewed and statements regarding any findings, facts, deviations, deficiencies, conclusions, actions taken, and recommended actions to ensure future compliance. The report should be placed in the regulatory file (ICH, 2018, 2025).

Close-Out Visit

The close-out visit serves to perform a final review of regulatory documentation, drug accountability record forms, and record retention guidelines. This visit typically involves the PI, study staff, and OCRNs. It takes place after the study has concluded, the site's responsibilities have been met, and all data have been collected with the sponsor's database locked.

A close-out visit may occur before the study is finished in certain situations, such as if the sponsor determines that the site's enrollment was insufficient or there were numerous protocol or regulatory violations. Alternatively, the PI may request to terminate the study if they are leaving the research site and no other investigator is available to take over their responsibilities. At the close-out visit, the monitor will ensure the following (Ness, n.d):

- Confirm that all original CRFs are retrieved and queries completed.
- Destroy or return all extra CRFs.
- Review the site's regulatory binder to ensure consistency with the sponsor's master file.
- Ensure that all study supplies have been returned or properly disposed.
- Ensure that all biologic samples have been shipped or that backup samples have been destroyed.
- Ensure that the PI has provided the IRB with the final study report.

The National Cancer Institute as a Study Sponsor

As an IND sponsor, NCI follows the same regulations as other study sponsors, including those related to study monitoring and auditing. It is among the most prominent sponsors of publicly funded cancer clinical trials. Since 2014, NCI has used the National Clinical Trials Network (NCTN) to coordinate and support NCI-funded cancer clinical trials worldwide (NCI, 2019; NCI Cancer Therapy Evaluation Program [CTEP], 2025). On-site monitoring has been active since 1982 and includes all trials conducted by NCTN. NCI allows for off-site and remote monitoring and auditing. However, sites must be able to provide remote access to the EHR system and other means of communication with the NCI monitor and auditor (NCI CTEP, 2023b).

The Clinical Trials Monitoring Branch (CTMB) is responsible for on-site or remote auditing of all clinical trials sponsored by CTEP and the Division of Cancer Treatment. CTMB oversees the Clinical Trial Monitoring Service (CTMS) and the contractor who conducts the audits (e.g., Theradex®). It sets guidelines and standards for the conduct of clinical trials to ensure data quality and compliance with regulatory requirements for clinical research (NCI CTEP, 2020).

Cooperative groups (e.g., Alliance for Clinical Trials in Oncology, ECOG-ACRIN Cancer Research Group, NRG Oncology, SWOG, Children's Oncology Group) monitor trial compliance at research sites in several ways, including a central review of major elements (e.g., pathology, radiation therapy, surgery, investigational agent administration). The protocol chair reviews CRFs, and the statistical office reviews research participant eligibility and response. Data quality control software is available for data management and statistical centers to help identify and correct inconsistencies and inaccuracies in submitted data. Cooperative groups conduct their on-site audits, overseen by a combination of central staff and group members, with direct oversight by CTMB. Typically, a CTMB staff member will attend NCI audits. On-site or remote audits are conducted, on average, once every three years or more frequently for high-accruing sites (NCI CTEP, 2023a).

For early-phase CTEP studies, protocol compliance is assessed by CTMS. Research sites conducting phase 0 (exploratory IND), phase 1, and early phase 2 studies submit data to CTMS on an ongoing basis (i.e., every two weeks). CTMS reviews data carefully for compliance with the protocol and requests clarifications if data are missing or do not appear to flow logically. Reports are provided periodically to the investigator and CTEP. According to the CTMS monitoring guidelines, contractors (e.g., Theradex) conduct on-site visits three times per year, consisting of two data visits and one annual review (NCI CTEP, 2023b). For more information on CTEP early-phase study monitoring, see *NCI Guidelines for Monitoring the Experimental Therapeutics Clinical Trials Network* (ETCTN) *and Other Early Phase CTMS-Monitored Studies* (NCI CTEP, 2025b).

When reporting results, NCI auditors use the ratings "Acceptable," "Acceptable Needs Follow-Up," or "Unacceptable." If the results are rated less than acceptable, the institution must provide a written response, including corrective actions, to ensure future compliance. Auditors have various action options when dealing with problems identified during on-site audits. In most cases, the measures are intended to be constructive and educational. However, the action options can include probation, issuance of a warning letter, suspension of patient enrollment privileges, repeat audits, removal of access to investigational agents, or termination of a grant or contract (NCI CTEP, 2023a, 2023b).

Internal Audits at the Investigational Site

Large research sites often have an office dedicated to clinical trial management, with an internal protocol compliance component. These offices are established to support investigators with regulatory submissions, data management, and study coordination and serve as a compliance safeguard for the institution. Community hospitals and private practices may hire independent auditors to monitor compliance. Because many entities may audit a clinical study site, it makes sense to have personnel dedicated to assisting with the numerous outside audits conducted annually and to perform internal audits of trials that do not undergo routine auditing (i.e., investigator-initiated trials). Such a protocol compliance group would focus on educating site faculty and staff on the local, state, and federal regulations governing their clinical research. This group would also serve as the primary point of contact for addressing compliance-related questions. Oversight of the clinical trials office would be performed by an institutional administrator or by a medical director.

Typically, any of the research site's protocols are subject to an internal audit conducted by the protocol compliance group. Most audit programs use a risk-based approach and are often described in the data safety monitoring plan for the site. Some factors considered when developing an audit plan may include the complexity of the study design, the study end points, the number of sites of the study, the study population (e.g., seriously ill, vulnerable), and the experience level of the PI (FDA, 2013).

An example of how a program could function is as follows:

A protocol is chosen for audit, and then a representative number of trial participant cases are reviewed (e.g., 10% of all enrolled trial participants). The associated regulatory documents are also subject to audit. After the audit, an audit report is generated and distributed to study personnel and the protocol PI. A point-by-point response to the audit report is submitted to the office, and a general corrective action plan is implemented to prevent any mistakes from being repeated.

Education is the key to these internal audits. Focusing on the positive aspects of the study conduct is essential, and correcting problems before they become routine is critical.

Human Research Protection Program Audits

Many IRB offices have independent quality assurance teams that conduct routine or random audits of approved research protocols to ensure the protection of research participants, compliance, and integrity of studies (Rutgers University Office for Research, 2025). This is due in part to the Association for the Accreditation of Human Research Protection Programs' accreditation requirements, which exceed the requirements of international laws and guidelines overseeing the protection of humans in research (Rutgers University Office for Research, 2024; Seda, 2023). Quality assurance teams work with the IRB staff and institutional officials to promote and maintain ethical research conduct and compliance with state and federal regulations, federal guidance, institutional policies, and best practices for human research protection (Rutgers University Office for Research, 2025). The quality assurance teams evaluate and improve human protection and Human Research Protection Program activities through oversight, monitoring, and educational initiatives.

Routine reviews, generally performed at the investigator's site, include a review of research documentation, a tour of the study's facilities, and a review of study-related procedures. Information is gathered through interviews, observations, and review of records. Study selection for routine reviews may be random or based on particular research aspects (e.g., special populations, risk level, investigational drugs, devices) and typically draws from a list of all active protocols. Any study involving research participants, including medical and nonmedical studies, may be selected for review. At the end of the review, an exit interview is conducted with the study team, including the PI and OCRNs. During this interview, the findings are discussed, and the study staff can ask questions or clarify any points. A report of the findings is reviewed by the IRB, typically at a full board meeting, and a decision, such as no further action, a clarification memo, or a debriefing memo with a corrective action plan, is sent back to the study chair (Rutgers University Office for Research, 2024).

How to Prepare for an Audit

Auditors prepare for an audit by reviewing the protocol, the site's internal standard operating procedures, applicable regulations, and sponsor guidelines. These preparations ensure the informed and efficient use of time and resources and certify an audit result that enhances site staff knowledge and compliance. Similarly, the research team must also prepare for an audit to facilitate the visit and, ideally, achieve a positive audit outcome. Once the research team has been notified of an upcoming audit, they should follow the steps outlined in Figure 34-4. To prepare for the audit, the research team should have the following readily available: regulatory

- Determine the nature (i.e., for-cause, routine) and the scope of the audit. What protocols will be reviewed? How long will the auditors be on-site?
- Notify all parties (as applicable) when initially contacted so that each can prepare for the visit, as necessary (e.g., the investigational pharmacy, the institutional review board, and all research team members).
- Obtain pertinent audit information such as the number of auditors who will conduct the audit, the approximate times the auditors will work each day, whether an exit interview will occur after the audit, and, if so, who will be required to attend.
- Follow the institution's standard operating procedures.
- If the audit is to be done on-site, schedule a quiet room with enough space to accommodate the auditors comfortably. The room should ideally be located near a copier and a restroom. A computer should also be made available for the auditors to view online medical records, x-rays and other imaging results, online protocol versions, consent documents, and data forms. If more than one sponsor is auditing simultaneously, it may be necessary to secure two rooms to prevent disclosing any confidential or proprietary information.
- If the audit is performed remotely, ensure that auditors have access to all necessary items (e.g., electronic health records, eRegulatory files) well in advance of the visit. Set up an initial meeting and an end-of-audit meeting (e.g., Webex, Zoom, Microsoft Teams) and invite all applicable staff members to those meetings (e.g., principal investigator, study team, oncology clinical research nurse, pharmacy).
- Allow access to all study-related areas and participants' medical records, including inpatient, outpatient, and physician's office records. Sites using electronic health records must understand how monitors access relevant records online and obtain the necessary permissions in advance. Alternatively, they can print all desired participant records.
- Study staff should pre-review all research records (medical and regulatory) for any missing documentation.
- If time allows, conduct an internal data review with the assistance of the research team before the audit.

FIGURE 34-4 | Preparing for an Audit

Note. Based on information from Ness, n.d.

files, informed consent documents, drug accountability records, and research participant records. Additionally, if the audit is to be conducted remotely, it is essential to ensure that the auditors have access to the EHR and any other necessary electronic resources to complete the audit remotely.

Regulatory Files

The regulatory files are reviewed to ensure that regulatory compliance is appropriately maintained throughout the study. They should be current, organized, complete, and accurate to facilitate the review of the regulatory documents. The files should contain all versions of the protocol and consent documents, including a copy of the initially approved protocol. The file should also contain all IRB correspondence (to and from the IRB), IRB-approved materials, and associated submissions (including the initial protocol and consent forms, amendments, and annual continuing reviews), along with the IRB roster and meeting minutes, as applicable. The file should include adverse event reports, along with evidence that these events were correctly reported to the IRB and the sponsor. Also contained in the file is a sponsor correspondence section (to and from the sponsor) (FDA, 2010; ICH, 2018, 2025; Ness, 2016). Refer to Chapter 32 for more information on maintaining a regulatory file.

Informed Consent Documents

All IRB-approved consent versions will be reviewed to verify that they contain all required elements of informed consent as mandated by 45 Code of Federal Regulations (C.F.R.) § 46.116 (General Requirements of Informed Consent, 2017) and 21 C.F.R. § 50.25 (Elements of Informed Consent, 1981). The auditors will review the consent versions to ensure that they reflect the appropriate risks, tests, and procedures for each version period. Original signed informed consent documents will be reviewed to verify that all blanks (i.e., dates and signatures) have been properly completed and that an informed consent document exists for each participant enrolled in the study. The auditors will ask the investigator and research team, including OCRNs, questions about the consent process to ensure that participants are properly informed, such as the following (FDA, 2010; ICH, 2018, 2025):

- Were patients introduced to the concept of clinical trials and then presented with all available treatment options, including research participation?
- Was consent obtained prior to the initiation of any research-related procedures?
- Was a copy of the consent given to the participant to take home?
- Was the entire consent process documented in the patient's medical record?
- Was a revised consent signed when new information became available that might affect the participant's willingness to participate in the trial?
- Was the correct version of the consent used for the appropriate time frame?

Drug Accountability Records

Accountability records for investigational agents, as well as for any other drugs supplied by the sponsor for the trial, will be subject to audit (FDA, 2010; ICH, 2018, 2025). The investigational pharmacist should be notified of any pending audit, as the auditors will most likely visit the pharmacy, either on-site or remotely.

Drug accountability records, often referred to as drug accountability record forms, are compared to shipment records to ensure that the drugs were properly received and logged at the site. If products were transferred from one office to another or were shipped back to the sponsor, those records will be compared to verify product accountability. A research participant registration log should correlate with the drug dispensing records. The auditor must ensure that all enrolled participants received the proper drug and dosage from the appropriate shipment, as per the protocol, and, conversely, that no patient other than those registered for the trial received study-supplied products. The auditor must verify that commercial supplies and investigational supplies are used appropriately and not interchanged.

The auditor will visit the pharmacy to ensure that the location is secure and that access to the area is restricted to authorized personnel only. If investigational products are present in the pharmacy at the time of the audit, the auditor will count the remaining drugs to confirm the amount indicated on the inventory records (Ness, n.d.).

Trial Participant Records

The auditor will compare the data collection forms (e.g., CRFs, serious adverse event report forms) or, if using remote data entry, sponsor-supplied data printouts against the participant's medical records (both inpatient and outpatient) to verify reporting accuracy and that no omissions occurred in the reported data. This document review enables the auditor to assess how well the research staff adhered to the protocol requirements: Were the proper tests ordered and obtained? Were adverse events reported and in a timely fashion? Specifically, the following will be reviewed in detail (FDA, 2010; ICH, 2018, 2025):

- Trial participant enrollment procedures: Was the first trial participant enrolled after IRB approval?
- Trial participant selection: Was each trial participant eligible for the trial?
- Informed consent
- Trial participant data
  - Inclusion and exclusion criteria
  - Protocol treatment administration records: Were treatments held or modified as required by the protocol?
  - Tumor response: Was the response documented at the appropriate timepoints and using the methods outlined in the protocol?

- Toxicities and adverse events: Were they reported appropriately (e.g., to the sponsor, IRB) as required by the protocol?
- Laboratory results
- Reasons for trial participant withdrawal
- Follow-up data

Close-Out Meeting

A close-out meeting is typically held with the research team, including the protocol PI, the regulatory coordinator, OCRNs, study coordinators, and the data manager. Positive audit findings should be highlighted at this meeting, and any deficiencies discovered will be discussed. The research team needs to take notes and write down suggestions made to develop a meaningful and informed audit response later. The auditor may suggest corrective actions or wait until input from the sponsor, IRB, or agency is obtained to include it in the audit report. The auditor may also provide the PI, OCRNs, and other members of the research team with a written summary of findings or missing materials before leaving the site and will subsequently send a more formal written follow-up. The PI and the research team must respond to any report generated by addressing all audit findings.

Summary

Audits, inspections, and monitoring visits are essential to ensure that the data generated during a clinical trial are reliable, all relevant regulations governing clinical trials are adhered to, and participants' rights, safety, and welfare are protected. Regardless of their names or classifications, these should be considered educational tools that educate research teams on the proper and ethical conduct of clinical trials. The ultimate goal of oncology clinical research should be to ensure the rights of human research participants, generate meaningful data, and conduct clinical trials ethically, all while striving to find treatments that will ultimately improve the lives of patients with cancer and those at high risk of developing cancer.

Key Points

- Preparation for all types of on-site or remote visits (e.g., audits, inspections, monitoring visits) is essentially the same.
- Multiple entities, such as the FDA, study sponsor, or internal auditor, may conduct an audit.
- Auditor and research team preparation before the visit leads to the most effective encounter.
- For-cause audit findings require the research team to provide specific responses and implement any necessary corrective actions to ensure future compliance with applicable regulations.

The author would like to acknowledge Ellen A. Patricia, MS, CIP, and Sandra A. Meadows, MPH, CIP, for their contribution to this chapter that remains unchanged from the previous edition of this book.

References

Anantha, M. (2019). Are you ready to handle an FDA Form 483? *Association of Clinical Research Professionals.* https://acrpnet.org/2019/11/21/are-you-ready-to-handle-an-fda-form-483

Coquia, S.F. (2023). *Clinical investigator site inspections—What to expect* [PowerPoint slides]. U.S. Food and Drug Administration Clinical Investigator Training Course. https://www.fda.gov/media/175400/download?attachment

Elements of Informed Consent, 21 C.F.R. § 50.25 (1981). https://www.ecfr.gov/current/title-21/chapter-I/subchapter-A/part-50/subpart-B/section-50.25

General Requirements of Informed Consent, 45 C.F.R. § 46.116 (2017). https://www.ecfr.gov/current/title-45/subtitle-A/subchapter-A/part-46/subpart-A/section-46.116

International Council for Harmonisation of Technical Requirements for Pharmaceuticals for Human Use. (2018). *E6(R2) Good clinical practice: Integrated addendum to ICH E6(R1).* https://www.fda.gov/media/93884/download

International Council for Harmonisation of Technical Requirements for Pharmaceuticals for Human Use. (2025). *ICH harmonised guideline: Guideline for good clinical practice: E6(R3).* https://database.ich.org/sites/default/files/ICH_E6%28R3%29_Step4_FinalGuideline_2025_0106.pdf

Meeker-O'Connell, A. (2023). *Integrating quality into clinical trials* [PowerPoint slides]. U.S Food and Drug Administration Clinical Investigator Training Course. https://www.fda.gov/media/175399/download?attachmentd

National Cancer Institute. (2019). *NOCRN: NCI's National Clinical Trials Network.* https://dctd.cancer.gov/research/networks

National Cancer Institute. (2024). *Clinical research coordinator orientation and resource manual.* https://ccrod.cancer.gov/confluence/download/attachments/69992615/CRC%20Orientation%20and%20Resource%20Manual%20Final%2020260326%20.pdf?version=1&modificationDate=1726252266753&api=v2

National Cancer Institute Cancer Therapy Evaluation Program. (2020). *Clinical trials monitoring branch (CTMB).* https://ctep.cancer.gov/branches/ctmb/default.htm

National Cancer Institute Cancer Therapy Evaluation Program. (2023a). *NCI guidelines for auditing clinical trials for the NCI National Clinical Trials Network (NCTN) program including NCI Community Oncology Research Program (NCORP) and NCORP research bases.* https://ctep.cancer.gov/branches/ctmb/clinicalTrials/docs/NOCRN_Auditing_Guidelines.pdf

National Cancer Institute Cancer Therapy Evaluation Program. (2023b). *NCI guidelines for monitoring the Experimental Therapeutics Clinical Trials Network (ETOCRN) and other early phase CTMS-monitored studies.* https://ctep.cancer.gov/branches/ctmb/clinicalTrials/monitoring_etOCRN_ctms.htm

National Cancer Institute Cancer Therapy Evaluation Program. (2025a). *Brief overview of NCI's National Clinical Trials Network.* https://ctep.cancer.gov/initiativesPrograms/nOCRN.htm

National Cancer Institute Cancer Therapy Evaluation Program. (2025b). NCI guidelines for monitoring the Experimental Therapeutics Clin*ical Trials Network (ETCTN) and other early phase CTMS-monitored studies.* https://dctd.cancer.gov/research/ctep-trials/for-sites/etctn-monitoring.pdf

Ness, E. (n.d.). *Monitoring and auditing of clinical trials* [PowerPoint slides]. https://ccrod.cancer.gov/confluence/download/attachments/71041052/Monitoring_auditing.pdf

Ness, E. (2016, February 29). *Quality management in clinical research* [Video]. YouTube. https://youtu.be/5e7hwmaauS4?si=IGUE_NPun8xqxL_9

Ohio State University. (n.d.). *Audits.* https://ccts.osu.edu/content/audits

Peepliwal, A.K. (2023). *Clinical trial project management.* Elsevier Science and Technology. https://shop.elsevier.com/books/clinical-trial-project-management/peepliwal/978-0-443-13627-6

Rutgers University Office for Research. (2024). *Investigator manual: A guide to human research protection in research 1.002 (HRP-103).* https://research.rutgers.edu/sites/default/files/2025-01/1-002-hrp-103-sop-investigator-manual-a-guide-to-hrpp.pdf

Rutgers University Office for Research. (2025). *HRPP Quality Assurance Team.* https://research.rutgers.edu/faculty-staff/compliance/human-research-protection/hrpp-quality-assurance-team

Seda, M. (2023, January 6). *Rutgers earns prestigious accreditation from the Association for the Accreditation of Human Research Protection Programs.* https://research.rutgers.edu/news/rutgers-earns-prestigious-accreditation-association-accreditation-human-research-protection

U.S. Food and Drug Administration. (n.d.). *Inspections.* https://datadashboard.fda.gov/oii/cd/inspections.htm

U.S. Food and Drug Administration. (2010). *Information sheet guidance for IRBs, clinical investigators, and sponsors: FDA inspections of clinical investigators.* https://www.fda.gov/media/75185/download

U.S. Food and Drug Administration. (2013). *Oversight of clinical investigations—A risk-based approach to monitoring.* https://www.fda.gov/regulatory-information/search-fda-guidance-documents/oversight-clinical-investigations-risk-based-approach-monitoring

U.S. Food and Drug Administration. (2020a). *Compliance program guidance manual.* https://www.fda.gov/media/75927/download

U.S. Food and Drug Administration. (2020b). *FDA bioresearch monitoring information.* https://www.fda.gov/inspections-compliance-enforcement-and-criminal-investigations/compliance-actions-and-activities/fda-bioresearch-monitoring-information

U.S. Food and Drug Administration. (2023a). *Inspection questions and answers.* https://www.fda.gov/inspections-compliance-enforcement-and-criminal-investigations/inspection-basics/inspection-questions-and-answers

U.S. Food and Drug Administration. (2023b). *Remote interactive evaluations of drug manufacturing and bioresearch monitoring facilities.* https://www.fda.gov/regulatory-information/search-fda-guidance-documents/remote-interactive-evaluations-drug-manufacturing-and-bioresearch-monitoring-facilities

U.S. Food and Drug Administration. (2024a). *Conducting remote regulatory assessments: Questions and answers–draft guidance for industry.* https://www.fda.gov/media/160173/download

U.S. Food and Drug Administration. (2024b). *Inspections database frequently asked questions.* https://www.fda.gov/inspections-compliance-enforcement-and-criminal-investigations/inspection-references/inspections-database-frequently-asked-questions#classification

U.S. Food and Drug Administration. (2024c). *Types of FDA inspections.* https://www.fda.gov/inspections-compliance-enforcement-and-criminal-investigations/inspection-basics/types-fda-inspections

U.S. Food and Drug Administration. (2025a). *Chapter 48: Bioresearch monitoring.* https://www.fda.gov/media/75909/download

U.S. Food and Drug Administration. (2025b). *Investigations operations manual 2025.* https://www.fda.gov/media/166525/download?attachment

U.S. Food and Drug Administration. (2025c). *Warning letters.* https://www.fda.gov/inspections-compliance-enforcement-and-criminal-investigations/compliance-actions-and-activities/warning-letters

SECTION VIII. Professional Development for Oncology Clinical Research Nurses

CHAPTER 35

Oncology Clinical Research Nurse Education

Rita Musanti, PhD, APN-BC, AOCNP®

Introduction

Oncology clinical research nurses (OCRNs) practice in a complex environment that requires knowledge, skills, and abilities to care for research participants and to coordinate and execute a clinical trial on behalf of a principal investigator (Kunhunny & Salmon, 2017; Xing et al., 2024). The pathway to attaining these necessary traits and competently performing the OCRN role is usually traversed through on-the-job training and short professional development courses, often offered by an OCRN's employer (Scott et al., 2013). Professional practice educational scope and standards throughout the history of the literature, such as those from the American Nurses Association (ANA) and the Oncology Nursing Society (ONS), emphasize that the registered nurse "seeks knowledge and competence that reflects current nursing practice and promotes futuristic thinking" (ANA, 2021; Lubejko & Wilson, 2019, p. 58).

This chapter will identify various professional development activities and resources for OCRNs and provide a tool for tracking educational activities.

Futuristic Thinking for Oncology Clinical Research Nurses

Futuristic thinking is embedded in clinical trial research, and OCRNs gain an understanding of advances in research methodology, drug development, and participant care through trial-specific educational sessions offered or mandated by trial sponsors (Scott et al., 2013). OCRNs must stay informed about socioeconomic, cultural, and ethical developments related to nursing and research professional practice, as these also impact participant care and the execution of protocols. For example, an update to the 2011 Institute of Medicine (now the National Academy of Medicine) report, *The Future of Nursing 2020–2030: Charting a Path to Achieve Health Equity,* emphasized the need for nurses to be prepared to address social determinants of health and achieve health equity (Hassmiller & Wakefield, 2022).

This focus on awareness and competence to promote health equity is consistent with the U.S. Food and Drug Administration's position of increasing participant diversity in clinical trials as a key component to advancing health equity (Hassmiller & Wakefield, 2022; U.S. Food and Drug Administration, 2020). The commitment to maintaining current competencies and clinical knowledge reflects the expectation that OCRNs engage in lifelong learning. This includes regularly evaluating their practice in alignment with national and ONS professional standards, state nurse practice acts, relevant regulatory requirements, and role-specific performance expectations.

Likewise, the ANA (2021) education competency (Standard 13. Standards of Professional Practice) addresses the nurse's need to identify areas for learning and personal growth through self-reflection, communication and shared experiences and ideas with peers, and maintenance of records to support learning activities. The assessment of learning needs is tied to the OCRN's role definition, which can vary widely depending on the worksite (McCabe & Ness, 2021). The *Oncology Clinical Research Nurse Competencies* were developed to define the OCRN role and provide a model for orientation and continuing education (ONS & Oncology Nursing Certification Corporation [ONCC], 2024). A joint publication by ANA and ONS in 2010, this documentation was updated in 2024 by ONS and ONCC.

The OCRN Competency Model Framework is based on the well-established concept that skill acquisition evolves and that structured and targeted education, lived experiences, self-evaluation, as well as peer, preceptor, or mentor support move an individual from novice to expert (Benner, 1982; Dreyfus & Dreyfus, 1980). Role-related behaviors are defined through nine domains (ONS & ONCC, 2024; see Figure 35-1).

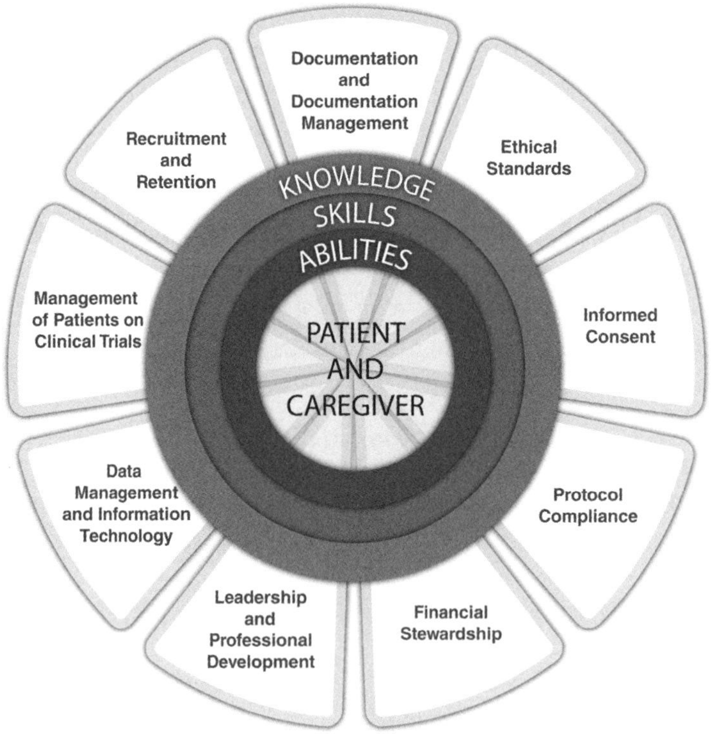

FIGURE 35-1 | Oncology Clinical Research Nurse Competency Model Framework

Note. From *Oncology Clinical Research Nurse Competencies* (p. 6), by Oncology Nursing Society & Oncology Nursing Certification Corporation, 2024. https://www.ons.org/sites/default/files/2025-01/ocrn-competencies-rebrand.pdf. Copyright 2024 by Oncology Nursing Society. Reprinted with permission.

The model identifies behaviors that start at level 1 and progress to level 2. The competency for specific domains inherent in the OCRN role is outlined in the competency document. It can be used for self-evaluation purposes and in the design of curricula for OCRN orientation and continuing education. OCRN professional education aligned with these competencies will advance the standardization of the role, foster recognition of its contributions, and facilitate the development of career pathways.

Professional Development for Oncology Clinical Research Nurses

Various formal and informal learning activities are available to promote the professional development of OCRNs. Such activities can be simple (e.g., reading professional journals) or complex (e.g., preparing a manuscript for publication, completing a certificate or master's program in clinical research management or regulatory compliance). OCRNs must stay current with practice and research trends by reading the relevant literature. Recommendations for journals of interest are listed in Figure 35-2. Each journal offers the reader a range of topics related to oncology and clinical research.

New digital technologies have enabled nursing professionals to access additional learning resources (see Table 35-1). Several agencies have developed electronic mailing lists that deliver real-time updates of federal regulations and guidelines, such as the U.S. Food and Drug Administration (www.fda.gov/drugs) and the U.S. Department of Health and Human Services Office for Human Research Protections (www.hhs.gov/ohrp/education-and-outreach/index.html).

Oncology Nursing Focus	Clinical Research Focus
• *Cancer Nursing* • *Clinical Journal of Oncology Nursing* • *European Journal of Oncology Nursing* • *Journal of Clinical Oncology* • *Journal of Gynecologic Oncology Nursing* • *Journal of Pediatric Oncology Nursing* • *Journal of the Advanced Practitioner in Oncology* • *Oncology Nursing Forum* • *Seminars in Oncology Nursing*	• *Applied Clinical Trials* • *Clinical and Translational Science* • *Clinical Research Practitioner* • *Clinical Trials: Journal of the Society for Clinical Trials* • *Contemporary Clinical Trials* • *Journal of Clinical Research Best Practices* • *SOCRA Source* • *The Monitor*

FIGURE 35-2 | Recommended Journals

TABLE 35-1 | Categories of Learning Technology

Type of Technology	Description
Artificial intelligence	Artificial intelligence can include educational games, adaptive learning platforms, chatbots, and intelligent tutoring systems. It provides individualized support for learners and program planning for educators.
Augmented reality (AR) and virtual reality (VR)	This emerging technology creates an immersive experience that can be used in simulation and experiential learning, allowing nurses to practice tasks and engage in simulations for skill development.
Cloud computing	Cloud computing uses the internet to access software and information, eliminating the need for local storage of resources. This technology enables on-demand access to information and facilitates hyperlinking, allowing for improved cross-referencing and access to information.
E-learning	E-learning refers to the delivery of educational activities via electronic means. It removes barriers of time and space compared to a traditional classroom setting, improving access to on-the-job and just-in-time learning, as well as formal certificate- or degree-granting educational programs. E-learning creates a more personalized learning experience and can be provided synchronously, where all parties are on audio or video at the same time, or asynchronously, where individuals with access can view or listen at any time.
Video and multimedia	Video-enabled smart devices and high-speed internet connections can transmit educational content, engage nurses as they learn, foster peer-to-peer communication, and help nurses understand complex concepts and ideas. It includes social media platforms.

Professional Associations and Organizations

Professional oncology associations and research organizations hold annual conferences that feature educational activities covering a broad range of topics, in addition to regional and e-learning educational opportunities (see Table 35-2). OCRNs can enhance their professional development by submitting an abstract for an oral or poster presentation at an annual conference. Conference websites often provide details about the event and information related to abstract submission, including deadlines. For more information about abstract and poster development, see Chapter 37.

Academic and Certificate Programs

Highly trained research professionals are in high demand in the expanding clinical research environment, leading to the development of various graduate and certification programs. Some programs are offered in schools

TABLE 35-2 | Professional Research Organizations for Oncology Clinical Research Nurses

Organization	Description	Educational Opportunities
Association of Clinical Research Professionals www.acrpnet.org	Established in 1976 to provide educational and networking opportunities for research nurses and others who support clinical research and development More than 16,500 global members	• Annual meeting in the spring • Classroom courses • E-learning courses • Home study • Webinars
International Association of Clinical Research Nurses www.iacrn.org	Established in 2007 Defines, validates, and advances clinical research nursing More than 1,500 members with 50 chapters worldwide	• Annual meeting • Certification • E-learning courses • Home study • Webinars
Society of Clinical Research Associates www.socra.org	Provides educational programs and a forum for research professionals to exchange information More than 13,700 members from several countries	• Annual meeting in the fall • Classroom courses • E-learning courses

Note. Based on information from Association of Clinical Research Professionals, 2025; International Association of Clinical Research Nurses, n.d.; Society of Clinical Research Associates, 2025.

of nursing, whereas others are offered through schools of health science. Several programs are also available outside of the United States. The best way to find a program is to perform an internet search using the phrase "clinical research management program" and provide the country of interest (Ness et al., 2012). Most programs offer distance learning options, with average requirements of 32–36 credits for a master's degree and 12–15 semester units for a certificate.

Specialty Certification

Certification is the formal process that validates that an individual is competent in a given field. It is attained by application to a certifying body, such as ONS. The applicant must meet specific criteria in order to be certified, such as proof of degree-granting and continuing education, experience in the field, and achievement of passing scores on tests of knowledge, skills, and abilities.

When considering certification, OCRNs can pursue several paths, such as academic degrees, certification programs, and organization-based certification programs. Most commonly, clinical research–specific certification is obtained from a non-nursing professional research organization, such as the Association of Clinical Research Professionals (2025) or the Society of Clinical Research Associates (2025). Eligibility requirements for applying and maintaining these certifications include a comprehensive résumé and a current job description. Unique requirements exist for those who hold a college degree in clinical research or a related field. Both organizations have membership requirements and associated costs for initial and maintenance submissions.

ONCC (www.oncc.org) does not offer a certification for the OCRN role; however, it does offer certifications that validate subspecialty practice in general and advanced oncology nursing (Oncology Certified Nurse [OCN®] and Advanced Oncology Certified Nurse Practitioner [AOCNP®]; Advanced Oncology Certified Nurse [AOCN®; renewal only]), pediatric hematology (Certified Pediatric Hematology Oncology Nurse [CPHON®]; Certified Pediatric Oncology Nurse [CPON®; renewal only]), breast care nurse (Certified Breast Cancer Nurse [CBCN®]), blood and marrow transplant (Blood and Marrow Transplant Certified Nurse [BMTCN®]), and advanced oncology clinical nurse specialist (Advanced Oncology Certified Clinical Nurse Specialist [AOCNS®; renewal only]).

OCRNs must engage in professional development activities to support their lifelong learning journey and plan for certificate renewals. ONCC's Individual Learning Needs Assessment process enables nurses to identify learning needs and earn points through professional development activities. Using the LearningBuilder platform (www.oncc.org/what-learningbuilder), nurses can complete and submit a learning plan as part of a certification renewal via continuing education and practice hours or retesting. More information on ONCC is available online (www.oncc.org/sites/default/files/2025-01/RenewalManualEffective2025.pdf).

The International Association of Clinical Research Nurses (www.iacrn.org) offers the only nurse-specific certification (Clinical Research Nurse Certification Council, 2022). Eligibility requirements are submitted as a portfolio that includes validation of 4,000 hours within the OCRN role, 36 hours of continuing education over three years, and 50 points of professional activities, such as poster presentations, publications, and academic courses.

Educating Other Nurses

Sharing knowledge and expertise with another nurse or student is the responsibility of the professional nurse (ANA, 2021). This is often performed through precepting a student in an academic program or a new hire in an orientation program. Even an experienced oncology nurse who transitions to the role of an OCRN may feel like a novice and require a preceptor. Resources for the orientation of OCRNs are available at the ONS Communities website (www.ons.org/network-advocacy/member-connections/ons-communities). Mentoring can provide a valuable experience for both the mentor and mentee.

Professional Portfolio

A professional portfolio is a collection of significant information that demonstrates professional competencies and accomplishments. It provides visual support to acknowledge and assess an individual's professional skills, knowledge, and attitude. A portfolio either demonstrates best work (i.e., evidence of competence and expertise) or growth and development (i.e., monitor and guide personal and professional goals). A portfolio needs to be succinct, clear, and dynamic; it grows as the individual's career grows and requires ongoing maintenance. A two- to three-inch, three-ring binder with clear sheet protectors can be used to store materials as the professional gains experience (Caplan, et.al, 2013). Portfolios can be maintained electronically; several software programs are available and can be found by searching the keyword "e-portfolio software" online. Figure 35-3 provides an example of portfolio content and organization.

Summary

Becoming a lifelong learner is a key component of professional development standards for nursing. Remaining current in professional practice enables nurses to provide safe, evidence-based care in an ever-changing healthcare environment. Being abreast of policy and healthcare regulations, as well as new technologies, allows nursing to contribute to the design of healthcare systems that are equitable and resource-aligned for all patients.

Section 1: Introduction
- Résumé/curriculum vitae
- Copies of licenses and certifications
- Photo
- School transcripts/internships
- Career trajectories
- Mentor/mentee relationships

Section 2: Showcase Professional Accomplishments
- Evidence-based practice projects
- Research
- Sample presentations
- Sample publications
- Committee membership and activities
- Professional society memberships and accomplishments
- Professional development logs
- Awards

Section 3: Complimentary
- Accolades
- Thank-you letters
- Recommendations

Section 4: Volunteer Service
- Professional organization membership and activities
- Community service
- Photos
- News clippings

FIGURE 35-3 | Sample Content for a Professional Portfolio

Note. Based on information from Shirey, 2009; Smith, 2011.

Key Points

- Nurses are lifelong learners.
- OCRNs are uniquely positioned to identify and assess learning needs in both oncology and clinical research.
- OCRNs can access professional practice learning opportunities through local, regional, and international venues, both in person and virtually.
- Maintaining a professional development log enables OCRNs to track and assess their professional development activities, supporting their lifelong learning journey.
- Maintaining a portfolio allows OCRNs to document their professional journey.

The author would like to acknowledge Elizabeth Ness, MS, RN, for her contribution to this chapter that remains unchanged from the previous edition of this book.

References

American Nurses Association. (2021). *Nursing: Scope and standards of practice* (4th ed.). https://www.nursingworld.org/practice-policy/scope-of-practice

Association of Clinical Research Professionals. (2025). *ACRP certification.* https://acrpnet.org/certification

Benner, P. (1982). From novice to expert. *American Journal of Nursing, 82*(3), 402–407. https://www.ncbi.nlm.nih.gov/pubmed/6917683

Capan, M.L., Ambrose, H.L., Burkett, M., Evangelista, T., Flook, D., & Straka, K. (2013). Nursing portfolio study: The use in annual performance reviews. *Journal for Nurses in Professional Development, 29*(4), 182–185. https://doi.org/10.1097/NND.0b013e31829aec0f

Clinical Research Nurse Certification Council. (2022). *Clinical research nurse certification.* https://www.crncc.org

Dreyfus, S.E., & Dreyfus, H.L. (1980). A five-stage model of the mental activities involved in directed skill acquisition. Defense Technical Information Center. https://apps.dtic.mil/sti/pdfs/ADA084551.pdf

Hassmiller, S.B., & Wakefield, M.K. (2022). The future of nursing 2020–2030: Charting a path to achieve health equity. *Nursing Outlook, 70*(6, Suppl. 1), S1–S9. https://doi.org/10.1016/j.outlook.2022.05.013

International Association of Clinical Research Nurses. (n.d.). *About IACRN.* https://iacrn.org/page-1863001

Kunhunny, S., & Salmon, D. (2017). The evolving professional identity of the clinical research nurse: A qualitative exploration. *Journal of Clinical Nursing, 26*(23–24), 5121–5132. https://doi.org/10.1111/jocn.14055

Lubejko, B.G., & Wilson, B.J. (2019). *Oncology nursing: Scope and standards of practice.* Oncology Nursing Society.

McCabe, M., & Ness, E. (Eds.). (2021). *Clinical research nursing core curriculum.* International Association of Clinical Research Nurses. https://www.iacrn.org/Publications

Ness, E., Parreco, L.K., Galassi, A., & O'Mara, A. (2012). Consider a career in clinical research. *American Nurse Today, 7*(11), 39–42. http://www.americannursetoday.com/consider-a-career-in-clinical-research

Oncology Nursing Society & Oncology Nursing Certification Corporation. (2024). *Oncology clinical research nurse competencies.* https://www.ons.org/sites/default/files/2025-01/ocrn-competencies-rebrand.pdf

Scott, K., White, K., & Roydhouse, J.K. (2013). Advancing the educational and career pathway for clinical trials nurses. *Journal of Continuing Education in Nursing, 44*(4), 165–170. https://doi.org/10.3928/00220124-20121217-38

Shirey, M.R. (2009). The nursing professional portfolio: Leveraging your talents. *Clinical Nurse Specialist, 23*(5), 241–244. https://doi.org/10.1097/NUR.0b013e3181b207af

Smith, L. (2011). Showcase your talents with a career portfolio. *Nursing, 42*(7), 54–56. https://doi.org/10.1097/01.NURSE.0000398641.62631.8e

Society of Clinical Research Associates. (2025). *CCRP certification quick facts.* https://www.socra.org/certification/certification-program/ccrp-certification-quick-facts

U.S. Food and Drug Administration. (2020). *Enhancing the diversity of clinical trial populations—Eligibility criteria, enrollment practices, and trial designs: Guidance for industry.* https://resource.nlm.nih.gov/9918249008406676

Xing, Y., Wang, X., Zhang, C., Yuan, W., Chen, X., & Luan, W. (2024). Characteristics and duties of clinical research nurses: A scoping review. *Frontiers in Medicine, 11,* 1333230. https://doi.org/10.3389/fmed.2024.1333230

CHAPTER 36

Mentorship

Rose Ermete, BSN, RN, OCN®, CRN-BC, CCRP

Introduction

Oncology nurses transitioning to the subspecialty of clinical trials assume a variety of new roles and responsibilities. These responsibilities shift from the traditional nurse role to being part of a research team. Oncology staff nurses may possess a thorough knowledge of oncology and help coordinate care; however, in the role of oncology clinical research nurse (OCRN), they will need to be team leaders who incorporate the science and regulations behind the research into care coordination. Lönn et al. (2022) and Chan et al. (2020) found that nurses transitioning into the research field expressed a lack of knowledge related to regulations and terminology, as well as ethical dilemmas, and reported having no formal training or preparation for the role. The nurses who were interviewed expressed the need for a mentor to help them navigate through the various issues and conflicts they experienced. Nurses are frequently selected for these positions based on their clinical expertise; however, when they enter the research setting, they often become novices (Chan et al., 2020).

The role of the OCRN varies based on the practice location, patient population, and the expectations of management and the principal investigator. In many settings, OCRNs are responsible for more than the clinical aspects of patient care. Large academic settings tend to have more resources, allowing OCRNs to focus more on clinical aspects. However, smaller settings in the community or physician's offices tend to have fewer resources, meaning OCRNs may also be responsible for many other duties, such as data management, regulatory requirements, specimen collection and processing, and budgeting (American Nurses Association, 2024; Hansen et al., 2022; Jones et al., 2022). The various work settings and responsibilities add to the complexity of mentoring a novice OCRN or one moving to a new work setting.

This chapter will focus on mentorship, presenting it as a process for novice research nurses and other healthcare professionals to transition to the subspecialty of clinical trials. It will also explore how more established individuals may achieve their professional goals through mentorship.

The Transition to Oncology Clinical Research Nursing

Clinical research nursing is different from staff nursing and most other areas of practice. New OCRNs must learn to adapt to an environment of unfamiliar rules and regulations. Nurses evolve from being part of a team to navigating multiple relationships with various key partners (see Figure 36-1). Staff nursing tends to be task oriented; however, in research, OCRNs often provide direction and coordinate the plan of care. To function effectively, OCRNs must be team leaders with a thorough knowledge of oncology, as well as the science and regulations underlying the research. The focus must broaden from clinical issues surrounding the patient to how these issues affect the quality of study outcomes, future therapy, and, most importantly, patient safety (American Nurses Association, 2024; Hansen et al., 2022; Jones et al., 2022; Ness, 2020). This broader focus will provide OCRNs with an understanding that encompasses clinical trials and their associated processes.

Novice OCRNs may experience significant role confusion in attempting to navigate toward competency. Role confusion is a result of the varying activities and responsibilities that surround the OCRN profession. Coupled with increasingly complex studies, stringent regulations, ethical dilemmas, and the lack of training, novice OCRNs may feel overwhelmed (Gruber et al., 2020; Lavender & Croudass, 2019; Lönn et al., 2022). They also may become frustrated when faced with complex decisions that sometimes require them to balance fidelity to the study with the protection of the patient (Freel et al., 2023; Larkin et al., 2019). Larkin et al. (2019) found that clinical research nurses felt it would be helpful to have other clinical research nurses with whom to discuss issues.

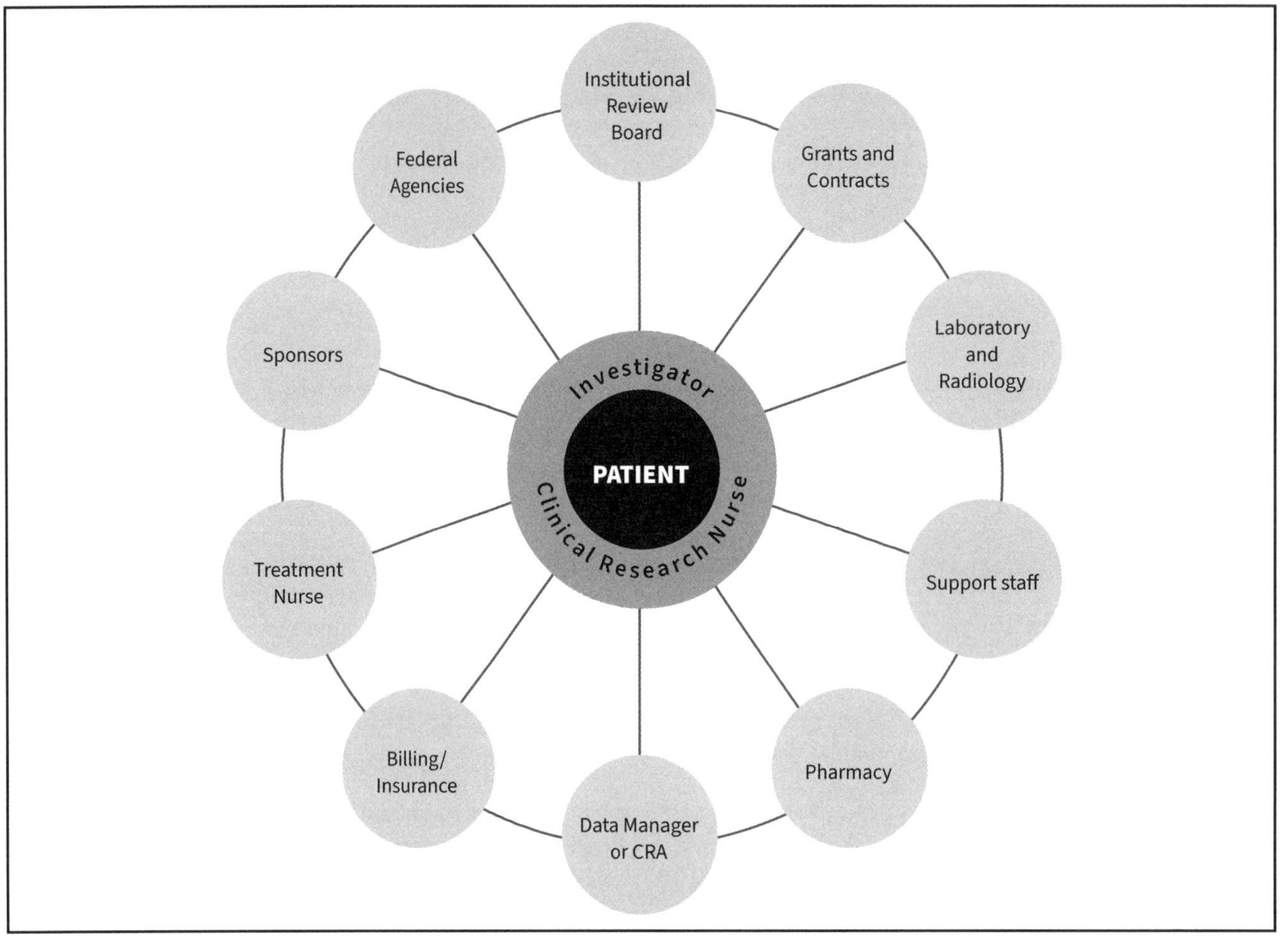

FIGURE 36-1 | The Oncology Clinical Research Nurse Role in the Coordination of Clinical Trial Activities

CRA—clinical research associate

Support staff includes, but is not limited to, dietitians, social workers, homecare nurses, medical assistants, navigators, and scheduling personnel.

Note. Based on information from American Nurses Association, 2024; Karam, 2021; Oncology Nursing Society & Oncology Nursing Certification Corporation, 2024.

From "Clinical Trials and Communicating Safety," by R.B. Ermete, 2012, *Clinical Journal of Oncology Nursing, 16*(1), p. 26. https://doi.org/10.1188/12.CJON.25-27. Copyright 2012 by Oncology Nursing Society. Adapted with permission.

Frustration and role confusion contribute to decreased job satisfaction, which can lead to the loss of potentially excellent OCRNs. Burnout, depression, and high rates of job dissatisfaction weaken the ability to retain nurses (Melnyk, Tan, Hsieh, Gawlik, et al., 2021; Shah et al., 2021). Mentoring new nurses increases job satisfaction, encourages retention, and improves patient safety (Freel et al., 2023; Hookmani et al., 2021; Knapke et al., 2022; Melnyk, Tan, Hsieh, & Gallagher-Ford, 2021). It provides novice nurses with knowledge, skills, and core values while reducing perceived barriers to their new roles (Chan et al., 2020; Evans et al., 2020). Mentoring can also aid a new nurse in transitioning to the subspecialty of clinical research nursing. Without support, nurses may explore other areas and abandon research nursing.

The statistics available on nursing shortages indicate potential issues in many nursing subspecialties. According to a 2022 survey, more than 25% of nurses reported planning to leave the nursing profession or retire within five years. Approximately 100,000 registered nurses and 34,000 licensed practical nurses left the workforce during the COVID-19 pandemic (Smiley et al., 2023). Freel et al. (2023) reported an average of 10 openings for every OCRN seeking employment. Fisher et al. (2021) noted that the cost to replace a clinical research coordinator has been estimated at $40,000–$60,000, based on hiring costs and employee onboarding time. Considering these statistics, there is a crucial need to develop new approaches and support experienced clinical research professionals (Freel et al., 2023), including those in the subspecialty of OCRN.

Mentoring the next generation of nurses is a professional obligation (Evans et al., 2020). In a budget-conscious environment, investing in a mentorship program may take a back seat to more pressing initiatives. However, studies demonstrate that when nurses are provided with mentorship opportunities, it benefits the institution through staff retention, the development of experienced nurses, and succession planning (Dirks, 2021; Evans et al., 2020) (see Figure 36-2). Experienced OCRNs can create a legacy by passing their knowledge and wisdom to the next generation. Through positive interaction with more experienced OCRNs, novices will better assimilate into their new role while strengthening the subspecialty of clinical research nursing.

Definition of Mentorship

The term *mentor* dates back to Greek mythology. When Odysseus left to fight in the Trojan War, he left his son, Telemachus, in the care of a trusted and wise friend, Mentor. Mentor not only raised Telemachus but also provided him with knowledge and guidance to prepare him for future responsibilities (Homer, trans. 1993).

Mentorship is a dynamic relationship between an experienced, trusted advisor (mentor) and a less experienced colleague (mentee) for the purpose of guiding the mentee toward personal and professional growth and experience in a profession (Chong et al., 2020; Hoover et al., 2020; Ng et al., 2020; Olaolorunpo, 2019; Van Patten & Bartone, 2019). It is not the same thing as a coach or preceptor. Coaching is a top-down process that involves specific skills training and goals required for a position. It occurs over a defined period and primarily benefits the apprentice (Byars-Winston & Dahlberg, 2019; Hussey & Campbell-Meier, 2020; Santiesteban et al., 2022). Precepting involves skills training during a planned orientation period where the preceptor serves as a clinical resource and assesses the competencies of new or transferred employees (Dirks, 2021; Kowalski, 2019).

In contrast, mentorship has a broader focus that is beyond organizational directives. It fosters a supportive environment that nurtures advancement toward self-development and professional growth. The focus is on the developmental needs and goals of the novice; however, the relationship is a reciprocal experience that empowers mentors and mentees to develop personally and professionally within a safe and collaborative environment. The relationship is typically long-lasting and evolves over time. Mentors challenge the mentee while offering guidance, insight, and opportunities that contribute to the mentee's personal and professional development (Byars-Winston & Dahlberg, 2019; Dirks, 2021; Gruber et al., 2020). This process not only contributes to the success of the mentee but also to the future success of the nursing profession (Evans et al., 2020; Nelson et al., 2024; Olaolorunpo, 2019).

- Staff retention
- Decreased cost for new hires
- Increased job satisfaction
- Increased employee productivity
- Improved patient outcomes
- Culture of safety
- Increased loyalty
- Improved communication and teamwork
- Improved reputation of organization
- Development of future leaders

FIGURE 36-2 | Benefits of Mentorship Programs to Institutions

Note. Based on information from Chan et al., 2020; Chong et al., 2020; Dirks, 2021; Olaolorunpo, 2019.

Theoretical Frameworks for Mentoring

To understand the mentorship process, it is essential to establish a theoretical framework of mentoring. The concept of mentoring involves guiding or assisting others along a path to increased knowledge and professional growth. Several relevant learning theories exist that support this endeavor, such as Knowles' Adult Learning Theory, Kolb's Experiential Learning Theory, Bloom's Taxonomy, Benner's Novice to Expert Model, Bandura's Social Learning Theory, and Miller's Relational Cultural Theory.

Adult Learning Theory

Knowles' Adult Learning Theory focuses on the needs of the adult learner. These needs are described using the andragogical model (Knowles et al., 2020) (see Table 36-1). Adults need to know why they need to know something and how it will apply to their life situations. They also must be ready to learn. Learning occurs more easily if it coincides with the developmental tasks of the adult. Adult learners bring with them differences in past experiences that will influence their interpretation and internalization of the material taught. Adults are generally self-directed and motivated to learn through internal desires rather than external stimuli (Machynska & Boiko, 2020). This means that they will resist learning if it is perceived as enforcing the will or needs of others. These concepts should be considered when mentoring novice and advanced beginner OCRNs. Employing the andragogical model in mentorship allows the mentor to channel energy toward the mentee's professional growth and development.

Experimental Learning Theory

Kolb's Experiential Learning Theory focuses on the experiences of the person and how they relate to the learning environment and includes four steps (Nurunnabi et al., 2022). The first is the experience itself, followed by self-reflection to understand the outcome or meaning of the experience. Reflecting on the experience is of greater benefit to the learner than being instructed by someone else. In the next step, generalization, the person begins to form concepts or create generalized principles that may be used in similar circumstances. The last step, active experimentation, involves applying new knowledge in future situations (Nurunnabi et al., 2022).

TABLE 36-1 | The Andragogical Model

Concept	Description
The need to know	Why is learning this important?
The learner's self-concept	I am responsible for my own decisions (self-directed instead of teacher-directed).
The role of the learner's experience	What is the meaning of this experience?
Readiness to learn	Will this benefit my current role in society?
Orientation to learning	How will this help me to deal with problems I may have?
Motivation	How will this help me achieve job satisfaction, self-esteem, and a better quality of life?

Note. Based on information from Knowles et al., 2020; Machynska & Boiko, 2020.

Bloom's Taxonomy

Bloom's Taxonomy focuses on three domains of the learner. The cognitive domain is the most used and is how individuals develop thoughts and gain knowledge. The psychomotor domain refers to learning physical or hands-on skills. The third domain is affective, which involves individual values or attitudes toward learning (Hrebin et al., 2020).

Novice to Expert Model

Benner's (2000) Novice to Expert Model focuses on how a nurse progresses through five stages, from novice to expert, as they assimilate into a new role. These stages are related to experiences, situations, and the meaning they hold. The novice stage is when a nurse enters a new position with no prior experience. Here, the focus is on learning objective attributes or tasks without situational experience. The advanced beginner is the next stage, where the nurse demonstrates acceptable performance and has experienced real situations to identify recurring meaning. The third stage is competent, when a nurse has been at a job for typically two to three years and can recognize aspects of a situation and identify what needs attention and what can wait. Next is the proficient stage, when the nurse looks at situations in their entirety. They have learned from experience what to expect in any given situation and how to modify plans accordingly. The final stage is expert. An expert nurse with extensive experience possesses an intuitive understanding of situations and can pinpoint the precise cause of the problem. They are highly proficient and confident. Much of Benner's work has been grounded in the Dreyfus Skill Acquisition Model, recognizing experience and science as the foundation for the development of the nurse from novice to expert (Evans et al., 2020; Van Patten & Bartone, 2019).

Social Learning Theory

Bandura's Social Learning Theory emphasizes how individuals acquire knowledge and skills through observation. The mentor serves as a model for the mentee by displaying appropriate behaviors and professional development. There are four subprocesses in this learning theory (Legg, 2023):

- Attention is the act of observing the model behavior.
- Retention is the act of remembering the behavior.
- Reproduction is an active response to what was observed, such as replicating the behavior.
- Motivation refers to the factors that incentivize the mentee to exhibit the observed behavior. Mentors can assist with this process by providing reinforcement, such as positive incentives and feedback (Legg, 2023).

Another important aspect discussed by Bandura is self-efficacy, which refers to the confidence one has in their ability to perform a particular behavior. One's self-efficacy increases when one observes others who possess similar knowledge and expertise succeeding at a task. The theory is useful in mentoring, as it helps identify how the behaviors of mentors and mentees contribute to learning (Koutroubas & Galanakis, 2022).

Relational Cultural Theory

Miller's Relational Cultural Theory emphasizes growth through connections within relationships. Historically, mentoring in academia has focused on a top-down or hierarchical model. Conversely, Relational Cultural Theory fosters an equal relationship that involves mutuality, empathy, authenticity, and interdependence. This theory de-emphasizes power associated with position and recognizes that both parties have something valuable to contribute. Expertise is recognized as being fluid. The mentor must be willing to demonstrate their needs and vulnerability, and the mentee must recognize that they have experiences and knowledge that they can share (Fletcher & Ragins, 2007). The mentee and mentor are attuned to and trust each other, thereby promoting a safe environment in which to learn. Growth occurs through high-quality connections, where disconnections such as those based on gender, race, or culture are recognized and addressed, and power dynamics are avoided. This theory acknowledges diversity and fosters collaboration for success (Cannon et al., 2020; Lewis & Olshansky, 2016).

These principles will help mentors guide the training of mentees by providing the appropriate opportunities at the proper stage of learning. This allows the mentorship process to be focused on the mentee's needs rather than on an external entity. By allowing the new OCRN to explore and problem-solve with guidance and insight from a mentor, the mentee can build self-confidence and develop as a professional nurse.

Mentor Competencies

Seasoned OCRNs may have excellent clinical skills, but this does not necessarily make them good mentors. Mentors must have a balance of skills, attributes, and qualities. The literature demonstrates that mentor training fosters an effective mentoring experience (Byars-Winston & Dahlberg, 2019; Hookmani et al., 2021; Knapke et al., 2022). An inadequate mentor can be detrimental to a potentially good OCRN. Mentors, therefore, should be chosen who do not exhibit unhealthy traits (see Figure 36-3). Mentorship training should promote the development of behaviors known to have a positive effect on mentoring. There are several competencies described in the literature for mentors and mentees. Although there does not appear to be extensive research or agreement on these, theoretical frameworks can be used to guide the mentoring process.

Several tools in the literature have demonstrated reliability in identifying common characteristics associated with an effective mentoring relationship. Some of these tools include the Mentor Evaluation Tool (Yukawa et al., 2020), the Mentor Competence Instrument (Mikkonen et al., 2022), the Mentoring Process Scale (Tolan et al., 2020), and the Mentor Effectiveness Scale (McBride et al., 2019). These characteristics impact the outcome of the mentoring process. They can be grouped by similar intent and function into the three domains of learning in Bloom's Taxonomy: cognitive, psychomotor, and affective. For the purposes of measuring competency, the psychomotor domain will focus on the skill of communication (see Figure 36-4).

The cognitive domain refers to those attributes of knowledge and expertise. Knowledge develops over time and with experience. Expert nurses demonstrate the ability to intuitively analyze situations and apply evidence-based practice and critical thinking (Benner, 2000). Mentors should be considered experts in their clinical area; however, being an expert does not necessarily equate to being a good mentor. Other cognitive abilities contribute to the development of a proficient mentor, such as knowing how to formulate goals, demonstrating professional integrity, providing guidance on professional issues, assessing understanding, stimulating reflection, and serving as a role model (Byars-Winston & Dahlberg, 2019; Yukawa et al., 2020).

- Distancing behavior or neglectful
- Unapproachable or intimidating
- Unreliable—violate confidentiality
- Unload work or tasks on mentees not related to their goals
- Misappropriation of the mentee's work
- Conflicts of interest
- Manipulative or controlling
- Bullying or jealousy of the mentee's achievements

FIGURE 36-3 | Toxic Mentors

Note. Based on information from Byars-Winston & Dahlberg, 2019; Dirks, 2021; McBride et al., 2019; Ng et al., 2020.

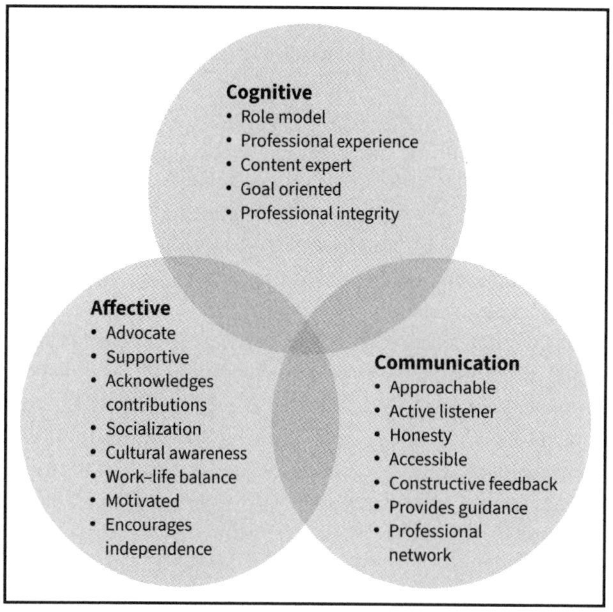

FIGURE 36-4 | The Balance of Mentor Competencies

Note. Based on information from McBride et al., 2019; Mikkonen et al., 2022; Olaolorunpo, 2019; Tolan et al., 2020; Veliverronena, 2023; Yukawa et al., 2020.

Effective communication is crucial to the success and fulfillment of the mentoring relationship (Ng et al., 2020). A mentor needs to be accessible and approachable for communication to occur. Poor communication negatively affects learning and growth, whereas effective communication is a core competency in mentoring (Byars-Winston & Dahlberg, 2019; Dirks, 2021; Olaolorunpo, 2019; Yukawa et al., 2020). A key element of communication is active listening, which includes paraphrasing, reflecting feelings, and asking relevant open-ended questions (Kluger & Itzchakov, 2022). A mentor should never assume that they know more about a stated problem than the mentee does. The ability to listen to what the mentee has to say without interjecting opinions or judgments promotes understanding and avoids bias (Byars-Winston & Dalhberg, 2019).

Providing feedback and access to resources are important aspects of communication. Assessment and evaluation are necessary to identify areas of strength and opportunities for improvement (Byars-Winston & Dahlberg, 2019). Feedback should not be berating or judgmental; instead, it should be constructive. Constructive feedback or critiques have been identified as desired by mentees. The mentor must also promote the professional advancement of the mentee by assisting with the development of a professional network, thereby providing access to resources and experiences that the mentor may not be able to provide (McBride et al., 2019; Mikkonen et al., 2022; Nguyen et al., 2024; Tolan et al., 2020; Yukawa et al., 2020). Effective communication and access to other professionals provide a solid framework for positive change to occur.

Addressing conflict is another aspect of communication. The mentor must understand how to address conflict to maintain positive and effective interactions. Negative outcomes are more likely to occur if conflict is not managed appropriately. The mentor must keep an open mind and refrain from making personal judgments. When addressing problems, opinions must not be confused with facts. The mentee must have the opportunity to elucidate the rationale without the mentor creating assumptions about what may have occurred. "I" statements should be used in place of "you" statements when confronting negative behavior. For example, the statement "I am concerned that the case report forms were submitted without verifying the data against the medical record" is preferable to the statement "You did not review all the source documents before completing the case report forms." "I" statements acknowledge the thoughts and feelings behind the mentor's comments. "You" statements put the novice on the defensive (Rogers et al., 2018). When a person is defensive, attention is diverted away from the genuine issues. The mentor must keep the conversation focused on the present situation, as the past is irrelevant to the current situation. By addressing conflict effectively, the mentor helps the novice develop the skills necessary to manage future problems and advance professionally.

The affective domain encompasses those attributes that contribute to the psychosocial support of the mentee. Good mentors foster a professional relationship with the mentee's interests in mind. They create a nonjudgmental and nurturing environment where the mentee feels safe to share their thoughts and ideas (Dirks, 2021; Olaolorunpo, 2019). Competent mentors advocate for their mentees, acknowledge contributions, provide motivation, and encourage creativity and confidence (Byars-Winston & Dahlberg, 2019; McBride et al., 2019; Tolan et al., 2020; Yukawa et al., 2020). Providing emotional support in managing stress and conflict is also essential (Dirks, 2021). Recognizing diversity and exhibiting multicultural humility demonstrates the mentor's ability to learn and be sensitive to the needs of the mentee (Ahmadmehrabi et al., 2021; Byars-Winston & Dahlberg, 2019; Gruber et al., 2020). Mentors will not always have all the answers for every situation. McBride et al. (2019) found that mentees often valued having more than one mentor. Having access to multiple mentors provides diverse forms of support and removes the expectation that the mentor must be all-knowing to be competent (Byars-Winston & Dahlberg, 2019; McBride et al., 2019).

The Mentoring Relationship

The success of mentoring is rooted in a relationship that is based on mutual trust and respect (Beitere-Selegovska, 2023; Nelson et al., 2024). Olaolorunpo (2019) found that shared values, reciprocity, clear expectations, mutual respect, and personal connection characterized successful mentoring relationships. Choosing a compatible mentor who exhibits these characteristics in a relationship is important (Dirks, 2021; Manuel & Poorsattar, 2021). There are two types of similarities to consider when matching a mentor and a mentee: surface-level (e.g., age, gender, race, ethnicity) and deep-level similarities (e.g., attitudes, goals, interests, values, problem-solving styles). Several studies have demonstrated that mentees may prefer to have mentors with similar surface-level attributes; however, deep-level similarities predict interpersonal comfort and appear to be related to positive outcomes (Byars-Winston & Dahlberg, 2019). Each person in a mentoring relationship has certain responsibilities, as well as unique qualities that they bring to the relationship. The mentee and mentor must understand their responsibilities to cultivate a successful relationship (see Figure 36-5). Mentoring relationships can also vary in their degree of formality or informality. A number of organizations can assist in finding a mentor (see Table 36-2).

The literature presents several models for the development of a mentoring relationship, including the Mentoring Up Theory (Hale & Phillips, 2019) and Kram's Mentoring Theory (Stoeger et al., 2021). Each has a different name for each stage, but all reflect a similar transition process. After identifying an appropriate mentor and mentee, the first step is for the two individuals to come together. This has been called the initiation or seeding stage, a period during which individuals get to know each other. Identifying similar attitudes, values, beliefs, and personality traits is important in laying the foundation for a positive relationship (Hale & Phillips, 2019; Stoeger et al., 2021).

During the opening stage, goals and objectives are established, and boundaries are discussed. Through reciprocal interactions, where the mentor responds to the needs

Mentees
- Demonstrate a willingness to learn.
- Identify initial learning goals.
- Seek and be open to feedback.
- Arrive prepared and on time.
- Take an active role in learning (self-directed).
- Reflect critically before and after meetings (active listener).
- Follow through on commitments or renegotiate them as needed.

Mentors
- Treat the mentee as a colleague.
- Have reasonable expectations of the mentee.
- Help the mentee to develop an appropriate learning plan.
- Facilitate professional and personal growth.
- Assist in identifying resources and experiences.
- Provide support and encouragement.
- Provide feedback.
- Allocate time and energy.
- Follow through on commitments or renegotiate them as needed.

FIGURE 36-5 | Mentee and Mentor Responsibilities

Note. Based on information from Byars-Winston & Dahlberg, 2019; Evans et al., 2020; Gruber et al., 2020; Veliverronena, 2023.

TABLE 36-2 | Additional Resources for Mentoring

Resource	Website
Academy of Medical-Surgical Nurses: Mentoring	www.amsn.org/Learning-Development/Mentoring
American Nurses Association Mentoring Program	https://community.ana.org/pages/mentorprogram?ssopc=1
Center for the Improvement of Mentored Experiences in Research: Mentor Curricula and Training	https://cimerproject.org/entering-mentoring
Consortium for Research on Emotional Intelligence in Organizations: Emotional and Social Competence Inventory	www.eiconsortium.org/measures/eci_360.html
iMentoring	www.mentoringgroup.com
International Association of Clinical Research Nurses: Leadership Program	www.iacrn.org/iacrn-leadership-program
Kentucky Nurses Association Mentoring Toolkit	https://kentucky-nurses.nursingnetwork.com/nursing-news/175977-mentoring-tool-kit-robert-wood-johnson-and-aarp
MentorNet	www.mentornet.net
National League for Nursing Mentoring Tool Kit [login required]	www.nln.org/docs/default-source/default-document-library/nln-mentoring-toolkit-2022.pdf
National Research Mentoring Network	https://nrmnet.net
Oncology Nursing Society: Teach and Mentor	www.ons.org/career-development/teach-mentor
Pew Research Center: Internet, Broadband Fact Sheet	www.pewresearch.org/internet/fact-sheet/internet-broadband
Robert Wood Johnson Foundation: The Mentoring Toolkit and Handbook	www.newcareersinnursing.org/resources/mentoring-toolkit-and-handbook.html
Together	www.togetherplatform.com
University of Washington: I-Tech: Clinical Mentoring Toolkit	www.go2itech.org/resources/clinical-mentoring-toolkit

of the mentee, the likelihood of a successful relationship is assessed (Hale & Phillips, 2019). A lack of awareness of one's role can lead to misunderstandings and trigger unhealthy communication. Differences in expectations can undermine the mentoring relationship and negatively influence the learning experience. Expectations should be clear from the start of the relationship (Manuel & Poorsattar, 2021). Figure 36-6 provides a template for an individual development plan that can be used at the outset to clarify expectations.

In the next stage, known as cultivating or laddering, the mentoring process unfolds (Hale & Phillips, 2019; Stoeger et al., 2021). The mentee's professional and personal goals are addressed through shared interactions that stimulate and challenge the mentee. The mentor provides support, guidance, and opportunities that lead to the attainment of confidence and independence (Hale & Phillips, 2019).

During the subsequent equalizing or separation stage, a transformation of the relationship occurs, where the two become colleagues or peers. The mentor and mentee become equal in terms of professional ability. The frequency of interaction decreases, and autonomy increases as communication becomes more collaborative. Mentors remain available and continue to be in contact, but more as colleagues than as mentors (Hale & Phillips, 2019; Stoeger et al., 2021).

The last stage, reframing or redefinition, is a contemplative process. (Hale & Phillips, 2019; Stoeger et al., 2021). The relationship may or may not continue, but it often evolves into a long-term collegial friendship. Mentees reflect on the significance of the relationship and its contribution to their professional development (Hale & Phillips, 2019; Stoeger et al., 2020). The mentee becomes part of the mentor's network and may also become a mentor themselves.

Mentee: ______ Home: ______ Work: ______ Mobile: ______ Texting: ☐ Yes ☐ No Email: ______ Preferred method of contact: ______ Are there any disabilities that need special accommodation? ☐ Yes ☐ No	Mentor: ______ Home: ______ Work: ______ Mobile: ______ Texting: ☐ Yes ☐ No Email: ______ Preferred method of contact: ______ Are there any disabilities that need special accommodation? ☐ Yes ☐ No
This agreement sets the parameters of the voluntary mentoring relationship. It should be completed during the first discussion to provide clarification of expectations from both parties. Both parties should sign and get a copy of the form.	
Goals	
1.	1.
2.	2.
3.	3.
Expectations	
What will be the nature of assessments?	☐ Self ☐ Mutual
Values, Attitudes, Interests (personal and professional)	
Boundaries	
How often will you meet? ☐ Weekly ☐ Monthly ☐ Other	
Where will you meet?	How long will meetings be:
Who is responsible for scheduling meetings? ☐ Mentee ☐ Mentor ☐ Other:	
Preferred type of meeting? ☐ Face to face ☐ Email ☐ Video chat ☐ Phone ☐ Other:	
If a meeting must be canceled, how should you be notified?	
Are there times or days that you should not be contacted?	
Mentee:	Mentor:
Conflicts of Interest and Confidentiality	
• This relationship is strictly confidential, and content of meetings will remain between the mentor and mentee. • The mentor and mentee have affirmed that there are no conflicts of interest and that products, papers, projects, etc., developed through this relationship by the mentee are the intellectual property of the mentee, unless stated otherwise in this agreement. • Both parties agree to a no-fault conclusion of the mentoring relationship.	
Other Comments/Agreements:	
Signature and date:	Signature and date:

FIGURE 36-6 | Sample Mentorship Agreement Template

The literature confirms that individuals who have been mentored are more likely to mentor others, thereby continuing the legacy (McBride et al., 2019).

The age of the OCRN workforce has been gradually shifting, with many seasoned OCRNs nearing retirement. As of 2025, Millennials (those born between 1980 and 2000) account for 75% of the workforce (Waljee et al., 2020). They are already in the workforce and value a work–life balance. The primarily day-shift, weekend-free schedules of clinical trial offices could attract these nurses to the OCRN role. This generational group has life experiences and expectations that differ from those of Baby Boomers or Generation X. Mentors will need to consider these differences to minimize misunderstandings.

Millennials have grown up with instantaneous information and have an innate aptitude for technology, which has led to their expectation of immediate feedback. They may also expect their mentor to be available for regular informal meetings (Waljee et al., 2020). They are more accustomed to working collaboratively in groups where learning is interactive and diverse. They are not intimidated by a lack of experience and value purpose over process (Bittner, 2019; Waljee et al., 2020). Mentors will need to consider these behaviors when planning a mentoring relationship with this group of OCRNs.

Virtual Mentoring

Mentoring can occur in various settings, including formal programs or informal arrangements with a colleague. Social distancing during the COVID-19 pandemic led to an increase in the use of virtual or e-mentoring, indicating that the mentoring process will likely continue to use technology for the foreseeable future (Mineva et al., 2023; Murray et al., 2022). E-mentoring employs a virtual platform to facilitate mentoring relationships (Nguyen et al., 2024). This technology encompasses email, synchronized chats, webcams, videoconferencing, captioning, and digital note-taking (Chong et al., 2020; Mullen & Klimaitis, 2021; Mutiarin et al., 2023; Rollnik-Sadowska & Ryciuk, 2023). Virtual technology can provide access to resources, thereby maintaining the mentoring relationship when face-to-face interaction is not possible (Mutiarin et al., 2023).

Virtual mentoring can offer many advantages and disadvantages (see Figure 36-7). For one, technology allows for flexible, time-efficient meetings and eliminates space availability issues. Meetings can also be recorded or transcripts provided if a group meeting is missed or if there are accessibility or language barriers (Chong et al., 2020; McReynolds et al., 2020; Mineva et al., 2023; Nguyen et al., 2024). This type of mentoring takes the mentee far beyond local resources, allowing relationships to be more global and providing access to mentors that would typically be impossible to encounter. Virtual mentoring is not limited by boundaries of geography, hierarchy, or time. Studies have demonstrated that virtual mentoring can also provide opportunities for career and psychosocial support when local mentors are unable to meet the mentees' needs or exhibit negative mentoring behaviors (Byars-Winston & Dahlberg, 2019; Volkova, 2023).

Advantages	Disadvantages
• Allows for more global relationships without boundaries – Geography – Hierarchy – Time and flexibility – Eliminates space availability • Cost-effective • Less judgmental • Reduces gender and racial discrimination • Provides generational adaptation for younger nurses • Can be recorded or transcripts generated	• Requires a stable internet connection • Depends on the technical and administrative capacity of the host organization • May slow down the development of relations • Individual weariness in sharing their personal environment • Lack of nonverbal communication • Misinterpretation of information • Lacks warm human connection • Lack of confidentiality with internet • Generational issues with technology

FIGURE 36-7 | Advantages and Disadvantages of Virtual Mentoring

Note. Based on information from McReynolds et al., 2020; Mullen & Klimaitis, 2021; Nguyen et al., 2024; Veliverronena, 2023.

Virtual mentoring can also present challenges. A reliable mechanism of electronic communication and the ability to solve technical problems are necessary. Maintaining a personal touch without face-to-face contact is difficult to achieve (Ahmadmehrabi et al., 2021; Kumar et al., 2023; Mullen & Klimaitis, 2021). With the loss of nonverbal clues and personal connections, meanings may often be misinterpreted.

O'Dowd et al. (2020) discussed several studies on virtual communication and found that interactions are often superficial and lacking in engagement, which can make virtual communication less conducive to effective learning. However, Tinoco-Giraldo et al. (2020) found an increase in the development of skills and abilities, learning potential, interpersonal relations, and communication skills within the e-mentoring environment. Blended mentoring, where face-to-face engagement is complemented with electronic technology, potentially provides timely and personalized support and fosters improved rapport. Beitere-Selegovska (2023) discussed several studies that demonstrated that mentors with high emotional intelligence are better equipped to understand how a remote mentee is feeling and are more effective at adapting to both remote and in-person settings. More data are needed to understand the effect of this blended approach to mentoring (Chong et al., 2020; Veliverronena, 2023).

McReynolds et al. (2020) and Yiorka and Taliadorou (2023) recommended several considerations when preparing for a virtual mentoring session. First, a reliable internet connection is needed, along with a web camera. The camera is essential to facilitate face-to-face interaction. It should also be positioned on the screen where the interaction takes place to ensure adequate eye contact and engagement. Avoiding distractions, such as cell phones, is pertinent. Phones should be placed in silent mode. Appearance is important; wearing appropriate dress and having an uncluttered room can minimize distractions. Several platforms (e.g., Zoom, Microsoft Teams) offer template backgrounds that can be used. If possible, a quiet room should be selected to avoid interruptions and to prevent uninvolved people from overhearing the conversations, thereby maintaining confidentiality. If using Zoom, a room should be password-protected to avoid "Zoom bombing," or the risk of unauthorized individuals entering the call. An agenda should also be prepared in advance to keep the meeting on schedule and be mindful of everyone's time.

O'Dowd et al. (2020) discussed the use of proper "netiquette," including behaviors such as not eating or reading emails during meetings, focusing on the conversation, reexamining assumptions about intentions, and dealing with misunderstandings. A mentor who is accustomed to phone or in-person communication may struggle with texting, emojis, or acronyms (Volkova, 2023). Acronyms can be confusing, and emoticons can be misconstrued as mockery; therefore, their use should be limited (Mutiarin et al., 2023).

Virtual mentoring has been described positively in the literature; however, further studies are needed to evaluate its effectiveness. It remains a flexible means of interaction. If used appropriately, it can generate and nurture the mentoring relationship. There are many virtual mentoring programs available to OCRNs (see Table 36-3).

As technology continues to advance, novel methods of e-mentoring are emerging. One of the latest innovations is artificial intelligence (AI), which involves the utilization of algorithms—sets of programmed rules—to analyze large amounts of data. This enables computers to reason and perform cognitive functions similar to those of humans (Ferrari et al., 2022). There are several platforms available that use AI to match mentors and mentees, as well as develop learning plans, assist with writing, set reminders, schedule meetings, evaluate progress, translate or provide captions from meetings, and evaluate progress in the mentoring relationship (Bagai & Mane, 2023; Gupta & Rathore, 2020; Murray et al., 2022). AI-based mentoring has the advantage of eliminating the time and guesswork involved in finding a mentor while also providing personalized assistance 24 hours a day from anywhere (Bagai & Mane, 2023).

Despite these benefits, several important factors must be considered. These platforms require personal data to develop an individualized plan. Whenever data are shared over the internet, concerns about privacy and security arise (Bagai & Mane, 2023; Kobis & Mehner, 2021). The design of the algorithms determines the effectiveness of the resulting AI. If the rules used are flawed, the results could be biased (Bagai & Mane, 2023; Kobis & Mehner, 2021; Treasure et al., 2022). Another limitation of AI is the lack of a human connection; AI cannot replicate the emotional intelligence and empathy that are essential for a successful mentoring relationship (Bagai & Mane, 2023; Gupta & Rathore, 2020). Personal or emotional issues that occur may not be addressed adequately; therefore, AI should be used to facilitate or enhance mentorship rather than serve as a standalone program. Mentoring with AI is still considered a relatively new concept. Although several applications using this technology are available, the validity of their effectiveness has not been determined. Studies on the ethical and other issues of AI in mentorship are scarce, and further research is needed to understand its contributions and effectiveness in mentorship (Kobis & Mehner, 2021).

Mentorship and the Future

Mentoring benefits the mentor, the mentee, and the profession. The mentee gains valuable experience as they progress toward and attain professional goals. Through mentoring, the mentor creates a personal legacy that makes a positive contribution to the profession. Mentorship is important to the future of the nursing profession. OCRNs must continue to nurture and encourage new and less-experienced colleagues. Experienced OCRNs must also provide support and guidance for innovative ideas, as these new ideas pave the way for change. Without change, the subspecialty of clinical research nursing cannot advance. Without advancement, growth cannot occur. Without growth, the OCRN role—and the nursing profession—will not survive.

Summary

OCRNs work in a variety of settings and assume diverse roles; their responsibilities differ from those of traditional staff nurses. Successfully taking on these unique responsibilities can be aided by a mentoring relationship. Through mentorship, novice and advanced beginner OCRNs can assimilate into the role and grow professionally. Many opportunities for mentoring exist both locally and through various organizations. Novice nurses are best served by mentors who have effective communication skills and available time for mentoring, demonstrate professionalism, and encourage professional growth and development. More experienced OCRNs should consider becoming mentors to help guide novices and sustain the continued growth of the profession.

TABLE 36-3 | Virtual Mentoring Platforms

Platform	Type	Virtual Mentoring Features
Zoom	Audio and video call application	Waiting room feature, calendar integration, multi-screen share, free basic interface, chat feature
Skype	Audio and video call application	Messaging, screen sharing, recording capabilities; can call phones; free basic interface
Trello	Project management tool	Free for basic service; simple sharing of tasks including calendar and deadlines
Slack	Collaboration software	Organized chat conversations by topics; team members can share files; face-to-face or chat options
BlueJeans	Videoconferencing application	Audio or videoconferencing option, scheduling and productivity tools
X	Social media platform	Tweet threading for themed information sharing; mentorship extended to broad group of followers; direct messaging option
Facebook	Social media platform	Information sharing, direct messaging option, option to join mentoring groups
WeChat	Messaging application	Overseas favorite
WhatsApp	Messaging application	End-to-end encryption
QQ	Messaging application	Most popular video/chatting app in China; connects internationally and has both phone and computer interfaces
LINE	Messaging application	Video and text messaging, games, voice calls
KakaoTalk	Messaging application	Video and text messaging, file sending, remote logout for PC version, voice calls, calendar

Note. From "The Art of Virtual Mentoring in the Twenty-First Century for STEM Majors and Beyond," by M.R. McReynolds, C.M. Termini, A.O. Hinton, B.L. Taylor, Z. Vue, S.C. Huang, … C.S. Carter, 2020, *Nature Biotechnology, 38*(12), p. 1478. https://doi.org/10.1038/s41587-020-00758-7. Copyright 2020 by Springer Nature America. Reprinted with permission.

Key Points

- Mentorship fosters a supportive environment that nurtures advancement toward self-development and professional growth.
- Mentorship can contribute to decreased stress and increased OCRN retention.
- Nurses have a responsibility to mentor the next generation.
- Mentoring provides a significant return on investment to institutions and the nursing profession.
- Proper training of potential mentors is vital to the success of the relationship.
- Generational differences should be considered when planning a relationship.
- Virtual mentoring is a viable option to supplement the mentoring process.

References

Ahmadmehrabi, S., Farlow, J.L., Wamkpah, N.S., Esianor, B.I., Brenner, M.J., Valdez, T.A., … Francis, H.W. (2021). New age mentoring and disruptive innovation—Navigating the uncharted with vision, purpose and equity. *JAMA Otolaryngology Head and Neck Surgery, 147*(4), 389–394. http://doi.org/10.1001/jamaoto.2020.5448

American Nurses Association. (2024). *Clinical research nursing: Scope and standards of practice* (2nd ed.). Author.

Bagai, R., & Mane, V. (2023). Designing an AI-powered mentorship platform for professional development: Opportunities and challenges. *International Journal of Computer Trends and Technology, 71*(4), 108–114. https://doi.org/10.14445/22312803/IJCTT-V71I4P114

Beitere-Selegovska, Z. (2023). E-mentoring program's evaluation. In *E-mentoring: Theory and Practice.* (pp. 126–147). Bialystok University of Technology. https://www.researchgate.net/publication/377815506

Benner, P. (2000). *From novice to expert: Excellence and power in clinical nursing practice.* Prentice Hall.

Bittner, A. (2019). Mentoring millennials for nursing leadership. *Nursing, 49*(10), 53–56. https://doi.org/10.1097/01.NURSE.0000580656.81188.ee

Byars-Winston, A., & Dahlberg, M.L. (Eds.). (2019). *The science of effective mentorship in STEMM.* National Academies Press. https://doi.org/10.17226/25568

Cannon, Y., Haiyasoso, M., & Tello, A. (2020). Relational aspects in research mentoring of women doctoral counseling students. *Journal of Creativity in Mental Health, 15*(3), 278–291. https://doi.org/10.1080/15401383.2019.1689213

Chan, E.Y., Glass, G.F., & Phang, K.N. (2020). Evaluation of a hospital-based nursing research and evidence-based practice mentorship program on improving nurses' knowledge, attitudes, and evidence-based practice. *Journal of Continuing Education in Nursing, 51*(1), 46–52. https://doi.org/10.3928/00220124-20191217-09

Chong, J.Y., Ching, A.H., Renganathan, Y., Lim, W.Q., Toh, Y.P., Mason, S., & Krishna, L.K.R. (2020). Enhancing mentoring experiences through e-mentoring: A systematic scoping review of e-mentoring programs between 2000 and 2017. *Advances in Health Sciences Education: Theory and Practice, 25*(1), 195–226. https://doi.org/10.1007/s10459-019-09883-8

Dirks, J.L. (2021). Alternative approaches to mentoring. *Critical Care Nurse, 41*(1), e9–e16. https://doi.org/10.4037/ccn2021789

Evans, M.M., Kowalchik, K., Riley, K., & Adams, L. (2020). Developing nurses through mentoring: It starts in nursing education. *Nursing Clinics of North America, 55*(1), 61–69. https://doi.org/10.1016/j.cnur.2019.10.006

Ferrari, L., Mari, V., Capelli, G., & Spolverato, G. (2022). Mentorship and early career mentorship. *Artificial Intelligence Surgery, 2,* 177–185. https://doi.org/10.20517/ais.2022.16

Fisher, E., Thomas, R.S., Higgins, M.K., Williams, C.J., Choi, I., & McCauley, L.A. (2021). Finding the right candidate: Developing hiring guidelines for screening applicants for clinical research coordinator positions. *Journal of Clinical and Translational Science, 6*(1), e20. https://doi.org/10.1017/cts.2021.853

Fletcher, J.K., & Ragins, B.R. (2007). Stone Center Relational Cultural Theory: A window on relational mentoring. In B.R. Ragins & K.E. Kram (Eds.), *The handbook of mentoring at work: Theory, research and practice* (pp. 373–393). Sage. https://doi.org/10.4135/9781412976619.n15

Freel, S.A., Snyder, D.C., Bastarache, K., Jones, C.T., Marchant, M.B., Rowley, L.A., ... Landis, S.P. (2023). Now is the time to fix the clinical research workforce crisis. *Clinical Trials, 20*(5), 457–462. https://doi.org/10.1177/17407745231177885

Gruber, J., Borelli, J.L., Prinstein, M.J., Clark, L.A., Davila, J., Gee, D.G., ... Weinstock, L.M. (2020). Best practices in research mentoring in clinical science. *Journal of Abnormal Psychology, 129*(1), 70–81. https://doi.org/10.1037/abn0000478

Gupta, B., & Rathore, B. (2020). Mentoring in the post COVID-19 era. *UGC Care Group-1 Journal, 23*(4), 145–151. https://www.researchgate.net/publication/357031548_Mentoring_in_the_post_Covid_19_era

Hale, R.L., & Phillips, C.A. (2019). Mentoring up: A grounded theory of nurse-to-nurse mentoring. *Journal of Clinical Nursing, 28*(1–2), 159–172. https://doi.org/10.1111/jocn.14636

Hansen, B.R., Whitehouse, C.L., Nkimbeng, M., Beer, K., Mackintosh, K., Allgood, S., ... Wright, R. (2022). Capturing the value and core concepts of the clinical research nurse. *Journal of Research in Nursing, 27*(1–2), 32–47. https://doi.org/10.1177/17449871211073760

Homer. (1993). *The odyssey* (A. Cook, Trans.). W.W. Norton. (Original work published ca. 8th or 7th century B.C.E.)

Hookmani, A.A., Lalani, N., Sultan, N., Zubairi, A., Hussain, A., Hasan, B.S., & Rasheed, M.A. (2021). Development of an on-job mentorship program to improve nursing experience for enhanced patient experience of compassionate care. *BMC Nursing, 20*(1),175. https://doi.org/10.1186/s12912-021-00682-4

Hoover, J., Koon, A.D., Rosser, E.N., & Rao, K.D. (2020). Mentoring the working nurse: A scoping review. *Human Resources for Health, 18*(1), 52. https://doi.org/10.1186/s12960-020-00491-x

Hrebin, N., Hrabovska, S., Karkovska, R., & Vovk, A. (2020). Applying Benjamin Bloom's taxonomy ideas in adult learning. *Journal of Education Culture and Society, 11*(1), 61–72. https://doi.org/10.15503/jecs2020.1.61.72

Hussey, L., & Campbell-Meier, J. (2020). Are you mentoring or coaching? Definitions matter. *Journal of Librarianship and Information Science, 53*(3), 510–521. https://doi.org/10.1177/0961000620966651

Jones, C.T., Griffith, C.A., Fisher, C.A., Grinke, K.A., Keller, R., Lee, H., ... Turba, E. (2022). Nurses in clinical trials: Perceptions of impact on the research enterprise. *Journal of Research in Nursing, 27*(1–2), 50–65. https://doi.org/10.1177/17449871211073757

Karam, S. (2021, December 7). Nursing roles in clinical trials. *ONS Voice.* https://voice.ons.org/news-and-views/nursing-roles-in-clinical-trials

Kluger, A.N., & Itzchakov, G. (2022). The power of listening at work. *Annual Review of Organizational Psychology and Organizational Behavior, 9,* 121–146. http://doi.org/10.1146/annurev-orgpsych-012420-091013

Knapke, J.M., Jenkerson, M., Tsao, P., Freel, S., Fritter, J., Helm, S.L., ... Jones, C.T. (2022). Academic medical center clinical research professional workforce: Part 2—Issues in staff onboarding and professional development. *Journal of Clinical and Translational Science, 6*(1), e81. https://doi.org/10.1017/cts.2022.412

Knowles, M.S., Holton, E.F. Swanson, R.A., & Robinson, P.A. (2020). *The adult learner: The definitive classic in adult education and human resource development* (9th ed.). Routledge. https://doi.org/10.4324/9780429299612

Kobis, L., & Mehner, C. (2021). Ethical questions raised by AI-supported mentoring in higher education. *Frontiers in Artificial Intelligence, 4,* 62450. https://doi.org/10.3389/frai.2021.624050

Koutroubas, V., & Galanakis, M. (2022). Bandura's social learning theory and its importance in the organizational psychology context. *Journal of Psychology Research, 12*(6), 315–322. https://doi.org/10.17265/2159-5542/2022.06.001

Kowalski, K. (2019). Differentiating mentoring from coaching and precepting. *Journal of Continuing Education in Nursing, 50*(11), 493–494. https://doi.org/10.3928/00220124-20191015-04

Kumar, S., Roumell, E.A., & Bolliger, D.U. (2023). Faculty perceptions of e-mentoring doctoral dissertations: Challenges, strategies, and institutional support. *American Journal of Distance Education, 39*(2), 128–148. https://doi.org/10.1080/08923647.2023.2213137

Larkin, M.E., Beardslee, B., Cagliero, E., Griffith, C.A., Milaszewski, K., Mugford, M.T., ... Witte, E.R. (2019). Ethical challenges experienced by clinical research nurses: A qualitative study. *Nursing Ethics, 26*(1), 172–184. https://doi.org/10.1177/0969733017693441

Lavender, V., & Croudass, A. (2019). The role of the nurse in supporting cancer clinical trials. *British Journal of Nursing, 28*(4), S14–S17. https://doi.org/10.12968/bjon.2019.28.4.S14

Legg, R.S. (2023). When enactive learning went missing, vicarious learning became a must. *Theory Into Practice, 62*(3), 245–254. https://doi.org/10.1080/00405841.2023.2226557

Lewis, C., & Olshansky, E. (2016). Relational-cultural theory as a framework for mentoring in academia: Toward diversity and growth-fostering collaborative scholarly relationships. *Mentoring and Tutoring: Partnership in Learning, 24*(5), 383–398. https://doi.org/10.1080/13611267.2016.1275390

Lönn, B.B., Hörnsten, A., Styrke, J., & Hajdarevic, S. (2022). Transitioning to the clinical research nurse role—A qualitative descriptive study. *Journal of Advanced Nursing, 78*(11), 3817–3829. https://doi.org/10.1111/jan.15397

Machynska, N., & Boiko, H. (2020). Andragogy—The science of adult education: Theoretical aspects. *Journal of Innovation in Psychology, Education and Didactics, 24*(1), 25–34. https://epale.ec.europa.eu/sites/default/files/eded.pdf

Manuel, S.P., & Poorsattar, S.P. (2021). Mentoring up: Twelve tips for successfully employing a mentee-driven approach to mentoring relationships. *Medical Teacher, 43*(4), 384–387. https://doi.org/10.1080/0142159X.2020.1795098

McBride, A.B., Campbell, J., & Deming, K. (2019). Does having been mentored affect subsequent mentoring? *Journal of Professional Nursing, 35*(3),156–161. https://doi.org/10.1016/j.profnurs.2018.11.003

McReynolds, M.R., Termini, C.M., Hinton, A.O., Jr., Taylor, B.L., Vue, Z., Huang, S.C., ... Carter, C.S. (2020). The art of virtual mentoring in the twenty-first century for STEM majors and beyond. *Nature Biotechnology, 38*(12), 1477–1482. https://doi.org/10.1038/s41587-020-00758-7

Melnyk, B.M., Tan, A., Hsieh, A.P., & Gallagher-Ford, L. (2021). Evidence-based practice culture and mentorship predict EBP implementation, nurse job satisfaction, and intent to stay: Support for the ARCC® Model. *Worldviews on Evidence-Based Nursing, 18*(4), 272–281. https://doi.org/10.1111/wvn.12524

Melnyk, B.M., Tan, A., Hsieh, A.P., Gawlik, K., Arslanian-Engoren, C., Braun, L.T., ... Wilbur, J.E. (2021). Critical care nurses' physical and mental health, worksite wellness support, and medical errors. *American Journal of Critical Care, 30*(3), 176–184. https://doi.org/10.4037/ajcc2021301

Mikkonen, K., Tomietto, M., Tuomikoski, A.M., Kaučič, B.M., Riklikiene, O., Vizcaya-Moreno, F., ... Kääriäinen, M.M. (2022). Mentors' competence in mentoring nursing students in clinical practice: Detecting profiles to enhance mentoring practices. *Nursing Open, 9*(1), 593–603. https://doi.org/10.1002/nop2.1103

Mineva, K., Jecheva, V., & Baltov, M. (2023). E-mentoring: Past, present & future. In *E-mentoring: Theory and practice* (pp. 7–23). Bialystok University of Technology. https://www.researchgate.net/publication/377815506

Mullen, C.A., & Klimaitis, C.C. (2021). Defining mentoring: A literature review of issues, types, and applications. *Annals of the New York Academy of Sciences, 1483*(1), 19–35. https://doi.org/10.1111/nyas.14176

Murray, S.A., Shuler, H., Spencer, E.C., & Hinton, A. (2022). Mentoring future science leaders to thrive. *Trends in Pharmaceutical Science, 43*(6), 457–460. https://doi.org/10.1016/j.tips.2022.03.012

Mutiarin, D., Manaf, H.A., Man, M.N., Kasiwi, A.N., & Nurjanah, A. (2023). Analysis of e-mentoring platform for future leaders' development: A comprehensive literature review. *ES3 Web of Conferences, 440,* 03021. https://doi.org/10.1051/e3sconf/202344003021

Nelson, J.D., Dunn, M.E., & Strekalova, Y.A. (2024). Pilot implementation of a co-mentoring circles program for the clinical research professionals: Evidence for formative evaluation and logic model. *Journal of Clinical and Translational Science, 8*(1), e21. https://doi.org/10.1017/cts.2023.712

Ness, E. (2020). The oncology clinical research nurse study coordinator: Past, present, and future. *Asia-Pacific Journal of Oncology Nursing, 7*(3), 237–242. https://doi.org/10.4103/apjon.apjon_10_20

Ng, Y.X., Koh, Z.Y.K., Yap, H.W., Tay, K.T., Tan, X.H., Ong, Y.T., ... Krishna, L. (2020). Assessing mentoring: A scoping review of mentoring assessment tools in internal medicine between 1990 and 2019. *PLOS ONE, 15*(5), e0232511. https://doi.org/10.1371/journal.pone.0232511

Nguyen, L., Tomy, S., Pardede, E. (2024). Enhancing collaborative learning and e-mentoring in a smart education system in higher education. *Computers, 13*(1), 28. https://doi.org/10.3390/computers13010028

Nurunnabi, A.S.M., Rahim, R., Alo, D., Mamun, A.A., Kaiser, A.M., Mohammad, T., & Sultana, F. (2022). Experiential learning in clinical education guided by the Kolb's Experiential Learning Theory. *International Journal of Human and Health Sciences, 6*(2), 155–160. https://doi.org/10.31344/ijhhs.v6i2.438

O'Dowd, R., Sauro, S., & Spector-Cohen, E. (2020). The role of pedagogical mentoring in virtual exchange. *TESOL Quarterly, 54*(1), 146–172. https://doi.org/10.1002/tesq.543

Olaolorunpo, O. (2019). Mentoring in nursing: A concept analysis. *International Journal of Caring Sciences, 12*(1), 142–148. https://www.internationaljournalofcaringsciences.org/docs/16_olorufremi_12_1.pdf

Oncology Nursing Society & Oncology Nursing Certification Corporation. (2024). *Oncology clinical research nurse competencies.* https://www.ons.org/sites/default/files/2025-01/ocrn-competencies-rebrand.pdf

Rogers, S.L., Howieson, J., & Neame, C. (2018). I understand you feel that way, but I feel this way: The benefits of I-language and communicating perspective during conflict. *PeerJ, 6,* e4831. https://doi.org/10.7717/peerj.4831

Rollnik-Sadowska, W., & Ryciuk, U. (2023). E-mentoring in the era of industry 4.0—Changes in the human resource management. In *E-mentoring: Theory and practice* (pp. 39–57). Bialystok University of Technology. https://www.researchgate.net/publication/377815506

Santiesteban, L., Young, E., Tiarks, G.C., Boemi, M.G., Patel, R.K., Bauckman, K.A., ... Rajput, V. (2022). Defining advising, coaching, and mentoring for student development in medical education. *Cureus, 14*(7), e27356, https://doi.org/10.7759/cureus.27356

Shah, M.K., Gandrakota, N., Cimiotti, J.P., Ghose, N., Moore, M., & Ali, M.K. (2021). Prevalence of and factors associated with nurse burnout in the US. *JAMA Network Open, 4*(2), e2036469. https://doi.org/10.1001/jamanetworkopen.2020.36469

Smiley, R.A., Allgeyer, R.L., Shobo, Y., Lyons, K.C., Letourneau, R., Zhong, E., ... Alexander, M. (2023). The 2022 national nursing workforce survey. *Journal of Nursing Regulation, 14*(1, Suppl. 2), S1–S90. https://doi.org/10.1016/S2155-8256(23)00047-9

Stoeger, H., Balestrini, D.P., & Ziegler, A. (2021). Key issues in professionalizing mentoring practices. *Annals of the New York Academy of Sciences, 1483*(1), 5–18. https://doi.org/10.1111/nyas.14537

Tinoco-Giraldo, H., Torrecilla Sánchez, E.M., & García-Peñalvo, F.J (2020). E-mentoring in higher education: A structured literature review and implications for future research. *Sustainability, 12*(11), 4344. https://doi.org/10.3390/su12114344

Tolan, P.H., McDaniel, H.L., Richardson, M., Arkin, N., Augenstern, J., & Duboi, D.L. (2020). Improving understanding of how mentoring works: Measuring multiple intervention processes. *Journal of Community Psychology, 48*(6), 2086–2107. https://doi.org/10.1002/jcop.22408

Treasure, A.M., Hall, S.M., Lesko, I., Moore, D., Sharan, M., van Zaanen, M., ... van der Walt, A. (2022). Ten simple rules for establishing a mentorship program. *PLoS Computational Biology, 18*(5), e1010015. https://doi.org/10.1371/journal.pcbi.1010015

Van Patten, R.R., & Bartone, A.S. (2019). The impact of mentorship, preceptors, and debriefing on the quality of program experiences. *Nurse Education in Practice, 35,* 63–68. https://doi.org/10.1016/j.nepr.2019.01.007

Veliverronena, L. (2023). E-mentoring issues, effects, opportunities—profession development. In *E-mentoring: Theory and practice* (pp. 58–77). Bialystok University of Technology. https://www.researchgate.net/publication/377815506

Volkova, J. (2023). E-mentoring relationship. In *E-mentoring: Theory and practice* (pp. 24–38). Bialystok University of Technology. https://www.researchgate.net/publication/377815506

Waljee, J.F., Chopra, V., & Saint, S. (2020). Mentoring millennials. *JAMA, 323*(17), 1716–1717. https://doi.org/10.1001/jama.2020.3085

Yiorka, S., & Taliadorou, A. (2023). Tips for e-mentors. In *E-mentoring: Theory and practice* (pp. 148–159). Bialystok University of Technology. https://www.researchgate.net/publication/377815506

Yukawa, M., Gansky, S.A., O'Sullivan, P., Teherani, A., & Feldman, M.D. (2020). A new mentor evaluation tool: Evidence of validity. *PLOS ONE, 15*(6), e0234345. https://doi.org/10.1371/journal.pone.0234345

CHAPTER 37

Publishing Guidance for Oncology Clinical Research Nurses

Crystal D. Chu, PhD, RN

Introduction

Clinical research that is ethically sound moves science forward. Clinical trials may help determine the most beneficial therapeutic interventions, establish new best practices for screening and detection of cancer, or identify interventions that improve the quality of life for patients and their families. However, if the results of clinical trials are not published and shared with the medical, nursing, and local communities, vital knowledge that could help people is lost.

This chapter will discuss the benefits of publishing as an oncology clinical research nurse (OCRN), detailing what to write, how to write, and how to receive authorship credit for writing and study coordination, as well as how to maintain integrity in writing. Although much of the information imparted is general and not specific to OCRNs, wherever possible, it will be directed to their publishing needs.

Why Publish?

Nurses, particularly OCRNs, have a unique perspective and voice when it comes to clinical practice and nursing science. By harnessing that perspective, OCRNs can offer new insights into clinical practice, patient experience, and quality of life, as well as innovative ways to improve evidence-based practice. By publishing, nurses gain and share new knowledge, help improve patient care, advance the nursing profession, and reach new career advancements (Cleveland Clinic, 2024; Oermann et al., 2019). According to Oermann (2022, p. 4), there are five main reasons for nurses to publish: "(a) to share ideas and expertise with other nurses; (b) to disseminate evidence and the findings of nursing research studies; (c) for promotion, tenure, and other personnel decisions; (d) for development of one's own knowledge and skills; and (e) for personal satisfaction." Furthermore, OCRNs have the opportunity and responsibility to provide nurses in clinical, educational, and research settings with information about multiple aspects of clinical trials. Possible topics that OCRNs may address in publications are listed in Figure 37-1.

Abstract, Poster, Article, or Other Publications

Once OCRNs determine the topic to develop and have checked for institutional policies regarding publishing, the next step is to decide whether the topic would be best suited

- Results of a clinical trial (e.g., study drug, device, randomized controlled trial)
- Insights into the use of study drug or device
- Symptom clusters identified while caring for patients receiving a study drug
- Patient beliefs and misconceptions about study drug or device
- Adverse events in patients receiving study drug
- Nursing interventions to prevent or manage adverse events in patients receiving a study drug
- Patient education required while being treated with a study drug or device
- Patients' reports on adverse events during and after study drug therapy
- Study of nursing care satisfaction of patients receiving a study drug
- Disease process treated with a study drug or device
- Relationship of demographic age, gender, or weight with an adverse effect of a study drug
- Case study of a patient's experience from treatment with a study drug or device
- New black box warnings for a previously approved drug or device

FIGURE 37-1 | Possible Topics for Oncology Clinical Research Nurses to Publish

Note. Oncology clinical research nurses should review their local or institutional publication policies before submitting abstracts or manuscripts for publication.

as an abstract for a conference, a poster presentation, an article in a noted journal, or a chapter in a book or similar publication. Each has value and unique characteristics, as well as qualities that overlap with one another.

Abstract

Regardless of whether the topic will be further developed into a poster presentation or an article, the starting point for disseminating research findings is an abstract. An abstract is a self-contained statement that provides a summary of the research, an overview of the facts, and highlights of the author's work (Ness, 2024). An abstract can be further developed, if selected, as a podium presentation at a conference, a poster presentation, or a summary of an article. Depending on the topic, an abstract can be categorized as clinical, research, evidence-based, quality improvement, or a creative solution to a gap in clinical care (Ness, 2024).

Conference Abstracts

Professional organizations typically announce a call for abstracts at annual meetings. If selected, a conference abstract is usually published in conference proceedings. Conference abstracts may be submitted as a podium presentation or a poster and typically range from 200 to 500 words (Hayakawa & Barrows, 2022). Because conferences may differ in expectations, it is essential to review the abstract criteria closely for each submission to ensure a successful outcome. It is also important to consider the target audience and adjust the abstract accordingly (Hayakawa & Barrows, 2022). OCRNs may consider submitting abstracts to the Oncology Nursing Society, Society of Clinical Research Associates, Association of Clinical Research Professionals, and International Association of Clinical Research Nurses. Depending on the clinical research area, there may be more professional organizations or conferences to consider. The four Cs of writing an abstract can ensure that it is a success (International Association of Clinical Research Nurses, 2013, p. 25):

- Complete: Covers the major parts of the project
- Concise: Contains no excess wordiness or unnecessary information
- Clear: Readable, well-organized, and not too jargon-laden
- Cohesive: Flows smoothly between the parts

Before submitting a conference abstract, OCRNs should confirm with their supervisor that they will be able to attend the conference, what costs the employer will cover, and whether they will be able to use work time for any conference-related activities or if the abstract development will be completed outside of work hours. Depending on the conference, the professional organization may also provide funding for attendees. For example, the Oncology Nursing Society offers ONS Congress® Scholarships to support travel arrangements for selected nurses to attend its annual meeting (Oncology Nursing Foundation, 2024).

Article Abstracts

Typically, conference abstracts offer a strong foundation for an article. OCRNs considering an article should determine the most appropriate journal for the topic and adjust the abstract accordingly to the audience. Slightly differing from the conference abstract, an article abstract is a "brief, comprehensive summary of the contents of the paper" (American Psychological Association [APA], 2020, p. 13). Abstracts should be accurate, concise, and nonevaluative (i.e., informational and reporting the facts without adding bias or opinion). An article abstract, typically 250 words, may be written in paragraph form and separated into sections (e.g., Objective, Method, Results, Conclusions) (APA, 2020).

A publisher's website will have formatting procedures in its guidelines for authors that specify what is expected to be in an abstract or article. It is important to include only information from the article in an abstract and to adhere to other requirements of the publisher, such as word count, font size, and deadlines (Ness, 2024). CONSORT (Consolidated Standards of Reporting Trials) for Abstracts can help OCRNs construct an abstract for reporting randomized controlled trials within the constraints of a publisher (Hopewell et al., 2025). This 30-item checklist can be applied to a randomized controlled trial report in a journal or conference abstract. Examples of abstracts and their contents are summarized in Table 37-1.

Poster

Posters are a visual means of presenting primary research results, clinical reports, and other information at meetings or conferences. Most professional organizations will provide details and possibly a recommended template if an abstract is selected for a poster presentation. Traditional printed research posters are large, ranging in size from 4 feet wide by 3 feet tall to 6 feet wide by 4 feet tall. Some organizations may request an e-poster, which requires specific dimension specifications depending on the virtual platform (Wood & Mowery, 2024). The poster instructions may be found on a conference website or sent directly to the lead poster author. A poster is a visual representation of the research, and it should minimize text by using simple, brief bullet points, provide a clean visual design, and feature easy-to-view graphics. Fonts should be consistent in style and size, with the largest font used for the poster title (between 50- to 85-point font), the second largest for section titles (30- to 40-point font), and the smallest for text (no smaller than 24-point font). Recommended fonts to use are Arial, Calibri, Verdana, Times New Roman, or Helvetica (Wood & Mowery, 2024). To reduce the amount of text on the poster, a QR code can be added to link the viewer to a reference list, additional data analysis or findings, or to provide the author's contact information rather than using business cards (Wood & Mowery, 2024).

E-posters may also include a brief recording, allowing individuals to listen to an overview of the project if they are

TABLE 37-1 | What to Include in an Abstract

Type of Abstract	Components
Research or randomized controlled trial	• Background or problem statement • Participant characteristics, trial registration, funding • Trial design, methods, randomization, blinding, outcomes • Results, randomized numbers, sample size, recruitment, data analysis (including effect sizes and confidence intervals), outcomes, harms • Conclusion with applications and future research considerations
Literature review or meta-analysis	• Background or problem statement • Search methodology, eligibility criteria, Preferred Reporting Items for Systematic Reviews and Meta-Analyses (PRISMA) diagram • Conclusions and limitations • Implications for practice
Case study	• Subject and characteristics • Intervention to resolve a problem • Implications for clinical practice and future research
Evidence-based practice	• Introduction, background, or problem statement that may be in the form of PICOT (Population, Intervention, Comparison, Outcome, and Time) • Methods • Results • Significance and implications • Discussion • Conclusion

Note. Based on information from American Psychological Association, 2020; Hayakawa & Barrows, 2022; Ness, 2024.

unable to attend the scheduled poster session. The recording is typically around two minutes, either a blank visual or a clear image of the person speaking, and should sound professional. It is a good idea to write a script and rehearse before submitting the final recording (Wood & Mowery, 2024).

The information on the poster should be presented similarly to an abstract with sections such as Introduction or Background, Methods, Analysis, Results, and Conclusions (Wood & Mowery, 2024). The poster should flow aesthetically and be easily understood. It is advised to create a draft and receive feedback from others on content, visuals, and readability (Wood & Mowery, 2024). If the poster is in a traditional format that requires printing, then it is essential to schedule printing time, prepare for printing costs, and consider logistics (e.g., a poster transport tube) for delivering the poster to the conference (Wood & Mowery, 2024).

Creating an Article From an Abstract or Poster

An abstract or poster for a conference may be developed into an article at a later date and serve as an outline to get started. It is important to determine which aspects of the research to elaborate on and to identify a target journal that may be interested in publishing a full article related to the topic. Once a journal is identified (some conferences have a journal that may accept a full article of a recent poster or abstract presentation), it is time to outline the entire paper.

To begin, use the title of the abstract or poster as the first draft of the article, adding headings and subheadings to guide the writing and make the article easy to read. Next, identify the key concepts and bullet points that can be expanded to detailed findings, discussions, and a conclusion. Each journal has criteria and guidelines for organizing an article, but most typically follow a similar flow, including an Abstract, Introduction, Methods, Results, and Conclusions (Tume et al., 2021). Taking the next step to prepare an article from a recent abstract or poster presentation is an excellent way for OCRNs to build upon work already completed.

Articles

An article is a composite of written ideas about a topic that is communicated to a specific audience via a print or online journal. It should be written in the author's distinctive voice or style of writing; reading it out loud will help the author decide if it sounds authentic. OCRNs must identify a target journal that is the best fit and has the most relevant audience for their topic or research study. Each journal will have specific author guidelines that need to be followed. These typically include topics to write about; article length (e.g., word limit, page limit); use of abbreviations; reference style (e.g., APA); use of tables, photos, and illustrations; format to be used (e.g., double-spaced, one-inch margins); and how to prepare and submit a manuscript. A letter of inquiry may be the first step in determining whether the target journal is interested in the topic. Also, journals may have special requests for topics related to recent conferences or special editions.

OCRNs may also have the opportunity to expand an accepted abstract or poster if the journal is publishing a conference edition. They should visit a journal's website to locate information about a letter of inquiry and guidelines. For example, the Oncology Nursing Society website features a page designed for authors interested in submitting a manuscript to the *Oncology Nursing Forum* (www.ons.org/onf/authors). It addresses submissions and financial disclosures and provides a detailed section on manuscript preparation.

OCRNs should be aware that several layers or levels of peer review may be involved once the final draft of an article or abstract is completed, particularly if a contractual agreement exists with the study's sponsor. The same peer review process is also standard with book projects and other similar publications. Therefore, OCRNs need to schedule preparation, writing, and revision time accordingly.

To increase the likelihood of an article being accepted for publication, OCRNs should select a journal that targets the audience for whom the article is written. For example, communicating implications for practice has a different focus than articles published in a research journal. Types of articles that OCRNs might be interested in publishing are listed in Table 37-2.

Book Chapter Authorship

The Oncology Nursing Society and similar organizations also offer opportunities to turn abstracts into lengthier book chapters or individual book titles for specialized publications. This submission process is similar to that of a peer-reviewed journal, with interested potential authors able to submit their curriculum via email or a submission form.

Interested authors can find more information on how they may contribute to an Oncology Nursing Society book publication by visiting www.ons.org/resources-book-authors-and-editors. This webpage offers documentation on how to prepare and submit a manuscript, format references and citations, seek permissions on tables and figures, and write using evidence-based practice and subject matter experts. Checklists for these steps and additional revisions are also included.

Guidelines for Reporting Research Results

Specific reporting guidelines are available for various study designs that authors should follow when preparing their manuscripts. Many of the guidelines are specific to particular types of health research reports. Enhancing the QUAlity and Transparency Of health Research (EQUATOR) is a comprehensive summary of guidelines for authors of systematic reviews and other relevant documents (www.equator-network.org) (see Table 37-3).

OCRNs may be asked to assist in manuscript preparation for studies they coordinate, such as providing demographic or adverse event data. Understanding how to use CONSORT guidelines will help ensure that OCRNs report randomized controlled trials completely, accurately, ethically, and without bias (Schulz et al., 2010). To increase transparency in randomized controlled trials, the CONSORT guidelines expanded in scope to include early-phase clinical trials and reporting on harms and outcomes (Hopewell et al., 2025). Guidelines for reporting research results enable authors to describe the research and methodology in detail, conveying important information to readers, peers, reviewers, and editors (International Committee of Medical Journal Editors [ICMJE], 2025). See Figure 37-2 for advice on getting research published.

TABLE 37-2 | Types of Articles That Oncology Clinical Research Nurses Might Publish

Article Type	Definition
Case study	A summary of the care of a single patient (real or hypothetical) to propose a resolution for a defined problem
Clinical	A description of content applicable to clinical practice
Evidence based	A review and integration of knowledge and scientific evidence to improve clinical practice and patient outcomes
Literature review	Documentation of a systematic review or meta-analysis
Research or empirical studies	Report of an original research study, including an introduction, method and analysis, results, and conclusions

Note. Based on information from American Psychological Association, 2020; Roush, 2017.

Authorship

Authorship, or recognizing the person or people who wrote an article, abstract, poster, or book chapter, is a visual way to document who made significant contributions to and is accountable for these publications (APA, 2020; ICMJE, 2025). When starting a collaborative writing project, to guarantee proper authorship is to (a) discuss plans for what (articles or abstracts) should be written at the end of a project before the project begins, (b) document it in an agreement, and (c) follow the agreement.

ICMJE recommends that those listed as authors participate sufficiently and accept accountability for the work they have contributed. It requires that authors contributing to ICMJE member journals meet the criteria. However, many national and international journals require adherence to the ICMJE criteria for authorship before publishing an article (ICMJE, 2025). To best determine credit and authorship, ICMJE recommends that authorship be based on the following four criteria (ICMJE, 2025, p. 2):

- Substantial contributions to the conception or design of the work; or the acquisition, analysis, or interpretation of data for the work
- Drafting the work or reviewing it critically for important intellectual content
- Final approval of the version to be published
- Agreement to be accountable for all aspects of the work in ensuring that questions related to the accuracy or integrity of any part of the work are appropriately investigated and resolved

To find the latest version of the *Recommendations for the Conduct, Reporting, Editing, and Publication of Scholarly Work in Medical Journals*, visit www.ICMJE.org.

TABLE 37-3 | Examples of Reporting Guidelines for Writing Research Articles

Type of Article/Source of Guideline	Guidelines	Website
Diagnostic accuracy studies	STARD	www.stard-statement.org
Health research	EQUATOR	www.equator-network.org Lists all reporting guidelines for health research
Literature reviews	STARLITE	www.ncbi.nlm.nih.gov/pmc/articles/PMC1629442
Observational studies	STROBE	http://strobe-statement.org
Randomized trials	SPIRIT-CONSORT 2025	www.consort-spirit.org
Systematic reviews and meta-analyses	PRISMA	www.prisma-statement.org
U.S. National Library of Medicine	Research Reporting Guidelines and Initiatives by Organization	www.nlm.nih.gov/services/research_report_guide.html Lists the major biomedical research reporting guidelines as well as editorial style guides for writing research reports or other publications

EQUATOR—Enhancing the QUAlity and Transparency Of health Research; PRISMA—Preferred Reporting Items for Systematic Reviews and Meta-Analyses; SPIRIT-CONSORT—Standard Protocol Items: Recommendations for Interventional Trials-CONsolidated Standards Of Reporting Trials; STARD—Standards for the Reporting of Diagnostic Accuracy Studies; STARLITE—sampling strategy, type of study, approaches, range of years, limits, inclusion and exclusions, terms used, electronic sources; STROBE—Strengthening the Reporting of Observational Studies in Epidemiology

Note. Based on information from Booth, 2006; Page et al., 2021; Schulz et al., 2010; U.S. National Library of Medicine, 2023.

Authorship is generally conveyed with a byline, a line usually located at the beginning of an article that notes the person's or people's names and affiliations, or group authorship where multiple authors are credited, possibly under a single group name (APA, 2020; ICMJE, 2025). The lead author of an article or abstract is generally agreed upon before writing. It may be the individual who suggested the topic, one who has expertise or interest in the topic, or one who represents a group, such as the president of a special interest group in an organization. The corresponding author is the person to whom all correspondence for the publication is directed. They coordinate to handle all editorial and publishing issues and assume responsibility for the publication, including accuracy (e.g., data, facts), integrity, and the determination of contributions to the publication (e.g., authorship) (ICMJE, 2025).

Individuals who are not contributors to the project and do not meet the ICMJE criteria for authors should be listed under acknowledgments (ICMJE, 2025). For example, a nurse who recruits patients for a clinical trial but does not conduct the research, contribute to the research process, or take public responsibility for the integrity of the research should be acknowledged but not cited as an author. Additionally, any use of artificial intelligence should be reported in the acknowledgment section. Furthermore, authors should report how artificial intelligence was used (i.e., writing assistance, data collection or analysis, or figure generation) (ICMJE, 2025).

Order of Authors

The authors often establish the order of authors in an article's byline before the project begins. It is common practice for the principal contributor (who does the most work) to be listed first, followed by the other authors according to their level of contribution (APA, 2020). OCRNs who are the coordinators of a clinical trial should request inclusion in the byline and writing process from the principal investigator or sponsor before the trial begins, with a written agreement outlining their responsibilities. Other arrangements, such as a lead author and coauthors in alphabetical order, may be agreed upon if one or more authors have published prolifically or are mentors and are content to give front-position author placement to other, less experienced authors.

Authorship in Multicenter Clinical Trials

Multicenter research has several advantages over single-center research, including faster accrual rates, less scientific

- Use an accurate, short, and interesting title.
- Follow the journal's author guidelines.
- Check that the flow of the manuscript is logical.
- Explain the methodology and results thoroughly.
- Use your own words and develop a compelling scientific presentation of your work.

FIGURE 37-2 | Advice for Publishing Research

Note. Based on information from Huston & Choi, 2017.

misconduct, and greater generalizability of the results (Dulhunty et al., 2011). Multicenter authorship, on the other hand, can be a source of conflict if a plan for authorship is not developed beforehand and a hundred or more contributors want to be recognized in the byline. All authors of multicenter trials must meet ICMJE criteria (2025) for authorship. No universally accepted guidelines exist, leaving researchers and sponsors to determine a best approach individually.

Authorship Agreement or Policy

Historically, the verbal agreement of a lead author, principal investigator, or project lead for an evidence-based project was sufficient to confer authorship. Today, however, a written agreement should be signed before a project is started to avoid misconceptions and conflict. The agreement should delineate the project tasks, workload division, tasks that earn authorship credit, and the order in which authors will be listed (APA, 2020; DeTora et al., 2022). Although this may not be a critical issue when OCRNs decide to write an article for a nursing journal about adverse events related to a study drug, it can take on tremendous importance when one considers that the study was planned and performed by investigators, research nurses, clinical research assistants, statisticians, pharmacists, sponsor employees or contractors, and other members of the research team (DeTora et al., 2022). By doing so, they will protect their contributions to the research process.

Company-Sponsored Medical Research

Representative members of the International Society for Medical Publication Professionals developed the Good Publication Practice (GPP) guidelines (version 2022) to assist authors of research reports sponsored by companies in writing manuscripts that are ethical and unbiased (DeTora et al., 2022). The GPP 2022 guidelines are designed for authors writing articles for company-sponsored research in peer-reviewed journals and presentations for scientific meetings (DeTora et al., 2022). Topics covered in GPP 2022 are listed in Figure 37-3.

- Publication types
- Publication professional roles and professional development
- Ethical principles
- Publication plans
- Publication working groups
- Authorship and contributorship determination
- Publication process
- Documentation guidelines
- Expert reviewers

FIGURE 37-3 | Topics Addressed in the Good Publication Practice Guidelines for Communicating Company-Sponsored Research

Note. Based on information from DeTora et al., 2022.

The GPP 2022 guidelines are important for OCRNs who are coordinating a clinical trial sponsored by a company, as they may be involved in writing or contributing to an article or abstract for presentation at a conference. In that case, OCRNs would be expected to adhere to the GPP 2022 guidelines, presenting their topic in an ethical and unbiased manner while crediting the sponsor or company.

Although it is ideal for OCRNs to document an agreement in writing that describes how authorship will be determined in a single-site or multicenter clinical trial and what method will be used to assign contributors to a manuscript (DeTora et al., 2022), it may be more common for them to know the publication policy of the institution or sponsor, discuss with the principal investigator writing a nursing article, and share nursing implications with peers. If there is no institutional or sponsor-driven policy for publication, OCRNs may be wholly dependent on the professional relationship they share with the principal investigator.

Acknowledgments

Acknowledgments are used to credit all project contributors who do not meet the criteria for authorship, such as statisticians, technical personnel, department chairs, data collectors, supervisors, medical writers, sponsoring companies or agencies, funding agencies, and artificial intelligence programs (DeTora et al., 2022; ICMJE, 2025). Generally, written permission must be obtained from the individuals being acknowledged to confirm their understanding that readers may interpret their acknowledgment as an endorsement of everything stated in the article (ICMJE, 2025). Acknowledgments may have predetermined placement in an article or book based on publisher guidelines, usually on the front two pages or the last page. Acknowledgments for poster presentations are typically found in italics at the end of the poster.

Medical Writers

Medical writers are proficient in scientific writing and often collaborate with doctors, researchers, and other subject matter experts to create documents that describe research findings, product usage, and other medical information (American Medical Writers Association, 2024). If an OCRN is coordinating a clinical trial sponsored by a pharmaceutical company, they may need to collaborate with a medical writer who is a company employee. In a 2017 joint position statement, the American Medical Writers Association, the European Medical Writers Association, and the International Society for Medical Publication Professionals described the appropriate role of professional medical writers in the development of medical and scientific publications. Within the statement, they agreed to follow GPP guidelines, ICMJE recommendations, and CONSORT reporting guidelines with the expectation that they receive an acknowledgment from the company providing support and that the medical writer receives recognition as a coauthor if ICMJE authorship requirements are met (American Medical Writers Association et al., 2017, DeTora et al., 2022, ICMJE, 2025).

Writing With Integrity

Writing with integrity is the moral and ethical responsibility of every author. It means taking the time and effort to produce an original work and guaranteeing the originality of that work to the publisher. It also means ensuring the accuracy of scientific knowledge and giving credit to others when their work is used (APA, 2020).

Plagiarism

One of many definitions of plagiarism is "the act of presenting the words, ideas, or images of another as your own; it denies authors or creators of content the credit they are due" (APA, 2022, para. 1).

One example of plagiarism is the practice of duplicate publishing. This occurs when an article is published in a journal as original when, in fact, a similar article has been published elsewhere in print or online, and the previous article is not credited (ICMJE, 2025). Not only are ideas and data misrepresented as being original, but they may also inadvertently lead to double counting of data, resulting in an inappropriate weighting of results (ICMJE, 2025). Plagiarism is not necessarily intentional. Unintentional plagiarism may occur as a result of something as simple as not citing or improperly citing a reference. It is essential to carefully plan and review writing, along with incorporating appropriate citations, to avoid plagiarism of any kind.

Preventing plagiarism is more time consuming than complicated (Klimaszewski, 2012). An author should have a clear understanding of the topic before writing, write using their own words, use quotation marks when direct phrases are copied, accurately cite sources, and give proper acknowledgment to those who contributed to the work (Jitani et al., 2024). See Table 37-4 for more suggestions about how to prevent plagiarism by using citations.

Paraphrasing

Paraphrasing is taking someone else's ideas or works and restating them in one's own words. Reading to understand the content well enough to paraphrase it accurately without changing the author's meaning is time consuming, but it is the best way to avoid unintentional plagiarism (Hilliard et al., 2023). Paraphrasing requires an in-text citation (adding the page number of the original work is suggested) and a complete reference in the reference list or bibliography (APA, 2020).

TABLE 37-4 | Preventing Plagiarism With Citations

Material Used	Action
Ideas or data (print or online)	Cite the source properly in the text. Add websites, dates of posting or updates, and digital object identifiers (DOIs) to the reference list.
Public domain content (print or online)	Cite the source properly in the text. Add websites, dates of posting or updates, and DOIs to the reference list.
Copyrighted material that qualifies as fair use (print or online)	Cite the source properly in the text. Add websites, dates of posting or updates, and DOIs to the reference list.
Copyrighted material that does not qualify as fair use (print or online)	Obtain permission for use. Cite the source as directed by the copyright holder. Use quotation marks in text but not in figures and tables. Add to the reference list in the form directed by the copyright holder. Submit approval for use to the editor and publisher.

Note. Based on information from American Psychological Association, 2020; U.S. Copyright Office, n.d.-a, n.d.-b.

Summarizing

Summarizing is different from paraphrasing in that it involves using one's own words to shorten an original idea. It is helpful to read the content, take separate notes, and return later to review and summarize the notes. The intent is to preserve, rather than change, the original meaning in a shortened version, written in the voice of the person writing the summary (Purdue University, n.d.). Summarizing requires a citation in the text and a complete reference in the reference list or bibliography.

Quoting

Quoting is copying the words of another word-for-word and should be limited whenever possible. Quotes of 40 words or less can be enclosed in quotation marks and accompanied by added text, including the page number. If a page number is not available on the internet, the paragraph number should be cited after the year (APA, 2020). If a larger quote of more than 40 words is required, it is recommended not to use quotation marks and to start the text on a new line. This also requires the citation to include the author's name, the publication year, and the page number (APA, 2020). Quoting requires accuracy in copying, quotation marks or block quotation format, an in-text citation with the page or paragraph number of the original passage, and a complete reference in the reference list or bibliography.

Citations

Reference citations provide readers with evidence about when scientific, literary, or other contributions were published (APA, 2020). When an article is cited, it implies that the author read and reflected upon the work of those contributors. Citations enable readers to return to the work of others that influenced or supported an author's ideas, theories, or scientific or creative work (APA, 2020). Reasons to cite references are listed in Figure 37-4.

If the information is not an original thought, then it must be cited. Information found on the internet is either copyrighted or in the public domain. Regardless of copyright status, information from the internet should always include attribution to the original authors, similar to citations for books, journals, or any other source.

Copyrighted material is indicated by the symbol © or the word or abbreviation *Copyright* or *Copr*, along with the year of copyright and the copyright owner's name (U.S. Copyright Office, n.d.-a). Permission must be obtained to reprint or adapt (i.e., change) a figure or table from material that is copyrighted. Permissions must be submitted to the publisher at the time the manuscript is submitted. For more detailed information about copyright, visit www.copyright.gov.

An exception to copyright law is the fair use doctrine, which allows for the reproduction of a short passage of copyrighted material (text) for research, scholarship, criticism, comment, teaching, and news reporting without requiring permission (U.S. Copyright Office, n.d.-b). For example, an OCRN may quote a short passage from a copyrighted work to clarify or validate an observation and will not need to request permission from the copyright owner to do so. However, the material used must have quotation marks and a proper reference citation.

Information in the public domain (i.e., government or government-funded publications and material for which a copyright has been lost, not renewed, or expired) may be used without permission and with the proper citation (U.S. Copyright Office, n.d.-a). For example, if an OCRN elects to use a figure from a government website or a short passage from a website without a copyright, they may do so as long as the source is cited in the text of the manuscript and the reference list or bibliography.

- Give credit for ideas, theories, words, or creations.
- Stimulate critical thinking about the original work.
- Provide evidence for conclusions.
- Validate an argument.
- Show where the research being reported was obtained.
- Protect oneself from plagiarism and establish credibility.

FIGURE 37-4 | Reasons to Cite References

Note. Based on information from Middlebury Libraries, n.d.

Summary

OCRNs have an opportunity to offer a unique perspective to advancing clinical research and practice. Furthermore, OCRNs must acknowledge their responsibility to provide pertinent information about clinical trials, particularly regarding advancements in patient care, innovative interventions, or topics related to ethical considerations in research. There are many opportunities for publication, and often, the best place to start is with an abstract. Using institutional or professional organization support systems can help a beginner gain the guidance and mentorship needed to get started. Coauthoring with an experienced OCRN or other seasoned authors can also provide an excellent learning experience while gaining traction in becoming published. In addition to promoting professional growth and disseminating new knowledge to peers in the healthcare community, OCRNs can serve as an extension of the patient voice to advocate for and advance clinical trial equity. Regardless of the OCRN research area or interests, various pathways to publication can be embraced.

Key Points

- Nurses can add valuable insight across all actions associated with writing.
- Writers should always write with integrity and without bias.
- Reading written material out loud can help confirm natural flow as if speaking.
- By keeping the target audience in mind, writing can be explicitly directed to the intended reader.
- All policies, guidelines, and instructions should be followed from the journal or conference website.
- To avoid plagiarism, references should be included for anything that is not common knowledge or an original thought.
- To make writing unique and free from potential plagiarism, writers should learn to paraphrase content in their own words.
- Primary references should be cited, even if the information is found in a secondary source.
- Articles, abstracts, and poster presentations all contribute to the translation of research to clinical practice.

The author would like to acknowledge Angela D. Klimaszewski, MS, RN, for her contribution to this chapter that remains unchanged from the previous edition of this book.

References

American Medical Writers Association. (2024). *Ultimate guide to becoming a medical writer.* https://info.amwa.org/ultimate-guide-to-becoming-a-medical-writer#what_is_medical_writing

American Medical Writers Association, European Medical Writers Association, & International Society for Medical Publication Professionals. (2017). *AMWA-EMWA-ISMPP joint position statement on the role of professional medical writers.* https://www.ismpp.org/assets/docs/Inititives/amwa-emwa-ismpp%20joint%20position%20statement%20on%20the%20role%20of%20professional%20medical%20writers_january%202017.pdf

American Psychological Association. (2020). *Publication manual of the American Psychological Association* (7th ed.). https://apastyle.apa.org/products/publication-manual-7th-edition

American Psychological Association. (2022). *Plagiarism.* https://apastyle.apa.org/style-grammar-guidelines/citations/plagiarism

Booth, A. (2006). "Brimful of STARLITE": toward standards for reporting literature searches. *Journal of the Medical Library Association, 94*(4), 421–429, e205. http://www.ncbi.nlm.nih.gov/pmc/articles/PMC1629442

Cleveland Clinic. (2024, October 25). *The power of publishing your clinical and research work.* https://consultqd.clevelandclinic.org/the-power-of-publishing-your-clinical-and-research-work

DeTora, L.M., Toroser, D., Sykes, A., Vanderlinden, C., Plunkett, F.J., Lane, T., ... Citrome, L. (2022). Good Publication Practice (GPP) guidelines for company-sponsored biomedical research: 2022 update. *Annals of Internal Medicine, 175*(9). https://doi.org/10.7326/M22-1460

Dulhunty, J.M., Boots, R.J., Paratz, J.D., & Lipman, J. (2011). Determining authorship in multicenter trials: A systematic review: Authorship in multicenter trials. *Acta Anaesthesiologica Scandinavica, 55*(9), 1037–1043. https://doi.org/10.1111/j.1399-6576.2011.02477.x

Hayakawa, J., & Barrows, J. (2022). How to write an abstract for poster or podium submission. *Pediatric Nursing, 48*(6), 308–310. https://doi.org/10.62116/PNJ.2022.48.6.308

Hilliard, W., Hobbs, S., & Jimenez, R. (2023). Exploring plagiarism. *Nursing, 53*(9), 35–39. https://doi.org/10.1097/01.NURSE.0000942848.64158.dc

Hopewell, S., Chan, A.-W., Collins, G.S., Hróbjartsson, A., Moher, D., Schulz, K.F., ... Boutron, I. (2025). CONSORT 2025 statement: Updated guideline for reporting randomized trials. *JAMA, 333*(22), 1998–2005. https://doi.org/10.1001/jama.2025.4347

Huston, P., & Choi, B. (2017). A guide to publishing scientific research in the health sciences. *Canada Communicable Disease Report, 43*(9), 169–175. https://doi.org/10.14745/ccdr.v43i09a01

International Association of Clinical Research Nurses. (2013, June 1). *Writing a conference abstract: Tips for success* [PowerPoint slides]. https://iacrn.org/Resources/Documents/2013%20Conference/Abstract%20Development%20V5.pdf

International Committee of Medical Journal Editors. (2025). *Recommendations for the conduct, reporting, editing, and publication of scholarly work in medical journals (Updated April 2025).* https://www.icmje.org/icmje-recommendations.pdf

Jitani, A., Mandal, P.K., & Jajodia, E. (2024). Publication of medical research without plagiarism – How to achieve it? *Journal of Hematology and Allied Sciences, 3*(3), 88–92. https://doi.org/10.25259/JHAS_1_2023

Klimaszewski, A. (2012). Preventing plagiarism. *Oncology Nursing Forum, 39*(6), 525–527. https://doi.org/10.1188/12.ONF.525-527

Middlebury Libraries. (n.d.). *Citation and style guide.* https://middlebury.libguides.com/citation/cite

Ness, E. (2024). *Writing conference abstracts: Tips for success.* https://ccrod.cancer.gov/confluence/download/attachments/283017573/PD%20Series_Abstracts_March%202024.pdf?version=1&modificationDate=1709917505310&api=v2

Oermann, M.H. (2022). *Writing for publication in nursing* (5th ed.). Springer. https://doi.org/10.1891/9780826177865

Oermann, M.H., Chinn, P.L., Carter-Templeton, H., & Nicoll, L.H. (2019). The importance of nursing in nursing publications. *Nurse Author and Editor, 29*(3), 1–6. https://doi.org/10.1111/j.1750-4910.2019.tb00043.x

Oncology Nursing Foundation. (2024). *Funding for nurses.* https://onsfoundation.org/funding-nurses

Page, M.J., McKenzie, J.E., Bossuyt, P.M., Boutron, I., Hoffmann, T.C., Mulrow, C.D., ... Moher, D. (2021). The PRISMA 2020 statement: An updated guideline for reporting systematic reviews. *BMJ, 372,* n71. https://doi.org/10.1136/bmj.n71

Purdue University. (n.d.). *Best practices to avoid plagiarism.* https://owl.purdue.edu/owl/avoiding_plagiarism/best_practices.html

Roush, K. (2017). What types of articles to write. *American Journal of Nursing, 117*(5), 68–71. https://doi.org/10.1097/01.NAJ.0000516278.97098.02

Schulz, K.F., Altman, D.G., Moher, D., & CONSORT Group. (2010). CONSORT 2010 statement: Updated guidelines for reporting parallel group randomized trials. *BMJ, 340,* c332. https://doi.org/10.1136/bmj.c332

Tume, LN., Vollam, S., & Trapani, J. (2021). How to convert your conference abstract into a paper for *Nursing in Critical Care. Nursing in Critical Care, 26*(Suppl.), 4–5. https://doi.org/10.1111/nicc.12691

U.S. Copyright Office. (n.d.-a). *FAQ definitions.* https://www.copyright.gov/help/faq/faq-definitions.html

U.S. Copyright Office. (n.d.-b). *FAQ fair use.* https://www.copyright.gov/help/faq/faq-fairuse.html

U.S. National Library of Medicine. (2023). *Research reporting guidelines and initiatives: By organization.* https://www.nlm.nih.gov/services/research_report_guide.html

Wood, E.B., & Mowery, B. (2024). Creating a conference poster. *Pediatric Nursing, 50*(1), 40–50. https://doi.org/10.62116/PNJ.2024.50.1.40

Index

The letter *f* after a page number indicates that relevant content appears in a figure; the letter *t*, in a table

D

E

F

V

W